Prioritization & Clinical Judgment
for NCLEX-RN®

SECOND EDITION

Prioritization & Clinical Judgment
for NCLEX-RN®
SECOND EDITION

Christi D. Doherty DNP, MSN, RNC-OB, CNE
Assistant Professor
American Sentinel University
Aurora, Colorado

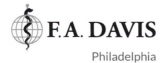
F.A. DAVIS

Philadelphia

F. A. Davis Company
1915 Arch Street
Philadelphia, PA 19103
www.fadavis.com

Printed in the United States of America

Last digit indicates print number: 10 9 8 7 6 5 4 3 2 1

Acquisitions Editor: Jacalyn C. Sharp
Content Project Manager: Sean P. West
Electronic Project Editor: Sandra A. Glennie
Illustration and Design Manager: Carolyn O'Brien

As new scientific information becomes available through basic and clinical research, recommended treatments and drug therapies undergo changes. The author(s) and publisher have done everything possible to make this book accurate, up to date, and in accord with accepted standards at the time of publication. The author(s), editors, and publisher are not responsible for errors or omissions or for consequences from application of the book, and make no warranty, expressed or implied, in regard to the contents of the book. Any practice described in this book should be applied by the reader in accordance with professional standards of care used in regard to the unique circumstances that may apply in each situation. The reader is advised always to check product information (package inserts) for changes and new information regarding dose and contraindications before administering any drug. Caution is especially urged when using new or infrequently ordered drugs.

Library of Congress Cataloging-in-Publication Data

Names: Doherty, Christi D., author.
Title: Prioritization & clinical judgment for NCLEX-RN® / Christi D.
  Doherty.
Other titles: Prioritization and clinical judgment for NCLEX-RN®
Description: Second edition. | Philadelphia : F.A. Davis, [2020] | Includes
  bibliographical references and index.
Identifiers: LCCN 2019046737 (print) | LCCN 2019046738 (ebook) | ISBN
  9780803697232 (paperback) | ISBN 9780803697263 (ebook)
Subjects: MESH: Nursing Assessment | Nursing Care | Health Priorities |
  Clinical Decision-Making | Examination Question
Classification: LCC RT48 (print) | LCC RT48 (ebook) | NLM WY 18.2 | DDC
  616.07/5--dc23
LC record available at https://lccn.loc.gov/2019046737
LC ebook record available at https://lccn.loc.gov/2019046738

Thank you to all the nursing students, nursing faculty, and nursing colleagues I have had the privilege to work with during my career. Thank you to Jacalyn Sharp, Acquisitions Editor at F. A. Davis, and your team for the support and guidance on this project. Finally, thank you to Kathy Colgrove for your mentorship and friendship.

This book is dedicated to my mother, Ellen Shomette, who showed me that hard work and perseverance could make dreams come true; to my mother-in-law, Clara June Doherty, RN, who lived her life with such kindness and generosity, an inspiration for self-improvement every day; and to my husband and best friend, Kevin Doherty, thank you for all the support and encouragement in all my endeavors. You make everything worthwhile.

—Christi D. Doherty

Contributor

Kevin D. Doherty, BS, RDCS, RDMS, RVT
Cardiovascular Sonographer
Baylor Scott and White Heart and Vascular Hospital
Dallas, Texas

Reviewers

Anna M. Bruch, RN, MSN
Nursing Professor
Illinois Valley Community College
Oglesby, Illinois

Lisa Peden, RN, MSN
Associate Professor of Nursing
Dalton State College
Dalton, Georgia

Deborah J. Pumo, MS, EdD, RN
Professor
Illinois Valley Community College
Oglesby, Illinois

Table of Contents

Introduction to Prioritization & Clinical Judgment for NCLEX-RN®

1

Each problem that I solved became a rule which served afterwards to solve other problems.

—Rene Descartes

This book is designed to assist the student throughout nursing school and in taking nursing examinations, particularly the NCLEX-RN® exam, for licensure as a registered nurse (RN). *Prioritization & Clinical Judgment for NCLEX-RN®* focuses on assisting students to improve and enhance their clinical judgment skills. Clinical judgment involves the nurse's ability to acquire information, analyze the data, recognize relevant findings, make inferences in a clinical situation, and implement appropriate nursing interventions. This ability requires a combination of knowledge, logical reasoning, and intuition. The nurse must implement appropriate nursing interventions and evaluate the client's response. Other aspects included in the application of clinical judgment involve complex nursing tasks such as setting priorities for client care, delegating nursing tasks, and managing clients and staff. Clinical judgment is necessary in all nursing practice areas including medical, surgical, critical care, obstetric, pediatric, geriatric, rehabilitation, home health, mental health nursing, inpatient, and outpatient health-care settings.

Clinical judgment questions involving critical thinking, management, prioritizing, and delegation are some of the most difficult questions for the student and new graduate to answer because there is no reference book available to find the correct answers for each individual scenario. Determining the answers to these types of questions requires knowledge of basic scientific principles, standards of care, pathophysiology, psychosocial behaviors, leadership qualities, and the ability to think critically. This book is designed to challenge students to hone their clinical judgment abilities in a variety of nursing situations. Each question provides the student with detailed rationales for correct and incorrect responses. Many of the questions include a helpful tip, termed a "Clinical Judgment Guide," to assist the student with identifying what the questions are asking, recognizing the relevant data in the question stem, and selecting the correct response. It is considered poor test taking to read rationales for the incorrect answers. By doing this, students often will remember reading the rationale, but not if the rationale was for the correct or incorrect answer.

Prioritization & Clinical Judgment for NCLEX-RN® contains numerous questions regarding a variety of nursing areas and roles. Each of the next 12 chapters (Chapters 2 to 13) contain 70 questions in a related field and an additional 10-question clinical scenario. Chapter 14 contains unfolding case studies that require detailed examination and assessment of clients with different illnesses or injuries in multiple health-care settings. A Comprehensive Examination with answers and rationales is also included for each field of nursing. It is important for the test taker to note that practice questions and tests are valuable in preparing for an examination, but there is no substitute for studying the material.

THE NATIONAL COUNCIL OF STATE BOARDS OF NURSING (NCSBN) TEST PLAN FOR QUESTIONS

The National Council of State Boards of Nursing (NCSBN) provides a test plan that helps test takers prepare for the examination and assists nursing faculty in developing test questions for the NCLEX-RN®. Table 1–1 indicates the breakdown of content on the NCLEX-RN®. Clinical judgment skills are necessary for the nurse to function competently in each content area. The Client Needs category of the Safe and Effective Care Environment section includes content in management of care, safety, and infection control. Content included in the management of care section guides and directs nursing care that enhances the health-care delivery setting to protect clients and health-care personnel. Specific content includes but is not limited to advance directives, advocacy, case management, client rights, collaboration with the interdisciplinary team, delegation, establishing priorities, ethical practice, informed consent, information technology, and performance improvement. Other topics include legal rights and responsibilities, referrals, resource management, staff education, supervision, confidentiality and information security, and continuity of care. Content included in the safety and infection control section is used to guide the nurse with purposeful protection of the client and others from health and environmental risks. Specific content includes but is not limited to reporting requirements, security procedures, verification of appropriateness of treatment orders, and infection control measures. The questions in this book follow the NCLEX-RN® test plan.

CLINICAL JUDGMENT GUIDE

Nurses* base their decisions on many different principles in order to arrive at a course of action. Among the basic guidelines to apply in nursing practice—and in answering test questions—are the nursing process and Maslow's Hierarchy of Needs.

TABLE 1–1   Client Needs Categories and Percentage of Items (April 2019)

Client Needs	Percentage of Items
Safe and Effective Care Environment	
• Management of Care	17%–23%
• Safety and Infection Control	9%–15%
Health Promotion and Maintenance	6%–12%
Psychosocial Integrity	6%–12%
Physiological Integrity	
• Basic Care and Comfort	6%–12%
• Pharmacological and Parenteral Therapies	12%–18%
• Reduction of Risk Potential	9%–15%
• Physiological Adaptation	11%–17%

Source: The National Council of State Boards of Nursing, Chicago, IL, with permission.

---

* In this book, the term "nurse," unless otherwise specified, refers to a licensed RN. An RN can assign tasks to an LPN or delegate to a UAP, which may be known under other terms such as "medical assistant" or "nurse's aide." An LPN can delegate tasks to a UAP. Each state will have specific regulations that govern what duties or tasks can be delegated or assigned to each of these types of personnel.
The term "health-care provider," as used in this book, refers to a client's primary provider of medical care. It includes physicians (including osteopathic physicians), nurse practitioners (NPs), and physician assistants (PAs). Depending on state regulations, many NPs and some PAs have prescriptive authority for at least some categories of prescribed drugs.

The Nursing Process

One of the basic guidelines to apply in nursing practice is the nursing process, which consists of five steps—assessment, nursing diagnosis, planning, intervention, and evaluation—that are usually completed in a systematic order. Assessment is the first step. If a priority setting question asks the test taker which step to implement first, the test taker should first look at assessment.

EXAMPLE

> The nurse is caring for a client diagnosed with congestive heart failure who is currently reporting dyspnea. Which intervention should the nurse implement **first?**
>
> 1. Administer furosemide IV pyelogram (IVP).
> 2. Check the client for adventitious lung sounds.
> 3. Ask the respiratory therapist to administer a treatment.
> 4. Notify the health-care provider (HCP).
>
> **Answer: 2**
> Checking for adventitious lung sounds is assessing the client to determine the extent of the client's breathing difficulties causing the dyspnea.

There are numerous words, such as "check," that can be used to indicate assessment. The test taker should not discard an option because the word "assess" or "assessment" is not used. Alternatively, the test taker shouldn't assume that an option is correct merely because the word "assess" is used. The test taker must also be aware that the assessment data must match the problem stated in the stem, regardless of terminology. The nurse must assess for the correct information. If option 2 in the previous example said, "Assess urinary output," it would not be a correct option even though it includes the word "assess," because urinary output is not related to heart failure or breathing difficulties. In addition, the test taker should be aware that assessment is not always the correct answer when the question asks which should be done first. Suppose, for example, that the previous question had listed option 3 as "Apply oxygen via nasal cannula at 2 liters per minute." In that case, assessment would not come first. The nurse would first attempt to relieve the client's distress and then assess.

When a question asks what a nurse should do next, the test taker should determine from the information given in the question which steps in the nursing process have been completed and then choose an option that matches the next step in the nursing process.

EXAMPLE

> The client diagnosed with peptic ulcer disease has a blood pressure of 88/42, an apical pulse of 132, and respirations of 28. The nurse documents the nursing diagnosis "altered tissue perfusion related to decreased circulatory volume." Which intervention should the nurse implement **first?**
>
> 1. Notify the laboratory to draw a type & crossmatch.
> 2. Assess the client's abdomen for tenderness.
> 3. Insert an 18-gauge catheter and infuse lactated Ringer's.
> 4. Check the client's pulse oximeter reading.
>
> **Answer: 3**
>
> 1. Notifying the laboratory for a type and crossmatch would be an appropriate intervention because the client is showing signs of hypovolemia, but it is not the first intervention because it would not directly support the client's circulatory volume.
> 2. The stem of the question has provided enough assessment data to indicate the client's problem of hypovolemia. Further assessment data are not needed.
> 3. **The vital signs indicate hypovolemia, which is a life-threatening emergency that requires a nursing intervention to support the client's circulatory volume. The nurse can do this by infusing lactated Ringer's solution.**
> 4. A pulse oximeter reading would not support the client's circulatory volume.

The nurse has assessed the client and formulated a nursing diagnosis. The next step in the nursing process is implementation. The nurse should proceed to a nursing intervention appropriate for the situation. This type of question is designed to determine if the test taker can set priorities in client care.

Maslow's Hierarchy of Needs

If the test taker has looked at the question and the nursing process does not assist the test taker in determining the correct option, then a tool such as Maslow's Hierarchy of Needs (Fig. 1–1) should be utilized. Note, the bottom of the pyramid—physiological needs—represents the top priority in instituting nursing interventions. If a question asks the test taker to determine which is the priority intervention and a physiological need is listed among the options, then that is the priority. If a physiological need is not listed, safety and security take priority, and so on up the pyramid.

TYPES OF QUESTIONS

Most of the questions on the NCLEX-RN® are multiple choice. Clinical judgment questions often involve prioritizing client care, delegating staff tasks, and managing issues related to clients and staff. These questions may include interpreting medication administration records (MARs) or laboratory values, determining when notifying the primary HCP is a priority, and choosing which tasks can be assigned to a licensed practical nurse (LPN) or unlicensed assistive personnel (UAP) and which must be performed by an RN.

Some questions on the NCLEX-RN® are termed "alternate-format questions" and include choosing more than one option that correctly answers a question, ranking procedures or actions in correct order, drop-and-drag questions, and fill-in-the-blank questions.

EXAMPLE

> The nurse is assigning tasks to the UAP. Which is an appropriate delegation to the UAP? **Select all that apply.**
>
> 1. Check the area around an incisional wound for redness.
> 2. Help a client with an upper limb cast to eat.
> 3. Assist a client recovering from a hysterectomy to walk to the bathroom.
> 4. Explain to a client being discharged how to empty and clean the colostomy bag.
> 5. Transport a client with a suspected fractured tibia to the x-ray department.
>
> **Correct answers are 2, 3, and 5.**
>
> 1. Checking the area around a wound is an assessment. An RN cannot delegate assessment, teaching, evaluation, medications, or care of an unstable client to a UAP.
> 2. **The UAP can assist a client with a cast to eat.**
> 3. **The UAP can assist a stable client to the bathroom.**
> 4. Explaining colostomy care is a teaching intervention. An RN cannot delegate assessment, teaching, evaluation, medications, or care of an unstable client to a UAP.
> 5. **The UAP can transport a client to the x-ray department.**

Prioritizing Questions and Setting Priorities

In test questions that ask the nurse which action to take first, two or more of the options will be appropriate nursing interventions for the situation described. When choosing the correct answer, the test taker must decide which intervention should occur *first* in a sequence of events or which intervention directly impacts the situation.

With a question that asks which client the nurse should assess first, the test taker should first look at each option and determine if the signs or symptoms the client is exhibiting are normal or expected for the disease process; if so, the nurse does not need to assess that particular client first. Second, if two or more of the options state signs or symptoms that are not

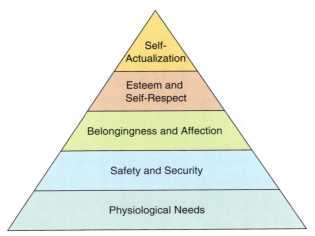

Figure 1–1. Maslow's Hierarchy of Needs

normal or expected for the disease process, then the test taker should select the option that has the greatest potential for a poor outcome. Each option should be examined carefully to determine the priority by asking these questions:

- Is the situation life threatening or life altering? *If yes, this client is the highest priority.*
- Is the situation unexpected for the disease process? *If yes, then this client may be the priority.*
- Is the data presented abnormal? *If yes, then this client may be the priority.*
- Is the situation expected for the disease process and not life threatening? *If yes, then this client may be—but probably is not—the priority.*
- Is the situation or data normal? *If yes, this client can be seen last.*

On a computerized test, such as the NCLEX-RN® exam, the test taker must make a decision before advancing to the next question.

Delegating and Assigning Care

Although each state has its own Nursing Practice Act, there are some general guidelines that apply to all professional nurses.

- When delegating to a UAP, the nurse may not delegate any activity that requires nursing clinical judgment. These activities include assessing, teaching, evaluating, administering medications to any client, and the care of any unstable client.
- When assigning care to an LPN, the RN can assign the administration of some medications but cannot assign assessing, teaching, or evaluating any client and cannot delegate the care of an unstable client.

Management Decisions

The nurse is frequently called upon to make decisions about staffing, movement of clients from one unit to another, or handling conflicts as they arise. Some general guidelines for answering questions in this area include the following:

- The most experienced nurse gets the most critical client.
- A graduate nurse can care for any client with supervision.
- The most stable client can move or be discharged, whereas the most unstable client must move to the intensive care unit (ICU) or stay in the ICU.

When the nurse must make decisions regarding a conflict among nursing staff, a good rule to follow is to involve the chain of command. The primary nurse should directly address a conflict with a peer (another primary nurse) or a subordinate unless the situation is illegal (such as stealing drugs). The primary nurse should use the chain of command in situations that address superiors (a manager or director of nursing). In this case, the nurse should discuss the situation with the next in command above the superior.

General Test-Taking Guidelines

A few common test-taking guidelines should be utilized for the examination.

- Read the entire question and identify keywords, such as time frames, age, sex, marital status, disease or condition, symptoms, and so on.
- All HCP orders needed to perform a listed intervention are already written, unless otherwise stated.
- Make an educated guess.
- Absolutes, such as "all" or "every," are usually not correct.
- When selecting an answer, choose a client-centered option before equipment.
- According to the NCSBN, "select-all-that-apply" questions can have one correct response, more than one correct response, or all responses correct. No minimum or maximum number of responses are required. There are no partially correct answers.
- Answer "select-all-that-apply" questions by evaluating if each answer is true or false. Each option stands alone.
- The RN does not delegate assessment, teaching, evaluation, or an unstable client to an LPN or UAP. The RN does not assign a task to a staff member that is not within his or her scope of practice.
- If the client is in distress, do not assess; instead, do something.

For general information on how to prepare for an examination and on the types of questions used in nursing examinations, refer to *Fundamentals Success: A Q&A Review Applying Critical Thinking to Test Taking* by Patricia Nugent, RN, MA, MS, EdD, and Barbara Vitale, RN, MA.

PUTTING THE PIECES TOGETHER

The nurse is required to acquire information, analyze the data, and make inferences based on the available information. Sometimes this process is relatively easy and at other times the pieces of available information and data do not seem to fit. This is precisely where clinical judgment guides decision making and nursing actions.

Cardiovascular Management

2

When you do the common things in life in an uncommon way, you will command the attention of the world.

—George Washington Carver

QUESTIONS

1. The nurse on the cardiac unit has received the shift report from the outgoing nurse. Which client should the nurse assess **first?**
   1. The client who has just been brought to the unit from the emergency department (ED) without any reported symptoms
   2. The client who received pain medication 30 minutes ago for chest pain that was a level 3 on a 1-to-10 pain scale
   3. The client who had a cardiac catheterization in the morning and has palpable pedal pulses bilaterally
   4. The client who has been turning on the call light frequently and stating her care has been neglected

2. The nurse on the cardiac unit is preparing to administer medications after receiving the morning change-of-shift report. Which medication should the nurse administer **first?**
   1. The cardiac glycoside to the client who has an apical pulse of 58
   2. The loop diuretic to a client with a serum K$^+$ level of 3.2 mEq/L
   3. The antidysrhythmic to the client in ventricular fibrillation
   4. The calcium-channel blocker to the client who has a blood pressure of 110/68

3. Which client should the telemetry nurse assess **first** after receiving the a.m. shift report?
   1. The client diagnosed with deep vein thrombosis who has an edematous right calf
   2. The client diagnosed with mitral valve stenosis who has heart palpitations
   3. The client diagnosed with arterial occlusive disease who has intermittent claudication
   4. The client diagnosed with congestive heart failure who has pink frothy sputum

4. The RN charge nurse is making assignments for clients on a cardiac unit. Which client should the RN charge nurse assign to a new graduate nurse (GN)?
   1. The 44-year-old client diagnosed with a myocardial infarction
   2. The 65-year-old client diagnosed with unstable angina
   3. The 75-year-old client scheduled for a cardiac catheterization
   4. The 50-year-old client reporting chest pain

5. The RN charge nurse is making assignments for a 30-bed cardiac unit staffed with three registered nurses (RNs), three licensed practical nurses (LPNs), and three unlicensed assistive personnel (UAPs). Which assignment is **most** appropriate by the charge nurse?
   1. Assign an RN to perform all sterile procedures.
   2. Assign an LPN to give all IV medications.
   3. Assign a UAP to complete the a.m. care.
   4. Assign an LPN to write the care plans.

6. The nurse on a cardiac unit is discussing a client with the case manager. Which information should the nurse share with the case manager?
   1. Discuss personal information the client shared with the nurse in confidence.
   2. Provide the case manager with any information that is required for continuity of care.
   3. Explain that client confidentiality prevents the nurse from disclosing information.
   4. Ask the case manager to get the client's permission before sharing information.

7. The RN staff nurse assesses erratic electrical activity on the telemetry reading while the client is talking to the nurse on the intercom system. Which task should the nurse instruct the UAP to implement?
   1. Call a Code Blue immediately.
   2. Check the client's telemetry leads.
   3. Find the nurse to check the client.
   4. Remove the telemetry monitor.

8. The RN charge nurse on the cardiac unit has to float a nurse to the emergency department for the shift. Which nurse should be floated to the emergency department?
   1. The nurse who has 4 years of experience in the operating room
   2. The nurse who just transferred from critical care to the cardiac unit
   3. The nurse with 1 year of experience on the cardiac unit who has been on a week's sick leave
   4. The nurse who has worked in the gastrointestinal lab for 2 years and in the cardiac unit for 3 years

9. The cardiac nurse is preparing to administer 1 unit of blood to a client. Which interventions should the nurse implement? **Rank in order of priority.**
   1. Infuse the unit of blood at 20 gtts/min the first 15 minutes.
   2. Check the unit of blood and the client's blood band with another nurse.
   3. Initiate Y-tubing with normal saline via an 18-gauge angiocatheter.
   4. Assess the client's vital signs and lung sounds and assess for a rash.
   5. Obtain informed consent for the blood administration from the client.

10. The RN charge nurse in the cardiac critical care unit is making rounds. Which client should the nurse see **first?**
   1. The client diagnosed with coronary artery disease who is reporting that the nurses are being rude and won't answer the call lights
   2. The client diagnosed with an acute myocardial infarction who has an elevated creatinine phosphokinase-cardiac muscle (CPK-MB) level
   3. The client diagnosed with atrial fibrillation on an oral anticoagulant who has an International Normalized Ratio (INR) of 2.8
   4. The client 2 days postoperative coronary artery bypass who is being transferred to the cardiac unit

11. The nurse is preparing to administer digoxin 0.25 mg IVP to a client in severe congestive heart failure who is receiving $D_5W/0.9$ NaCL at 25 mL/hr. **Rank in order of performance.**
   1. Administer the medication over 5 minutes.
   2. Dilute the medication with normal saline.
   3. Draw up the medication in a tuberculin syringe.
   4. Check the client's identification band.
   5. Clamp the primary tubing distal to the port.

12. The client is in the cardiac intensive care unit on dopamine and BP increases to 210/130. Which intervention should the intensive care nurse implement **first?**
    1. Discontinue the client's dopamine.
    2. Notify the client's health-care provider.
    3. Administer hydralazine intravenously.
    4. Assess the client's neurological status.

13. The RN charge nurse is making client assignments in the cardiac critical care unit. Which client should be assigned to the **most** experienced nurse?
    1. The client diagnosed with acute rheumatic fever carditis who refuses to stay on bedrest
    2. The client who has the following ABG values: pH, 7.35; Pao$_2$, 88; Paco$_2$, 44; Hco$_3$, 22
    3. The client who is showing multifocal premature ventricular contractions (PVCs)
    4. The client diagnosed with angina who is scheduled for a cardiac catheterization

14. The primary cardiac RN staff nurse is delegating tasks to the unlicensed assistive personnel (UAP). Which delegation task **warrants** intervention by the RN charge nurse of the cardiac unit?
    1. The UAP is instructed to bathe the client who is on telemetry.
    2. The UAP is requested to obtain a bedside glucometer reading.
    3. The UAP is asked to assist with a portable chest x-ray.
    4. The UAP is told to feed a client diagnosed with dysphagia.

15. The nurse is administering medications to clients in the cardiac critical care area. Which client should the nurse **question** administering the medication?
    1. The client receiving a calcium channel blocker who is drinking a glass of grapefruit juice
    2. The client receiving a beta-adrenergic blocker who has an apical heart rate of 62 bpm
    3. The client receiving nonsteroidal anti-inflammatory drugs (NSAIDs) who has just finished eating breakfast
    4. The client receiving an oral anticoagulant who has an International Normalized Ratio (INR) of 2.8

16. The charge nurse on the cardiac unit is counseling a staff nurse because the nurse has clocked in late multiple times for the 7:00 a.m. to 7:00 p.m. shift. Which conflict resolution uses the **win-win** strategy?
    1. The charge nurse terminates the staff nurse as per the hospital policy so that a new nurse can be transferred to the unit.
    2. The charge nurse discovers that the staff nurse is having problems with child care; therefore, the charge nurse allows the staff nurse to work a 9:00 a.m. to 9:00 p.m. shift.
    3. The charge nurse puts the staff nurse on probation with the understanding that the next time the staff nurse is late to work it will result in termination.
    4. The staff nurse asks another employer to talk to the charge nurse to explain that he or she is a valuable part of the team.

17. Which client warrants **immediate** intervention by the nurse?
    1. The client diagnosed with pericarditis who has chest pain with inspiration
    2. The client diagnosed with mitral valve regurgitation who has a thready peripheral pulse
    3. The client diagnosed with Marfan syndrome who has pectus excavatum
    4. The client diagnosed with atherosclerosis who has slurred speech and drooling

18. The UAP working in a long-term care facility notifies the RN staff nurse that the client diagnosed with congestive heart failure who is on a low-sodium diet is reporting that the food is inedible. Which intervention should the RN staff nurse implement **first?**
    1. Have the family bring food from home for the client.
    2. Check to see what the client has eaten in the past 24 hours.
    3. Tell the client that a low-sodium diet is important for this diagnosis.
    4. Ask the dietitian to discuss food preferences with the client.

19. The RN charge nurse on the cardiac unit is making shift assignments. Which client should be assigned to the **most** experienced nurse?
    1. The client diagnosed with mitral valve stenosis
    2. The client diagnosed with asymptomatic sinus bradycardia
    3. The client diagnosed with fulminant pulmonary edema
    4. The client diagnosed with acute atrial fibrillation

20. The evening nurse in a long-term care facility is preparing to administer medications to a client diagnosed with atrial fibrillation. Which medication should the nurse **question** administering?

Client: Mr. A Date: Today	Allergies: Penicillin Diagnosis: Atrial Fibrillation	
Medication	0701–1900	1901–0700
Warfarin 5 mg PO daily		1800 INR: 3.4 today
Metoclopramide 5 mg PO tid	0900 DN 1300 DN	1800
Docusate PO bid	0900 DN	1800
Atorvastatin PO daily		1800
Nurse Name/Initials	Day Nurse RN/DN	Night Nurse RN/NN

    1. Warfarin
    2. Metoclopramide
    3. Docusate
    4. Atorvastatin

21. The RN staff nurse and the UAP enter the client's room and discover that the client is unresponsive. Which action, according to the American Heart Association (AHA) guidelines, should the RN staff nurse assign to the UAP **first?**
    1. Ask the UAP to check whether the client is asleep.
    2. Tell the UAP to perform cardiac compressions.
    3. Instruct the UAP to get the crash cart.
    4. Request the UAP to put the client in a recumbent position.

22. The elderly client on a cardiac unit has a do not resuscitate (DNR) order written. Which interventions should the nurse implement? **Select all that apply.**
    1. Continue to care for the client's needs as usual.
    2. Place a DNR identification armband on the client.
    3. Refer the client to a hospice organization.
    4. Limit visitors to two at a time, so as not to tire the client.
    5. Remove telemetry monitors from the client.

23. The nurse is initiating discharge teaching to a 68-year-old male client who had quadruple coronary bypass surgery. Which **priority** question should the nurse ask the client?
    1. "Are you sexually active?"
    2. "Can you still drive your car?"
    3. "Do you have pain medications at home?"
    4. "Do you know when to call your HCP?"

24. The LPN informs the clinic RN that the client diagnosed with atrial fibrillation has an INR of 4.5. Which intervention should the clinic RN implement?
    1. Tell the LPN to notify the clinic health-care provider (HCP).
    2. Instruct the LPN to assess the client for abnormal bleeding.
    3. Obtain a STAT electrocardiogram on the client.
    4. Take no action because this INR is within the normal range.

25. The RN staff nurse at a disaster site is triaging victims when a woman states, "I am a certified nurse aide. Can I do anything to help?" Which action should the RN staff nurse implement?
    1. Request the woman to please leave the area.
    2. Ask the woman to check the injured clients.
    3. Tell the woman to try and keep the victims calm.
    4. Instruct the woman to help the paramedics.

26. The cardiac clinic RN staff nurse hears the UAP tell the client, "You have gained over 15 pounds since your last visit." The scale is located in the open office area. Which action should the clinic RN staff nurse implement?
    1. Tell the UAP in front of the client to not comment on the weight.
    2. Ask the UAP to put the client in the room and take no action.
    3. Explain to the UAP, in private, that this is an inappropriate comment and violates the HIPAA.
    4. Report the UAP to the director of nurses of the clinic.

27. The nurse on the cardiac unit is discussing case management with a client who asks, "Why do I need a case manager for my heart disease?" Which statements are **most** appropriate for the nurse to respond? **Select all that apply.**
    1. "Case management helps contain the costs of your health care."
    2. "It will help enhance your quality of life with a chronic illness."
    3. "It decreases the fragmentation of care across many health-care settings."
    4. "Case management is a form of health insurance for clients diagnosed with chronic illnesses."
    5. "We try to provide quality care along the health-care continuum."

28. The client diagnosed with arterial hypertension has been taking a calcium channel blocker, a loop diuretic, and an ACE inhibitor for 3 years. Which statement by the client would **warrant** intervention by the nurse?
    1. "I have to go to the bathroom a lot during the morning."
    2. "I get up very slowly when I have been sitting for a while."
    3. "I do not salt my food when I am cooking it but I add it at the table."
    4. "I drink grapefruit juice every morning with my breakfast."

29. The RN director of nurses in the cardiac clinic is counseling an unlicensed assistive personnel (UAP) in the clinic who returned late from her lunch break seven times in the past 2 weeks. Which conflict resolution uses the **win-lose** strategy?
    1. The UAP explains she is checking on her ill mother during lunch, and the nurse allows her to take a longer lunch break if she comes in early.
    2. The director of nurses offers the UAP a transfer to the emergency weekend clinic so that she will be off during the week.
    3. The director of nurses terminates the UAP, explaining that all staff must be on time so that the clinic runs smoothly.
    4. The UAP is placed on 1-month probation, and any further occurrences will result in termination from this position.

30. The RN cardiac clinic nurse has told the unlicensed assistive personnel (UAP) twice to change the sharps container in the examination room, but it has not been changed. Which action should the nurse implement **first**?
    1. Tell the UAP to change it immediately.
    2. Ask the UAP why the sharps container has not been changed.
    3. Change the sharps container as per clinic policy.
    4. Document the situation and place a copy of the documentation in the employee file.

31. The wife of a client calls the clinic and tells the nurse her husband is having chest pain but won't go to the hospital. Which action should the nurse implement **first**?
    1. Instruct the wife to call 911 immediately.
    2. Tell the wife to have the client chew an aspirin.
    3. Ask the wife what the client had to eat recently.
    4. Request that the husband talk to the clinic physician.

32. The home health (HH) nurse received phone messages from the agency secretary. Which client should the nurse contact **first**?
    1. The client diagnosed with hypertension who is reporting a BP of 148/92
    2. The client diagnosed with cardiomyopathy who has a pulse oximeter reading of 93%
    3. The client diagnosed with congestive heart failure who has edematous feet
    4. The client diagnosed with chronic atrial fibrillation who is having chest pain

33. The client is diagnosed with end-stage congestive heart failure. The nurse finds the client lying in bed, short of breath, unable to talk, and with buccal cyanosis. Which intervention should the nurse implement **first**?
    1. Assist the client to a sitting position.
    2. Assess the client's vital signs.
    3. Call 911 for the paramedics.
    4. Auscultate the client's lung sounds.

34. The home health (HH) nurse is visiting a client diagnosed with congestive heart failure. The client has an out-of-hospital do not resuscitate (DNR) order, has stopped breathing, and has no pulse or blood pressure. The client's family is at the bedside. Which intervention should the HH nurse implement **first**?
    1. Contact the agency's chaplain.
    2. Pronounce the client's death.
    3. Ask the family to leave the bedside.
    4. Call the client's funeral home.

35. The cardiac nurse received laboratory results on the following clients. Which client warrants **immediate** intervention from the nurse?
    1. The client who has an INR of 2.8
    2. The client who has a serum potassium level of 3.8 mEq/L
    3. The client who has a serum digoxin level of 2.6 mg/dL
    4. The client who has a glycosylated hemoglobin of 6%

36. The home health (HH) nurse is completing the admission assessment for an obese client diagnosed with a myocardial infarction with comorbid type 1 diabetes and arterial hypertension. Which **priority** intervention should the nurse implement?
    1. Encourage the client to walk 30 minutes a day.
    2. Request an HH-registered dietitian to talk to the client.
    3. Refer the client to a cardiac rehabilitation unit.
    4. Discuss the client's need to lose 1 to 2 pounds a week.

37. The home health (HH) nurse is preparing for the initial visit to a client diagnosed with congestive heart failure. Which intervention should the HH nurse implement **first**?
    1. Prepare all the needed equipment for the visit.
    2. Call the client to arrange a time for the visit.
    3. Review the client's referral form and pertinent data.
    4. Make the necessary referrals for the client.

38. Which information should the experienced home health (HH) nurse discuss when orienting a new nurse to HH nursing? **Select all that apply.**
    1. If the client or family is hostile or obnoxious, call the police.
    2. Carry the HH care agency identification in a purse or wallet.
    3. Visits can be scheduled at night with permission from the agency.
    4. Inform the agency of the times of the client's scheduled visits.
    5. Report unsafe environments to the HH agency.

39. The home health (HH) aide tells the HH nurse that the grandson of the client she is caring for asked her out on a date. Which statement is the HH nurse's **best** response?
    1. "I am so excited for you; he seems like a very nice young man."
    2. "You should not go out with him as long as she is a client of our agency."
    3. "I think you should tell the director of the HH care agency about this date."
    4. "You should never date someone you meet while taking care of a client."

40. The cardiac nurse is teaching the client diagnosed with congestive heart failure. Which teaching interventions should the nurse discuss with the client? **Select all that apply.**
    1. Notify the health-care provider (HCP) if the client gains more than 2 lb in 1 day.
    2. Keep the head of the bed elevated when sleeping.
    3. Take the loop diuretic once a day before going to sleep.
    4. Teach the client which foods are high in sodium and should be avoided.
    5. Perform isotonic exercises at least once a day.

41. The nurse is administering medications on a cardiac unit. Which medication should the nurse **question** administering?
    1. Warfarin to a client with a PT of 14 and an INR of 1.6 mg/dL
    2. Digoxin to a client with a potassium level of 3.3 mEq/L
    3. Atenolol for the client with an aspirate aminotransferase (AST) of 18 U/L
    4. Lisinopril for the client with a serum creatinine level of 0.8 mg/dL

42. The nurse is providing end-of-life care to the client diagnosed with cardiomyopathy who is in hospice. Which **priority** assessment intervention should the hospice nurse implement?
    1. Assess the client's spiritual needs.
    2. Assess the client's financial situation.
    3. Assess the client's support system.
    4. Assess the client's medical diagnosis.

43. The husband of the client diagnosed with infective endocarditis and who has a do not resuscitate (DNR) order tells the nurse, "My wife is not breathing." Which intervention should the RN staff nurse implement **first?**
    1. Contact the client's health-care provider (HCP).
    2. Notify the Rapid Response Team.
    3. Stay with the client and her husband.
    4. Instruct the UAP to perform postmortem care.

44. The hospice nurse is triaging phone calls from clients. Which client should the nurse contact **first?**
    1. The client whose family reports the client is not eating
    2. The client who wants to rescind the out-of-hospital DNR
    3. The client whose pain is not being controlled with the current medications
    4. The client whose urinary incontinence has caused a stage 1 pressure ulcer

45. The hospice nurse is working with a volunteer. Which task could the nurse delegate to the volunteer? **Select all that apply.**
    1. Sit with the client while he or she reminisces about life experiences.
    2. Give the client a sponge bath and rub lotion on the bony prominences.
    3. Provide spiritual support for the client and family members.
    4. Check the home to see that all necessary medical equipment is available.
    5. Assist with light housekeeping chores and meal preparation.

46. The RN staff nurse delegates postmortem care to the unlicensed assistive personnel (UAP). The UAP tells the nurse she has never performed postmortem care. Which statement is the **best** response by the RN staff nurse to the UAP?
    1. "It can be uncomfortable. I will go with you and show you what to do."
    2. "The client is already dead. You cannot hurt him now."
    3. "There is nothing to it; it is just a bed bath and change of clothes."
    4. "Don't worry. You can skip it this time, but you need to learn what to do."

47. The unlicensed assistive personnel (UAP) tells the RN staff nurse the client is reporting chest pain. Which task should the RN staff nurse delegate to the UAP?
    1. Call the health-care provider (HCP) and report the client's chest pain.
    2. Give the client some acetaminophen while the nurse checks the client.
    3. Bring the electronic health record (EHR) to the client's room.
    4. Notify the client's family of the onset of chest pain.

48. The registered nurse (RN) and licensed practical nurse (LPN) are caring for a group of clients on a cardiac unit. Which nursing tasks can be assigned to the LPN? **Select all that apply.**
    1. Feed the client who has an IV in both forearms.
    2. Assess the client diagnosed with stage IV heart failure.
    3. Perform discharge teaching with the client who had a cardiac catheterization.
    4. Administer the intravenous piggyback (IVPB) ceftriaxone.
    5. Contact the health-care provider for a PRN acetaminophen order for a client.

49. The RN hospice nurse is discussing the client's care with the unlicensed assistive personnel (UAP). Which statement contains the **best** information about caring for a client diagnosed with end-stage heart failure who is dying?
    1. "Perform as much care for the client as possible to conserve his or her strength."
    2. "Do not get too attached to the client because it will hurt when he or she dies."
    3. "Be careful not to promise to withhold health-care information from the team."
    4. "The client may want to talk about his or her life, but you should discourage that."

50. The client on telemetry is showing ventricular tachycardia. Which action should the telemetry RN staff nurse delegate to the unlicensed assistive personnel (UAP)?
    1. Have the UAP call the operator and announce the code.
    2. Tell the UAP to answer the other call lights on the unit.
    3. Send the UAP to the room to start rescue breaths.
    4. Ask the family to step out of the room during the code.

51. The family member of the client experiencing a cardiac arrest refuses to leave the client's room. Which intervention should the administrative supervisor implement?
    1. Stay with the family member and explain what the team is doing.
    2. Call hospital security to escort the family member out of the room.
    3. Ask the health-care provider (HCP) whether the family member can stay.
    4. Ignore the family member unless he or she becomes hysterical.

52. The client presents to the emergency department with a report of chest pain but does not have the ability to pay for the services. Which action should the emergency department nurse implement **first?**
    1. Place the client on a telemetry monitor and assess the client.
    2. Call an ambulance to transfer the client to a charity hospital.
    3. Have the client sign a form agreeing to pay the bill.
    4. Ask the client why he chose to come to this hospital.

53. The nurse is caring for clients on a cardiac unit. Which client should the nurse assess **first?**
    1. The client diagnosed with angina who is reporting chest pain
    2. The client diagnosed with CHF who has bilateral 4+ peripheral edema
    3. The client diagnosed with endocarditis who has a temperature of 100°F
    4. The client diagnosed with aortic valve stenosis who has syncope

54. Which medication should the nurse administer **first** after receiving the morning shift report?
    1. The IVPB antibiotic to the client diagnosed with endocarditis admitted at 0530 today
    2. The antiplatelet medication to the client who had a myocardial infarction
    3. The coronary vasodilator patch to the client diagnosed with coronary artery disease
    4. The statin medication to the client diagnosed with atherosclerosis

55. The nurse in a critical care cardiac unit is administering medications to a client. Which intervention should the nurse implement **first?**
    1. Check the radial pulse before administering digoxin.
    2. Monitor the amiodarone level for the client receiving amiodarone.
    3. Obtain the latest PTT results on the client with a heparin drip.
    4. Check the liver function panel for the client receiving a dopamine drip.

56. The surgical nurse is admitting a client having heart surgery to the operating room. Which information would require the nurse to call a time-out? **Select all that apply.**
    1. The client is drowsy from the preoperative medication and drifts off to sleep.
    2. The consent form states mitral valve replacement and the client states aortic valve replacement.
    3. The EHR and client's armband state the client is allergic to the narcotic analgesic morphine.
    4. The client states his or her name and birth date as it appears on the EHR.
    5. The surgical procedure is beginning to start and the team (surgeon, anesthesiologist, and nurse) are present.

57. The nurse is administering medications at 1800 to a client and uses the following medication administration record (MAR). Which intervention should the nurse implement **first?**

Client's Name: CC	Allergies: NKDA	
Diagnosis: Heart Failure	Height: 68 inches	
Medication	0701–1900	1901–0700
Digoxin 0.125 mg PO daily	0900 DN	
Furosemide 40 mg IVP daily	0900 DN	
Cephalosporin 1800 500 mg PO every 6 hours	1200 DN	1800
Warfarin 5 mg PO daily		1800
Nurse Name/Initials	Day Nurse RN/DN	Night Nurse RN/NN

    1. Assess the client's potassium and digoxin levels.
    2. Monitor the client's partial thromboplastin level.
    3. Check the client's International Normalized Ratio (INR).
    4. Verify the client's name and ID number with the MAR.

58. The nurse is administering medications to clients on a cardiac unit. Which medication should the nurse **question** administering?
    1. Furosemide to a client who had a 320-mL output in 4 hours
    2. Enoxaparin to a client who had open-heart surgery
    3. Ticlopidine to a client being prepared for surgery
    4. Captopril to a client who has a BP of 100/68

59. The RN intensive care unit nurse and a UAP are caring for a client who has had a coronary artery bypass graft (CABG). Which nursing tasks should the RN staff nurse assign to the UAP? **Select all that apply.**
    1. Monitor the client's arterial blood gases.
    2. Re-infuse the client's blood using the cell saver.
    3. Assist the client to take a sponge bath.
    4. Change the client's saturated leg dressing.
    5. Empty the urinary catheter drainage bag.

60. The nurse is preparing to administer two units of PRBCs to a client diagnosed with congestive heart failure (CHF). Which HCP order should the nurse **question?**
    1. Administer each unit over 2 hours.
    2. Administer furosemide IVP once.
    3. Restrict the client's fluids to 1,000 mL per 24 hours.
    4. Have a complete blood count (CBC) done the following morning.

61. The elderly client on the cardiac unit was found on the floor by the bed. Which information should the nurse document in the client's EHR?
    1. Fell. No injuries noted. Incident report completed. HCP notified.
    2. Found on floor. No reports of pain. Able to move all extremities.
    3. States no one answered call light, so attempted to get up without help.
    4. Got out of bed without assistance and fell by the bedside.

62. The RN home health (HH) nurse is caring for an elderly client. Which nursing task should the RN delegate to the HH aide?
    1. Cook and freeze meals for the client.
    2. Assist the client to sit on the front porch.
    3. Take the client for outings to the store.
    4. Monitor the client's mental status.

63. The client is admitted to determine if the client is experiencing a myocardial infarction. The client is reporting substernal chest pain radiating to the left arm and jaw. Which intervention should the nurse implement **first?**
    1. Take the client's pulse, respirations, and blood pressure.
    2. Call for a STAT electrocardiogram and a troponin level.
    3. Place sublingual nitroglycerin 0.3 mg under the tongue.
    4. Notify the HCP that the client has pain.

64. The client on the cardiac unit has a cardiac arrest. Which is the administrative supervisor nurse's **first** intervention during the code?
    1. Begin to take notes to document the code.
    2. Make sure all the jobs are being done.
    3. Arrange for an intensive care unit bed.
    4. Administer the emergency medications.

65. Which client should the cardiac nurse assess **first** after receiving the p.m. shift report?
    1. The client who is completing the second unit of PRBCs
    2. The client who is crying after being informed of a terminal diagnosis
    3. The client who refused to eat the dietary tray but got food from home
    4. The client who became short of breath ambulating in the hallway

66. The nurse is caring for Mr. A.B., a client on a telemetry unit. At 0830 the client reports chest pain. Which medication should the nurse administer?

Client Name: Mr. A.B. Weight in pounds: 202	Account Number: 1122337 Weight in kg: 91.82		Height: 72 inches Date: Today	
Medication			**1901–0700**	**0701–1900**
Morphine sulfate 2 mg IVP every 1 hour PRN chest pain				
Oxycodone 7.5/acetaminophen 325 mg PO every 4 hours PRN pain			0030 NN 0545 NN	
Aluminum Hydroxide; Magnesium Hydroxide; Simethicone 30 mL PO PRN indigestion				
Nitroglycerin 0.4 mg SL every 5 minutes up to 3 tablets PRN chest pain				
Nitroglycerin transdermal cream 1/2 inch			2100 Remove	0900 Apply
Signature/Initials			Night Nurse RN/NN	Day Nurse RN/DN

1. One-half inch of nitroglycerin transdermally now
2. Morphine sulfate 2 mg IVP STAT
3. Oxycodone 7.5 mg/acetaminophen 325 mg PO now
4. Nitroglycerin 0.4 mg sublingual STAT

67. The charge nurse on a cardiac unit has received laboratory reports to assess. Which laboratory report is **priority** for the charge nurse to assess?
1. Ms. C.T., who is on a heparin drip

Client Name: C.T. Diagnosis: DVT Weight in kg: 60	Account Number: 2233669 Height: 66 inches Weight in pounds: 132	Allergies: NKDA
Laboratory Report		
Laboratory Test	**Client Value**	**Normal Value**
aPT	15	10–13 seconds
INR	1.4	2.0–3.0 (therapeutic value)
aPTT	56	25–35 seconds

2. Mr. R.S., who is scheduled for a coronary artery bypass graft (CABG) this morning

Client Name: R.S. **Diagnosis:** Coronary Artery Disease **Weight in pounds:** 248	**Account Number:** 8855992 **Allergies:** Sulfa **Height:** 73 inches **Weight in kg:** 112.73	
Laboratory Report		
Laboratory Test	**Client Value**	**Normal Value**
aPT	11	10–13 seconds
INR	1.0	2.0–3.0 (therapeutic value)
aPTT	34	25–35 seconds
WBC	5.9	4.5–11.1 (x 10^3/microL)
RBC	4.9	Male: 4.21–5.81 (10^6 cells/microL)
		Female: 3.61–5.11 (10^6 cells/microL)
Hemoglobin	13.5	Male: 14–17.3 g/dL
		Female: 11.7–15.5 g/dL
Hematocrit	44.2	Male: 42%–52%
		Female: 36%–48%
Platelets	292	140–400 (10^3/microL)

3. Ms. T.R., who had a cardiac cauterization 18 hours ago

Client Name: T.R. **Diagnosis:** Chest pain **Weight in kg:** 90.9	**Account Number:** 6655774 **Height:** 62 inches	**Allergies:** Penicillin **Weight in pounds:** 200
Laboratory Report		
Laboratory Test	**Client Value**	**Normal Value**
aPT	12	10–13 seconds
INR	1.0	2.0–3.0 (therapeutic value)
aPTT	29	25–35 seconds

4. Mr. J.E., who is being evaluated for a heart murmur

Client Name: J.E. **Diagnosis:** R/O Gallbladder Disease **Weight in kg:** 90	**Account Number:** 6251489 **Height:** 68 inches	**Allergies:** NKDA **Weight in pounds:** 198
Laboratory Report		
Laboratory Test	**Client Value**	**Normal Value**
aPT	9.8	10–13 seconds
INR	1.3	2.0–3.0 (therapeutic value)
aPTT	26	25–35 seconds
Platelet	392	140–400 (10^3/microL)

68. The nurse on a medical unit is making rounds after receiving the shift report. Which client should the nurse see **first? Rank in order of priority.**
    1. The 45-year-old client who reported having chest pain at midnight last night and received nitroglycerin (NTG) sublingually
    2. The 62-year-old client who is reporting that no one answered the call light for 2 hours yesterday
    3. The 29-year-old client diagnosed with septicemia who called to request more blankets because of being cold
    4. The 78-year-old client diagnosed with dementia whose daughter is concerned because the client is more confused today
    5. The 37-year-old client who has a stage 4 pressure sore and the dressing needs to be changed this morning

69. While ambulating in the hallway with the nurse, the client diagnosed with myocardial infarction reports chest pain. Which interventions should the nurse implement? **Select all that apply.**
    1. Administer nitroglycerin 0.4 mg sublingual STAT.
    2. Have the client walk back to the room.
    3. Take the client's vital signs.
    4. Place the client on supplemental oxygen.
    5. Ask the unit secretary to call the health-care provider for orders.

70. The nurse received an aPTT report on a client receiving heparin via continuous drip infusion. According to the report, the client's drip rate should be decreased by 100 units per hour. The heparin comes prepared as 25,000 units in 500 mL of fluid. The current rate of infusion is 26 mL per hour. At what rate should the nurse set the pump?

CARDIAC CLINICAL SCENARIO

The 7 a.m. to 7 p.m. RN charge nurse is on a 24-bed telemetry unit in a level II trauma center in an urban area. There are four RNs, two LPNs, two UAPs, two telemetry technicians, and one unit secretary working with the charge nurse. There are 20 culturally diverse clients in the unit.

1. Which client should the charge nurse assign to the **most** experienced RN on the unit?
   1. The elderly client diagnosed with atrial fibrillation who is receiving the first dose of dabigatran
   2. The 43-year-old client diagnosed with congestive heart failure who is coughing up pink, frothy sputum
   3. The 47-year-old client diagnosed with a myocardial infarction who is exhibiting occasional premature ventricular contractions
   4. The young adult client diagnosed with mitral valve prolapse who is reporting shortness of breath when sitting in the chair

2. The telemetry technician tells the primary nurse the 59-year-old client in room 420 has a flat line. Which intervention should the primary nurse implement **first?**
   1. Instruct the UAP to take the crash cart to room 420.
   2. Tell the telemetry technician to call the Rapid Response Team.
   3. Determine if the client has an apical pulse and blood pressure.
   4. Check to see if the client has the telemetry leads on the chest.

3. The RN primary nurse has instructed the unlicensed assistive personnel (UAP) to assist the elderly client in room 410 to the bathroom for a shower. Which action by the UAP **warrants** intervention by the RN primary nurse?
   1. The UAP did not notify the desk the telemetry was being removed.
   2. The UAP did not remove the electrodes from the client's chest.
   3. The UAP placed a bath chair in the shower for the client.
   4. The UAP stayed in the client's bathroom while the client showered.

4. The RN charge nurse is looking over the morning laboratory results. Which client **warrants** the RN charge nurse notifying the health-care provider (HCP)?
   1. The 65-year-old client receiving IVP digoxin who has a digoxin level of 2.4 mg/dL
   2. The middle age client receiving warfarin who has an INR of 1.2
   3. The 56-year-old client receiving furosemide who has a potassium level of 3.5 mEq/L
   4. The young adult client receiving nystatin who has a cholesterol level of 205

5. Which client should the RN charge nurse assign to the LPN?
   1. The 19-year-old client who was just admitted from the emergency department to the unit
   2. The 72-year-old client who is exhibiting supraventricular tachycardia on telemetry
   3. The middle age client who had a left femoral cardiac catheterization this morning
   4. The 61-year-old client who needs teaching concerning coronary artery disease

6. The RN charge nurse is entering the health-care provider's admissions orders into the EHR for a 67-year-old client being admitted for R/O myocardial infarction. Which HCP's order should the RN charge nurse **question?**
   1. Draw cardiac isoenzymes every 6 hours.
   2. Provide low-fat, low-cholesterol diet.
   3. Administer morphine IVP 2 mg every 5 minutes for chest pain.
   4. Schedule client for endoscopy in the a.m.

7. Which nursing task is **most** appropriate for the RN charge nurse to delegate to the UAP?
   1. Request the UAP to obtain the newly admitted client's weight.
   2. Ask the UAP to clean the room for the client who has been discharged.
   3. Tell the UAP to take the vital signs on the client who is hypovolemic.
   4. Instruct the UAP to discuss the low-fat, low-cholesterol diet with the client.

8. The 79-year-old client in room 412 is reporting severe chest pain of 10 on a 1-to-10 pain scale. Which intervention should the nurse implement **first?**
   1. Check the client's MAR for the last time medication was administered.
   2. Assess the client's apical pulse, blood pressure, and lung sounds.
   3. Administer a sublingual nitroglycerin to the client.
   4. Place oxygen via nasal cannula at 6 L/min.

9. The 70-year-old client is in ventricular tachycardia. Which intervention should the nurse implement **first?**
   1. Defibrillate the client.
   2. Assess the carotid pulse.
   3. Administer epinephrine IVP.
   4. Start cardiopulmonary resuscitation.

10. The RN charge nurse is completing discharge teaching for the 56-year-old client diagnosed with angina. Which statement indicates the client needs **more** teaching?
    1. "I must keep my nitroglycerin tablets in a dark bottle at all times."
    2. "I should walk at least 30 minutes at least three times a week."
    3. "I will decrease the number of cigarettes I smoke daily."
    4. "I am going to take one baby aspirin every day."

The correct answer number and rationale for why it is the correct answer are given in **boldface type**. Rationales for why the other possible answer options are incorrect also are given, but they are not in boldface type.

1. 1. **This client may or may not be stable. The client may have no reported symptoms at this time, but the nurse must assess this client first to determine whether the issue that brought the client to the ED has stabilized. This client should be seen first.**
   2. It is important for the nurse to assess for pain relief in a timely manner, but this client has been medicated and the pain was a 3. The nurse can evaluate the amount of pain relief after making sure that the ED admission is stable.
   3. This client has been back from the procedure and a bilateral pedal pulse indicates the client is stable; therefore, this client does need to be seen first.
   4. Psychological issues are important but not more so than a physiological issue, and the client admitted from the ED may have a physiological problem.

CLINICAL JUDGMENT GUIDE: The test taker should use some tool as a reference to guide the decision-making process. In this situation, Maslow's Hierarchy of Needs should be applied. Physiological needs have priority over psychosocial ones.

2. 1. The cardiac glycoside, such as digoxin, should not be administered unless the apical pulse is 60 or above.
   2. Because the client's serum K^+ level is already low, the nurse should question administering a loop diuretic.
   3. **The client in ventricular fibrillation is in a life-threatening situation; therefore, the antidysrhythmic, such as amiodarone, should be administered first.**
   4. The client's blood pressure is above 90/60, so the calcium-channel blocker can be administered but it is not a priority over a client who is in a life-threatening situation.

CLINICAL JUDGMENT GUIDE: The test taker should know which medications are priority, such as life-sustaining medications, insulin, and mucolytics (Carafate). These medications should be administered first by the nurse.

3. 1. The nurse would expect the client diagnosed with a deep vein thrombosis to have an edematous right calf, so the nurse would not need to assess this client first.
   2. The nurse would expect the client diagnosed with mitral valve stenosis to have heart palpitations (sensations of rapid, fluttering heartbeat).
   3. The nurse would expect the client diagnosed with arterial occlusive disease to have intermittent claudication (leg pain), so the nurse would not need to assess this client first.
   4. **The nurse would not expect the client diagnosed with congestive heart failure to have pink, frothy sputum because this is a sign of pulmonary edema. This client should be assessed first.**

CLINICAL JUDGMENT GUIDE: The test taker must determine which sign or symptom is not expected for the disease process. If the sign or symptom is not expected, then the nurse should assess the client first. This type of question determines if the nurse is knowledgeable of signs or symptoms of a variety of disease processes.

4. 1. This client is at high risk for complications related to necrotic myocardial tissue and will need extensive teaching; therefore, this client should not be assigned to a new graduate.
   2. Unstable angina means this client is at risk for life-threatening complications and should not be assigned to a new graduate.
   3. **A new graduate should be able to complete a pre-procedural checklist and get this client to the catheterization laboratory.**
   4. Chest pain means this client could be having a myocardial infarction and should not be assigned to a new graduate.

CLINICAL JUDGMENT GUIDE: When the test taker is deciding which client should be assigned to a new graduate, the most stable client should be assigned to the least experienced nurse.

5. 1. An LPN can perform sterile procedures such as inserting indwelling catheters and IV catheters. An RN should perform the functions that require nursing judgment, such as planning and evaluating the care of the clients.
   2. Although an LPN could administer most intravenous piggyback (IVPB) medications, only qualified RNs may administer intravenous push (IVP) medications and chemotherapy.

3. **A UAP is capable of performing the morning care. This is an appropriate nursing task to delegate.**
4. Writing a care plan for a client requires nursing judgment; therefore, an RN should be assigned this function.

CLINICAL JUDGMENT GUIDE: An RN cannot delegate assessment, teaching, evaluation, medications, or an unstable client to a UAP. Tasks that cannot be delegated are nursing interventions that require nursing clinical judgment. Remember, in most instances, options with the word "all" (options 1 and 2) can be eliminated because if the test taker can think of one time when some other level of licensure could safely perform the task, then the option automatically becomes wrong.

6. 1. Unless the information shared is directly connected to health-care issues, the nurse should not share confidential information with anyone else. The nurse should inform clients that information directly affecting the client's health care will be shared on a need-to-know basis only.
   2. **The case manager's job is to ensure continuity and adequacy of care for the client. This individual has a "need to know."**
   3. The case manager is part of the health-care team; therefore, information should be shared.
   4. The client gave permission when being admitted to the hospital for information to be shared among those providing care. The case manager does not need to obtain further consent.

CLINICAL JUDGMENT GUIDE: The test taker must be knowledgeable of the role of each member of the multidisciplinary health-care team as well as the Health Insurance Portability and Accountability Act (HIPAA) rules and regulations. These topics will be tested on the NCLEX-RN® exam.

7. 1. The telemetry strip indicates an artifact, so there is no need for the UAP or any staff member to call a Code Blue, which is used when someone has arrested.
   2. **The UAP should be instructed to check the telemetry lead placement; this reading cannot be ventricular fibrillation because the client is talking to the nurse over the intercom system. This telemetry is an artifact; therefore, the leads should be checked and the UAP can do this because the client is stable.**
   3. The UAP can take care of this problem; there is no need for the primary nurse to check the client based on the information provided.

4. The strip indicates an artifact, but there is no indication that the client should be removed from telemetry.

CLINICAL JUDGMENT GUIDE: An RN cannot delegate assessment, teaching, evaluation, medications, or an unstable client to a UAP. Tasks that cannot be delegated are nursing interventions requiring nursing clinical judgment.

8. 1. The nurse who just has surgical nursing experience would not be the choice to float to the emergency department.
   2. **The nurse with critical care experience would be the best choice to float to the emergency department.**
   3. The nurse just returning from sick leave would not be a good choice to send to the emergency department, which may be very busy at times.
   4. This nurse has not had experience in critical care; therefore, this nurse would not be the best choice to float to the emergency department.

CLINICAL JUDGMENT GUIDE: The nurse needs to know management issues for the NCLEX-RN®. The nurse with experience in certain areas of nursing would be most appropriate to float to the areas with related types of clients, such as critical care and the emergency department.

9. Correct order is 5, 4, 3, 2, 1.
   5. **The nurse must first obtain informed consent before administering the blood product.**
   4. **The nurse needs to complete the pretransfusion assessment including assessing for any signs of allergic reaction before administering the unit of blood.**
   3. **The blood must be hung with Y-tubing and normal saline, and an 18-gauge angiocatheter is preferred.**
   2. **The nurse must check the unit of blood from the laboratory with another nurse and with the client's blood band.**
   1. **During the first 15 minutes, the blood transfusion must be administered slowly to determine if the client is going to have an allergic reaction.**

CLINICAL JUDGMENT GUIDE: This is an alternate type of question included in the NCLEX-RN® test plan. The nurse must be able to perform skills in the correct order. Obtaining informed consent and assessment should always be the first interventions.

10. 1. The charge nurse is responsible for all clients. At times it is necessary to see clients diagnosed with a psychosocial need before other clients who have situations that are expected and are not life threatening.
2. An elevated CPK-MB, cardiac isoenzyme, level is expected in a client diagnosed with an acute myocardial infarction; therefore, the charge nurse would not see this client first.
3. The INR is within the normal limits of 2 to 3; therefore, this client does not need to be assessed first.
4. This client is being transferred to the cardiac unit; therefore, the client is stable and does not require the charge nurse to see this client first.

CLINICAL JUDGMENT GUIDE: The test taker must determine if any of the assessment data is normal or abnormal for the client's diagnosis. If the data is abnormal, then this client should be seen first. If the physiological data is normal, then a client diagnosed with a psychosocial problem is the client the nurse should assess first.

11. **Correct order is 3, 2, 4, 5, 1.**
3. **Because this is a lower amount than 1 mL, the nurse should draw this medication up in a 1-mL tuberculin syringe to ensure accuracy of dosage.**
2. **The nurse should dilute the medication with normal saline to help decrease pain during administration and maintain the IV site longer. Administering 0.25 mg of digoxin in 0.5 mL is very difficult, if not impossible, to push over 5 full minutes, which is the manufacturer's recommended administration rate. If the medication is diluted, it is easier for the nurse to administer the medication over 5 minutes.**
4. **The nurse must check two identifiers according to the Joint Commission safety guidelines.**
5. **The nurse should clamp the tubing between the port and the primary IV line so that the medication will enter the vein, not ascend up the IV tubing.**
1. **Cardiovascular and narcotic medications are administered over 5 minutes.**

CLINICAL JUDGMENT GUIDE: This is an alternate type of question that is included in the NCLEX-RN® test plan. The nurse must be able to perform skills in the correct order.

12. 1. **The nurse should first discontinue the medication dopamine, a vasoconstrictor,** that is causing the increase in the client's blood pressure before doing anything else.
2. The nurse should notify the HCP but not before taking care of the client's elevated blood pressure.
3. The client may need a vasopressor hydralazine medication to decrease the blood pressure but the nurse should first discontinue the medication causing the elevated blood pressure.
4. The nurse must first decrease the client's blood pressure before assessing the client.

CLINICAL JUDGMENT GUIDE: The test taker should remember that when the client is in distress, do not assess. The nurse must intervene and take care of the client. If any of the options are assessment data the HCP will need or an intervention that will help the client, then the test taker should not select the option to notify the HCP.

13. 1. The client diagnosed with rheumatic heart fever is expected to have carditis and should be on bedrest. The nurse needs to talk to the client about the importance of being on bedrest but this client is not in a life-threatening situation and does not need the most experienced nurse.
2. These ABG values are within normal limits; therefore, a less experienced nurse could care for this client.
3. **Multifocal PVCs are an emergency and are possibly life threatening. An experienced nurse should care for this client.**
4. A cardiac catheterization is a routine procedure and would not require the most experienced nurse.

CLINICAL JUDGMENT GUIDE: The test taker must determine which client is the most unstable and would require the most experienced nurse, thus making this type of question an "except" question. Three clients are either stable or have non–life-threatening conditions.

14. 1. All clients in the ICU are on telemetry, and the UAP could bathe the client. This would not warrant intervention by the charge nurse.
2. The UAP can perform glucometer checks at the bedside, and there is nothing that indicates the client is unstable. This would not warrant intervention by the charge nurse.
3. The UAP can assist with helping the client sit up for a portable chest x-ray as long as the UAP is not pregnant and wears a shield.
4. **This client is at risk for choking and is not stable; therefore, the charge nurse should intervene and not allow the UAP to feed this client.**

CLINICAL JUDGMENT GUIDE: This is an "except" question. The test taker could ask which task is appropriate to delegate to the UAP; three options would be appropriate to delegate and one would not be. Remember, the RN cannot delegate assessment, teaching, evaluation, medications, or an unstable client to the UAP.

15. 1. **The client receiving a calcium channel blocker should avoid grapefruit juice because it can cause the CCB to rise to toxic levels. Grapefruit juice inhibits cytochrome P450-3A4 found in the liver and the intestinal wall. This inhibition affects the metabolism of some drugs and can, as is the case with CCBs, lead to toxic levels of the drug. For this reason, the nurse should investigate any medications the client is taking if the client drinks grapefruit juice.**
    2. The apical heart rate should be greater than 60 beats/minute before administering the medication; therefore, the nurse would not question administering this medication.
    3. Nonsteroidal anti-inflammatory drugs (NSAIDs) should be taken with foods to prevent gastric upset; therefore, the nurse would not question administering this medication.
    4. The INR therapeutic level for warfarin (Coumadin), an anticoagulant, is 2 to 3; therefore, the nurse would not question administering this medication.

CLINICAL JUDGMENT GUIDE: The test taker must be knowledgeable of medications. In most scenarios, there is no test-taking hint to help the test taker when answering medication questions except common nursing interventions, such as do not administer cardiac medications if client has AP lower than 60 or BP lower than 90/60, do not administer medications with grapefruit juice or antacids, or administer most medications with food to prevent GI distress.

16. 1. This is a win-lose strategy wherein, during the conflict, one party (charge nurse) exerts dominance and the other (staff nurse) submits.
    2. **This is a win-win strategy that focuses on goals and attempts to meet the needs of both parties. The charge nurse keeps an experienced nurse and the staff nurse keeps his or her position. Both parties win.**
    3. This is negotiation in which the conflicting parties give and take on the issue. The staff nurse gets one more chance and the charge nurse's authority is still intact.

4. This is not an example of a win-win strategy and is not an appropriate action for the staff nurse to take. The opinion of the staff should not influence the charge nurse's action.

CLINICAL JUDGMENT GUIDE: There will be management questions on the NCLEX-RN®. In many instances, there is no test-taking strategy; the nurse must be knowledgeable of management issues.

17. 1. The client diagnosed with pericarditis is expected to have chest pain with inspiration; therefore, this client does not warrant immediate intervention.
    2. The client diagnosed with mitral valve regurgitation is expected to have thready peripheral pulses and cool, clammy extremities. Therefore, this client does not warrant immediate intervention.
    3. The client diagnosed with Marfan syndrome is expected to have a chest that sinks in or sticks out, known as funnel chest or pectus excavatum; therefore, this client does not warrant immediate intervention.
    4. **Slurred speech and drooling are signs of a cerebrovascular accident (stroke) and is not normal for a client diagnosed with atherosclerosis; therefore, this client should be assessed first.**

CLINICAL JUDGMENT GUIDE: The test taker should ask, "Is the assessment data normal for the disease process?" If it is normal for the disease process, the nurse would not need to intervene; if it is not normal for the disease process, then this warrants intervention by the nurse.

18. 1. The family may be allowed to bring in food occasionally from home, but what they bring may not adhere to a low-sodium diet, and the family should not be required to provide three meals per day for the client. This is the facility's responsibility.
    2. **Assessing the client's intake will help the nurse to determine the extent of the client's dissatisfaction with the food. This is the first intervention.**
    3. This may be true but does not help the client adjust to a lack of sodium in the diet.
    4. A referral to the dietitian should be made after the nurse fully assesses the situation.

CLINICAL JUDGMENT GUIDE: Assessment is the first step of the nursing process, and the test taker should use the nursing process or some other systematic process to assist in determining priorities.

19. 1. The client diagnosed with mitral valve stenosis can live with this diagnosis and it is not a life-threatening condition.
2. The client diagnosed with asymptomatic sinus bradycardia is stable and, because the client is not exhibiting any signs or symptoms, this client does not need to be assigned to the most experienced nurse.
3. **A client diagnosed with fulminant pulmonary edema is experiencing an acute, life-threatening problem. The most experienced nurse should be assigned to this client.**
4. A client diagnosed with acute atrial fibrillation is not in a life-threatening situation; therefore, this client would not be assigned to the most experienced nurse.

CLINICAL JUDGMENT GUIDE: The test taker must determine which client is the most unstable and would require the most experienced nurse, thus making this type of question an "except" question. Three clients are either stable or have non–life-threatening conditions.

20. 1. **The client's International Normalized Ratio (INR) is 3.4. The therapeutic range is 2 to 3 for a client diagnosed with atrial fibrillation. This client is at risk for bleeding. The nurse should hold the medication and discuss the warfarin (Coumadin) with the HCP.**
2. Metoclopramide (Reglan) is used to stimulate gastric emptying. Nothing in the stem or the MAR indicates a problem with administering this medication. The nurse would administer this medication.
3. Docusate (Colace) is a stool softener. Nothing in the stem or the MAR indicates a problem with administering this medication. The nurse would administer this medication.
4. Atorvastatin (Lipitor) is a lipid-lowering medication. Nothing in the stem or the MAR indicates a problem with administering this medication. The nurse would administer this medication.

CLINICAL JUDGMENT GUIDE: This is an alternate type question included in the NCLEX-RN® test plan. The test taker must be able to read a medication administration record (MAR), be knowledgeable of medications, and be able to make a decision as to the nurse's most appropriate intervention.

21. 1. The first step in cardiopulmonary resuscitation according to the American Heart Association (AHA) guidelines is to establish unresponsiveness by "shaking and shouting." If the client does not respond to being shaken, then the nurse can proceed to the next step, which is to "look, listen, and feel" for breaths. This is assessment and, according to AHA guidelines, the UAP could perform this function if alone. However, the nurse should assess the client before a UAP.
2. Administering chest compressions is performed after establishing unresponsiveness and lack of respiration.
3. **The nurse can tell the UAP to get the crash cart while the nurse assesses the client. This is the best task to assign the UAP at this time because this client may be unstable; until that is determined, the nurse should not delegate any client care.**
4. The nurse should place the client in the recumbent position before attempting to perform chest compressions; the nurse should send the UAP for help and the crash cart.

CLINICAL JUDGMENT GUIDE: This is an "except" question. The test taker could ask which task is appropriate to delegate to the UAP; three options would be appropriate to delegate and one would not be. Remember, the RN cannot delegate assessment, teaching, evaluation, medications, or an unstable client to the UAP.

22. Correct answers are 1 and 2.
1. **The nurse should care for the client as if the DNR order was not on the EHR. A DNR order does not mean the client no longer wishes treatment. It means the client does not want CPR or to be placed on a ventilator if the client's heart stops beating.**
2. **The information about the DNR status should be communicated to other healthcare personnel by placement of a special armband on the client or a similar form of designation.**
3. The client has a DNR order, but this does not imply that there may be 6 months or less life expectancy for the client. (Hospice care may be requested for clients with a fewer than 6-month life expectancy.) An order for hospice must be written by the attending healthcare provider before making this referral.
4. The client should be allowed as many visitors as the hospital policy allows.
5. A DNR order does not indicate that the client does not want cardiac telemetry monitoring or other diagnostic procedures.

CLINICAL JUDGMENT GUIDE: This is an alternate type of question included in the NCLEX-RN®. The nurse must be able to select all the options

that answer the question correctly. There are no partially correct answers. The NCLEX-RN® test plan includes nursing care that is ruled by legal requirements. The nurse must be knowledgeable of these issues.

23. **1. The nurse should be aware that sexual activity is important to most adults and should not decide that the client is not sexually active because of a client's age. The nurse should provide instructions regarding sexual activity before the client is discharged. This is the question that should be asked because many clients may be embarrassed to bring up the subject.**
   2. The client should not drive a motor vehicle until released to do so by the health-care provider (HCP). This is not an appropriate question at this time.
   3. The client should be discharged with a prescription for oral pain medications to be taken as directed by the surgeon. The nurse should not encourage the client to use old medications the client may have at home. This is not an appropriate question.
   4. The nurse is providing discharge instructions and should tell the client when to call the health-care provider (HCP). This is not an appropriate question.

CLINICAL JUDGMENT GUIDE: The NCLEX-RN® test plan includes sexuality under Health Promotion and Maintenance with the goal to assist the client to achieve optimal health. The nurse should assess and educate the client on sexuality issues following surgery.

24. **1. The LPN can contact the HCP and give pertinent information. The INR is high (therapeutic is 2 to 3), and the HCP should be informed.**
   2. The RN cannot assign assessment to an LPN.
   3. The INR is elevated, but this will not affect the client's atrial fibrillation. The client is at risk for abnormal bleeding, not a life-threatening dysrhythmia.
   4. The normal INR is 2 to 3; therefore, some action should be implemented.

CLINICAL JUDGMENT GUIDE: The nurse cannot assign assessment, teaching, evaluation, or an unstable client to an LPN. The LPN can transcribe HCP orders and can call them on the phone to obtain orders for a client.

25. 1. In a disaster, the nurse should utilize as many individuals as possible to help control the situation; therefore, this is an inappropriate intervention.
   2. The unlicensed assistive personnel (UAP) cannot assess clients; therefore, this is not an appropriate action.
   3. The unlicensed assistive personnel (UAP) have the ability to keep the victims calm; therefore, this is an appropriate action. This action is not critical to the safety of the victims.
   4. The paramedics do not need civilians assisting them as they stabilize and transport the victims. This is not an appropriate action.

CLINICAL JUDGMENT GUIDE: The test taker must be knowledgeable of the role of each member of the multidisciplinary health-care team as well as HIPAA rules and regulations. These topics will be tested on the NCLEX-RN® examination.

26. 1. The clinic nurse should not correct the UAP in front of the client. This is embarrassing to the UAP and makes the client uncomfortable.
   2. The clinic nurse must correct the UAP's behavior. The client's weight gain should not be announced in the office area so that all staff, clients, and visitors can hear. This is a violation of confidentiality.
   3. The clinic nurse should correct the UAP's behavior, but it should be done in private and with an explanation as to why the action is inappropriate. This is a violation of confidentiality because the scale is located in the office area and any client or visitor passing by, as well as other staff members, can hear the comment.
   4. The clinic nurse should handle this situation. If the UAP's behavior shows a pattern of behavior, then it should be reported to the director of nurses.

CLINICAL JUDGMENT GUIDE: In any business, including a health-care facility, arguments or discussions of confidential information should not occur among staff of any level where the customers—in this case, the clinic clients—can hear it or see it.

27. Correct answers are 1, 2, 3, and 5.
   1. Case managers help coordinate health care between multiple sources of health care attempting to contain health-care cost.
   2. The case manager is a client advocate and helps with communication between the

client and health-care providers, which, it is hoped, enhances the client's quality of life.

3. **The case manager coordinates outpatient care and inpatient care and helps with referrals for the client.**

4. Case management is not a form of health insurance.

5. **The case manager is involved in assessing, planning, facilitating, and advocating for health services for a client, which, it is hoped, provide quality care. Trying to coordinate this is often exhausting and frustrating for the client and family.**

CLINICAL JUDGMENT GUIDE: The test taker must be knowledgeable of the role of each member of the multidisciplinary health-care team as well as HIPAA rules and regulations. These topics will be tested on the NCLEX-RN® examination. This is an alternate type question wherein the test taker must select all appropriate options to receive credit for a correct answer.

28. 1. If the client takes the loop diuretic in the morning, then going to the bathroom frequently in the morning would not warrant intervention.

2. Rising from a sitting position slowly helps prevent orthostatic hypotension, which is a potential side effect of all the medications. This statement would not warrant intervention.

3. This statement indicates the client is adhering to a low-sodium diet, as he should be. No intervention is warranted.

4. **Grapefruit juice can cause calcium channel blockers to rise to toxic levels. Grapefruit juice inhibits cytochrome P450-3A4 found in the liver and intestinal wall. This statement warrants intervention by the nurse.**

CLINICAL JUDGMENT GUIDE: The test taker must be knowledgeable of medications. In most scenarios, there is no test-taking hint to help the test taker when answering medication questions except common nursing interventions, such as do not administer cardiac medications if the client has an AP less than 60 or BP less than 90/60, do not administer medications with grapefruit juice or antacids, or administer most medications with food to prevent GI distress.

29. 1. This is a win-win strategy that focuses on goals (to have adequate staff) and attempts to meet the needs of both parties. The director

of nurses keeps an experienced nurse, and the UAP keeps her position. Both parties win.

2. This is a possible win-win strategy in which both parties win. The UAP keeps her job, and the director of nurses can hire a UAP who will be able to work the assigned hours.

3. **This is a win-lose strategy during which the conflict shows one party (the director of nurses) exerts dominance and the other party (UAP) must submit and loses.**

4. This is a negotiation in which the conflicting parties give and take on the issues. The UAP gets one more chance, and the director of nurse's authority is still intact.

CLINICAL JUDGMENT GUIDE: There will be management questions on the NCLEX-RN®. In many instances, there is no test-taking strategy; the nurse must be knowledgeable of management issues.

30. 1. A full sharps container is a violation of Occupational Health and Safety Administration (OSHA) regulations, and because the UAP has not changed it after being asked twice, a third request is not necessary.

2. The nurse should discuss why the sharps container has not been changed, but it is not the first intervention.

3. **A full sharps container is a violation of OSHA regulations and may result in a $25,000 fine. The nurse should first take care of this situation immediately and then discuss it with the UAP. This is modeling appropriate behavior.**

4. The situation should be documented because the UAP was told twice, but documentation is not the first intervention.

CLINICAL JUDGMENT GUIDE: The NCLEX-RN® test plan includes nursing care that is ruled by legal requirements. The nurse must be knowledgeable of these issues. The nurse may have to take action first and then take further action if necessary.

31. 1. The wife should call 911, but the American Heart Association recommends chewing a baby aspirin at the onset of chest pain.

2. **The American Heart Association (AHA) recommends the client having chest pain chew an aspirin to help decrease platelet aggregation. This is the first intervention the clinic nurse should tell the wife to do. The client is in distress; therefore, the nurse should have the wife do something.**

3. This question could be asked to determine whether the pain is secondary to a gallbladder attack or gastric irritation, but this is not the first intervention.
4. The clinic physician could possibly talk to the client while the wife is getting an aspirin, but this is not the first intervention.

CLINICAL JUDGMENT GUIDE: The test taker should apply the nursing process when the nurse asks the question, "Which intervention should be implemented first?" If the client is in distress, do not assess; if the client is in distress, do something.

32. 1. This blood pressure—148/92—is elevated, but it would not be life threatening for someone diagnosed with hypertension; therefore, the nurse would not contact this client first.
2. A pulse oximeter reading of 93% is low but still within normal limits, and a client diagnosed with cystic fibrosis, a chronic respiratory condition, would be expected to have a chronically low oxygen level. This client would not need to be contacted first.
3. The client diagnosed with CHF would be expected to have edematous feet; this client would not need to be contacted first.
4. **The client diagnosed with chronic atrial fibrillation is at risk for pulmonary emboli, a potentially life-threatening complication. Chest pain is a common symptom of pulmonary embolism. The nurse should contact this client first.**

CLINICAL JUDGMENT GUIDE: When deciding which client to assess first, the test taker should determine whether the signs or symptoms the client is exhibiting are normal or expected for the client situation. After eliminating the expected option, the test taker should determine which situation is more life threatening.

33. 1. **The nurse's first intervention is to assist the client to a sitting position to decrease the workload of the heart by decreasing venous return and maximizing lung expansion. This will, it is hoped, help relieve the client's respiratory distress.**
2. The nurse should assess the client's vital signs, but the first intervention is to help the client breathe.
3. The nurse should contact the paramedics if the client does not improve after being placed in a sitting position, but this is not the nurse's first intervention.

4. The nurse should auscultate the client's lungs, but the first intervention is to help the client breathe more easily.

CLINICAL JUDGMENT GUIDE: The nurse should remember that if a client is in distress and the nurse can do something to relieve the distress, that action should be done first, before assessment. The test taker should select an option that directly helps the client's condition.

34. 1. The HH nurse can contact the agency's chaplain to provide spiritual support for the client's family, but the first intervention is to pronounce the client's death.
2. **Nurses in home health have been given the authority to pronounce death for clients who are on service and if death is imminent. This intervention should be implemented first.**
3. The family should be able to stay at the bedside, but if for some reason they need to leave, the nurse asking them to leave is not the first intervention. The nurse can assess the apical pulse with the family at the bedside.
4. The client's funeral home needs to be contacted, but it is not the nurse's first action, and often the family will call the funeral home.

CLINICAL JUDGMENT GUIDE: The NCLEX-RN® test plan includes nursing care that is ruled by legal requirements. The nurse must be knowledgeable of these issues. The nurse must be aware of the rules and regulations of the various areas of nursing.

35. 1. The therapeutic range for INR is 2 to 3; therefore, this client would not need to be contacted first.
2. The client's serum potassium level is within the normal range—3.5 to 5.3 mEq/L. Therefore, this client would not need to be contacted first.
3. **The client's digoxin level is higher than the therapeutic level for digoxin, which is 0.5 to 2 ng/dL. This client should be contacted first to assess for signs or symptoms of digoxin toxicity.**
4. The glycosylated hemoglobin, which is the average of blood glucose levels over 3 months, should not be more than 8%. This client, with a level of 6%, does not need to be contacted.

CLINICAL JUDGMENT GUIDE: The test taker must know normal laboratory data.

36. 1. The client should be encouraged to exercise, but it should be in a supervised setting such as a cardiac rehabilitation unit because the client has diabetes and hypertension.
2. The client should adhere to a low-fat, low-cholesterol, carbohydrate-counting diet, but this is not the priority intervention. The client needs to be in a supervised setting, and diet teaching is included in cardiac rehabilitation.
3. **Cardiac rehabilitation includes progressive exercise, diet teaching, and classes on modifying risk factors. This supervised setting would be the priority intervention for this client when the client is discharged from HH.**
4. The client should lose weight slowly, but the priority intervention for this client would be a referral to a supervised setting where the client can lose weight slowly and safely.

CLINICAL JUDGMENT GUIDE: The test taker must be knowledgeable of the role of each member of the multidisciplinary health-care team as well as HIPAA rules and regulations. These topics will be tested on the NCLEX-RN® examination.

37. 1. The nurse should prepare the needed equipment, but it is not the nurse's first intervention.
2. The nurse should call and arrange a time convenient for the visit, but the nurse should first review the client referral so the nurse is aware of the need for the visit.
3. **The nurse should review the client's referral form and other pertinent data concerning the client's condition first before taking any further steps. The nurse may need to contact the referring agency if the information is unclear or if important information is missing. This is assessment.**
4. The nurse will not know which referrals will be needed until after the first visit.

CLINICAL JUDGMENT GUIDE: Assessment is the first step of the nursing process, and the test taker should use the nursing process or some other systematic process to assist in determining priorities. The client is not in distress because he or she is at home.

38. Correct answers are 4 and 5.
1. If the client or family is intoxicated, hostile, or obnoxious, the nurse should leave and reschedule the visit. There is no need to call the police unless the nurse thinks he or she will be hurt.

2. The HH nurse should wear the agency identification on the shirt or blouse; it should be visible to anyone talking to the nurse.
3. To be eligible for HH visits, the client must be homebound, and all visits should be done in the daylight hours as a safety precaution.
4. **The agency should be informed of the schedule so the nurse can be located if the nurse does not return when expected.**
5. **The HH nurse should report unsafe work environments to the HH agency. The agency should be proactive in providing support for HH nurses caring for clients in an unsafe situation.**

CLINICAL JUDGMENT GUIDE: This is an alternate type of question included in the NCLEX-RN®. The nurse must be able to select all the options that answer the question correctly. There are no partially correct answers. The test taker must be knowledgeable of all the various areas of nursing and the role of each member of the multidisciplinary health-care team, as well as HIPAA rules and regulations. These topics will be tested on the NCLEX-RN® examination.

39. 1. This is professional boundary crossing. Even though the grandson is not the client, he is related to the client. The HH aide should not go out with him.
2. **This statement protects the HH aide. This is professional boundary crossing. The employee should not date any relatives of the client because this may pose a conflict of interest. The HH aide should wait until the client is no longer on service.**
3. The nurse's best response is to tell the HH aide the facts about dating relatives of clients. The director would tell the HH aide the same information.
4. The HH aide could date the grandson when the client is no longer on service. So this statement is not the nurse's best response.

CLINICAL JUDGMENT GUIDE: There will be management questions on the NCLEX-RN®. In many instances, there is no test-taking strategy; the nurse must be knowledgeable of management issues. Boundary crossing is a very important area of which every nurse must be aware.

40. Correct answers are 1, 2, 4, and 5.
1. **A 2-lb weight gain indicates the client is retaining fluid and should contact the HCP. This is an appropriate teaching intervention.**

2. **Keeping the head of the bed elevated will help the client breathe easier; therefore, this is an appropriate teaching intervention.**
3. The loop diuretic should be taken in the morning to prevent nocturia. This is not an appropriate teaching intervention.
4. **Sodium retains water. Telling the client to avoid eating foods high in sodium is an appropriate teaching intervention.**
5. **Isotonic exercise, such as walking or swimming, helps tone the muscles, and discussing this with the client is an appropriate teaching intervention.**

CLINICAL JUDGMENT GUIDE: This is an alternate type of question included in the NCLEX-RN®. The nurse must be able to select all the options that answer the question correctly. There are no partially correct answers.

41. 1. The INR is not at a therapeutic level yet; the nurse should administer warfarin (Coumadin), an anticoagulant medication.
    2. **This potassium level is very low. Hypokalemia potentiates dysrhythmias in clients receiving digoxin (Lanoxin), a cardiac glycoside. This nurse should discuss potassium replacement with the HCP before administering this medication.**
    3. An aspartate aminotransferase (AST) test measures the amount of this enzyme in the blood. The enzyme is part of the liver function panel. The normal is 14 to 20 U/L for males and 10 to 36 U/L for females.
    4. Creatinine level is reflective of renal status. Normal is 0.61 to 1.21 mg/dL (males) and 0.51 to 1.11 mg/dL (females).

CLINICAL JUDGMENT GUIDE: The test taker must know normal laboratory data.

42. 1. Assessment of the client's spiritual needs in end-of-life issues is a key consideration but is the chaplain's responsibility when he or she is a member of the hospice team.
    2. The client's financial situation can be assessed, but it is not a priority over the client's spiritual needs when death is near.
    3. **The client's support system is the priority assessment for the hospice nurse. The client will be cared for in the home and the nurse must know who is available to help the client.**
    4. The client's medical diagnosis is important when addressing the grieving process, but there is nothing the nurse can do about the medical diagnosis, which is why assessing,

supporting, and addressing the client's spiritual needs will be carried out before the medical diagnosis.

CLINICAL JUDGMENT GUIDE: The test taker must be knowledgeable of all the various areas of nursing and the role of each member of the multidisciplinary health-care team, as well as HIPAA rules and regulations. These topics will be tested on the NCLEX-RN® examination.

43. 1. The client's HCP will need to determine time of death, but it is not the nurse's first intervention.
    2. The Rapid Response Team would not be notified because the client has a DNR.
    3. **The nurse should stay with the client and her husband and not make any life-rescuing interventions while the client is dying. The husband should not be left alone.**
    4. The UAP can perform postmortem care but it is not the first intervention when the client's husband tells the nurse his wife has quit breathing.

CLINICAL JUDGMENT GUIDE: A do not resuscitate (DNR) is a written physician's order instructing health-care providers not to attempt CPR. A new term recently introduced is "allow natural death" (AND), which may be more acceptable to clients and their families. The nurse cannot legally perform CPR on a client who has a DNR.

44. 1. This client should be seen, but a client who is terminally ill and is refusing to eat is not an emergency situation.
    2. The client has a right to rescind the out-of-hospital DNR, but paperwork is not a priority over a client who is in pain.
    3. **One of the main goals of hospice is pain and symptom control. This client should be seen first so that appropriate pain control can be obtained immediately.**
    4. A stage 1 pressure ulcer must be assessed and treatment started but this is not a priority over pain control.

CLINICAL JUDGMENT GUIDE: The nurse can use Maslow's Hierarchy of Needs to determine which client to assess first. Pain is a physiological need.

45. Correct answers are 1 and 5.
    1. **Encouraging the client to review his or her life experiences assists the client to come to a closure of his or her life. This is an important intervention the volunteer can perform.**
    2. This is the job of the UAP, not the volunteer.
    3. This is the job of the chaplain, not the volunteer.

4. This is the job of the nurse or occupational therapist, not the volunteer.
5. **The hospice volunteer can assist with light housekeeping chores, meal preparation, running errands, and other tasks.**

CLINICAL JUDGMENT GUIDE: When the test taker is deciding which options are appropriate tasks to delegate or assign, the test taker should choose the tasks that allow each staff member to function within his or her full scope of practice. Do not assign a task to a staff member that falls outside the staff member's or volunteer's expertise.

46. 1. **The nurse should provide instruction and support to the UAP. This is the best response.**
2. This is a callous statement and does not help the UAP learn to provide postmortem care.
3. This is not hearing the UAP's concern.
4. The nurse should assist the UAP to learn to perform the duties of a UAP, not circumvent the workload.

CLINICAL JUDGMENT GUIDE: The nurse cannot delegate any task in which the UAP admits to not being able to perform. Delegation means the nurse is responsible for the UAP's actions; therefore, the nurse must also intervene if the UAP is performing unsafely.

47. 1. If the HCP is called, the nurse should perform this task, not the UAP. A UAP cannot take a telephone order; only a licensed nurse can take telephone orders.
2. The UAP cannot administer a medication, not even acetaminophen (Tylenol).
3. **The nurse should immediately go to the client's room and assess the client. Sometimes the nurse may need to access the client's EHR and review the medication administration record (MAR) to assist in the assessment of findings. The UAP can bring a computer or tablet that contains the electronic health record (EHR) to the client's room.**
4. The UAP should not be asked to relay such information. This is the nurse's or HCP's responsibility.

CLINICAL JUDGMENT GUIDE: When the test taker is deciding which option is the most appropriate task to delegate or assign, the test taker should choose the task that allows each staff member to function within his or her full scope of practice. Do not assign a task to a staff member that requires a higher level of expertise than that staff member has. Conversely, do not assign a task to a

staff member when that task could be performed by a staff member with a lower level of expertise.

48. **Correct answers are 1, 4, and 5.**
1. **The LPN can feed a client who is stable but unable to feed himself or herself because of medical equipment. This is an appropriate task to assign.**
2. The nurse cannot assign assessment. This is the inappropriate task to assign to the LPN.
3. The LPN should not perform discharge teaching for a client. This is an inappropriate task to assign to the LPN.
4. **The LPN can administer a routine IVPB antibiotic ceftriaxone (Rocephin) medication.**
5. **The LPN can contact the health-care provider for a PRN analgesic medication for a client. This is an appropriate task to assign.**

CLINICAL JUDGMENT GUIDE: The nurse cannot assign assessment, teaching, evaluation, or an unstable client to an LPN. The LPN can call HCPs on the phone to obtain orders for a client.

49. 1. The UAP should encourage the client to remain independent as long as possible. If the client is unable to perform activities of daily living (ADLs), then the UAP should perform the tasks.
2. This may be true, but the UAP cannot and should not distance himself or herself from the clients. The UAP should maintain a professional relationship with the clients.
3. **This is an important statement for the UAP to understand. If information revealed to the UAP is necessary to provide appropriate care to the client, then the information must be shared on a need-to-know basis with the health-care team.**
4. Clients should be encouraged to discuss their life because life review may help clients accept their death.

CLINICAL JUDGMENT GUIDE: The test taker must be knowledgeable of the role of each member of the multidisciplinary health-care team as well as HIPAA rules and regulations. These topics will be tested on the NCLEX-RN® examination.

50. 1. The nurse in the client's room notifies the hospital operator of a code situation.
2. **Answering the call lights of the other clients on the unit can be delegated to the UAP.**
3. In a hospital, the respiratory therapist assumes the responsibility for ventilations.

4. The nursing supervisor is responsible for requesting the family to leave the room. The UAP does not have the authority to make this request.

CLINICAL JUDGMENT GUIDE: When the test taker is deciding which option is the most appropriate task to delegate or assign, the test taker should choose the task that allows each member of the staff to function within his or her full scope of practice. Do not assign a task to a staff member that requires a higher level of expertise or that a staff member with a lower level of expertise could perform.

51. 1. **If the family is not causing a disruption in the code, the family member should be allowed to stay in the room with the supervisor remaining near the family member. Explaining why the interventions are being implemented will help the client to survive. The supervisor should be ready to escort the family member out of the code if the family member becomes disruptive.**
    2. This will cause ill will on the part of the family and could result in the filing of a needless lawsuit.
    3. The HCP is busy with the care of the client. This is not the time to ask an HCP a question the supervisor can handle.
    4. Ignoring the family member could cause a problem; the supervisor should be proactive in managing the situation.

CLINICAL JUDGMENT GUIDE: The nurse should always try and support the client or the family's request if it does not violate any local, state, or federal rules and regulations. This is the test taker's best decision if unsure of the correct answer.

52. 1. **Federal law requires that clients presenting to an emergency department must be assessed and treated without regard to payment. The nurse should initiate steps to assess the client.**
    2. The nurse must assess the client. If a transfer is made, it will be after the client has been stabilized and the receiving hospital has accepted the transfer.
    3. Federal law requires that clients presenting to an emergency department must be assessed and treated without regard to payment. The hospital will attempt to recover the costs after the client has been treated.
    4. This is irrelevant information.

CLINICAL JUDGMENT GUIDE: The NCLEX-RN® test plan includes nursing care that is ruled by legal requirements. The nurse must be knowledgeable of these issues.

53. 1. **The client diagnosed with angina should be asymptomatic; when the client is reporting chest pain, this is abnormal data. Therefore, this client should be assessed first. Remember Maslow's Hierarchy of Needs identifies physiological needs as a priority and pain is a priority.**
    2. In a client diagnosed with CHF, 4+ edema is expected. The nurse would not need to assess this client first.
    3. The client diagnosed with endocarditis is expected to have a fever. The nurse would not need to assess this client first.
    4. The client diagnosed with aortic valve stenosis has the classic triad of syncope, angina, and exertional dyspnea; therefore, this client would not be assessed first.

CLINICAL JUDGMENT GUIDE: The test taker must determine which sign or symptom is not expected for the disease process. If the sign or symptom is not expected, then the nurse should assess the client first. This type of question is posed to determine whether the nurse is knowledgeable of the signs or symptoms of a variety of disease processes.

54. 1. **First-dose intravenous antibiotic medications are priority medications and should be administered within 1 to 2 hours of when the order was written. This should be the first medication administered.**
    2. Antiplatelet medication, aspirin, is not a priority medication.
    3. A coronary vasodilator patch, nitroglycerin, is not a priority medication.
    4. Most statin medications that decrease cholesterol levels should be administered in the evening when the enzyme for cholesterol metabolism is at its highest peak.

CLINICAL JUDGMENT GUIDE: The test taker should know which are priority medications, such as life-sustaining medications, insulin, and mucolytics (Carafate). As the rationale explains, antibiotic therapy should be initiated as soon as possible; a delay could cause death of the client.

55. 1. The nurse checks an apical pulse, not a radial pulse, before administering digoxin, a cardiac glycoside.

2. There is no serum amiodarone level; therefore, the nurse cannot implement this intervention.

3. **Intravenous heparin increases the client's partial thromboplastin time and causes an anticoagulant effect. The nurse should always be aware of the client's most current PTT levels when therapeutic heparin is being administered.**

4. The nurse should monitor the client's renal function and creatinine level, not the liver function.

CLINICAL JUDGMENT GUIDE: The nurse must be aware of interventions that must be implemented before administering medications. The nurse must know what to monitor before administering medications because untoward reactions and possibly death can occur.

56. **Correct answers are 2 and 5.**
    1. The client would be expected to be drowsy after a narcotic preoperative medication. The nurse would not need to call a time-out for this client.
    2. **Whenever there is a discrepancy on the EHR or with what the client says, the nurse should call an immediate time-out until the situation has been resolved.**
    3. The client's allergy must be documented on the client's EHR and identification band; therefore, this would not warrant a time-out.
    4. Because this is what is supposed to happen, the nurse would not need to call a time-out.
    5. **A time-out is standard procedure before surgical procedures and should include vital team members such as the surgeon, anesthesiologist, and nurse.**

CLINICAL JUDGMENT GUIDE: The NCLEX-RN® test plan includes nursing care that is ruled by the current safety measures and familiarization with the National Patient Safety Goals. The nurse must be knowledgeable of these goals.

57. 1. The day shift nurse should check the client's potassium and digoxin levels before administering the digoxin (Lanoxin). The digoxin has been administered for the day.
    2. A partial thromboplastin time is monitored for IV heparin, not warfarin (Coumadin).
    3. **The nurse should monitor the INR before administering warfarin (Coumadin). The therapeutic level for warfarin is 2 to 3.**
    4. This should be done immediately before administering the medication at the bedside.

CLINICAL JUDGMENT GUIDE: This is an alternate type question included in the NCLEX-RN® test plan. The test taker must be able to read a medication administration record (MAR), be knowledgeable of medications, and be able to make a decision as to the nurse's most appropriate intervention.

58. 1. The loop-diuretic furosemide (Lasix) should be administered to the client who has an adequate urinary output.
    2. The anticoagulant enoxaparin (Lovenox) is prescribed to prevent deep vein thromboses (DVT) in clients who are immobile, such as a postsurgical client.
    3. **The nurse should not administer ticlopidine (Ticlid), an antiplatelet medication, to a client going to surgery because this will increase postoperative bleeding. The nurse should hold this medication and discuss this with the surgeon.**
    4. The client's blood pressure is within an acceptable range. The nurse should administer the ACE inhibitor captopril (Capoten).

CLINICAL JUDGMENT GUIDE: The nurse must be knowledgeable of interventions when administering medications to clients undergoing surgery; for example, the client should not receive any PO medications or should not receive any medications that could increase bleeding.

59. **Correct answers are 3 and 5.**
    1. The nurse and respiratory therapist, not the UAP, are responsible for monitoring the ABGs.
    2. Infusion of blood and blood products, even the client's own, cannot be delegated to a UAP.
    3. **The UAP can assist with hygiene needs; this is one of the main tasks that may be delegated to UAPs.**
    4. The nurse must assess the surgical site for bleeding, infection, and healing. The UAP cannot perform assessments.
    5. **The UAP can perform repetitive tasks such as emptying the urinary catheter drainage (Foley) bag.**

CLINICAL JUDGMENT GUIDE: This is an alternate type of question included in the NCLEX-RN®. The nurse must be able to select all the options that answer the question correctly. There are no partially correct answers. An RN cannot delegate assessment, teaching, evaluation, medications, or an unstable client to a UAP. Tasks that cannot be delegated are nursing interventions requiring nursing clinical judgment.

60. 1. **The nurse should administer a unit of blood over the greatest length of time possible (4 hours) to a client diagnosed with CHF to prevent fluid volume overload. The nurse should question this order.**
   2. Administering the loop diuretic furosemide (Lasix) to a client diagnosed with CHF who is receiving blood is an appropriate order. The nurse would not question this HCP order.
   3. Restricting fluids to a client diagnosed with CHF is an appropriate order depending on the severity of the client's condition. The nurse would not question this order, especially when administering IV fluids to the client.
   4. The HCP should evaluate the effects of the two units of blood. The nurse would not question this HCP order.

CLINICAL JUDGMENT GUIDE: When the stem asks the nurse to determine which health-care provider's order to question, the test taker needs to realize this is an "except" question. Three of the options are appropriate for the HCP to prescribe and one is not appropriate for the client's disease process or procedure.

61. 1. The nurse should not document that the client fell unless the nurse observed the client fall. The nurse should never write "incident report" in an EHR. An incident report can be called an occurrence report. This becomes a red flag to a lawyer.
   2. **The nurse should document exactly what was observed. This statement is the correct documentation.**
   3. This statement is not substantiated and should not be placed in the EHR.
   4. This statement is documenting something the nurse did not observe, a fall.

CLINICAL JUDGMENT GUIDE: The nurse must be able to document nursing care safely; it includes accurate, timely documentation; it meets professional, legislative, and agency standards; it facilitates communication between nurses and other health-care providers; and it is comprehensive.

62. 1. Cooking and cleaning are jobs that can be arranged through some home health agencies, but these jobs would be done by a housekeeper, not by the UAP.
   2. **The home health aide is responsible for assisting the client with activities of daily living and transferring from the bed to**

the chair. Sitting outside is good for the client and is a task that can be delegated to the home health aide.
   3. This is boundary crossing by the UAP and could create legal difficulties if the UAP had an accident.
   4. This is assessment and cannot be delegated to a UAP.

CLINICAL JUDGMENT GUIDE: When the test taker is deciding which option is the most appropriate task to delegate or assign, the test taker should choose the task that allows each staff member to function within his or her full scope of practice. Do not assign a task to a staff member that falls outside the staff member's or volunteer's expertise. Remember the RN cannot delegate assessment, teaching, evaluation, medications, or an unstable client to the UAP.

63. 1. If the client is in distress, assessment is not the first intervention if there is an action the nurse can take to relieve the distress. The nurse should administer the nitroglycerin first.
   2. Calling for an electrocardiogram and troponin level should be implemented but not before administering the nitroglycerin.
   3. **Placing nitroglycerin under the client's tongue may relieve the client's chest pain and provide oxygen to the heart muscle. This is the nurse's first intervention.**
   4. Notification of the HCP can be done after the nurse has stabilized the client.

CLINICAL JUDGMENT GUIDE: The nurse should remember that if a client is in distress and the nurse can do something to relieve the distress, that action should be done first, before assessment. The test taker should select an option that directly helps the client's condition.

64. 1. The supervisor can take notes documenting the code until relieved, but the supervisor needs to be free to supervise the code and coordinate room assignments and staffing.
   2. **The first intervention for the supervisor is to ensure that all the jobs in the code are being filled.**
   3. This is the responsibility of the supervisor, but it is not the first intervention.
   4. The supervisor can administer medications, but the supervisor needs to be flexible to complete the duties of the supervisor.

CLINICAL JUDGMENT GUIDE: The test taker must be knowledgeable of the role of each member of

the multidisciplinary health-care team as well as HIPAA rules and regulations. These topics will be tested on the NCLEX-RN® examination. The administrative manager is responsible for the other members of the health-care team.

65. 1. This client is being treated, and if the blood is almost finished, then it can be assumed that the client is tolerating the blood without incident.
    2. **The client has been given devastating news. When all the information in the options is expected and not life threatening, then psychological issues have priority. This client should be seen first.**
    3. The client has eaten. The nurse could arrange for the dietitian to consult with the client about food preferences, but this client does not need to be assessed first.
    4. Dyspnea on exertion is not a priority if the client is exerting himself or herself.

CLINICAL JUDGMENT GUIDE: The test taker must determine if the assessment data is normal or abnormal for the client's diagnosis or situation. If the data is abnormal then this client should be seen first. If the data is normal then a client diagnosed with a psychosocial problem is the client the nurse should assess first.

66. 1. This medication could be administered but it will not have as rapid an impact as the SL dose.
    2. Nitroglycerin (NTG) is administered first because it will dilate the vessels and resolve the cause of the chest pain. If the chest pain still is present after three (3) NTG then the morphine should be administered.
    3. Oxycodone and acetaminophen will not address the chest pain specifically.
    4. **The nurse should administer the medication that will have the most rapid onset and directly resolve the problem. Nitroglycerin is a potent vasodilator and will dissolve rapidly under the tongue (sublingually).**

CLINICAL JUDGMENT GUIDE: This is an alternate type question included in the NCLEX-RN® test plan. The test taker must be able to read a medication administration record (MAR), be knowledgeable of medications, and be able to make a decision as to the nurse's most appropriate intervention.

67. 1. A client diagnosed with a DVT on a heparin drip should have an aPTT in this range. The charge nurse should make sure that the drip

is maintaining the client in the therapeutic range, but the safety of the client going to surgery is the first priority.
    2. **This client is scheduled for surgery this morning; therefore, the charge nurse must make sure that he is stable for the procedure and notify the surgeon if there is any reason to question the safety of the client having the procedure this morning.**
    3. This client is post-procedure so, unless there is a situation that arises from the nurse's assessment, this client is not a priority.
    4. A heart murmur is not life threatening, although it can be associated with other disease processes. This client is not a priority.

CLINICAL JUDGMENT GUIDE: This is an alternate type of question included in the NCLEX-RN® test plan. The test taker must be able to read an EHR, be knowledgeable of laboratory data, and be able to make a decision as to the nurse's most appropriate action.

68. Correct order is 3, 1, 4, 2, 5.
    3. **This client may be chilling, indicating a potential rise in temperature. The nurse should assess the client and the temperature to see if interventions should be initiated based on a progression of the septicemia.**
    1. **This client should be assessed to be sure that the client is stable because there was chest pain during the last shift.**
    4. **The nurse should assess the client next because although confusion is expected, the nurse must determine whether any new situation is occurring.**
    2. **This client has a psychosocial need but it must be addressed and steps implemented to resolve the problem.**
    5. **A dressing change can take some time to complete. This is a physiological situation but not a life-threatening one and the nurse should see this client when he or she has time to perform the dressing change.**

CLINICAL JUDGMENT GUIDE: This is an alternate type of question which requires the nurse to assess clients in order of priority. This requires the nurse to evaluate each client's situation and determine which situations are life threatening, which situations are expected for the client's situation, or which client has a psychosocial problem.

69. **Correct answers are 1, 3, and 4.**
    1. **Nitroglycerin tablets are vasodilators that are administered to dilate the coronary vessels and provide oxygen to the heart muscle.**
    2. The client should be made to sit down immediately. Exercise is the probable cause of the chest pain; therefore, the activity should immediately stop.
    3. **The nurse should assess the client's vital signs as part of the assessment of the client's current situation.**
    4. **Supplemental oxygen will assist in getting higher concentrations of oxygen to the heart muscle.**
    5. A unit secretary cannot take orders; only a nurse should discuss the client with the health-care provider.

CLINICAL JUDGMENT GUIDE: This is an alternate type of question included in the NCLEX-RN®. The nurse must be able to select all the options that answer the question correctly. There are no partially correct answers.

70. **Answer: 24 mL per hour.**
    25,000 divided by 500 mL = 50 units of heparin per mL.
    26 (current rate) × 50 = 1,300 units of heparin currently infusing.
    1,300 − 100 = 1,200 units of heparin needed as new infusion rate.
    1,200 divided by 50 = 24 mL per hour to infuse.

CLINICAL JUDGMENT GUIDE: This is an alternate type of question included in the NCLEX-RN®. The nurse must know how to perform math calculations.

CARDIAC CLINICAL SCENARIO ANSWERS AND RATIONALES

The correct answer number and rationale for why it is the correct answer are given in **boldface type**. Rationales for why the other possible answer options are incorrect also are given, but they are not in boldface type.

1. 1. Dabigatran (Pradaxa) is a medication specifically prescribed to prevent clotting in clients who have atrial fibrillation. Any nurse could administer the first dose of the medication; it would not have to be the most experienced nurse.
   2. **Pink, frothy sputum indicates pulmonary edema, which is a serious complication of CHF; therefore, the most experienced nurse should be assigned this client.**
   3. Occasional premature ventricular contractions are experienced by most individuals and this client would not require the most experienced nurse.
   4. Clients diagnosed with mitral valve prolapse exhibit signs of congestive heart failure; therefore, SOB is expected and the most experienced nurse should not be assigned to this client.

2. 1. The crash cart would need to be brought to the room if the client was coding, but first the nurse should determine if the client's leads are on the chest.
   2. The Rapid Response Team is called if the client is in a potentially life-threatening situation and the nurse must first determine if the leads are on the client.
   3. The nurse should assess the client's vital signs, but because the telemetry technician reports the client is flatlined the nurse should first check if the leads are in place on the chest.
   4. **The RN primary nurse should first determine if the client's telemetry leads are in place on the chest. If the leads are off then it will show as a flat line at the telemetry station. The telemetry technician cannot leave the station.**

3. 1. **This warrants intervention because the telemetry technician needs to know if the client's telemetry is being removed so the technician won't think the client is in asystole.**
   2. The electrodes attached to the client's chest do not have to be removed when the client showers, so this would not warrant intervention. The telemetry must be removed, not the electrodes.

3. Placing a bath chair in the shower is an appropriate intervention so the client won't get tired during the shower; this would not warrant intervention.
4. The UAP should stay near the client in the shower in case the client needs assistance; this would not warrant intervention.

4. 1. **The therapeutic digoxin level is 0.5 to 2.0 mg/dL; therefore, the charge nurse should notify the client's HCP because this is above the therapeutic level.**
2. The therapeutic INR level is 2 to 3; therefore, the charge nurse would not notify the HCP.
3. The normal potassium level is 3.5 to 5.3 mEq/L, so the charge nurse would not notify the HCP.
4. Normal cholesterol level is below 200 mg/dL, but 205 mg/dL is not life threatening and would not warrant notifying the HCP.

5. 1. This client must have an admission assessment completed and the charge nurse cannot assign assessment to an LPN.
2. The client diagnosed with SVT will need intravenous adenosine; therefore, this client should not be assigned to an LPN.
3. **The LPN could care for a client who has had a diagnostic test; this would be an appropriate client assignment.**
4. The charge nurse cannot assign teaching to the LPN.

6. 1. The client would need to have cardiac isoenzymes to determine if a myocardial infarction has occurred; therefore, this HCP order would not be questioned.
2. The client probably has coronary artery disease, and a low-fat, low-cholesterol diet would be expected.
3. Intravenous morphine is the drug of choice for chest pain; therefore, this order would not be questioned.
4. **An endoscopy is not a usual diagnostic test for a client diagnosed with R/O myocardial infarction; therefore, the charge nurse should question this order.**

7. 1. **The UAP can obtain the client's weight. The nurse cannot delegate assessment, teaching, evaluation, medications, or an unstable client.**
2. The custodial or housekeeping department is responsible for cleaning the room, not the UAP.
3. The nurse cannot delegate assessment, teaching, evaluation, medications, or an

unstable client. A client who is hypovolemic is not stable; therefore, this task cannot be delegated.
4. The nurse cannot delegate assessment, teaching, evaluation, medications, or an unstable client. Discussing the diet is teaching, which cannot be delegated to a UAP.

8. 1. The nurse can check the MAR but it is not the first intervention when the client is having acute chest pain. Remember, the nurse does not treat paperwork.
2. When the client is in distress the nurse should not assess. The nurse should treat the client's pain immediately; therefore, this is not the first intervention.
3. **The nurse should treat the pain, so administering sublingual nitroglycerin, a coronary vasodilator, is the nurse's first intervention.**
4. The nurse should administer oxygen but not before addressing the client's chest pain first.

9. 1. The nurse must first determine if the client has a pulse. If the client does not have a pulse then the nurse must defibrillate the client. If the client has a pulse then the nurse should not defibrillate the client.
2. **The nurse must determine if the client has a pulse or not before taking any further action; therefore, this is the nurse's first intervention.**
3. This is the first medication administered during a code, but the nurse first determines if the client has a pulse.
4. This is appropriate intervention if the client has no pulse, but the nurse first determines if the client has a pulse.

10. 1. Nitroglycerin tablets lose efficacy when exposed to sunlight; therefore, keeping the tablets in a dark bottle indicates the client understands the teaching.
2. A sedentary lifestyle is a modifiable risk factor for atherosclerosis, which causes angina, so walking three times a week is an appropriate intervention.
3. **This is a modifiable risk factor; the client must stop smoking altogether. Decreasing the number of cigarettes a day indicates the client needs more teaching.**
4. A daily aspirin will help prevent platelet aggregation; therefore, this indicates the client understands the discharge teaching.

Peripheral Vascular Management

3

Not everything that can be counted counts, and not everything that counts can be counted.

—Albert Einstein

QUESTIONS

1. The nurse has finished receiving the morning change-of-shift report. Which client should the nurse assess **first?**
   1. The client diagnosed with arterial occlusive disease who has intermittent claudication
   2. The client on strict bedrest who is reporting calf pain and has a reddened calf
   3. The client who reports low back pain when lying supine in the bed
   4. The client who is upset because the food doesn't taste good and is cold all the time

2. The nurse is caring for clients on a vascular disorder unit. Which laboratory data warrant **immediate** intervention by the nurse?
   1. The PTT of 98 seconds for a client diagnosed with deep vein thrombosis (DVT)
   2. The hemoglobin of 14.4 for a client diagnosed with Raynaud's phenomenon
   3. The white blood cell (WBC) count of 11,000 for a client diagnosed with a stasis venous ulcer
   4. The triglyceride level of 312 mmol/L in a client diagnosed with hypertension (HTN)

3. The unlicensed assistive personnel (UAP) tells the RN staff nurse the client has a blood pressure of 78/46 and a pulse of 116 using a vital signs machine. Which intervention should the nurse implement **first?**
   1. Notify the health-care provider immediately.
   2. Have the UAP recheck the client's vital signs manually.
   3. Place the client in the Trendelenburg position.
   4. Assess the client's cardiovascular status.

4. The RN charge nurse on a vascular unit is working with a new unit secretary. Which statement concerning laboratory data is **most** important for the charge nurse to tell the unit secretary?
   1. "Be sure to inform me of any lab information that is called in to the unit."
   2. "Make sure to confirm all lab reports are in the EHR (electronic health record)."
   3. "Do not take any laboratory reports over the telephone."
   4. "Verify all telephone reports by calling back to the lab."

5. The nurse is preparing to administer medications to clients on a vascular unit. Which medication should the nurse **question** administering?
   1. Vitamin K to a client with an International Normal Ratio (INR) of 2.8
   2. Propranolol to a client diagnosed with arterial hypertension
   3. Nifedipine to a client diagnosed with Raynaud's disease
   4. Enalapril to a client with a sodium level of 138 mEq/L

6. The nurse has received the shift report. Which client should the nurse assess **first**?
   1. The client diagnosed with a deep vein thrombosis who is reporting dyspnea and coughing
   2. The client diagnosed with Buerger's disease who has intermittent claudication
   3. The client diagnosed with an aortic aneurysm who has an audible bruit
   4. The client diagnosed with acute arterial ischemia who has bilateral palpable pedal pulses

7. The client diagnosed with atherosclerosis tells the clinic nurse her stomach hurts after she takes her morning medications. The client is taking a calcium channel blocker, a daily acetylsalicylic acid, and a statin. The medications have not changed during the past year. Which intervention should the nurse implement **first**?
   1. Assess the client for abnormal bleeding.
   2. Instruct the client to stop taking the acetylsalicylic acid.
   3. Recommend the client take an enteric-coated acetylsalicylic acid.
   4. Instruct the client to notify the HCP.

8. The RN nurse educator on a vascular unit is discussing delegation guidelines to a group of new graduates (GN). Which statement from the group indicates the need for **more** teaching?
   1. "The UAP will be practicing on my brand-new nursing license."
   2. "I will still retain accountability for what I delegate to the UAP."
   3. "I must make sure the UAP to whom I delegate is competent to perform the task."
   4. "When I delegate, I must follow up with the UAP and evaluate the task."

9. The nurse is reviewing the literature to identify evidence-based practice research that supports a new procedure using a new product when changing the central line catheter dressing. Which research article would **best** support the nurse's proposal for a change in the procedure?
   1. The article in which the study was conducted by the manufacturer of the product used
   2. The research article that included 10 subjects participating in the study
   3. The review-of-literature article that cited ambiguous statistics about the product
   4. The review-of-literature article that cited numerous studies supporting the product

10. The RN staff nurse and the unlicensed assistive personnel (UAP) are caring for clients on a vascular unit. Which task is **most** appropriate for the nurse to delegate?
    1. Provide indwelling catheter care to a client on bedrest.
    2. Evaluate the client's 8-hour intake and output.
    3. Give a bath to the client who is third-spacing.
    4. Administer a cation-exchange resin enema to a client.

11. The RN staff nurse asks the UAP to apply the sequential compression devices (SCDs) to a client who is on strict bedrest. The UAP tells the nurse that she has never done this procedure. Which action would be a **priority** for the RN to take?
    1. Tell another UAP to put the SCDs on the client.
    2. Demonstrate the procedure for applying the SCDs.
    3. Perform the task and apply the SCDs to the client.
    4. Request the UAP watch the video demonstrating this task.

12. The RN staff nurse in the vascular critical care unit is working with a LPN who was pulled to the unit because of high census. Which task is **most** appropriate for the nurse to assign to the LPN?
    1. Assess the client who will be transferred to the medical unit in the morning.
    2. Administer a unit of blood to the client who is 1 day postoperative.
    3. Hang the bag of heparin for a client diagnosed with a pulmonary embolus.
    4. Assist the HCP with the insertion of a client's Swan-Ganz catheter.

13. The nurse is administering 1 unit of packed red blood cells to a client. Fifteen minutes after initiation of the blood transfusion, the client becomes restless and reports itching on the trunk and arms. Which intervention should the nurse implement **first?**
    1. Assess the client's vital signs.
    2. Notify the HCP.
    3. Maintain a patent IV line.
    4. Stop the transfusion at the hub.

14. The staff nurse on a vascular disorder unit asks the RN charge nurse, "What should I be looking for when I read a research article?" Which response indicates the charge nurse understands how to read a nursing research article? **Select all that apply.**
    1. "You should be able to determine why the research was done."
    2. "You should look to find out how much money was used for the study."
    3. "You should evaluate which research method was used for the study."
    4. "You should read the method section to find out what setting was used."
    5. "You should find information about how the data was collected for the study."

15. The nurse calls the HCP for an order for pain medication for a client who is 2 days postoperative aortic aneurysm repair. The HCP gives the nurse an order for "meperidine 50 mg IVP now and then every 4 hours as needed." Which action should the nurse implement **first?**
    1. Enter the order in the EHR with the words "per telephone order (TO)."
    2. Request another nurse to verify the HCP's order on the phone.
    3. Read back the order to the HCP before hanging up the phone.
    4. Call the pharmacy to add the medication to the MAR.

16. The charge nurse on the vascular unit is reviewing laboratory blood work. Which result **warrants** intervention by the charge nurse?
    1. The client whose INR is 2.3
    2. The client whose H&H is 11 g/dL and 36%
    3. The client whose platelet count is 65,000 per mL of blood
    4. The client whose red blood cell count is 4.8×10^6 cells/microL

17. A client on the vascular unit tells the day shift primary nurse that the night nurse did not answer the call light for almost 1 hour. Which statement would be **most** appropriate by the day shift primary nurse?
    1. "The night shift often has trouble answering the lights promptly."
    2. "I am sorry that happened and I will answer your lights promptly today."
    3. "I will notify my charge nurse to come and talk to you about the situation."
    4. "There might have been an emergency situation so your light was not answered."

18. The nurse is preparing to administer a unit of packed red blood cells to an elderly client who is 1-day postoperative abdominal aortic aneurysm. Which interventions should the nurse implement? **Rank in order of performance.**
    1. Obtain the unit of blood from the blood bank.
    2. Start an IV access with normal saline at a keep-open rate.
    3. Have the client sign the permit to receive blood products.
    4. Check the unit of blood with another nurse at the bedside.
    5. Initiate the transfusion at a slow rate for 15 minutes.

19. The elderly client diagnosed with deep vein thrombosis is reporting chest pain during inhalation. Which intervention should the nurse implement **first?**
    1. Ask the HCP to order a STAT lung scan.
    2. Place oxygen on the client via nasal cannula.
    3. Prepare to administer intravenous heparin.
    4. Tell the client not to ambulate and remain in bed.

20. Which laboratory data should the nurse in the long-term care unit notify the health-care provider about?
    1. The client receiving digoxin who has a digoxin level of 2.6
    2. The client receiving enoxaparin who has a PT of 12.9 seconds
    3. The client receiving ticlopidine who has a platelet count of 160,000
    4. The client receiving furosemide who has a potassium level of 4.2 mEq/L

21. The occupational nurse is caring for the client who just severed two fingers from the right hand. Which intervention should the occupational nurse implement **first?**
    1. Place the severed fingers in a sterile cloth and then in an ice chest.
    2. Instruct the client to elevate the right arm over the heart.
    3. Don non-sterile gloves on both hands.
    4. Apply direct pressure to the right radial pulse.

22. The RN clinic nurse is making assignments to the staff. Which assignment or delegation is **most** appropriate?
    1. Request the LPN to escort the client to the examination room.
    2. Ask the unlicensed assistive personnel (UAP) to prepare the room for the next client.
    3. Instruct the RN to administer the tetanus shot to the client.
    4. Tell the clinic secretary to call in a new prescription for a client.

23. The client tells the RN charge nurse that the unlicensed assistive personnel (UAP) did not know how to take a blood pressure. Which action should the charge nurse implement **first?**
    1. Discuss the client's comment with the UAP.
    2. Retake the BP and inform the client of the BP reading.
    3. Explain that the UAP knows how to take a BP reading.
    4. Ask the UAP to demonstrate taking a BP reading.

24. Which medication is **most** appropriate for the RN staff nurse to assign to the LPN to administer?
    1. The intravenous push antiemetic to the client who is nauseated and vomiting
    2. The subcutaneous low-molecular-weight heparin to the client diagnosed with a pulmonary embolus
    3. The oral pentoxifylline to the client who has intermittent claudication
    4. The sublingual nitroglycerin to the client who is reporting chest pain

25. The clinic nurse is assessing a client who is reporting right leg calf pain. The right calf is edematous and warm to the touch. Which intervention should the nurse implement **first?**
    1. Notify the clinic HCP immediately.
    2. Ask the client how long the leg has been hurting.
    3. Complete a neurovascular assessment on the leg.
    4. Place the client's right leg on two pillows.

26. The fire alarm starts going off in the family practice clinic. Which action should the nurse take **first?**
    1. Determine whether there is a fire in the clinic.
    2. Evacuate all the people from the clinic.
    3. Immediately call 911 and report the fire.
    4. Instruct clients to stay in their rooms and close the doors.

27. The unlicensed assistive personnel (UAP) tells the RN clinic nurse, "One of the medical interns asked me out on a date. I told him no but he keeps asking." Which statement is the nurse's **best** response?
    1. "I will talk to the intern and tell him to stop."
    2. "Did anyone hear the intern asking you out?"
    3. "He asks everyone out; that is just his way."
    4. "You should inform the clinic's director of nurses."

28. The clinic nurse overhears another staff nurse telling the pharmaceutical representative, "If you bring us lunch from the best place in town, I will make sure you get to see the HCP." Which action should the clinic nurse take?
    1. Tell the pharmaceutical representative the staff nurse's statement was inappropriate.
    2. Report this behavior to the clinic's director of nurses immediately.
    3. Do not take any action and wait for the food to be delivered.
    4. Inform the HCP of the staff nurse's and pharmaceutical representative's behavior.

29. The home health (HH) nurse in the office is notified the client on warfarin has an International Normalized Ratio (INR) of 3.8. Which action should the HH nurse implement **first?**
    1. Document the result of the INR in the client's EHR.
    2. Contact the client and ask whether or not she has any abnormal bleeding.
    3. Notify the client's health-care provider of the INR results.
    4. Schedule an appointment with the client to draw another INR.

30. The home health (HH) nurse is caring for a client diagnosed with arterial hypertension who has had a cerebrovascular accident. Which **priority** intervention should the nurse discuss with the client when teaching about arterial hypertension?
    1. Discuss the importance of the client adhering to a low-salt diet.
    2. Explain the need for the client to take antihypertensive medications as prescribed.
    3. Tell the client to check and record his or her blood pressure readings daily.
    4. Encourage the client to walk at least 30 minutes three times a week.

31. Which action by the unlicensed assistive personnel (UAP) indicates to the RN staff nurse the UAP **understands** the correct procedure for applying compression stockings to the client recovering from a pulmonary embolus? **Select all that apply.**
    1. The UAP instructs the client to sit in the chair when applying the stockings.
    2. The UAP can insert one finger under the proximal end of the stocking.
    3. The UAP ensures the toe opening is placed on the top side of the feet.
    4. The UAP checked to make sure the client's toes were warm after putting the stockings on.
    5. The UAP applies lotion to the legs immediately before applying the stockings.

32. The home health (HH) nurse enters the yard of a client and is bitten on the leg by the client's dog. Which intervention should the nurse implement **first?**
    1. Clean the dog bite with soap and water and apply antibiotic ointment.
    2. Obtain the phone number and contact the client's veterinarian.
    3. Contact the HH care agency and complete an occurrence report.
    4. Ask the client whether the dog has had all the required vaccinations.

33. The nurse on the vascular unit is caring for a client diagnosed with arterial occlusive disease. Which statement by the client warrants **immediate** intervention by the nurse?
    1. "My legs start to hurt when I walk to check my mail."
    2. "My legs were so cold I had to put a heating pad on them."
    3. "I hang my legs off the side of my bed when I sleep."
    4. "I noticed that the hair on my feet and up my leg is gone."

34. The home health (HH) nurse has completed a home assessment on a client and finds out there are no smoke detectors in the home. The client tells the nurse they just cannot afford them. Which action should the nurse implement **first**?
    1. Purchase at least one smoke detector for the client's home.
    2. Notify the HH care agency social worker to discuss the situation.
    3. Ask the client whether a family member could buy a smoke detector.
    4. Contact the local fire department to see if they can provide smoke detectors for the client.

35. The nurse is admitting a 72-year-old female client and notes multiple bruises on the face, arms, and legs along with possible cigarette burns on her upper arms. The client states she fell on an ashtray and doesn't want to talk about it. Which nursing intervention is the **priority**?
    1. Document the objective findings in the client's EHR.
    2. Tell the client she must talk about the situation with the nurse.
    3. Report the situation to the Adult Protective Services.
    4. Take photographs of the bruises and cigarette burns.

36. The nurse is admitting a client diagnosed with deep vein thrombosis (DVT) in the right leg. Which statement by the client warrants **immediate** intervention by the nurse?
    1. "I take a baby acetylsalicylic acid every day at breakfast."
    2. "I have ordered myself a medical alert bracelet."
    3. "I eat spinach and greens at least twice a week."
    4. "I got a new recliner so I can elevate my legs."

37. The male client diagnosed with peripheral vascular disease tells the nurse, "I know my foot is really bad. My doctor told me I don't have any choice and I must have an amputation, but I don't want one." Which action supports the nurse being a client advocate?
    1. Support the medical treatment, and recommend the client have the amputation.
    2. Recommend the client talk to his spouse and children about his decision.
    3. Explain to the client that he has a right to a second opinion if he doesn't want an amputation.
    4. Tell the client she will go with him to discuss his decision with the doctor.

38. The RN charge nurse observes the unlicensed assistive personnel (UAP) crying after the death of a client. Which is the charge nurse's **best** response to the UAP?
    1. "If you cry every time a client dies, you won't last long on the unit."
    2. "It can be difficult when a client dies. Would you like to take a break?"
    3. "You need to stop crying and go on about your responsibilities."
    4. "Did you not realize that clients die in a health-care facility?"

39. The nursing staff confronts the hospice nurse overseeing the care of a client in a long-term care facility. The nursing staff wants to send the client, who is diagnosed with gangrene of the left leg secondary to peripheral occlusive disease, to the hospital for treatment. Which intervention should the nurse implement **first**?
    1. Check with the client to see whether or not the client wants to go to a hospital.
    2. Explain that the client can be kept comfortable at the long-term care facility.
    3. Discuss the hospice concept of comfort measures only with the staff.
    4. Call a client care conference immediately to discuss the conflict.

40. The client diagnosed with an abdominal aortic aneurysm died unexpectedly, and the nurse must notify the significant other. Which statement by the nurse is the **best** over the telephone?
    1. "I am sorry to tell you, but your loved one has died."
    2. "Could you come to the hospital? The client is not doing well."
    3. "The HCP has asked me to tell you of your family member's death."
    4. "Do you know whether the client wished to be an organ donor?"

41. The nurse has been pulled from a medical unit to work on the vascular unit for the shift. Which client should the charge nurse assign to the medical unit nurse?
1. The client with the femoral-popliteal bypass who has paraesthesia of the foot
2. The client diagnosed with an abdominal aortic aneurysm who is reporting low back pain
3. The client newly diagnosed with chronic venous insufficiency who needs teaching
4. The client diagnosed with varicose veins who is reporting deep, aching pain of the legs

42. The charge nurse in the vascular intensive care unit assigns three clients to the staff nurse. The staff nurse thinks this is an unsafe assignment. Which action should the staff nurse implement **first?**
1. Refuse to take the assignment and leave the hospital immediately.
2. Tell the supervisor that he or she is concerned about the unsafe assignment.
3. Document his or her concerns in writing and give it to the supervisor.
4. Take the assignment for the shift but turn in his or her resignation.

43. At 2230, the nurse is preparing to administer pain medication to a client who rates his pain as a 4 on the numeric pain scale. Which medication should the nurse administer?

Client: M. C.	Allergies: Ibuprofen	
Date: Today	Diagnosis: Chronic vein insufficiency	
Medication	**0701–1900**	**1901–0700**
Morphine sulfate 2 mg IVP q 2 hours prn	0930 DN	
Promethazine 12.5 mg IVP q 4 hours prn	1845 DN	
Prochlorperazine 5 mg PO tid prn		
Hydrocodone 5 mg PO q 4–6 hours prn	1730 DN	
Ibuprofen 600 mg PO q 3–4 hours prn		
Nurse Name/Initials	Day Nurse RN/DN	Night Nurse RN/NN

1. Administer morphine 2 mg IVP.
2. Administer promethazine 12.5 mg IVP.
3. Administer hydrocodone 5 mg PO.
4. Administer ibuprofen 600 mg PO.

44. The matriarch of a family has died on the vascular unit. The family tells the nurse the daughter is coming to the hospital from a nearby city to see the body. Which intervention should the nurse implement?
1. Plan to allow the daughter to see the client in the room.
2. Take the client to the morgue for the daughter to view.
3. Request the family call the daughter and tell her not to come.
4. Explain to the daughter that the unit is too busy for family visitation.

45. The unit manager on the vascular unit is planning a change in the way postmortem care is provided. Which is the **first** step in the change process?
1. Collect data.
2. Identify the problem.
3. Select an alternative.
4. Implement a plan.

46. The nurse is preparing to administer the third unit of packed red blood cells (PRBCs) to a client diagnosed with a ruptured aortic aneurysm. Which interventions should the nurse implement? **Select all that apply.**
1. Hang a bag of D_5NS to keep open (TKO).
2. Change the blood administration set.
3. Check the client's current vital signs.
4. Assess for allergies to blood products.
5. Obtain a blood warmer for the blood.

47. The RN staff nurse and the unlicensed assistive personnel (UAP) are caring for clients on a vascular unit. Which task should the nurse delegate to the UAP?
  1. Apply bilateral sequential compression devices to the client diagnosed with deep vein thrombosis.
  2. Accompany the client diagnosed with thromboangiitis obliterans outside to smoke a cigarette.
  3. Elevate the leg of the client who is 1 day postoperative femoral-popliteal bypass.
  4. Perform Doppler studies on the client diagnosed with right upper extremity lymphedema.

48. The RN charge nurse on a vascular postsurgical unit observes a new graduate (GN) telling an elderly client's spouse not to push the client's patient-controlled analgesia (PCA) pump button. Which action should the charge nurse implement?
  1. Encourage the visitor to push the button for the client.
  2. Ask the nurse to step into the hallway to discuss the situation.
  3. Discuss the hospital protocol for the use of PCA pumps.
  4. Continue to perform the charge nurse's other duties.

49. Which client should the nurse assess **first** after receiving the shift report?
  1. The client with a right above-the-knee amputation who is reporting right foot pain
  2. The client diagnosed with arterial hypertension who is reporting a severe headache
  3. The client diagnosed with lymphedema who has 4+ pitting edema of the left lower leg
  4. The client diagnosed with gangrene of the right foot who has a foul-smelling discharge

50. The RN staff nurse observes an LPN crushing nifedipine XL before administering the medication to a client diagnosed with arterial hypertension who has difficulty swallowing pills. Which intervention should the nurse implement **first?**
  1. Tell the LPN to take the client's blood pressure.
  2. Take no action because this is appropriate behavior.
  3. Show the LPN where to find pudding for the client.
  4. Tell the LPN this medication cannot be crushed.

51. A 90-year-old male client was recently widowed after more than 60 years of marriage. The client was admitted to a long-term care facility and is refusing to eat. Which intervention is an example of the ethical principle of autonomy?
  1. Place a nasogastric feeding tube and feed the client.
  2. Discuss why the client does not want to eat anymore.
  3. Arrange for the family to bring food for the client.
  4. Allow the client to refuse to eat if he wants to.

52. The nurse is admitting a client diagnosed with an abdominal aortic aneurysm who is a member of the Church of Jesus Christ of Latter-Day Saints (Mormon). Which action by the nurse indicates cultural sensitivity to the client?
  1. The nurse does not insist on administering a blood transfusion.
  2. The nurse pins the client's amulet to the client's pillow.
  3. The nurse keeps the client's undershirt on during the bath.
  4. The nurse notifies the client's curandero of the admission.

53. Which client should the nurse on the vascular unit assess **first** after receiving the shift report?
  1. The client diagnosed with lymphedema whose ABG results are pH 7.33, Pao_2 89, $Paco_2$ 47, HCO_3 25
  2. The client diagnosed with Raynaud's phenomenon who has bluish cold upper extremities
  3. The client diagnosed with chronic venous insufficiency who has an ulcerated area on the right foot
  4. The client receiving intravenous heparin infusion who has a PTT of 78

54. The RN charge nurse of a long-term care facility is making assignments. Which client should be assigned to the **most** experienced unlicensed assistive personnel (UAP)?
1. The client diagnosed with arterial occlusive disease who must dangle the legs off the side of the bed
2. The client diagnosed with congestive heart failure who is angry about the family not visiting
3. The client with an above the knee amputation who needs a full body lift to get in the wheelchair
4. The client diagnosed with Buerger's disease who is particular about the way things are done

55. The client reports chest pain on deep inspiration. Which intervention should the nurse implement **first?**
1. Place the client on oxygen.
2. Assess the client's lungs.
3. Notify the respiratory therapist.
4. Assess the client's pulse oximeter reading.

56. Which of the staff nurse's personal attributes is an important consideration for the unit manager when discussing making an experienced nurse a preceptor for new graduates? **Select all that apply.**
1. The nurse's need for the monetary stipend
2. The nurse's ability to organize the work
3. The ability of the nurse to interact with others
4. The quality of care the nurse provides
5. The nurse's willingness to be a preceptor

57. The nurse just received the a.m. shift report. Which client should the nurse assess **first?**
1. The client who is 6 hours post-op vein ligation who has absent pedal pulses
2. The client diagnosed with deep vein thrombosis who is reporting calf pain
3. The client diagnosed with Raynaud's disease who has throbbing and tingling in the extremities
4. The client diagnosed with Buerger's disease who has intermittent claudication of the feet and arms

58. The intensive care unit nurse is calculating the total intake for a client diagnosed with hypertensive crisis. The client has received 950 mL of D_5W, 2 IVPB of 100 mL of 0.9% NS, 16 ounces of water, 8 ounces of milk, and 6 ounces of chicken broth. The client has had a urinary output of 2,200 mL. What is the total intake for this client?

> [   ]

59. The nurse is teaching the client diagnosed with arterial occlusive disease. Which statement indicates the client needs **more** teaching?
1. "I will wash my legs and feet daily in warm water."
2. "I should buy my shoes in the afternoon."
3. "I must wear knee-high stockings."
4. "I should not elevate my legs."

60. The RN staff nurse is caring for clients on a vascular unit. Which nursing task is **most** appropriate to delegate to an unlicensed assistive personnel (UAP)?
1. Tell the UAP to obtain the glucometer reading of the client who is dizzy and lightheaded.
2. Request the UAP to elevate the feet of the client diagnosed with chronic venous insufficiency.
3. Ask the UAP to take the vital signs of the client who has numbness of the right arm.
4. Instruct the UAP to administer a tap water enema to the client diagnosed with an aorta aneurysm.

61. A client is 2 days postoperative abdominal aortic aneurysm repair. Which data require **immediate** intervention from the nurse?
1. The client refuses to take deep breaths and cough.
2. The client's urinary output is 300 mL in 8 hours.
3. The client has hypoactive bowel sounds.
4. The client's vital signs are T 98, P 68, R 16, and BP 110/70.

62. The nurse is caring for clients on a vascular surgical floor. Which client should be assessed **first**?
1. The client who is 2 days postoperative right below-the-knee amputation who has phantom pain in the right foot
2. The client who is 1 day postoperative abdominal aortic aneurysm who is reporting numbness and tingling of both feet
3. The client diagnosed with superficial thrombophlebitis of the left arm who is reporting tenderness to the touch
4. The client diagnosed with arterial occlusive disease who is reporting calf pain when ambulating down the hall

63. The nurse is caring for a client receiving heparin sodium via constant infusion. The heparin protocol reads to increase the IV rate by 100 units/hour if the PTT is fewer than 50 seconds. The current PTT level is 46 seconds. The heparin comes in 500 mL of D_5W with 25,000 units of heparin added. The current rate on the IV pump is 20 mL per hour. At what rate should the nurse set the pump?

64. The unlicensed assistive personnel (UAP) is caring for a client diagnosed with chronic venous insufficiency. Which action would warrant **immediate** intervention from the RN staff nurse?
1. The UAP assists the client to apply compression stockings.
2. The UAP elevates the client's leg while sitting in the recliner.
3. The UAP assists the client to the bathroom for a.m. care.
4. The UAP is cutting the client's toenails after soaking the client's feet in tepid water.

65. The nurse has just received the a.m. shift report. Which client would the nurse assess **first**?
1. The client diagnosed with a venous stasis ulcer who is refusing to eat the high-protein meal
2. The client diagnosed with varicose veins who is refusing to wear thromboembolic hose
3. The client diagnosed with arterial occlusive disease who is refusing to elevate his or her legs
4. The client diagnosed with deep vein thrombosis who is refusing to stay in the bed

66. At 1000 a client who has had femoral-popliteal bypass surgery on the right leg is reporting severe right upper quadrant pain of 10 out of 10 on the pain scale. Based on the information in the following chart, what should the nurse do for the client?

Client Name: B.A. Weight in pounds: 220	Account Number: 0101223 Weight in kg: 100		Height: 72 inches Date: Today
Medication		1901–0700	0701–1900
Morphine sulfate 2 mg IVP every 4 hours prn pain		0445 NN	0845 DN
Oxycodone 7.5/acetaminophen 325 mg PO every 3 hours prn pain		0030 NN 0545 NN	
Aluminum hydroxide; magnesium hydroxide; simethicone 30 mL PO prn indigestion			
Nitroglycerin 0.4 mg SL every 5 minutes up to 3 tablets prn Chest pain			
Signature/Initials		Night Nurse RN/NN	Day Nurse RN/DN

1. Administer the oxycodone and acetaminophen PO.
2. Help the client to practice guided imagery for the pain.
3. Call the surgeon for an increase in pain medication.
4. Administer a dose of morphine to the client.

67. The client on a surgical unit is scheduled to receive an antibiotic piggyback for 1 hour. The piggyback is prepared in 150 mL of solution. At what rate should the nurse set the piggyback if the administration set delivers 20 drops per mL?

[ ]

68. The client in the day surgical unit is scheduled to have vein ligation on the right leg. The client states, "I am having surgery on my left leg." Which intervention should the nurse implement **first?**
1. Have the client sign the surgical operative permit.
2. Assess the client's neurological status.
3. Ask when the client last took a drink of water or ate anything.
4. Call a time-out until clarifying which leg is having the vein ligation.

69. The 63-year-old client is diagnosed with an abdominal aortic aneurysm. On which area of the figure should the nurse place a stethoscope to assess for a bruit?

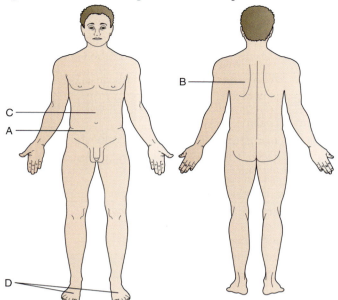

1. A
2. B
3. C
4. D

70. The male post-op femoral-popliteal bypass client notifies the desk via the intercom system he has fallen and is now bleeding. Which interventions should the nurse implement? **Rank in order of performance.**
1. Apply pressure directly to the bleeding site.
2. Notify the surgeon of the fall and the bleeding.
3. Redress the site with a sterile dressing.
4. Assist the client to a recumbent position in the bed.
5. Make out an occurrence report and document the fall.

PERIPHERAL VASCULAR DISEASE CLINICAL SCENARIO

The 7 p.m. to 7 a.m. RN charge nurse is on a 32-bed medical unit in a large suburban, multidisciplinary hospital. There are three primary nurses: one RN who has been a nurse on the unit for 12 years, another RN who has been a nurse on the unit for 1 year, and a new graduate nurse (GN). There are three UAPs. The clients are demographically diverse and range in stay from 24-hour observation to multiple days.

1. The nurse with 12 years of experience just received the a.m. shift report. Which client should the nurse assess **first?**
   1. The noncompliant middle-aged client diagnosed with coronary artery disease who has a BP of 170/100
   2. The obese young adult client diagnosed with deep vein thrombosis who is reporting calf pain
   3. The client with tobacco addiction diagnosed with arterial occlusive disease who has intermittent claudication
   4. The disruptive elderly client diagnosed with aortic abdominal aneurysm who has low back pain

2. Which assessment data would warrant **immediate** intervention by the RN charge nurse for the middle-aged client diagnosed with arterial occlusive disease?
   1. The client has decreased hair on his or her calf.
   2. The client has no palpable dorsal pedal pulse.
   3. The client has paralysis and parasthesia.
   4. The client hangs his or her legs off the side of the bed.

3. The RN with 12 years of experience and the unlicensed assistive personnel (UAP) are caring for an elderly client who is 4 hours postoperative right femoral-popliteal by-pass surgery. Which nursing task should the RN delegate to the UAP?
   1. Check the client's pedal pulse with the Doppler.
   2. Assist the client to ambulate down the hall.
   3. Review the client's neurovascular assessment.
   4. Elevate the client's leg on two pillows.

4. Which interventions should the RN charge nurse discuss with the elderly client diagnosed with atherosclerosis? **Select all that apply.**
   1. Take a low dose acetylsalicylic acid daily.
   2. Eat a low-fat, low-cholesterol diet.
   3. Maintain a sedentary lifestyle as much as possible.
   4. Decrease all foods high in fiber.
   5. Walk 30 minutes a day at least 3 days a week.

5. The client is 2 days postoperative abdominal aortic aneurysm. Which intervention should the nurse with 1 year of experience implement **first** when making initial rounds?
   1. Auscultate the client's bowel sounds.
   2. Assess the client's surgical dressing.
   3. Encourage the client to splint the incision.
   4. Monitor the client's intravenous therapy.

6. The middle-aged client is diagnosed with a small abdominal aortic aneurysm. Which statement by the client indicates to the RN with 1 year of experience the client needs more discharge teaching?
   1. "I should not lift more than 5 pounds for at least 4 to 6 weeks."
   2. "I attend a support group to help me quit smoking."
   3. "I will need to wear a truss at all times after the surgery."
   4. "If I get a temperature of 101°F or higher I will call my doctor."

7. The new graduate nurse (GN) is assigned the following clients. Which client should the GN assess **first?**
   1. The client who is 4 days postoperative abdominal surgery and is reporting abdominal pain when ambulating
   2. The client who 1 day postoperative femoral-popliteal repair has a 3+ posterior tibial pulse
   3. The client who had an abdominal aortic repair who had a urine output of 150 mL in the last 8 hours
   4. The client diagnosed with deep vein thrombosis who is reporting being unable to get out of the bed

8. The new graduate nurse (GN) is caring for a client receiving heparin sodium via constant infusion. The heparin protocol reads to decrease the IV rate by 100 units/hour if the PTT is between 78 to 90 seconds. The current PTT level is 85 seconds. The heparin comes in 500 mL of D_5W diagnosed with 25,000 units of heparin added. The current rate on the IV pump is 18 mL per hour. At what rate should the GN set the pump?

9. The unlicensed assistive personnel (UAP) is caring for the middle-aged client diagnosed with chronic venous insufficiency. Which action would warrant **immediate** intervention by the new graduate nurse (GN)?
   1. The UAP is elevating the client's legs on two pillows.
   2. The UAP is massaging the client's calf muscles.
   3. The UAP is instructing the client to stay in the bed.
   4. The UAP is calculating the client's shift intake and output.

10. An 80-year-old client is being discharged home after having surgery to débride a chronic venous ulcer on the right ankle. Which referral is appropriate for the RN charge nurse to make?
    1. Hospice
    2. Home health
    3. Physical therapist
    4. Cardiac rehabilitation

The correct answer number and rationale for why it is the correct answer are given in **boldface type**. Rationales for why the other possible answer options are incorrect also are given, but they are not in boldface type.

1. 1. Intermittent claudication is a symptom of arterial occlusive disease; therefore, this client does not need to be assessed first.
   2. **The client diagnosed with calf pain could be experiencing deep vein thrombosis (DVT), a complication of immobility, which may be fatal if a pulmonary embolus occurs; therefore, this client should be assessed first.**
   3. The client experiencing low back pain when sitting in a chair should be assessed but not before the client diagnosed with suspected DVT.
   4. The nurse should address the client's concern about the food, but it is not a priority over a physiological problem.

CLINICAL JUDGMENT GUIDE: When deciding which client to assess first, the test taker should determine whether the signs or symptoms the client is exhibiting are normal or expected for the client situation. After eliminating the expected options, the test taker should determine which situation is more life threatening.

2. 1. **Therapeutic levels for PTT should be 11/2 to 2 times the normal value, which is 39 seconds; therefore, this client is at risk for bleeding. The prolonged PTT indicates the client is receiving heparin (drug of choice to treat DVT). The nurse should stop the infusion and follow the facility protocol.**
   2. The hemoglobin is within normal range and the client diagnosed with Raynaud's disease does not have a problem with bleeding.
   3. The WBC count is elevated (normal is 4,500 to 11,100), but it would be elevated in a client who has an infection such as venous stasis ulcer.
   4. The nurse should notify the HCP on rounds of any laboratory data that are abnormal but not immediately life threatening. The triglyceride level is high, but it will take weeks to months of a heart healthy diet, exercise, and possibly medications to lower this level.

CLINICAL JUDGMENT GUIDE: When a question asks for immediate intervention, the test taker must decide whether there is an intervention the nurse can implement immediately or whether the HCP must be notified. If the data are abnormal, but not life threatening, then the option can be eliminated as a possible correct answer.

3. 1. The nurse should first assess the client to determine the status before notifying the HCP.
   2. The unlisted assistive personnel (UAP) has notified the nurse of a potentially serious situation. The nurse must first assess the client before taking any action.
   3. The nurse might place the client in the Trendelenburg position once cardiovascular shock is determined.
   4. **The nurse should immediately go to the client's room to assess the client.**

CLINICAL JUDGMENT GUIDE: Any time the nurse receives information about a client (who may be experiencing a complication) from another staff member, the nurse must assess the client. The nurse should not make decisions about the client's needs based on another staff member's information.

4. 1. **Because laboratory values called into a unit usually include critical values, the charge nurse should tell the unit secretary "to inform me of any laboratory information that is called in immediately." The charge nurse must evaluate this information immediately.**
   2. Posting laboratory results in the EHR is the responsibility of the laboratory staff, not the unit secretary.
   3. This is unrealistic because laboratory data are important information that must be called in to a unit when there is a critical value so that immediate action can be taken for the client's welfare. The secretary must know how to process the information.
   4. The unit secretary should verify the information by repeating back the information at the time of the call, not by making a second telephone call to the laboratory.

CLINICAL JUDGMENT GUIDE: The test taker must be knowledgeable of the roles of all members of the multidisciplinary health-care team, as well as HIPAA rules and regulations. The nurse must ensure the health-care team member knows appropriate actions to take in specific situations. These will be tested on the NCLEX-RN®.

5. 1. **Vitamin K (AquaMephyton), a vitamin, is the antidote for warfarin (Coumadin) overdose and is administered to a client when his or her INR level is above the**

therapeutic 2–3; therefore, the nurse should question administering this medication.

2. Propranolol (Inderal), a beta-adrenergic, is administered to clients diagnosed with hypertension; therefore, the nurse would not question administering this medication.
3. Nifedipine (Procardia), a calcium channel blocker, reduces the number of vasospastic attacks in clients diagnosed with Raynaud's disease; therefore, the nurse would not question administering this medication.
4. Enalapril (Vasotec), an angiotensin-converting enzyme (ACE) inhibitor, is administered to clients diagnosed with diabetes to help prevent diabetic nephropathy. The nurse would not question administering this medication.

CLINICAL JUDGMENT GUIDE: The nurse must be aware of interventions that must be implemented before administering medications. The nurse should know what to monitor before administering medications because untoward reactions and possibly death can occur.

6. 1. **This client is exhibiting signs and symptoms of a potentially fatal complication of DVT—pulmonary embolism. The nurse should assess this client first.**
   2. Intermittent claudication of the feet, hands, and arms is a symptom of Buerger's disease; therefore, this client should not be assessed first.
   3. The client diagnosed with an aortic aneurysm is expected to have an audible bruit and does not indicate any life-threatening condition; therefore, this client does not need to be assessed first.
   4. The client diagnosed with acute arterial ischemia should have unpalpable pedal pulses to be considered a medical emergency; therefore, this client does not need to be assessed first.

CLINICAL JUDGMENT GUIDE: The test taker must determine which sign or symptom is not expected for the disease process. If the sign or symptom is not expected, then the nurse should assess the client first. This type of question is determining if the nurse is knowledgeable of the signs or symptoms of a variety of disease processes.

7. 1. **Because the client has been on the daily acetylsalicylic acid (aspirin) for more than a year, the nurse should assess for bleeding by asking questions such as, "Do your gums bleed after brushing teeth?" or "Do you notice blood when you blow your nose?"**

2. Because acetylsalicylic acid (aspirin) can cause gastric distress, the nurse could instruct the client to stop taking it; however, because this is a daily medication being used as an antiplatelet agent, the nurse should provide information that would allow the client to continue the medication.
3. The nurse should realize the stomach discomfort is probably secondary to daily acetylsalicylic acid (aspirin), and enteric-coated acetylsalicylic acid (aspirin) would be helpful to decrease the stomach discomfort and allow the client to stay on the medication, but the nurse should first assess the client for bleeding.
4. Because acetylsalicylic acid (aspirin) is not a prescription medication, the nurse can recommend a different form of acetylsalicylic acid (aspirin), such as one that is enteric coated. However, if the enteric-coated acetylsalicylic acid (aspirin) does not relieve the pain, the HCP should then be notified.

CLINICAL JUDGMENT GUIDE: Assessment is the first step of the nursing process and the test taker should use the nursing process or some other systematic process to assist in determining priorities.

8. 1. **This statement indicates the new graduate needs more teaching because the nurse is responsible for delegating the right task to the right individual. Absolutely no one works on the nurse's license but the nurse holding the license.**
   2. The nurse does retain accountability for the task delegated; therefore, the new graduate does not need more teaching.
   3. The nurse must make sure the unlicensed assistive personnel (UAP) is able to perform the task safely and competently; therefore, the new graduate does not need more teaching.
   4. The nurse must make sure the delegated task was completed correctly; therefore, the new graduate does not need more teaching.

CLINICAL JUDGMENT GUIDE: An RN cannot delegate assessment, teaching, evaluation, medications, or an unstable client to a UAP. Tasks that cannot be delegated are nursing interventions requiring nursing clinical judgment. The nurse must be aware of delegation rules and regulations.

9. 1. The manufacturer of a product would provide biased information and would not provide the best data to support a change proposal.
   2. Research studies with a limited number of participants indicate the need for further

research and would not be the best research to support a change proposal.

3. Research should provide clear statistical data that support the research problem or hypothesis.

4. **The more research articles there are that support a change proposal, the more valid is the information, which increases the possibility for change to be considered by the health-care facility.**

CLINICAL JUDGMENT GUIDE: The NCLEX-RN® test plan includes nursing care based on evidence-based practice. The nurse must be knowledgeable of nursing research.

10. 1. **The unlicensed assistive personnel (UAP) can clean the perineal area of a client who is on bedrest and who has an indwelling catheter. Because the client is stable, this nursing task could be delegated to the UAP.**

2. The UAP can obtain the client's intake and output, but the nurse must evaluate the data to determine whether interventions are needed or whether interventions are effective.

3. A client who is third-spacing is unstable and in a life-threatening situation; therefore, the nurse cannot delegate the UAP to give this client a bath.

4. This is a medication enema, and the UAP cannot administer medications. In addition, if a cation-exchange resin enema is ordered, the client is unstable and has an excessively high serum potassium (K^+) level.

CLINICAL JUDGMENT GUIDE: An RN cannot delegate assessment, teaching, evaluation, medications, or an unstable client to a UAP. Tasks that cannot be delegated are nursing interventions requiring nursing clinical judgment.

11. 1. Although the nurse could request another unlicensed assistive personnel (UAP) to perform the task, this is not the best action because the nurse should demonstrate applying SCDs so that the UAP can learn how to complete the task.

2. **This is the priority action because the nurse will ensure the UAP knows how to apply SCDs correctly, thereby enabling the nurse to delegate the task to the UAP successfully in the future.**

3. The nurse could do the task, but if the UAP is not shown how to do it, then the UAP will not be able to perform the task the next time it is delegated.

4. The UAP could watch a video demonstrating this task, but the priority action is that the nurse should demonstrate SCD application to the UAP.

CLINICAL JUDGMENT GUIDE: The nurse cannot delegate any task in which the UAP admits to not being able to perform. It is the nurse's responsibility to know what can be delegated and when. The nurse may have to complete the task if the UAP is not competent to do so.

12. 1. The nurse should not assign assessment of a client to an LPN even if the client is stable.

2. The LPN cannot initiate administration of blood; therefore, this task must be completed by the nurse.

3. **The LPN can administer medications; therefore, the LPN could hang a bag of heparin on an IV pump to this client.**

4. The nurse must assess for dysrhythmias during the insertion, and the nurse assisting the HCP should be experienced in inserting the line. An LPN pulled from another unit should not be assigned this task.

CLINICAL JUDGMENT GUIDE: The nurse cannot assign assessment, teaching, evaluation, or an unstable client to an LPN. The LPN can call HCPs on the phone to obtain orders for a client.

13. 1. The client is having signs or symptoms of a blood transfusion reaction. The nurse must stop the transfusion immediately and then assess the client's vital signs.

2. The HCP needs to be notified, but not before the nurse stops the blood transfusion.

3. The nurse should maintain a patent IV so that medications can be administered, but this is not the first intervention.

4. **Any time the nurse suspects the client is having a reaction to blood or blood products, the nurse should stop the infusion at the spot closest to the client and not allow any more of the blood to enter the client's body. This is the nurse's first intervention.**

CLINICAL JUDGMENT GUIDE: The nurse should remember: If a client is in distress and the nurse can do something to relieve the distress, it should be done first, before assessment. The test taker should select an option that directly helps the client's condition.

14. **Correct answers are 1, 3, 4, and 5.**

1. **A research article should answer the question "Why?": Why was the research**

done? This statement indicates the charge nurse understands how to read a research article.

2. The cost of the research is not pertinent when reading a research article and determining whether the research supports evidence-based practice. This statement indicates the charge nurse does not understand how to read a research article.

3. **A research article should answer the question "What?": What research method was used? This statement indicates the charge nurse understands how to read a research article.**

4. **A research article should answer the question "Where?": In what setting was the research conducted? This statement indicates the charge nurse understands how to read a research article.**

5. **A research article should give information about how the data was collected. This statement indicates the charge nurse understands how to read a research article.**

CLINICAL JUDGMENT GUIDE: The NCLEX-RN® test plan includes nursing care based on evidence-based practice. The nurse must be knowledgeable of nursing research.

15. 1. The nurse should enter the order in the EHR and document "per telephone order," but this is not the nurse's first intervention.
2. The nurse does not need to have another nurse verify the HCP's telephone order.
3. **The Joint Commission has implemented this requirement for all telephone orders. The nurse should document on the HCP's order for meperidine (Demerol) "repeat order verified."**
4. The nurse should send electronic or written confirmation of the order to the pharmacy but it is not the first intervention.

CLINICAL JUDGMENT GUIDE: The NCLEX-RN® test plan includes nursing care that is ruled by legal requirements as well as rules and regulations of the Joint Commission, Centers for Medicare & Medicaid Services, Centers for Disease Control and Prevention, and the Occupational Safety and Health Administration. The nurse must be knowledgeable regarding these standards.

16. 1. The therapeutic level for a client on warfarin (Coumadin) is an INR of 2 to 3; therefore, this client does not warrant intervention.
2. These hemoglobin or hematocrit levels are a little low but not so critical that this would

warrant intervention by the charge nurse.
3. **A platelet count of fewer than 100,000 per milliliter of blood indicates thrombocytopenia; therefore, this client warrants intervention by the charge nurse.**
4. This is a normal red blood cell count; therefore, the charge nurse would not need to intervene.

CLINICAL JUDGMENT GUIDE: The nurse must be knowledgeable of normal laboratory values. These values must be memorized and the nurse must be able to determine if the laboratory value is normal for the client's disease process or medications the client is taking.

17. 1. This statement is not supporting the night shift and makes the unit look bad. The nurse should not "bad-mouth" the night shift.
2. The nurse has no idea what happened that delayed answering the call light; it could have been a code or other type of life-threatening situation. The day shift primary nurse may not be able to answer the light in some certain situations and should not falsely reassure the client.
3. **The nurse should have someone come talk to the client who is in a position to then investigate what happened on the night shift and determine why this happened. The day shift primary nurse does not have this authority.**
4. This is negating the client's feeling, and the client does not need to know what was going on in the critical care unit.

CLINICAL JUDGMENT GUIDE: There will be management questions on the NCLEX-RN®. In many instances, there is no test-taking strategy for these questions; the nurse must be knowledgeable of management issues.

18. **Correct order is 3, 2, 1, 4, 5.**
3. **The client must agree to the risks and benefits of a blood transfusion before the nurse can administer the blood product. This is the first intervention.**
2. **The nurse has only 30 minutes from the time the blood is retrieved from the blood bank until the transfusion is initiated. The nurse should make sure the client has a patent IV access before obtaining the blood from the blood bank.**
1. **The nurse can obtain the unit of packed cells when the client has signed the permit and has a patent IV access.**
4. **The nurse should always check the blood product with another nurse at the client's**

bedside against the client's hospital identification band and blood bank crossmatch band.

5. After the nurse has followed the procedure to ensure the correct blood product is being administered, the transfusion of packed cells can be initiated with a second nurse. The blood is initiated at a slow rate—10 mL per hour for the first 15 minutes—so that the nurse can observe the client for potential complications.

CLINICAL JUDGMENT GUIDE: This is an alternate type of question included in the NCLEX-RN® test plan. The nurse must be able to perform skills in the correct order. Obtaining informed consent and performing an assessment should always be the first interventions.

19. 1. This should be an anticipated order if the nurse suspects a pulmonary embolus, but it is not the first intervention.
    2. The nurse should suspect the client has a pulmonary embolus, a complication of the thrombophlebitis. Pulmonary emboli decrease the oxygen supply to the body, and the nurse should immediately administer oxygen to the client.
    3. An anticoagulant infusion will be ordered for the client once it is determined that the client is experiencing a pulmonary embolus.
    4. Getting oxygen to the body is a priority; telling the client not to ambulate can be done after initiating the oxygen.

CLINICAL JUDGMENT GUIDE: Physiological problems have the highest priority when deciding on a course of action. If the client is in distress, then the nurse must intervene with a nursing action that attempts to alleviate or control the problem. The test taker should not choose a diagnostic test if there is an option that directly treats the client.

20. **1. The therapeutic level for digoxin is 0.5 to 2.0 ng/mL so this warrants notifying the HCP.**
    2. There is no serum blood level to monitor enoxaparin (Lovenox), which is a low-molecular-weight heparin administered to prevent deep vein thrombosis.
    3. The platelet level is within the normal level of 140,000 to 400,000, so this would not warrant notifying the HCP.
    4. The normal potassium level is 3.5 to 5.3 mEq/L, so this result would not warrant notifying the HCP.

CLINICAL JUDGMENT GUIDE: The nurse must be knowledgeable of normal laboratory values. These values must be memorized and the nurse must be able to determine if the laboratory value is normal for the client's disease process or for medications the client is taking.

21. 1. This is the correct procedure to help preserve the fingers so the surgeon can reattach the fingers, but is not the first intervention.
    2. Elevating the right arm will help decrease bleeding, but it is not the first intervention.
    3. The nurse should first put on non-sterile gloves to protect from getting any blood-borne diseases.
    4. Applying direct pressure is an appropriate intervention, but the first intervention is to apply gloves to protect the nurse.

CLINICAL JUDGMENT GUIDE: The test taker must remember: If the client is in distress, do not assess, but Standard Precautions take priority. The nurse must always put Standard Precautions as a priority when caring for all clients, especially when blood and body fluids are present.

22. 1. The unlicensed assistive personnel (UAP) could escort the client to the room so that the LPN could be assigned tasks that are within the LPN's scope of practice.
    2. The UAP can make sure the room is clear of the previous client's gown and equipment used with the previous client. The UAP can also make sure there are gowns, tongue blades, and additional equipment in the examination room.
    3. The LPN can administer medication; therefore, it would be more appropriate to assign this task to the LPN, so that the RN could be assigned tasks that are beyond the scope of practice of an LPN and within the RN scope of practice.
    4. The clinic secretary is unlicensed personnel and does not have the authority to call in a new prescription for a client.

CLINICAL JUDGMENT GUIDE: When the test taker is deciding which option is the most appropriate task to delegate or assign, the test taker should choose the task that requires each member of the staff to function within his or her full scope of practice. Do not assign a task to a staff member that requires a higher level of expertise than the staff member has, and do not assign a task to a staff member when the task could be delegated or assigned to a staff member with a lower level of expertise.

23. 1. The nurse should discuss the client's comment, but it is not the nurse's first intervention.
   2. **The nurse should first take the client's BP correctly and address the client's concern.**
   3. If the nurse's BP reading and the UAP's BP reading are close to the same, the nurse could reassure the client that the UAP does know how to take BP readings. However, this is not the nurse's first intervention.
   4. This is an appropriate action, but it is not the first intervention. The nurse is responsible for making sure the UAP has the ability to perform any delegated tasks correctly.

CLINICAL JUDGMENT GUIDE: The nurse should address client needs first, including answering the client's questions, verifying the client's vital signs, or assessing the client if the client is not in distress.

24. 1. Intravenous push medications cannot be assigned to an LPN. It is the most dangerous route for administering medication, and only an RN (or HCP) can perform this task.
   2. The client who is diagnosed with a pulmonary embolus is not stable; therefore, this medication is not the best medication to be assigned to the LPN.
   3. **Pentoxifylline (Trental) is a PO medication prescribed specifically to treat intermittent claudication. It increases erythrocyte flexibility and reduces blood viscosity.**
   4. The client may be having a myocardial infarction; therefore, this client is unstable and should not be assigned to an LPN.

CLINICAL JUDGMENT GUIDE: The test taker must determine which option is included within the LPN's scope of practice. LPNs are not routinely taught how to administer intravenous push medications. The test taker must also determine which client is the most stable, which makes this an "except" question. Three clients are either unstable or have potentially life-threatening conditions and should not be assigned to an LPN.

25. 1. **The nurse should realize the client probably has deep vein thrombosis, which is a medical emergency. The HCP should be notified immediately so the client can be started on IV heparin and admitted to the hospital.**
   2. This information may be needed, but the nurse should notify the HCP based on the signs or symptoms alone.

3. A neurovascular assessment should be completed, but not before notifying the HCP. The signs or symptoms alone indicate a potentially life-threatening condition.
   4. The client's leg should be elevated, but this is a potentially life-threatening emergency and the nurse should first call the HCP.

CLINICAL JUDGMENT GUIDE: The test taker needs to read all the options carefully before choosing the option that says, "Notify the HCP." If any of the options will provide information the HCP needs to know in order to make a decision, the test taker should choose that option. If, however, the HCP does not need any additional information to make a decision and the nurse suspects the condition is serious or life threatening, the priority intervention is to call the HCP.

26. 1. **The nurse should first determine whether there is a fire or whether someone accidentally or purposefully pulled the fire alarm. Because this is a clinic, not a hospital, the nurse should keep calm and determine the situation before taking action.**
   2. The nurse should not evacuate clients, visitors, and staff unless there is a real fire.
   3. The nurse should assess the situation before contacting the fire department.
   4. This is an appropriate intervention, but this is not the first intervention. The nurse should first assess to determine whether there is a fire.

CLINICAL JUDGMENT GUIDE: The nurse must be knowledgeable of emergency preparedness. Employees receive this information in employee orientation and are responsible for implementing procedures correctly. The NCLEX-RN® test plan includes questions on safe and effective care environment.

27. 1. The clinic nurse should allow the director to address sexual harassment allegations. This is a matter that should be handled legally.
   2. This is an appropriate question to ask when investigating sexual harassment allegations, but the clinic nurse should allow the director of nurses to pursue this situation.
   3. The clinic nurse is responsible for taking the appropriate action when sexual allegations are reported. This statement shows that the clinic nurse is not taking the allegations seriously and could result in disciplinary action against the nurse.

4. This is the most appropriate response because sexual harassment allegations are a legal matter. The clinic nurse implemented the correct action by making sure the unlicensed assistive personnel (UAP) reported the allegation to the director of nurses.

CLINICAL JUDGMENT GUIDE: There will be management questions on the NCLEX-RN®. In many instances, there is no test-taking strategy for these questions. The nurse must be knowledgeable of which management issues must comply with local, state, and federal requirements.

28. 1. The clinic nurse should not discuss the staff nurse's statement with the pharmaceutical representative because the staff member's behavior is unethical and could have repercussions. The clinic nurse should notify the director of nurses.
    2. **This behavior is unethical and is making promises that the staff nurse may or may not be able to keep. Because this situation includes the HCP, an outside representative, and the staff nurse, this situation should be reported to the director of nurses for further action.**
    3. This behavior must be reported. This is bribing the pharmaceutical representative and using a meeting with the HCP as the reward.
    4. The clinic nurse should maintain the chain of command and report this to the nursing supervisor, not to the HCP.

CLINICAL JUDGMENT GUIDE: There will be management questions on the NCLEX-RN®. In many instances, there is no test-taking strategy for these questions. The nurse must be knowledgeable of management issues.

29. 1. The nurse should document the results in the client's EHR, but this is not the nurse's first intervention.
    2. **The therapeutic value for INR is 2 to 3; levels higher than that increase the risk of bleeding. The nurse should first contact the client and determine whether she has any abnormal bleeding and then instruct the client to not take any more warfarin (Coumadin), an oral anticoagulant.**
    3. The nurse should notify the client's HCP, but the nurse should first determine whether the client has any abnormal bleeding so that it can be reported to the HCP.
    4. The client will need to have another INR drawn, but it is not the nurse's first intervention.

CLINICAL JUDGMENT GUIDE: Any time the nurse receives information from another source about a client who may be experiencing a complication, the nurse must assess the client. In this scenario, the nurse assesses the client by talking to him or her on the phone. The nurse should not make decisions about client needs unless the nurse talks to the client.

30. 1. A low-salt diet is used to treat arterial hypertension, but it is not the priority intervention.
    2. **The priority intervention for the client diagnosed with arterial hypertension is to take antihypertensive medications.**
    3. Taking and documenting blood pressure readings is important, but it does not treat the arterial hypertension; therefore, it is not the priority intervention.
    4. Walking will help decrease the client's high blood pressure in some situations, but it is not a priority.

CLINICAL JUDGMENT GUIDE: All options are plausible in questions that ask the test taker to identify a priority intervention. The test taker must identify the most important intervention.

31. **Correct answers are 2 and 4.**
    1. Stockings should be applied after the legs have been elevated for a period of time—when the amount of blood in the leg vein is at its lowest. Applying the stockings when the client is sitting in a chair indicates the UAP does not understand the correct procedure for applying compression stockings.
    2. **If a finger cannot be inserted under the proximal end of the stocking, the compression hose is too tight. By performing this test, the UAP demonstrated understanding of the correct procedure for applying the stockings.**
    3. The toe opening should be placed on the plantar side of the foot. Placing the toe opening on the top side of the foot indicates the UAP does not understand the correct procedure for applying compression stockings.
    4. **Warm toes mean the stockings are not too tight and there is good circulation. Checking that the toes are warm indicates the UAP HH aide understands the correct procedure for applying the compression stockings.**
    5. Lotions should not be applied immediately before putting on compression stockings. This indicates the UAP does not understand

the correct procedure for applying compression stockings.

CLINICAL JUDGMENT GUIDE: The nurse must ensure the UAP can perform any tasks that are delegated. It is the nurse's responsibility to evaluate the task, demonstrate, or teach the UAP how to perform the task.

32. 1. **The nurse should first take care of the bite and then determine whether the dog is up to date on the required vaccinations. The nurse should be concerned about the possibility of rabies.**
2. If the dog is not up to date on the required vaccinations, then the veterinarian should be notified to quarantine the dog to check for rabies.
3. The nurse should complete an occurrence report and document the dog bite. If the nurse must pay for anything concerning the dog bite, it should be covered by workers' compensation.
4. Besides an infection of the dog bite, the worst complication would be the nurse contracting rabies. If the dog is up to date on the required vaccinations, then this should not be a concern.

CLINICAL JUDGMENT GUIDE: The test taker should apply the nursing process when the question asks, "Which intervention should be implemented first?" If the client is in distress, do not assess; if the client is in distress, take action.

33. 1. This would not warrant immediate intervention because intermittent claudication, pain when walking, is the hallmark sign of arterial occlusive disease.
2. **This comment warrants immediate intervention because the client's legs have decreased sensation secondary to the arterial occlusive disease, and a heating pad could burn the client's legs without the client realizing it. The client should not use a heating pad to keep the legs warm.**
3. Hanging his or her legs off the bed helps increase the arterial blood supply to the legs, which, in turn, helps decrease the leg pain. This comment would not warrant immediate intervention by the nurse.
4. Hair growth requires oxygen, and the client has decreased oxygen to the legs; therefore, decreased hair growth would be expected and not require immediate intervention.

CLINICAL JUDGMENT GUIDE: When the question asks, "Which warrants immediate intervention?" it is an "except" question. Three of the comments indicate the client understands the

teaching and one indicates the client does not understand the teaching.

34. 1. The nurse cannot purchase supplies for the client. This is crossing a professional boundary.
2. The social worker does assist with financial concerns and referrals for the client, but purchasing smoke detectors is not within the social worker's scope of practice.
3. The nurse should not encourage the client to be dependent on family members for purchasing supplies for the client's home. This may be a possibility when all other avenues have been pursued.
4. **The nurse should contact the fire department. Many fire departments will supply and install smoke detectors for people who cannot afford them. The nurse should investigate this option first because it is the most immediate response to the safety need.**

CLINICAL JUDGMENT GUIDE: The nurse must be knowledgeable of emergency preparedness in the hospital as well as in the community. Employees receive this information in employee orientation and are responsible for implementing procedures correctly. The NCLEX-RN® test plan includes questions on a safe and effective care environment.

35. 1. The nurse should document the objective findings in the EHR, but this is not the priority intervention.
2. The nurse cannot force the client to talk about the situation.
3. **The bruises and burns should make the nurse suspect elder abuse, and the nurse is mandated by law to report this to Adult Protective Services.**
4. The nurse should let Adult Protective Services take pictures of the suspected abuse because there is a legal chain of custody that must be followed if the case goes to court.

CLINICAL JUDGMENT GUIDE: The NCLEX-RN® test plan includes nursing care that is ruled by legal requirements. The nurse is legally obligated to report possible child abuse or adult abuse. The nurse must be knowledgeable of these issues.

36. 1. **Acetylsalicylic acid (aspirin), an antiplatelet agent, puts the client at risk for bleeding. The client diagnosed with deep vein thrombosis will be on warfarin (Coumadin), an anticoagulant, which puts the client at risk for bleeding; therefore, this**

comment requires immediate intervention by the nurse.

2. The client should wear a medical alert bracelet to notify any emergency HCP of the client's condition and medication. This statement would not warrant immediate intervention.
3. Most books recommend not eating green, leafy vegetables that are high in vitamin K, because doing so is the antidote to Coumadin toxicity. The client would have to eat green, leafy vegetables more than twice a week to counteract the Coumadin; therefore, this comment would not warrant immediate intervention as much as the client's taking of daily acetylsalicylic acid (aspirin).
4. Elevating the client's legs would not warrant intervention by the nurse.

CLINICAL JUDGMENT GUIDE: This question asks the nurse to identify which statement warrants immediate intervention; this indicates three of the options are appropriate for the disease process or disorder and one is inappropriate. This is an "except" question, but it does not say all the options are correct "except."

37. 1. The nurse should be a client advocate and support the client's wishes, not support the HCP's recommendation even if it is best for the client.
2. Recommending the client talk to his family may be an appropriate action, but it does not support the nurse being a client advocate.
3. The client does have a right to a second opinion, but this action is not supporting the client's decision not to have an amputation, and thus is not client advocacy.
4. **This action shows the nurse being the client's advocate. Offering to go talk to the HCP about the amputation and making sure the HCP hears the client's opinion is being a client advocate. Another discussion may change the client's decision, but either way, client advocacy is supporting the client's decision.**

CLINICAL JUDGMENT GUIDE: There will be management questions on the NCLEX-RN® addressing client advocacy. A client advocate acts as a liaison between clients and health-care providers to help improve or maintain a high quality of health care.

38. 1. Crying at a death is a universal human response. Although the statement may be true, the nurse should recognize the UAP's

need for a short time to compose himself or herself.
2. **Hospital personnel are not immune to human emotions. The UAP needs a short time to compose himself or herself. The nurse should offer the UAP compassion. If this occurred with every death, the UAP could be counseled to transfer to a different area of the hospital.**
3. This is not accepting the UAP's feelings.
4. This is not accepting the UAP's feelings.

CLINICAL JUDGMENT GUIDE: There will be management questions on the NCLEX-RN®. In many instances, there is no test-taking strategy for these questions. The nurse must be knowledgeable regarding management issues.

39. 1. **Clients receiving hospice can decide to discontinue the service and resume standard health-care practices and treatments whenever they wish. The nurse should assess the client's wishes before continuing.**
2. This is true, but if the client wants to be treated, it is the client's decision. If the client does not want treatment, then the nurse should discuss the client's wishes with the long-term care facility staff.
3. If the client does not want treatment, then the nurse should discuss the client's wishes with the long-term care facility staff.
4. If the staff continues to try to get the client to accept futile treatment, a client conference should be called. This is not the first action for the hospice nurse because a client conference is a scheduled event and would not take place immediately.

CLINICAL JUDGMENT GUIDE: This question requires the test taker to have a basic knowledge of hospice and hospice goals. The nurse must also be aware of appropriate referrals.

40. 1. Telling the family over the telephone could cause the client's significant other to have an accident while driving to the hospital. The nurse should avoid disclosing this type of information over the telephone.
2. **This response allows the family or significant other to know there has been some incident, but it does not disclose the death. This is the best statement for the nurse at this time. The family will be able to arrive safely at the hospital before hearing the news their loved one has died.**
3. Telling the family over the telephone could cause the client to have an accident while

driving to the hospital. The nurse should avoid disclosing this type of information over the telephone.

4. This is a backward way of telling the family that the client died and should be avoided.

CLINICAL JUDGMENT GUIDE: There will be management questions on the NCLEX-RN®. In many instances, there is no test-taking strategy for these questions. The nurse must be knowledgeable regarding management issues.

41. 1. The client is experiencing a complication of the surgical procedure and should be assigned to a nurse who is more experienced in caring for clients diagnosed with vascular complications.

2. Low back pain could indicate a leaking abdominal aortic aneurysm and should not be assigned to a floating nurse. A more experienced vascular nurse should care for this client.

3. Because this client needs extensive teaching, this client should not be assigned to a floating nurse but a more experienced vascular nurse.

4. **The client diagnosed with varicose veins would be expected to have deep aching pain in the legs; therefore, the nurse who is being floated to the vascular unit could be assigned to this client.**

CLINICAL JUDGMENT GUIDE: The nurse should assign the most stable client to the least experienced nurse.

42. 1. Leaving the facility will make client care even more strained.

2. **The nurse should notify the supervisor that the nurse is concerned that the assignment will not allow the nurse to provide adequate care to any of the three clients. This is the first step the nurse should implement.**

3. This is the second step. The nurse should put his or her concerns in writing and present the documentation to the supervisor. In states that have a "safe harbor" clause in the Nursing Practice Act, this will prevent the nurse from losing his or her license should a poor outcome result from the assignment.

4. If the staffing continues to be unsafe, the nurse may choose to resign, but the resignation should follow accepted business practices.

CLINICAL JUDGMENT GUIDE: There will be management questions on the NCLEX-RN®. In

many instances, there is no test-taking strategy for these questions; the nurse must be knowledgeable of management issues. If the nurse thinks the assignment is a violation of the state's Nursing Practice Act, then the nurse must notify the supervisor immediately.

43. 1. Morphine is a potent narcotic analgesic. A 4 on the 1-to-10 pain scale is considered moderate pain and should be treated with a less potent pain medication.

2. Promethazine (Phenergan) is administered for nausea.

3. **Hydrocodone (Vicodin) is a narcotic analgesic that is less potent than morphine. It has been 5 hours since the hydrocodone was last administered, and no other pain medication has been required by the client. This is the best medication for moderate pain.**

4. Ibuprofen (Motrin) may be effective for moderate pain, but the client is allergic to ibuprofen. The nurse should tag the medical administration record (MAR) and EHR to notify the HCP to discontinue this medication.

CLINICAL JUDGMENT GUIDE: This is an alternate type question included in the NCLEX-RN® test plan. The test taker must be able to read a medication administration record (MAR), must be knowledgeable regarding medications, and must be able to make a decision as to the nurse's most appropriate intervention.

44. 1. **The daughter lives in a "nearby" city. The client should not be moved anywhere until the daughter arrives.**

2. A morgue is a difficult place to view a body. This could be appropriate if the daughter was going to take hours to days to get to the hospital.

3. Many people feel it is necessary to view the body. Not allowing the daughter time to view the body before transfer to a funeral home or the morgue could cause hurt feelings and impede the grieving process.

4. Many people feel it is necessary to view the body. Not allowing the daughter time to view the body before transfer to a funeral home or the morgue could cause hurt feelings and impede the grieving process.

CLINICAL JUDGMENT GUIDE: The nurse should always try and support the client's or family's request, if it does not violate any local, state, or federal rules and regulations. This is the test taker's best decision if unsure of the correct answer.

45. 1. **The change process can be compared with the nursing process. The first step of each process is to assess the problem. Assessment involves collecting the pertinent data that support the need for a change.**
2. The second step is to identify the problem or, in the nursing process, identify possible nursing diagnoses.
3. The third step is to select an alternative to implement to fix the problem. This is similar to choosing a specific nursing diagnosis.
4. The fourth step is to implement a plan of action. This is similar to implementing the nursing care plan.

CLINICAL JUDGMENT GUIDE: Assessment is the first step of the nursing process, and the test taker should use the nursing process or some other systematic process to assist in determining priorities.

46. **Correct answers are 2 and 3.**
1. The only solution compatible with blood is normal saline. Dextrose causes the blood to coagulate.
2. **The blood administration set is changed after every two units.**
3. **The nurse must assess the client's vital signs before every unit of blood is administered.**
4. The nurse should assess for allergies before administering medications. Before administering blood products, the nurse should assess to determine compatibility with the client's blood type. The client may have an incompatible blood type, but this is not an allergy.
5. A blood warmer is used when the client has identified cold agglutinins. This is not in the stem of the question.

CLINICAL JUDGMENT GUIDE: This is an alternate type of question included in the NCLEX-RN®. The nurse must be able to select all the options that answer the question correctly. There are no partially correct answers.

47. 1. The client diagnosed with a deep vein thrombosis is placed on strict bedrest and should not have any type of pressure on his or her calf, which may cause the clot to dislodge and cause a pulmonary embolus. This task should not be delegated to an unlicensed assistive personnel (UAP).
2. The number one intervention for a client diagnosed with thromboangiitis obliterans (Buerger's disease) is to stop smoking;

therefore, this task should not be elevated. The UAP should be on the unit caring for clients, not outside to allow a client to smoke.
3. **The leg should be elevated to prevent postoperative edema; therefore, this task could be delegated to the UAP.**
4. The UAP cannot perform Doppler studies; a trained technician must perform this test.

CLINICAL JUDGMENT GUIDE: An RN cannot delegate assessment, teaching, evaluation, medications, or an unstable client to a UAP. Tasks that cannot be delegated are nursing interventions requiring nursing clinical judgment.

48. 1. Only the client should activate the PCA pump. Allowing family or significant others to push the button places the client at risk for an overdose.
2. The nurse is acting appropriately; there is no reason to discuss the instructions further.
3. The nurse is acting appropriately; there is no reason to discuss the instructions further.
4. **The nurse is acting appropriately, and there is no reason to discuss the instructions further. The charge nurse should continue with other duties.**

CLINICAL JUDGMENT GUIDE: There will be management questions on the NCLEX-RN®. In many instances, there is no test-taking strategy for these questions; the nurse must be knowledgeable regarding management issues concerning personnel. The nurse is responsible for evaluating the behavior of subordinates when caring for clients.

49. 1. **This client may be having phantom pain, but it must be assessed and the client must be medicated. The nurse should assess this client first.**
2. The client's blood pressure must be taken to determine if the headache is because of hypertensive crisis, but it is not a priority for postoperative surgical pain.
3. The client diagnosed with lymphedema would be expected to have edema of the lower leg; therefore, the nurse would not assess this client first.
4. The client diagnosed with gangrene would be expected to have a foul-smelling discharge; therefore, this client would not be assessed first.

CLINICAL JUDGMENT GUIDE: When deciding which client to assess first, the test taker should determine whether the signs or symptoms the client is exhibiting are normal or expected for the client situation. After eliminating the expected option, the test taker should determine which situation is more life threatening.

50. 1. The LPN should not administer the medication if the client's BP is lower than 90/50, but this is not the first action the nurse should take.
2. This medication cannot be crushed and the nurse needs to intervene and correct the LPN's behavior.
3. The LPN should be shown where to find pudding or applesauce to mix in crushed medications, but this medication should not be crushed.
4. **The XL in the name of the medication nifedipine (Procardia XL) indicates that this medication is a sustained-release formulation and should not be crushed. The nurse should speak directly with the LPN to correct the behavior.**

CLINICAL JUDGMENT GUIDE: The nurse should be aware of interventions that must be implemented before administering medications. The nurse must know which medications cannot be crushed. The nurse is responsible for evaluating the behavior and actions of his or her subordinates.

51. 1. This is an example of paternalism or beneficence.
2. This is an example of beneficence.
3. This is an example of nonmalfeasance or beneficence.
4. **This is an example of autonomy.**

CLINICAL JUDGMENT GUIDE: The NCLEX-RN® test plan includes nursing care that addresses ethical principles, including autonomy, beneficence, justice, and veracity, to name a few.

52. 1. This would be culturally sensitive to a client who is a Jehovah's Witness.
2. Mormons do not wear amulets.
3. **The devout Mormon client wears a religious undershirt that should not be removed; this action indicates cultural sensitivity on the part of the nurse.**
4. Mormons do not consult curanderos. Some Hispanic cultures consult curanderos.

CLINICAL JUDGMENT GUIDE: The NCLEX-RN® test plan includes nursing care that addresses cultural diversity. The nurse needs to be aware of cultural differences.

53. 1. **These ABGs show respiratory acidosis, which needs immediate intervention;**
therefore, this client should be assessed first.
2. The client diagnosed with Raynaud's phenomenon would be expected to have bluish, cold upper extremities; therefore, the nurse would not need to assess the client first.
3. The client diagnosed with chronic venous insufficiency has ulceration on the feet; therefore, this nurse would not need to assess the client first.
4. The PTT is 1.5 to 2 times the normal; therefore, the nurse would not need to assess this client first. Normal PTT is 39 seconds; therefore, therapeutic PTT is 58 to 78.

CLINICAL JUDGMENT GUIDE: The test taker must determine which sign or symptom is not expected for the disease process. If the sign or symptom is not expected, then the nurse should assess the client first. This type of question determines if the nurse is knowledgeable regarding signs and symptoms of a variety of disease processes.

54. 1. The client diagnosed with arterial occlusive disease dangles the feet off the side of the bed to increase the blood supply to the legs; therefore, a less experienced unlicensed assistive personnel (UAP) could care for this client.
2. The nurse should be assigned to care for this client, who is angry about the family's not visiting, because the client requires assessment, nursing judgment, and therapeutic communication and intervention, which are not within the UAP's scope of practice.
3. **This client requires an experienced UAP who is skilled in client lifts, so the client is lifted safely and the UAP is not injured in the process. The most experienced UAP should be assigned this client.**
4. The experienced UAP could care for this client, but then other UAPs would not learn to care for the client. This client should be rotated through the UAPs so that all the UAPs can learn to care for the client who is particular about the way things are done.

CLINICAL JUDGMENT GUIDE: When the test taker is deciding which option is the most appropriate task to delegate or assign, the test taker should choose the task that allows each staff member to function within his or her full scope of practice. Remember: The RN cannot delegate assessment, teaching, evaluation, medications, or an unstable client to the UAP.

55. 1. **Chest pain on deep inspiration is a symptom of pulmonary embolism. The nurse should first place the client on oxygen.**
2. The first intervention is to provide the client with oxygen. The test taker should not assess when the client is in distress.
3. The respiratory therapist can be notified, but it is not the nurse's first intervention. The nurse should first address the client's needs.
4. The nurse should not select equipment over addressing the client's needs.

CLINICAL JUDGMENT GUIDE: The nurse should remember: If a client is in distress and the nurse can do something to relieve the distress, that should be done first, before assessment. The test taker should select an option that directly helps the client's condition.

56. Correct answers are 2, 3, 4, and 5.
1. Monetary need is not a good reason to select a nurse to become a preceptor.
2. **The nurse should be able to organize his or her own workload before becoming a role model for a new nurse. If the nurse is not organized, taking on new responsibilities will be very frustrating for the preceptor and for the preceptee.**
3. **The nurse who acts as a preceptor should have good people skills and be approachable.**
4. **The nurse should consistently provide quality care that others should emulate.**
5. **The nurse should be willing to take on this responsibility or the preceptor will resent the new nurse.**

CLINICAL JUDGMENT GUIDE: This is an alternate type of question included in the NCLEX-RN®. The nurse must be able to select all the options that answer the question correctly. There are no partially correct answers.

57. 1. **This client is experiencing neurovascular compromise and requires immediate attention. The client diagnosed with venous problems should have palpable pedal pulses. This procedure is for clients diagnosed with varicose veins.**
2. The calf pain is expected with a client diagnosed with deep vein thrombosis; therefore, the nurse would not assess this client first.
3. The client diagnosed with Raynaud's phenomenon has coldness and numbness in the vasoconstriction phase followed by throbbing, aching pain, tingling, and swelling in the hyperemic phase. The nurse would not see this client first because these are expected signs or symptoms.

4. Buerger's disease (thromboangiitis obliterans) is often confused with peripheral arterial disease (PAD). As the disease progresses, rest pain develops along with color and temperature changes in the affected limb or limbs.

CLINICAL JUDGMENT GUIDE: The test taker must determine which sign or symptom is not expected for the disease process. If the sign or symptom is not expected, then the nurse should assess the client first. This type of question determines if the nurse is knowledgeable regarding signs and symptoms of a variety of disease processes.

58. **Answer: 2,050 mL total intake.**
The urinary output is not used in this calculation. The nurse must add up both intravenous fluids and oral fluids to obtain the total intake for this client: 950 + 200 = 1,150 IV fluids; (1 ounce = 30 mL) 16 ounces × 30 mL = 480 mL, 8 ounces × 30 mL = 240 mL, 6 ounces × 30 mL = 180 mL; 480 + 240 + 180 = 900 oral fluids. Total intake is 1,150 + 900 = 2,050.

CLINICAL JUDGMENT GUIDE: This is an alternate type question included in the NCLEX-RN®. The nurse must be knowledgeable on how to perform math calculations.

59. 1. Cold water causes vasoconstriction and hot water may burn the client's feet; therefore, warm water should be used and the feet should be cleaned daily. This indicates the client understands the teaching.
2. Shoes should be purchased in the afternoon when the feet are the largest. This indicates the client understands the teaching.
3. **This statement indicates the client needs more teaching because knee-high stockings will further decrease circulation to the legs.**
4. The client should not elevate legs because it further decreases arterial blood flow to the legs. The client should dangle his or her legs off the side of the bed, which increases arterial blood flow to the lower extremities. This indicates that the client understands the teaching.

CLINICAL JUDGMENT GUIDE: When the question says "needs more teaching," it is an "except" question. Three of the comments indicate the client understands the teaching and one indicates the client does not understand the teaching.

60. 1. The nurse cannot delegate a client who is unstable to the unlicensed assistive personnel (UAP). The client is experiencing hypoglycemia and is not stable.

2. **The client is stable and elevating the feet is an appropriate intervention for a client diagnosed with venous problems; therefore, the UAP could assist this client.**
3. The nurse cannot delegate a client who is unstable to the UAP. The client has numbness of the right arm and should be assessed by the nurse.
4. The client diagnosed with an abdominal aortic aneurysm should not have any increased pressure in the abdomen because it may cause the aneurysm to rupture; therefore, this should not be implemented by anyone.

CLINICAL JUDGMENT GUIDE: This is an "except" question. The test taker could ask which task is appropriate to delegate to the UAP; three options would be appropriate to delegate and one would not be. Remember: The RN cannot delegate assessment, teaching, evaluation, medications, or an unstable client to the UAP.

61. 1. **The nurse needs to intervene because the client is at high risk for developing pneumonia, especially because of the abdominal incision.**
    2. The client must have 30 mL of urinary output every hour, and 300 mL in 8 hours is adequate urinary output. Clients who are postoperative AAA are at high risk for renal failure because of the anatomical location of the AAA near the renal arteries.
    3. The client should have hypoactive bowel sounds on the second day postoperative. The client was NPO before surgery and NPO until bowel sounds returned, so hypoactive bowel sounds would be expected.
    4. These vital signs are within normal limits and would not warrant immediate intervention by the nurse.

CLINICAL JUDGMENT GUIDE: The test taker should ask, "Are the assessment data normal for the disease process?" If they are normal for the disease process, then the nurse would not need to intervene; if they are not normal for the disease process, then this warrants intervention by the nurse.

62. 1. The nurse should assess the client's right foot pain, but not before a potentially life-threatening situation.
    2. **Parasthesia (numbness and tingling) indicates a graft occlusion from the surgical procedure, which is a potentially life-threatening complication; therefore, this client should be assessed first.**
    3. The most common cause of superficial thrombophlebitis is IV therapy, and tenderness to

the touch, redness, and warmth are expected. This is not a medical emergency; therefore, the nurse would not assess this client first.
4. The client diagnosed with arterial occlusive disease would be expected to have pain in the calf when ambulating, which is called intermittent claudication.

CLINICAL JUDGMENT GUIDE: When deciding which client to assess first, the test taker should determine whether the signs or symptoms the client is exhibiting are normal or expected for the client's situation. After eliminating the expected option, the test taker should determine which situation is more life threatening.

63. **Answer: 22 mL/hour.** To determine the rate, the test taker must first determine how many units are in each mL of fluid: 25,000 divided by 500 = 50 units of heparin in each mL of fluid, and 50 divided into 100 = 2, and 2 + 20 = 22.

CLINICAL JUDGMENT GUIDE: This is an alternate type of question included in the NCLEX-RN®. The nurse must be knowledgeable on how to perform math calculations.

64. 1. Compression stockings are used to treat chronic venous insufficiency; therefore, this action does not warrant intervention by the nurse.
    2. The client's legs should be elevated; therefore, this action would not warrant immediate intervention.
    3. The client can ambulate with assistance; therefore, this action does not warrant intervention.
    4. **The client should have a podiatrist cut his or her toenails. The unlicensed assistive personnel (UAP) should not do this because if the UAP accidently cuts the skin, it could cause a sore that may not heal, and then result in amputation of the extremity.**

CLINICAL JUDGMENT GUIDE: The nurse cannot delegate any task in which the UAP admits to not being able to perform. Delegation means the nurse is responsible for the UAP's actions; therefore, the nurse must intervene if the UAP is performing unsafely.

65. 1. The client diagnosed with a venous stasis ulcer should eat a diet high in protein (meat, beans, cheese, tofu), vitamin A (green, leafy vegetables), vitamin C (citrus fruits, tomatoes, cantaloupe), and zinc (meat, seafood). The nurse needs to talk to this client, but it is not a life-threatening condition or a complication; therefore, the client is not assessed first.

2. The client should wear thromboembolic hose, but this is not a life-threatening condition or a complication; therefore, the client does not have to be assessed first.
3. The client diagnosed with arterial occlusive disease should not elevate the feet because it further decreases oxygen to the extremity; therefore, this action is not required to be assessed by the nurse.
4. **The nurse should assess this client first because if the client does not stay in the bed, the clot in the calf muscle may dislodge and result in a pulmonary embolus. The client diagnosed with a DVT must be on bedrest.**

CLINICAL JUDGMENT GUIDE: The nurse must determine if the client's behavior is potentially unsafe for the client's disease process. If the client is putting himself or herself at risk, then the nurse must assess this client first.

66. 1. Oral pain medications provide relief for mild to moderate pain. A 10 is considered to be severe pain.
2. Guided imagery will not alleviate severe pain.
3. **If the current pain regimen is not working for this client, the nurse should notify the surgeon for an adjustment in the pain medication.**
4. It has only been 1 hour and 15 minutes since the pain medication was administered. It is too soon for the nurse to administer the morphine.

CLINICAL JUDGMENT GUIDE: This is an alternate type of question included in the NCLEX-RN® test plan. The test taker must be able to read a medication administration record (MAR), must be knowledgeable regarding medications, and must be able to make a decision as to the nurse's most appropriate intervention.

67. **Answer: 50 drops per minute.**
    150 mL ÷ 60 = 2.5 mL per minute to infuse
    2.5 × 20 = 50

CLINICAL JUDGMENT GUIDE: This is an alternate type question included in the NCLEX-RN®. The nurse must be knowledgeable on how to perform math calculations.

68. 1. The nurse needs to have the surgical operative permit signed by the client, but not until the discrepancy between what the operative permit says and what the client said is resolved.
2. The nurse can assess the client's neurological status, but not before calling a time out. Calling a time out is the priority intervention.

3. Determining if the client had anything by mouth is an appropriate intervention, but not a priority to clarifying which leg the surgical procedure will be performed on.
4. **The nurse must stop everything and clarify which leg will have the surgical procedure. This is the first and priority intervention the nurse must implement.**

CLINICAL JUDGMENT GUIDE: The NCLEX-RN® test plan includes nursing care administered by the current National Patient Safety Goals. The nurse must be knowledgeable regarding these goals.

69. 1. The abdominal bruit is located at the mid-abdominal area above the umbilicus.
2. The mid-scapula area is not an appropriate area to auscultate an abdominal aortic aneurysm.
3. **An abdominal aortic aneurysm is diagnosed when the client has an abdominal bruit. An abdominal bruit is a murmur that corresponds to the cardiac cycle. It is heard best with the diaphragm of the stethoscope, usually over the abdominal aorta.**
4. The nurse cannot auscultate a bruit on the feet.

CLINICAL JUDGMENT GUIDE: This is an alternate type question included in the NCLEX-RN®. It is a picture and the nurse must be able to point the curser at the appropriate area. It is called a hot spot.

70. **Correct order is 1, 4, 3, 2, 5.**
1. **The bleeding must be stopped. The nurse should don non sterile gloves and apply pressure to the bleeding site for a minimum of 5 minutes.**
4. **When the bleeding has stopped, the client can be assisted back to bed so a thorough assessment of the injuries can be performed.**
3. **The site should be redressed when possible to protect the wound from infectious organisms.**
2. **Once the nurse has been able to assess the client and has the client in a safe environment, then the nurse should notify the surgeon.**
5. **The occurrence should be noted on a report form and the appropriate hospital personnel notified, but this can be done after caring for the client.**

CLINICAL JUDGMENT GUIDE: This is an alternate type of question included in the NCLEX-RN®. The nurse must be able to place the interventions in order of priority. The nurse can use Maslow's Hierarchy of Needs to prioritize the interventions. Written documentation is the last action taken in an emergency or life-threatening situation.

CLINICAL SCENARIO ANSWERS AND RATIONALES

The correct answer number and rationale for why it is the correct answer are given in **boldface type**. Rationales for why the other possible answer options are incorrect also are given, but they are not in boldface type.

1. 1. The client has an elevated blood pressure, but it is not life threatening; therefore, the client does not need to be seen first.
   2. The client diagnosed with a DVT would be expected to be reporting calf pain; therefore, this client would not be seen first.
   3. The client diagnosed with peripheral vascular disease would be expected to have intermittent claudication; therefore, this client would not be seen first.
   4. **The client diagnosed with an AAA who has low back pain could have a leak, which could be life threatening; therefore, this client should be assessed first.**

2. 1. Increased hair loss occurs because of decreased oxygen to the lower extremities, but this is not life threatening; therefore, this information would not warrant immediate intervention.
   2. The client diagnosed with arterial occlusive disease would be expected to have an absent dorsal pedal pulse; therefore, this would not warrant immediate intervention.
   3. **Numbness, tingling, and inability to move his or her toes would warrant immediate intervention by the nurse. This indicates no arterial blood flow to the extremities.**
   4. The client hangs his or her legs off the bed to help increase arterial oxygen blood flow to the lower extremities. This would not warrant immediate intervention.

3. 1. The nurse cannot delegate assessment, teaching, evaluation, medications, or an unstable client to the UAP. Checking the pedal pulse is assessment.
   2. The client who is 4 hours postoperative leg surgery would not be able to ambulate down the hall. The client will be on bedrest for at least 24 hours.
   3. The nurse cannot delegate assessment, teaching, evaluation, medications, or an unstable client to the UAP.
   4. **The leg should be elevated to help decrease edema secondary to surgery; this can be delegated to a UAP.**

4. **Correct answers are 1, 2, and 5.**
   1. **A daily acetylsalicylic acid (aspirin) is recommended as an anticoagulant to clients diagnosed with atherosclerosis.**
   2. **A low-fat, low-cholesterol diet is recommended to help decrease plaque formation in the vessels.**
   3. Sedentary lifestyle is a "couch potato" lifestyle, which is not recommended for clients diagnosed with atherosclerosis.
   4. The client should eat foods high in fiber to help decrease his or her cholesterol level.
   5. **Walking is an excellent isotonic exercise, which is recommended to help lose weight, develop collateral circulation, and decrease stress.**

5. 1. The nurse should auscultate the bowel sounds, but the nurse should first assess the client's surgical incision, because the client is 2 days postoperative.
   2. **The nurse with 1 year of experience should first assess the surgical dressing to assess for bleeding or any type of drainage, then continue with the rest of the assessment, including bowel sounds, vital signs, and IV therapy.**
   3. The nurse should assess first, because it is the first part of the nursing process when the client is not in distress.
   4. Monitoring the intravenous therapy should be done by the nurse, but assessment is the first intervention.

6. 1. The client should not lift more than 5 pounds; doing so might cause the surgical incision to have dehiscence. This statement indicates the client understands the teaching.
   2. The number one factor for developing atherosclerosis and increased blood pressure is smoking cigarettes; therefore, the client must quit. This statement indicates the client understands the teaching.
   3. **A truss is a kind of surgical appliance used for clients diagnosed with a hernia. It provides support for the herniated area using a pad and belt arrangement to hold it in the correct position. This client would not be prescribed a truss; therefore, the client needs more discharge teaching.**
   4. The client should notify the health-care provider if there is an elevated temperature

because this indicates that the client has a postoperative infection. This statement indicates the client understands the teaching.

7. **1.** The new graduate nurse would expect the client to have pain in the surgical area and, though this client's pain needs to be assessed, it would not be assessed before a client in renal failure.
   2. The 3+ posterior tibial pulse indicates the blood supply to the foot is adequate and would not require the client to be seen first by the nurse.
   3. The client is going into renal failure (should be 30 mL/hr), which is a potentially life-threatening complication of AAA surgery; therefore, this client must be assessed first.
   4. The client report needs to be addressed, but not before a physiological, potentially life-threatening complication.

8. **Answer: 16 mL/hour.**
   To determine the rate, the test taker must first determine how many units are in each mL of fluid; 25,000 ÷ 500 = 50 units of heparin in each mL of fluid, and 50 divided into 100 = 2; 18 − 2 = 16.

9. **1.** The client should elevate the lower extremities to help decrease the edema and help the unoxygenated blood go up the inferior cava.
   2. Massaging the legs would not warrant intervention for this client; it would be inappropriate for a client diagnosed with deep vein thrombosis. Varicose veins will not dislodge a clot.
   3. The client diagnosed with varicose veins should not be on bedrest. The client should have bathroom privileges and up ad lib.
   4. The UAP can calculate the client's I&O, not evaluate the I&O.

10. **1.** Hospice is for a client whose health-care provider determines the client has fewer than 6 months to live. This client does not have this diagnosis.
    2. The home health nurse is an appropriate charge nurse referral for this client. The client's home should be assessed to determine if the client needs assistance in the home.
    3. The physical therapist addresses gait training and transferring.
    4. Cardiac rehabilitation helps clients who have had myocardial infarctions, cardiac bypass surgery, or congestive heart failure recover.

Respiratory Management 4

The best way to predict your future is to create it.

—Peter Drucker

QUESTIONS

1. The nurse on a medical unit has a client diagnosed with adventitious breath sounds, but the nurse is unable to determine the exact nature of the situation. Which multidisciplinary team member should the nurse consult **first?**
   1. The health-care provider
   2. The unit manager
   3. The respiratory therapist
   4. The case manager

2. The RN staff nurse is working with a licensed practical nurse (LPN) and an unlicensed assistive personnel (UAP) to care for a group of clients. Which nursing tasks can the RN delegate or assign? **Select all that apply.**
   1. The routine oral medications for the clients
   2. The bed baths and oral care
   3. Evaluating the client's progress
   4. Transporting a client to dialysis
   5. Administering scheduled vaccinations

3. Which client should the RN charge nurse assign to the new graduate (GN) on the respiratory unit?
   1. The client diagnosed with lung cancer who has rust-colored sputum and chest pain of 10 on a scale of 1 to 10
   2. The client diagnosed with atelectasis who is having shortness of breath and difficulty breathing
   3. The client diagnosed with tuberculosis who has a nonproductive cough and orange-colored urine
   4. The client diagnosed with pneumonia who has a pulse oximeter reading of 91% and has a CRT greater than 3 seconds

4. Which tasks are appropriate to assign to the unlicensed assistive personnel (UAP)? **Select all that apply.**
   1. Perform mouth care on the client diagnosed with pneumonia.
   2. Apply oxygen via nasal cannula to the client.
   3. Empty the trash cans in the clients' rooms.
   4. Take the empty blood bag back to the laboratory.
   5. Show the client how to ambulate on the walker.

5. Which client should the medical unit nurse assess **first** after receiving the shift report?
    1. The 84-year-old client diagnosed with pneumonia who is afebrile but getting restless
    2. The 25-year-old client diagnosed with influenza who is febrile and has a headache
    3. The 56-year-old client diagnosed with a left-sided hemothorax with tidaling in the water-seal compartment of the chest drainage system
    4. The 38-year-old client diagnosed with a sinus infection who has green drainage from the nose

6. The client who is 2 days postoperative following a left pneumonectomy has an apical pulse (AP) rate of 128 beats per minute and a blood pressure (BP) of 80/50 mm Hg. Which intervention should the nurse implement **first?**
    1. Notify the health-care provider (HCP).
    2. Assess the client's incisional wound.
    3. Prepare to administer dopamine.
    4. Increase the client's intravenous (IV) rate.

7. The client who is 1-day postoperative following chest surgery is having difficulty breathing, has bilateral rales, and is confused and restless. Which intervention should the nurse implement **first?**
    1. Assess the client's pulse oximeter reading.
    2. Notify the Rapid Response Team.
    3. Place the client in the Trendelenburg position.
    4. Check the client's surgical dressing.

8. The client in the postanesthesia care unit (PACU) has noisy and irregular respirations with a pulse oximeter reading of 89%. Which intervention should the PACU nurse implement **first?**
    1. Increase the client's oxygen rate via nasal cannula.
    2. Notify the respiratory therapist to draw arterial blood gases.
    3. Tilt the head back and push forward on the angle of the lower jaw.
    4. Obtain an intubation tray and prepare for emergency intubation.

9. The day surgery admission nurse is obtaining operative permits for clients having surgery. Which client should the nurse **question** signing the consent form?
    1. The 16-year-old married client who is diagnosed with an ectopic pregnancy
    2. The 39-year-old client diagnosed with paranoid schizophrenia
    3. The 50-year-old client who admits to being a recovering alcoholic
    4. The 84-year-old client diagnosed with chronic obstructive pulmonary disease (COPD)

10. The intensive care unit (ICU) nurse is caring for a client on a ventilator who is exhibiting respiratory distress. The ventilator alarms are going off. Which intervention should the nurse implement **first?**
    1. Notify the respiratory therapist.
    2. Ventilate with a manual resuscitation bag.
    3. Check the ventilator to resolve the problem.
    4. Auscultate the client's lung sounds.

11. The charge nurse on the critical care respiratory unit is evaluating arterial blood gas (ABG) values of several clients. Which client would require an **immediate** intervention by the charge nurse?

1. Mr. C.T., who is diagnosed with chronic obstructive pulmonary disease

Client Name: C.T.		Account Number: 2156669
Arterial Blood Gas Report		
Parameter	Client Value	Normal Range
pH	7.34	7.35–7.45
Po_2	70	80–95 mm Hg
Pco_2	55	35–45 mm Hg
Hco_3	24	22–26 mmol/L

2. Ms. L.D., who is diagnosed with acute respiratory distress syndrome

Client Name: L.D.		Account Number: 2377699
Arterial Blood Gas Report		
Parameter	Client Value	Normal Range
pH	7.35	7.35–7.45
Po_2	75	80–95 mm Hg
Pco_2	50	35–45 mm Hg
Hco_3	26	22–26 mmol/L

3. Ms. P.C., who is diagnosed with reactive airway disease

Client Name: P.C.		Account Number: 3004863
Arterial Blood Gas Report		
Parameter	Client Value	Normal Range
pH	7.48	7.35–7.45
Po_2	80	80–95 mm Hg
Pco_2	30	35–45 mm Hg
Hco_3	23	22–26 mmol/L

4. Mr. R.W., who is diagnosed with a pneumothorax

Client Name: R.W.		Account Number: 2758931
Arterial Blood Gas Report		
Parameter	Client Value	Normal Range
pH	7.41	7.35–7.45
Po_2	98	80–95 mm Hg
Pco_2	43	35–45 mm Hg
Hco_3	25	22–26 mmol/L

12. The primary nurse in the critical care respiratory unit is very busy. Which nursing task should be the nurse's **priority?**
   1. Assist the HCP with a sterile dressing change for a client with a left pneumonectomy.
   2. Obtain a tracheostomy tray for a client who is exhibiting air hunger.
   3. Review orders for a client diagnosed with cystic fibrosis who was transferred from the ED.
   4. Assess the client diagnosed with mesothelioma who is upset, angry, and crying.

13. The nurse is caring for a client diagnosed with flail chest who has had a chest tube for 3 days. The nurse notes there is no tidaling in the water-seal compartment. Which **initial** action should be taken by the nurse?
   1. Check the tubing for any dependent loops.
   2. Auscultate the client's posterior breath sounds.
   3. Prepare to remove the client's chest tubes.
   4. Notify the HCP that the lungs have re-expanded.

14. The client diagnosed with a right-sided pneumothorax had chest tubes inserted 2 hours ago. There is no fluctuation in the water-seal chamber of the chest drainage system (Pleur-evac). Which intervention should the nurse implement **first?**
   1. Assess the client's lung sounds.
   2. Check for any kinks in the tubing.
   3. Ask the client to take deep breaths.
   4. Turn the client from side to side.

15. Which client requires the **immediate** attention of the intensive care unit nurse?
   1. The client diagnosed with histoplasmosis who is having excessive diaphoresis and neck stiffness
   2. The client diagnosed with acute respiratory distress syndrome (ARDS) who has difficulty breathing
   3. The client diagnosed with pulmonary sarcoidosis who has a dry cough and mild chest pain
   4. The client diagnosed with asbestosis who has a productive cough and chest tightness

16. The client in the intensive care unit is on a ventilator. Which interventions should the nurse implement? **Select all that apply.**
   1. Ensure there is a manual resuscitation bag at the bedside.
   2. Monitor the client's pulse oximeter reading every shift.
   3. Assess the client's respiratory status every 2 hours.
   4. Check the ventilator settings every 4 hours.
   5. Collaborate with the respiratory therapist.

17. The unlicensed assistive personnel (UAP) is bathing the client diagnosed with adult acute respiratory distress syndrome (ARDS) who is on a ventilator. The bed is in the high position with the opposite side rail elevated. Which action should the ICU nurse take?
   1. Demonstrate the correct technique when giving a bed bath.
   2. Encourage the UAP to put the bed in the lowest position.
   3. Explain that the client on a ventilator should not be bathed.
   4. Give the UAP praise for performing the bath safely.

18. The female charge nurse on the respiratory unit tells the male nurse, "You are really cute and have a great body. Do you work out?" Which action should be taken by the male nurse if he thinks he is being sexually harassed?
   1. Document the comment in writing and tell another staff nurse.
   2. Ask the charge nurse to stop making comments such as this.
   3. Notify the clinical manager of the sexual harassment.
   4. Report this to the corporate headquarters office.

19. The client diagnosed with abdominal pain of unknown etiology has a nasogastric tube draining green bile and reports abdominal pain of 8 on a scale of 1 to 10. The client's arterial blood gas values are reported in the accompanying table. Which intervention should the nurse implement based on the client's ABGs?

Arterial Blood Gas Report		
Parameter	Client Value	Normal Range
pH	7.48	7.35–7.45
Po_2	98	80–95 mm Hg
Pco_2	36	35–45 mm Hg
Hco_3	28	22–26 mmol/L

    1. Assess the client to rule out any complications secondary to the client's pain.
    2. Determine the last time the client was medicated for abdominal pain.
    3. Check the amount of suction on the client's nasogastric tube.
    4. Administer intravenous sodium bicarbonate to the client.

20. The RN charge nurse in the intensive care unit asks a nurse to float from the medical/surgical unit to the ICU. Which client should the charge nurse assign to the float nurse?
    1. The client who is 3 hours postoperative lung transplant
    2. The client who has a central venous pressure of 13 cm H_2O
    3. The client who is diagnosed with bacterial pneumonia
    4. The client who is diagnosed with Hantavirus pulmonary syndrome

21. The client has arterial blood gas values of pH 7.38, Pao_2 77, $Paco_2$ 40, Hco_3 24. Which intervention should the critical care nurse implement?
    1. Administer oxygen 6 L/min via nasal cannula.
    2. Encourage the client to take deep breaths.
    3. Administer intravenous sodium bicarbonate.
    4. Assess the client's respiratory status.

22. The spouse of a client diagnosed with a terminal lung cancer asks the nurse, "How am I going to take care of the client when we go home?" Which action by the nurse is **most** appropriate?
    1. Notify the social worker about the spouse's concerns.
    2. Contact the hospital chaplain to talk to the spouse.
    3. Leave a note on the electronic health record (EHR) for the HCP to talk to the spouse.
    4. Reassure the spouse that everything will be all right.

23. The clinic nurse is scheduling a chest x-ray for a female client who may have pneumonia. Which question is **most** important for the nurse to ask the client?
    1. "Have you ever had a chest x-ray before?"
    2. "Can you hold your breath for a minute?"
    3. "Do you smoke or have you ever smoked cigarettes?"
    4. "Is there any chance you may be pregnant?"

24. The clinic nurse is returning phone messages from clients. Which client should the nurse contact **first?**
    1. The elderly client diagnosed with pneumonia who reports being dizzy when getting up
    2. The client diagnosed with cystic fibrosis who needs a prescription for pancreatic enzymes
    3. The client diagnosed with lung cancer on chemotherapy who reports nausea
    4. The client diagnosed with pertussis who reports coughing spells so severe that they cause vomiting

25. The client diagnosed with active tuberculosis tells the public health nurse, "I am not going to take any more medications. I am tired of them." Which statement is the nurse's **best** response?
    1. "You are tired of taking your tuberculosis medications."
    2. "You must take your TB medications. It is not an option."
    3. "You must discuss this with your health-care provider."
    4. "As long as you wear a mask, you do not have to take the meds."

26. The RN staff nurse is working in an outpatient clinic along with a licensed practical nurse (LPN). Which clients should the RN staff nurse assign to the LPN? **Select all that apply.**
    1. The client whose purified protein derivative (PPD) induration of the left arm is 14 mm
    2. The client diagnosed with pneumonia whose pulse oximeter reading is 90%
    3. The client diagnosed with acute bronchitis who has a chronic clear mucous cough and low fever
    4. The client diagnosed with reactive airway disease who has bilateral wheezing
    5. The client diagnosed with influenza reporting generalized muscle aches

27. The unlicensed assistive personnel (UAP) tells the RN clinic nurse that the client in Room 4 is "really breathing hard and can't seem to catch his breath." Which instruction should the nurse give to the UAP?
    1. Put 4 mL oxygen on the client.
    2. Sit the client upright in a chair.
    3. Go with the nurse to the client's room.
    4. Take the client's vital signs.

28. The clinic nurse is scheduling a 14-year-old client for a tonsillectomy. Which intervention should the clinic nurse implement?
    1. Obtain informed consent from the client.
    2. Send a throat culture to the laboratory.
    3. Discuss the need to cough and deep breathe.
    4. Request the laboratory to draw a PT and a PTT.

29. The client calls the clinic nurse and asks, "What is the best way to prevent getting influenza?" Which statement is the nurse's **best** response?
    1. "Take prophylactic antibiotics for 10 days after being exposed to influenza."
    2. "Stay away from large crowds and wear a scarf over your mouth during cold weather."
    3. "The best way to prevent getting influenza is to get a yearly flu vaccine."
    4. "You must eat three well-balanced meals a day and exercise daily to prevent influenza."

30. The clinic nurse is evaluating vital signs for clients being seen in the outpatient clinic. Which client would require **immediate** nursing intervention?
    1. The 10-month-old infant who has a pulse rate of 140 beats per minute
    2. The 3-year-old toddler who has a respiratory rate of 28 breaths per minute
    3. The 24-week gestational woman who has a BP of 142/96 mm Hg
    4. The 42-year-old client who has a temperature of 100.2°F (37.8°C)

31. The nurse is accidentally stuck with a needle used to administer an intradermal injection for a PPD. Which intervention should the nurse implement **first**?
    1. Complete the accident/occurrence report.
    2. Wash the area thoroughly with soap and water.
    3. Ask the client whether he or she has AIDS or hepatitis.
    4. Place an antibiotic ointment and bandage on the site.

32. The clinic nurse is reviewing laboratory results for clients seen in the clinic. Which clients require additional assessment by the nurse? **Select all that apply.**
    1. The client who has a hemoglobin of 9 g/dL and a hematocrit of 29%
    2. The client who has a WBC count of 9 x 10³/microL
    3. The client who has a serum potassium level of 4.8 mEq/L
    4. The client who has a serum sodium level of 125 mEq/L
    5. The client who has a cholesterol of 175 mg/dL and triglycerides of 125 mg/dL

33. A female client diagnosed with bacterial pneumonia is being admitted to the medical unit. The client's husband answers questions even though the nurse directly asks the client. The nurse suspects this may be because of a cultural issue. Which action should the nurse take?
    1. Ask the husband to allow his wife to answer the questions.
    2. Request the husband to leave the examination room.
    3. Continue to allow the husband to answer the wife's questions.
    4. Do not ask any further questions until the client starts answering.

34. The clinic nurse encounters a client who does not respond to verbal stimuli and initiates cardiopulmonary resuscitation (CPR). What should the nurse do? **Rank in order of performance.**
    1. Open the client's airway.
    2. Check the client's carotid pulse.
    3. Assess the client for unresponsiveness.
    4. Perform compressions at a 30:2 rate.
    5. Give two breaths with a CPR mask/face shield.

35. The RN home health nurse is visiting the client diagnosed with end-stage chronic obstructive pulmonary disease (COPD) while the unlicensed assistive personnel (UAP) is providing care. Which action by the UAP would **warrant** intervention by the RN home health nurse?
    1. Keeping the bedroom at a warm temperature.
    2. Maintaining the client's oxygen rate at 2 L/min.
    3. Helping the client sit in the orthopneic position.
    4. Allowing the client to sleep in the recliner.

36. Which task is **most** appropriate for the RN home health nurse to delegate to unlicensed assistive personnel (UAP)?
    1. Changing the client's subclavian dressing
    2. Reinserting the client's Foley catheter
    3. Demonstrating ambulation with a walker
    4. Getting the client up in a chair three times a day

37. In the local restaurant, the nurse overhears another hospital staff member talking to a friend about a client. The staff member discloses that the client was just diagnosed with lung cancer. What is the **most** appropriate action by the nurse?
    1. Do not approach the staff member in the restaurant.
    2. Ask the staff member not to discuss anything about the client.
    3. Contact the staff member's clinical manager and report the behavior.
    4. Tell the client that the staff member was discussing confidential information.

38. A 92-year-old client has a hospital bed in the home and is on strict bedrest. The unlicensed assistive personnel (UAP) cares for the client in the morning 5 days a week. Which statement indicates that the UAP **needs additional** education by the RN staff nurse?
    1. "I do not give her a lot of fluids so she won't wet the bed."
    2. "I perform passive range-of-motion exercises every morning."
    3. "I put her on her side so that there will be no pressure on her butt."
    4. "I do not pull her across the sheets when I am moving her in bed."

39. The home health client is diagnosed with chronic obstructive pulmonary disease. The unlicensed assistive personnel (UAP) tells the RN home health nurse that the client has trouble breathing when the client lies in a supine position. Which **priority** instruction should the RN provide to the UAP?
    1. To ensure the client's oxygen is in place correctly
    2. To allow the client to sleep in a recliner
    3. To allow a fan to blow on the client when lying in bed
    4. To have the client take slow, deep breaths

40. The wife of a client diagnosed as terminal is concerned that the client is not eating or drinking. Which is the home health nurse's **best** response?
    1. "I will start an IV if your husband continues to refuse to eat or drink."
    2. "You should discuss placing a feeding tube in your husband with the HCP."
    3. "This is normal at the end of life; the dehydration produces a type of euphoria."
    4. "You are right to be concerned. Would you want to talk about your worry?"

41. The client has just been told a medical condition cannot be treated successfully and the client has a life expectancy of about 6 months. To whom should the nurse refer the client at this time?
    1. A home health nurse
    2. The client's pastor
    3. A hospice agency
    4. The social worker

42. The hospice client asks the nurse, "What should I do about my house? My son and daughter are fighting over it." Which statement is the nurse's **best** response?
    1. "I think you should tell your children that you will leave the house to a charity."
    2. "I would sell the house and go on an extended vacation and spend the money."
    3. "What do you want to happen to your house? It is your decision."
    4. "Wait and let your children fight over the house after you are gone."

43. The nurse manager is communicating the results of the yearly performance evaluation with a nurse employee. Which information regarding communication styles is important to consider when talking with the employee? **Select all that apply.**
    1. Some nurses see the work from a global perspective focusing on feelings.
    2. Some nurses see the work environment from a logical, focused perspective.
    3. Some nurses ask many more questions than others and require specific answers.
    4. All nurses communicate similarly in a nursing environment.
    5. All nurses should keep an open mind when communicating with others in the workplace.

44. The newly hired nurse unit manager has identified that whenever a specific staff member is unhappy with an assignment, the entire unit has a bad day. Which action should the unit manager take to correct this problem?
    1. Determine why the staff member is unhappy.
    2. Discuss the staff member's attitude and the way it affects the unit.
    3. Place the staff member on a counseling record for the behavior.
    4. Suspend the staff member until the behavior improves.

45. The health-care facility where the nurse works uses e-mail to notify the staff of in-services and mandatory requirements. Which is important information for the nurse manager to remember when using e-mail to disseminate information?
    1. Give as much information as possible in each e-mail.
    2. Use e-mail for all communications with the staff.
    3. Use capital letters to get a point across with emphasis.
    4. Make the e-mail notices quick and easy to read.

46. At 1700, the HCP is yelling at the nursing staff because the early morning lab work is not available in the client's EHR. Which is the **most** appropriate response by the charge nurse?
1. Call the lab and have the lab supervisor talk with the HCP.
2. Discuss the HCP's complaints with the nursing supervisor.
3. Form a committee of lab and nursing personnel to fix the problem.
4. Tell the HCP to stop yelling and calm down.

47. The nurse is caring for a client who has a chest tube. What actions should the nurse perform? **Rank in order of performance.**
1. Assess the client's lung sounds.
2. Note the amount of suction being used.
3. Check the chest tube dressing for drainage.
4. Make sure that the chest tube is securely taped.
5. Place a bottle of sterile saline at the bedside.

48. The nurse is assessing clients on a respiratory unit. Which client should be the nurse's **first** priority?
1. The client diagnosed with bronchiectasis who has clubbing of the fingernails
2. The client diagnosed with byssinosis who reports chest tightness
3. The client diagnosed with cystic fibrosis who has a pulse oximeter reading of 91%
4. The client diagnosed with pneumoconiosis who has shortness of breath

49. The nurse is developing a nursing care plan for a client diagnosed with chronic obstructive pulmonary disease (COPD). What should be the client's **priority** nursing diagnosis?
1. Activity intolerance
2. Altered coping
3. Impaired gas exchange
4. Self-care deficit

50. The nurse assists with the insertion of a chest tube in a client diagnosed with a spontaneous pneumothorax. Which data indicates that the treatment has been **effective?**
1. The chest x-ray indicates consolidation.
2. The client has bilateral breath sounds.
3. The suction chamber has vigorous bubbling.
4. The client has crepitus around the insertion site.

51. The health-care provider ordered bumetanide to be administered STAT to a client diagnosed with pulmonary edema. After 4 hours, which assessment data indicates the client may be experiencing a **complication** of the medication?
1. The client develops jugular vein distention.
2. The client has bilateral rales and rhonchi.
3. The client reports painful leg cramps.
4. The client's output is greater than the intake.

52. The client involved in a motor vehicle accident is being prepped for surgery when the client asks the emergency department nurse, "What happened to my child?" The nurse knows the child is dead. Which statement is an example of the ethical principle of nonmaleficence?
1. "I will find out for you and let you know after surgery."
2. "I am sorry but your child died at the scene of the accident."
3. "You should concentrate on your surgery right now."
4. "You are concerned about your child. Do you want to talk?"

53. The new graduate has accepted a position at a facility that is accredited by The Joint Commission. Which statement describes the purpose of this organization?
    1. The Commission reviews facilities for compliance with standards of care.
    2. Accreditation by The Commission guarantees the facility will be reimbursed for care provided.
    3. Accreditation by The Commission reduces liability in a legal action against the facility.
    4. The Commission eliminates the need for Medicare to survey a hospital.

54. The client in a critical care unit has died. What action should the nurse implement **first?**
    1. Stay with the significant other.
    2. Gather the client's belongings.
    3. Perform post-mortem care.
    4. Ask about organ donation.

55. The nurse caring for client BC is preparing to administer medications. Based on the laboratory data given in this table, which intervention should the nurse implement?

Client Name: B.C.	Account Number: 55678-78	Allergies: Sulfa
Diagnosis: Deep Vein Thrombosis	Height: 70 inches	Weight: 150 pounds
Laboratory Report		
Laboratory Test	**Client Value**	**Normal Value**
PT	19.3	10–13 seconds
INR	1.7	2.0–3.0 (therapeutic)
PTT	53	34 seconds

    1. Administer warfarin IVP.
    2. Continue the heparin drip.
    3. Hold the next dose of warfarin.
    4. Administer the daily acetylsalicylic acid.

56. In the intensive care unit (ICU), the critical care nurse assesses a client diagnosed with an asthma attack who has a respiration rate of 10 and an oxygen saturation of 88%. Which intervention should the nurse implement **first?**
    1. Call a Rapid Response Team (RRT).
    2. Increase the oxygen to 10 LPM.
    3. Check the client's ABG results.
    4. Administer the fast-acting inhaler.

57. The client in the intensive care unit (ICU) has been on a ventilator for 2 weeks with an endotracheal tube in place. Which intervention should the nurse prepare the client for **next?**
    1. Transfer to a long-term care facility.
    2. Daily arterial blood gases.
    3. Removal of life support.
    4. Placement of a tracheostomy.

58. The nurse is teaching the parents of a child diagnosed with cystic fibrosis. Which information is **priority** to teach the parents?
    1. Explain that the child's skin tastes salty.
    2. Observe the consistency of the stools daily.
    3. Give pancreatic enzymes with every meal.
    4. Increase the intake of salt in the child's diet.

59. The UAP enters the elderly female client's room to give her a bath, but the client is watching her favorite soap opera and shakes her head "no." Which instructions should the RN staff nurse give to the UAP?
   1. Tell the UAP to complete the bath at this time.
   2. Have the UAP skip the client's bath for the day.
   3. Instruct the UAP to give the bath after the program.
   4. Document the attempt to give the bath as refused.

60. The nurse has been made the chairperson of a quality improvement committee. Which statement is an example of **effective** group process?
   1. The nurse involves all committee members in the discussion.
   2. The nurse makes sure all members of the group agree with the decisions.
   3. The nurse asks two of the committee members to do the work.
   4. The nurse does not allow deviation from the agenda to occur.

61. While the nurse is caring for a client on a ventilator, the ventilator alarm sounds. What is the **first** action taken by the nurse?
   1. Determine the ventilator alarm sounding.
   2. Notify the respiratory therapist.
   3. Assess the client's respiratory status.
   4. Ventilate the client using a manual resuscitation bag.

62. The client diagnosed with acute respiratory distress syndrome (ARDS) is having increased difficulty breathing. The arterial blood gas indicates an arterial oxygen level of 54% on O_2 at 10 LPM. Which intervention should the intensive care unit nurse implement **first?**
   1. Prepare the client for intubation.
   2. Bag the client with a bag/mask device.
   3. Call a Code Blue and initiate cardiopulmonary resuscitation (CPR).
   4. Start an IV with an 18-gauge catheter.

63. The nurse is reviewing Mr. A.W.'s arterial blood gas (ABG) results. Which intervention should the nurse implement **first?**

Client Name: A.W.		Account Number: 3785690
Arterial Blood Gas Report		
Parameter	Client Value	Normal Range
pH	7.34	7.35–7.45
Po_2	87	80–95 mm Hg
Pco_2	50	35–45 mm Hg
Hco_3	24	22–26 mmol/L

   1. Have the client turn, cough, and deep breathe.
   2. Place the client on oxygen via nasal cannula.
   3. Check the client's pulse oximeter reading.
   4. Notify the HCP of the ABG results.

64. The client is admitted to the emergency department with an apical pulse rate of 134, respiration rate of 28, BP of 92/56, and the skin is pale and clammy. What action should the nurse perform **first?**
   1. Type and crossmatch the client for PRBCs.
   2. Start two IVs with large-bore catheters.
   3. Obtain the client's history and physical.
   4. Check the client's allergies to medications.

65. The charge nurse of the respiratory care unit is making assignments. Which clients should be assigned to the intensive care nurse who is working on the respiratory care unit for the day? **Select all that apply.**
   1. The client who had four coronary artery bypass grafts 3 days ago
   2. The client who has anterior and posterior chest tubes after a motor vehicle accident
   3. The client who will be moved to the intensive care unit when a bed is available
   4. The client who has a do not resuscitate order and is requesting to see a chaplain
   5. The client who is on multiple intravenous drip medications that need to be titrated

66. The emergency department nurse is preparing to assist the surgeon to insert a chest tube in a client diagnosed with a right hemothorax. Which position is appropriate for the procedure?
   1. Have the client sit upright and bend over the bed table.
   2. Place the client in the left lateral recumbent position.
   3. Have the client sit on the side of the bed with the back arched similar to a Halloween cat.
   4. Place the client lying on the back with the head of the bed up 45 degrees.

67. The nurse is admitting a client diagnosed with pneumonia. Which health-care provider's order should be implemented **first?**
   1. 1,000 mL normal saline at 125 mL/hour
   2. Obtain sputum for Gram stain and culture
   3. Ceftriaxone 1,000 mg IVPB every 12 hours
   4. Ultrasonic nebulization treatment every 6 hours

68. The nurse is preparing to make rounds after receiving shift report. Which client should the nurse assess **first?**
   1. The client diagnosed with end-stage COPD reporting shortness of breath after ambulating to the bathroom
   2. The client diagnosed with a deep vein thrombosis who is requesting an anti-anxiety medication
   3. The client diagnosed with cystic fibrosis who has a sputum specimen to be taken to the laboratory
   4. The client diagnosed with an empyema who has a temperature of 100.8°F, pulse of 118, respiration rate of 26, and BP of 148/64

69. The respiratory unit nurse is calculating the shift intake and output for a client with right-sided chest tube. The client has received 1,500 mL of D_5W, IVPB of 100 mL of 0.9% NS, 12 ounces of water, 6 ounces of milk, and 4 ounces of chicken broth. The client has had a urinary output of 800 mL and chest drainage of 125 mL. What is the total intake and output for this client?

   [   ]

70. Which client should the RN charge nurse on the respiratory unit assign to the graduate nurse (GN) who just completed orientation?
   1. The client diagnosed with bronchiolitis who has a wheezy cough and rapid breathing
   2. The client diagnosed with pneumonia who has dull percussion and vocal fremitus
   3. The client diagnosed with a flail chest who has paradoxical movement of the chest wall
   4. The client diagnosed with reactive airway disease who has bilateral wheezing

RESPIRATORY CLINICAL SCENARIO

The RN charge nurse is on the respiratory unit in a level I adult, level II pediatric trauma hospital for the 7 a.m. to 7 p.m. shift. The staff includes three RNs, one LPN, and two UAPs for the socioeconomically diverse client population 16-bed unit.

1. The charge nurse is making shift assignments. Which client should be assigned to the **most** experienced RN?
    1. The elderly client diagnosed with pneumonia who has bilateral crackles and a pulse oximeter reading of 96%
    2. The client whose pulse oximeter reading keeps decreasing after receiving high levels of oxygen via nasal cannula
    3. The client who had a Caldwell Luc procedure 1 day ago and has purulent drainage on the drip pad
    4. The teenage client who had a tonsillectomy this morning who is reporting throat pain rated 8 on a pain scale of 1 to 10

2. The nursing home client diagnosed with a community-acquired pneumonia is being admitted to the unit. Which health-care provider's order should be implemented **first?**
    1. Administer ceftriaxone 50 mg IVPB every 24 hours.
    2. Apply oxygen 2 L via nasal cannula.
    3. Obtain a sputum specimen for culture and sensitivity.
    4. Place the elderly client in respiratory isolation.

3. The 50-year-old client diagnosed with an exacerbation of COPD and tobacco abuse is in respiratory distress. Which intervention should the nurse implement **first?**
    1. Place the client in the orthopneic position.
    2. Administer 6 L oxygen via nasal cannula.
    3. Assess the client's pulse oximeter reading.
    4. Notify the respiratory therapist.

4. Which client should the RN charge nurse assign to the licensed practical nurse (LPN)?
    1. The obese client who had a laryngectomy 2 days ago and has crepitus
    2. The client diagnosed with respiratory difficulty who is confused and keeps climbing out of bed
    3. The client with a productive cough and newly diagnosed with active tuberculosis who needs medication teaching
    4. The young adult client diagnosed with asthma who has a pulse oximeter reading of 90%

5. The RN charge nurse and the UAP are caring for the following clients. Which information provided by the UAP requires **immediate** intervention by the charge nurse?
    1. The client with a productive cough and diagnosed with active tuberculosis who is in respiratory isolation and has orange urine in the urinary catheter
    2. The middle age client who had a right upper lobectomy and is on a patient-controlled analgesia (PCA) pump, with level 4 pain on a scale of 1 to 10
    3. The client recovering from a fall and diagnosed with a left-sided pneumothorax who has 200 mL of blood in the collection chamber of the chest drainage system
    4. The 65-year-old client diagnosed with bacterial pneumonia who has an elevated temperature and chills

6. One of the RN charge nurse's staff nurses is preparing to administer a.m. medications to clients. Which medication should the nurse **question** administering to the client?
   1. Sucralfate for the diabetic client who has not had breakfast
   2. Digoxin to the elderly client with a digoxin level of 1.9 mg/dL
   3. Hanging the heparin bag for a client with a PT/PTT of 12.9/78
   4. The aminoglycoside antibiotic to the client with an elevated trough level

7. The edematous client is getting out of bed, becomes very anxious, and has a feeling of impending doom. The nurse reports these findings to the RN charge nurse. Which intervention should the charge nurse tell the nurse to implement **first** after placing the client in the high-Fowler's position?
   1. Administer oxygen via nasal cannula.
   2. Prepare the client for a ventilation/perfusion scan.
   3. Notify the client's health-care provider.
   4. Auscultate the client's lung sounds.

8. The postoperative client with a right-sided chest tube is reporting pain rated 6 on a pain scale of 1 to 10. Which intervention should the nurse implement **first?**
   1. Document the client's pain report in the nurse's notes.
   2. Instruct the client to take slow, deep breaths and exhale slowly.
   3. Assess the client's respiratory status and chest tube insertion site.
   4. Check the client's MAR to determine when the last pain medication was administered.

9. The RN charge nurse is discussing the care of a client with a right-sided chest tube secondary to a pneumothorax with a graduate nurse (GN). Which interventions should the charge nurse discuss with the graduate nurse? **Select all that apply.**
   1. Place the client in the high-Fowler's position.
   2. Assess the chest tube drainage system every shift.
   3. Maintain strict bedrest for the client.
   4. Ensure the tubing has no dependent loops.
   5. Mark the collection chamber for drainage every shift.

10. The RN charge nurse is making client assignments. Which client should the charge nurse assign to the LPN?
    1. The morbidly obese client who is suspected of having acute respiratory distress syndrome
    2. The recovering MVA client diagnosed with a hemothorax who needs two units of blood
    3. The postoperative client with chest tubes who has jugular vein distention and BP of 96/60
    4. The client with dyspnea who is scheduled for a bronchoscopy to R/O lung cancer

The correct answer number and rationale for why it is the correct answer are given in **boldface type.** Rationales for why the other possible answer options are incorrect also are given, but they are not in boldface type.

1. 1. The client's HCP should be consulted if the nurse determines a need, but at this time, the nurse should discuss the client with the respiratory therapist.
2. The unit manager may or may not be capable of helping the nurse assess a client diagnosed with adventitious breath sounds; therefore, this is not the first person the nurse should consult.
3. **Respiratory therapists assess and treat clients diagnosed with lung problems multiple times every day. Therefore, this is the best person to consult when the nurse needs help identifying a respiratory problem.**
4. The case manager is usually capable of maneuvering through the maze of health-care referrals, but is not necessarily an expert in lung sounds.

CLINICAL JUDGMENT GUIDE: The test taker must be knowledgeable regarding the role of all members of the multidisciplinary health-care team as well as HIPAA rules and regulations. These will be tested on the NCLEX-RN® examination.

2. Correct answers are 1, 2, 4, and 5.
1. **The LPN may be assigned to administer the routine oral medications to the clients.**
2. **Bed baths and oral care can be performed by the UAP.**
3. The nurse cannot delegate or assign tasks that require nursing judgment, such as evaluating a client's progress.
4. **The UAP can transport a client to dialysis.**
5. **The LPN may administer scheduled vaccinations.**

CLINICAL JUDGMENT GUIDE: This is an alternate type of question included in the NCLEX-RN®. The nurse must be able to select all the options that answer the question correctly. There are no partially correct answers. The nurse cannot delegate assessment, evaluation, teaching, or administration of medications to any client or the care of an unstable client to a UAP. Also, the nurse cannot assign assessment, evaluation, teaching, or tasks that require nursing judgment to an LPN.

3. 1. The client diagnosed with lung cancer is expected to have rust-colored sputum; however, reporting pain rated as a 10 warrants a more experienced nurse to assess the cause of the pain and medicate as needed.
2. The client diagnosed with atelectasis (collapsed lung) who is having difficulty breathing needs a more experienced nurse to assess the client. This client is not stable.
3. **The orange-colored urine is secondary to rifampin, an antitubercular medication, and a nonproductive cough is expected. Therefore, this client is stable and should be assigned to a new graduate nurse.**
4. The client is exhibiting respiratory compromise and is not stable. The pulse oximeter reading should be greater than 93% and the CRT should be fewer than 3 seconds.

CLINICAL JUDGMENT GUIDE: The charge nurse should assign the most stable client to the new graduate nurse. The test taker must determine which client is exhibiting expected signs or symptoms and this client should be assigned to the new graduate nurse. Clients exhibiting signs or symptoms not expected for the client should be assigned to a more experienced nurse.

4. Correct answers are 1 and 4.
1. **The UAP can perform mouth care on a client who is stable.**
2. Oxygen is a medication and the nurse cannot delegate medication administration to the UAP.
3. The housekeeping staff members empty trashcans, not the UAP. Remember not to assign tasks that should be done by another hospital department.
4. **The UAP can take the empty blood bag to the laboratory.**
5. The nurse cannot delegate teaching to the UAP.

CLINICAL JUDGMENT GUIDE: This is an alternate type of question included in the NCLEX-RN®. The nurse must be able to select all the options that answer the question correctly. There are no partially correct answers. The nurse should not delegate assessment, teaching, evaluation, medications, or an unstable client to the UAP.

5. 1. **Elderly clients diagnosed with pneumonia may not present with the "normal" symptoms, such as fever. The client's increased restlessness may indicate a decrease in oxygen to the brain. This client should be seen first.**

2. The client diagnosed with influenza would be expected to have an elevated temperature and a headache; therefore, this client would not need to be assessed first.
3. Tidaling in the water-seal compartment is expected; therefore, the nurse would not need to assess this client first.
4. Sinus drainage is to be expected in a client diagnosed with a sinus infection.

CLINICAL JUDGMENT GUIDE: The test taker must determine which sign or symptom is not expected for the disease process. If the sign or symptom is not expected, then the nurse should assess the client first. This type of question is determining if the nurse is knowledgeable regarding signs or symptoms of a variety of disease processes.

6. 1. The HCP should be notified, but this is not the first intervention. The HCP will require other information, such as how the incision looks and whether there is any bleeding that can be seen, before making any decisions. The nurse, therefore, should first provide emergency care to the client—in this case, support the client's circulatory system by increasing the IV rate—and then assess the client before reporting to the HCP.
2. The incisional wound should be assessed, but the priority is maintaining circulatory status because the client's vital signs indicate shock.
3. The client may require medication, such as dopamine, a vasopressor, to increase the blood pressure, but the client's circulatory system needs immediate support, which increasing the IV rate will provide. That, then, is the priority.
4. **Increasing the IV rate will provide the client with circulatory volume immediately. Therefore, this is the first intervention.**

CLINICAL JUDGMENT GUIDE: Remember: "If the client is in distress, do not assess." Situations such as those in this question require the nurse to intervene to prevent the client's status from deteriorating. Before selecting "notify the HCP" as the correct answer, the test taker must examine the other three options. If any of the other options contain data that will relieve the client's distress, prevent a life-threatening situation, or provide information the HCP will need to make an informed decision, then the test taker should eliminate the "notify the HCP" option.

7. 1. The client is in distress; therefore, the nurse should do something to help the client.
2. **The Rapid Response Team was mandated by The Joint Commission. It is a team of**

health-care professionals who respond to clients who are breathing but who the nurse thinks are in an emergency situation. A code is called if the client is not breathing.
3. The Trendelenburg position is used for a client who is in hypovolemic shock, so this would not be appropriate for a client in respiratory distress.
4. The stem of the question provides enough information to indicate the client is in distress, and assessing the surgical dressing will not help the client.

CLINICAL JUDGMENT GUIDE: The nurse must determine if the client is in distress; remember: if in distress do not assess. The nurse must intervene to help the client. Do not select equipment over the client's body. The NCLEX-RN® test plan includes nursing care that is ruled by the current National Patient Safety Goals. The nurse must be knowledgeable regarding these goals.

8. 1. Increasing the oxygen rate will not help open the client's airway, which is the first intervention. Oxygen can be increased after the airway is patent.
2. The respiratory therapist could be notified and arterial blood gases (ABGs) drawn if positioning does not increase the pulse oximeter reading, but this is not the first intervention.
3. **The client is exhibiting signs or symptoms of hypopharyngeal obstruction, and this maneuver pulls the tongue forward and opens the air passage.**
4. The client may need to be intubated if positioning does not open the airway, but this is not the first intervention.

CLINICAL JUDGMENT GUIDE: Physiological problems have the highest priority when deciding on a course of action. If the client is in distress, then the nurse must intervene with a nursing action that attempts to alleviate or control the problem. The test taker should not choose a diagnostic test if there is an option that directly treats the client.

9. 1. An emancipated minor under the age of 18 but married or independently earning his or her own living would not warrant the nurse's questioning whether she should sign the permit. "Married" indicates an independently functioning individual.
2. **An incompetent client cannot sign the consent form. An incompetent client is an individual who is not autonomous**

and cannot give or withhold consent, for example, individuals who are cognitively impaired, mentally ill, neurologically incapacitated, or under the influence of mind-altering drugs. The client may be able to sign the permit, but the nurse should question the client's ability to sign the permit because paranoid schizophrenia is a mental illness.

3. A recovering alcoholic is not considered incapacitated. If the client is currently under the influence of alcohol, then the permit could not legally be signed by the client.
4. The elderly client is considered competent until deemed incompetent in a court of law or meets the criteria to be considered incompetent.

CLINICAL JUDGMENT GUIDE: The NCLEX-RN® test plan includes nursing care that is ruled by legal requirements. The nurse must be knowledgeable regarding these issues.

10. 1. The nurse must first address the client's acute respiratory distress and then notify other members of the multidisciplinary team.
2. If the ventilator system malfunctions, the nurse must ventilate the client with a manual resuscitation bag (Ambu) until the problem is resolved. The nurse should determine whether he or she can remedy the situation by assessing the ventilator before beginning manual ventilations.
3. **The client is having respiratory distress and the ventilator is sounding an alarm; therefore, the nurse should first assess the ventilator to determine the cause of the problem and correct it because the client is totally dependent on the ventilator for breathing. This is one of the few situations wherein the nurse would assess the equipment before assessing the client.**
4. In most situations, assessing the client is the first intervention, but because the client is totally dependent on the ventilator for breathing, the nurse should first assess the ventilator to determine the cause of the alarms.

CLINICAL JUDGMENT GUIDE: The nurse must determine if the client is in distress; remember: if in distress do not assess. The nurse must intervene to help the client. In most situations the nurse should not select equipment over the client's body but because the ventilator is breathing for the client, the ventilator should be assessed first.

11. 1. Although these are abnormal ABG values, indicating respiratory acidosis, they are expected in a client diagnosed with COPD; therefore, the nurse would not need to see this client first.
2. The client diagnosed with ARDS would be expected to have a low arterial oxygen level; therefore, the nurse would not assess this client first.
3. **The ABG shows respiratory alkalosis; therefore, the nurse should assess this client first to determine if the client is hyperventilating, in pain, or has an elevated temperature.**
4. These are normal ABGs; therefore, the nurse would not need to assess this client first.

CLINICAL JUDGMENT GUIDE: The nurse must be knowledgeable regarding normal laboratory values. These values must be memorized and the nurse must be able to determine if the laboratory value is normal for the client's disease process or medications the client is taking.

12. 1. Changing the dressing is not a priority over a client who is in respiratory distress.
2. **The client who is exhibiting air hunger indicates respiratory distress; therefore, a tracheostomy tray should be obtained first.**
3. The reviewing of orders is important, but not more important than a client in respiratory distress.
4. The client who is angry and upset needs to be assessed but is not a priority over the client who is in respiratory distress.

CLINICAL JUDGMENT GUIDE: The nurse should use some tool as a reference to guide in the decision-making process. In this situation, apply Maslow's Hierarchy of Needs. Physiological needs have priority over psychosocial ones.

13. 1. After 3 days, the nurse should suspect that the lung has re-expanded. The nurse should not expect dependent loops to have caused this situation.
2. **After 3 days, the nurse should assess the lung sounds to determine whether the lungs have re-expanded. This would be the nurse's first intervention.**
3. This will be done if it is determined the lungs have re-expanded, but it is not the first intervention.
4. The nurse should notify the HCP if it is determined the lungs have re-expanded; a chest x-ray can be taken before removing the chest tubes.

CLINICAL JUDGMENT GUIDE: The nurse must determine if the client is in distress; remember: if in distress, do not assess. If the client is not in distress then the nurse should assess, the first part of the nursing process.

14. 1. The nurse should assess the client's breath sounds but not before determining why there is no tidaling in the water-seal chamber.
   2. **The nurse should first determine why there is no tidaling in the water-seal chamber. Because the client just had the chest tubes inserted, it is probably a kink or a dependent loop, or the client is lying on the tubing. The nurse should first check for this before taking any other action.**
   3. The nurse should encourage the client to take deep breaths and cough, which may push a clot through the tubing, but should not do so before checking for a kink.
   4. Turning the client side to side will not help determine why there is no tidaling in the water-seal compartment of the chest drainage system (Pleur-evac).

CLINICAL JUDGMENT GUIDE: When the test question asks the test taker to determine which intervention should be implemented first it means that all the options could be possible. This is one of the few times the nurse should check equipment before assessing the client.

15. 1. The client diagnosed with histoplasmosis would be expected to have excessive sweating and neck stiffness; therefore, this client would not be seen first. Histoplasmosis is an infection in the lungs caused by inhaling the spores of a fungus.
   2. **The client diagnosed with ARDS is expected to have difficulty breathing but of these four clients, the client diagnosed with breathing difficulty has priority. Apply Maslow's Hierarchy of Needs. ARDS is the sudden failure of the respiratory system. A person diagnosed with ARDS has rapid breathing, difficulty getting enough air into the lungs, and low blood oxygen levels.**
   3. The client diagnosed with pulmonary sarcoidosis would be expected to have a dry cough and mild chest pain; therefore, this client would not be seen first. In pulmonary sarcoidosis, small patches of inflamed cells can appear on the lungs' small alveoli,

bronchioles, or lymph nodes. The lungs can become stiff and may not be able to hold as much air as healthy lungs.
   4. The client diagnosed with asbestosis would be expected to have a productive cough and chest tightness; therefore, this client would not be seen first. Asbestosis is a disease that involves scarring of lung tissue because of breathing in asbestos fibers.

CLINICAL JUDGMENT GUIDE: The nurse should determine if the signs or symptoms the client is experiencing are expected or normal; if they are, then the client would not warrant immediate intervention. If all the clients have expected signs or symptoms, then apply Maslow's Hierarchy of Needs and oxygenation is priority.

16. Correct answers are 1, 3, 4, and 5.
   1. **There must be a manual resuscitation bag at the bedside in case the ventilator does not work appropriately. The nurse must use this to bag the client.**
   2. The pulse oximeter reading should be done more often than every shift.
   3. **The client's respiratory status should be assessed frequently—every 2 hours.**
   4. **The ventilator's settings should be monitored throughout the shift.**
   5. **The respiratory therapist is the member of the multidisciplinary team who is responsible for ventilators.**

CLINICAL JUDGMENT GUIDE: This is an alternate type of question included in the NCLEX-RN®. The nurse must be able to select all the options that answer the question correctly. There are no partially correct answers.

17. 1. This is the correct technique when bathing a client; therefore, the nurse does not need to demonstrate the correct technique to give a bath.
   2. The bed should be at a comfortable height for the UAP to bathe the client, not in the lowest position.
   3. All clients should receive a bath; therefore, this would not be an appropriate action for the nurse to take.
   4. **Part of the delegation process is to evaluate the UAP's performance and the nurse should praise any action on the part of the UAP that ensures the client's safety.**

CLINICAL JUDGMENT GUIDE: The nurse must ensure the unlicensed assistive personnel (UAP) can perform any tasks that are delegated. It is the nurse's responsibility to evaluate the task, demonstrate it, or teach the UAP how to perform the task.

18. 1. The male nurse should document the comment and tell other people, such as family, friends, and staff, but this is not the nurse's first intervention.
2. **The first action is to ask the person directly to stop. The harasser needs to be told in clear terms that the behavior makes the nurse uncomfortable and that he wants it to stop immediately.**
3. The male nurse could take this action, but it is not the first action.
4. This male nurse could take this action, but only if direct contact and the chain of command at the hospital do not stop the charge nurse's behavior.

CLINICAL JUDGMENT GUIDE: There will be management questions on the NCLEX-RN®. In many instances, there is no test-taking strategy; the nurse must be knowledgeable regarding management issues that must comply with local, state, and federal requirements.

19. 1. The client is in metabolic alkalosis, so this intervention is not appropriate for the client's ABGs.
2. The client is in metabolic alkalosis, so this intervention is not appropriate for the client's ABGs.
3. **The ABG indicates metabolic alkalosis, which could be caused by too much hydrochloric acid being removed via the NG tube. Therefore, the nurse should check the NG wall suction.**
4. Sodium bicarbonate is administered for metabolic acidosis, not metabolic alkalosis.

CLINICAL JUDGMENT GUIDE: The nurse must be knowledgeable regarding normal laboratory values. These values must be memorized and the nurse must be able to determine if the laboratory value is normal for the client's disease process or medications the client is taking.

20. 1. This client is critical and there is a possibility of organ rejection; therefore, this client should not be assigned to a float nurse.
2. The normal CVP is 4 to 10 cm H_2O and an elevated CVP indicates right ventricular failure or volume overload; therefore, this client should not be assigned to a float nurse.
3. **The float nurse from the medical unit is able to administer antibiotic therapy and complete respiratory assessments;**

therefore, this client would be the most appropriate client to assign to the float nurse.
4. Hantavirus pulmonary syndrome is a disease that results from contact with infected rodents or their urine, droppings, or saliva. HPS is potentially deadly. There is no specific treatment for HPS, and there is no cure. This client should be assigned to a more experienced nurse.

CLINICAL JUDGMENT GUIDE: The test taker must determine which client is most stable and assign that client to a float nurse. The clients who are more critical should be assigned to more experienced intensive care nurses.

21. 1. **The client's Pao$_2$ is below the normal level of 80 to 100; therefore, the nurse should administer oxygen.**
2. The client should take deep breaths if the client's Paco$_2$ is greater than 45.
3. The nurse should administer sodium bicarbonate if the client's Hco$_3$ is lower than 22.
4. The client needs oxygen because of the low arterial oxygen level; the client does not need a respiratory assessment.

CLINICAL JUDGMENT GUIDE: The nurse must be knowledgeable regarding normal laboratory values. These values must be memorized and the nurse must be able to determine if the laboratory value is normal for the client's disease process or medications the client is taking.

22. 1. **A social worker is qualified to assist the client with referrals to any agency or personnel that may be needed after the client is discharged home.**
2. The chaplain should be contacted if spiritual guidance is required, but the stem did not specify this need.
3. The HCP can talk to the spouse but will not be able to address the concerns of taking care of the client when discharged home.
4. This is false reassurance and does not address the spouse's concern after the client is discharged home. The nurse does not know whether everything is going to be all right.

CLINICAL JUDGMENT GUIDE: The test taker must be knowledgeable regarding the role of all members of the multidisciplinary health-care team as well as HIPAA rules and regulations. These will be tested on the NCLEX-RN® examination.

23. 1. The nurse could ask this question because the radiologist may need to compare the previous chest x-ray with the current one, but this is not the most important question.

2. The client will have to hold her breath when the chest x-ray is taken, but this is not the most important question.

3. Smoking or a history of smoking is pertinent to the diagnosis of pneumonia, but it is not the most important question.

4. **This is the most important question because if the client is pregnant, the x-rays can harm the fetus.**

CLINICAL JUDGMENT GUIDE: The test taker should realize that for any female client of child-bearing age, the most important questions or concerns will probably address the chance of pregnancy. Most medications and many diagnostic tests and treatments can harm the fetus.

24. 1. **The elderly client should be called first so that the nurse can determine whether the dizziness when getting up is the result of medication or some other reason. Orthostatic hypotension can be life threatening; therefore, this client may need to be assessed immediately.**

2. Ordering a prescription is not a priority over a client diagnosed with a physiological problem.

3. Nausea is often expected with chemotherapy; therefore, this client's phone call would not be returned before calling a client diagnosed with a potentially life-threatening problem.

4. Pertussis—known as whooping cough—is a serious, very contagious disease that causes severe, uncontrollable coughing fits. The coughing makes it difficult to breathe and often ends with a "whoop" noise. Because coughing spells are expected, the nurse would not call this client first.

CLINICAL JUDGMENT GUIDE: The test taker should apply some systematic approach when answering priority questions. All the clients are experiencing physiological problems, the first priority according to Maslow's Hierarchy of Needs. Once that is established, then the test taker should determine which physiological problem is most life threatening—in this case, dizziness when standing because of its possible cause, hypotension, which can be life threatening.

25. 1. This is a therapeutic response with the goal of having the client ventilate feelings. This is not appropriate for the client's comment. The nurse must give factual information.

2. **The client diagnosed with active TB must take the medication as prescribed for**

9 to 12 months. **If the client refuses to take the medication, a court order will be obtained to make the client take the medication because tuberculosis is a community threat.**

3. The nurse should provide factual information when possible and not "pass the buck" to the HCP.

4. This is not a true statement. The client must be on the prescribed medications.

CLINICAL JUDGMENT GUIDE: The nurse must be knowledgeable regarding diseases that pose a threat to the community. The nurse should provide factual information to the client.

26. **Correct answers are 3 and 5.**
1. An induration greater than 10 mm is positive for tuberculosis. This client needs to be assessed and followed up to rule out tuberculosis. This client should not be assigned to an LPN.

2. A pulse oximeter reading lower than 93% is life threatening; therefore, this client should not be assigned to an LPN.

3. **Acute bronchitis is an inflammation of the bronchial tubes, the major airways into the lungs. The client is exhibiting expected signs and symptoms; therefore, the LPN could care for this client.**

4. The client is exhibiting wheezing, an acute exacerbation of reactive airway disease. This client should be assigned to a nurse.

5. **Influenza is a viral infection of the respiratory system. The client is exhibiting generalized muscle aches, which is an expected symptom; therefore, the LPN could care for this client.**

CLINICAL JUDGMENT GUIDE: This is an alternate type of question included in the NCLEX-RN®. The nurse must be able to select all the options that answer the question correctly. There are no partially correct answers. The nurse should assign the LPN the clients who have the lowest level of need but for whom the task still remains in the LPN's scope of practice. The nurse cannot assign assessing, teaching, evaluating, or an unstable client to an LPN.

27. 1. The UAP cannot administer oxygen to a client. Oxygen is considered a medication.

2. The nurse should not depend on the UAP to care for the client who is experiencing a potentially life-threatening condition.

3. **This is the first intervention because the nurse must assess the client. Asking the UAP to accompany the nurse will allow**

the nurse to stay with the client while the UAP obtains any needed equipment.

    4. The nurse should immediately assess the client. The UAP does not have the knowledge or skills to care for the client experiencing shortness of breath.

CLINICAL JUDGMENT GUIDE: Any time the nurse receives information from another staff member about a client who may be experiencing a new problem, complication, or life-threatening problem, the nurse must assess the client. The nurse should not make decisions about client needs based on another staff member's information.

28. 1. The parent or guardian must sign the consent for surgery because the client is under the age of 18.

    2. The client has already been diagnosed with tonsillitis; therefore, a throat culture is not needed before surgery.

    3. The client should not cough after this surgery because it could cause bleeding from the incision site.

    4. A PT/PTT will assess the client for any bleeding tendencies. This is a priority before this surgery because bleeding is a life-threatening complication.

CLINICAL JUDGMENT GUIDE: The NCLEX-RN® test plan includes perioperative nursing care. The nurse must be knowledgeable regarding preoperative and postoperative care that is generic for all clients undergoing surgery.

29. 1. Influenza, or the flu, is a serious respiratory illness caused by a virus. Antibiotics are not prescribed to treat influenza.

    2. Staying away from large crowds and a scarf over the mouth are not the best ways to prevent getting influenza.

    3. Influenza, or flu, is a serious respiratory illness. It is easily spread from person to person and can lead to severe complications, even death. The best way to prevent influenza is to get a flu vaccine every year. The influenza virus is constantly changing. Each year, scientists work together to identify the virus strains that they believe will cause the most illness, and a new vaccine is made based on their recommendations.

    4. Three meals a day and daily exercise will help the client stay healthy in general but it is not the best way to prevent getting influenza.

CLINICAL JUDGMENT GUIDE: The nurse must be knowledgeable regarding immunizations for both children and adults. This is a knowledge-based

question that is included on the NCLEX-RN® examination.

30. 1. The normal pulse rate for a 1- to 11-month-old is 100 to 150. This client would not warrant immediate intervention.

    2. The normal respiratory rate for a toddler is 20 to 30. This client would not warrant immediate intervention.

    3. A 24-week gestational woman with a BP of 142/96 would warrant intervention because the average systolic BP should be between 90 and 140 mm Hg and the diastolic BP should be between 60 and 85 mm Hg. This BP could indicate gestational hypertension.

    4. This is an elevated temperature, but it would not warrant intervention from the nurse. This is not a potentially life-threatening temperature.

CLINICAL JUDGMENT GUIDE: The nurse must be knowledgeable regarding vital signs. This is basic nursing care that is tested on the NCLEX-RN®.

31. 1. The documentation of the accident must be completed but it is not a priority over caring for the wound first.

    2. The nurse should wash the area with soap and water and attempt to squeeze the area to make it bleed.

    3. The nurse should not ask this question directly to the client. The nurse could ask whether the client would agree to have blood drawn for testing, but not directly ask whether the client has AIDS or hepatitis.

    4. The puncture site would not require antibiotic ointment unless it is infected, which it wouldn't be immediately after the incident.

CLINICAL JUDGMENT GUIDE: The NCLEX-RN® test plan includes adhering to Standard Precautions when providing nursing care to clients. Remember: The nurse should always address the problem directly before completing documentation.

32. Correct answers are 1 and 4.

    1. The normal hemoglobin level is 11.7 to 15.5 g/dL (female) and 14 to 17.2 g/dL (male). Normal hematocrit is 36% to 48% (female) and 42% to 52% (male). This client's H&H is low. The nurse should contact the client and make an immediate appointment.

    2. The normal WBC count is 4.5 to 11.1×10^3/microL. This client's WBC count is within normal range and does not warrant intervention from the clinic nurse.

3. The normal serum potassium level is 3.5 to 5.3 mEq/L. This client's level is within normal range and does not warrant intervention from the clinic nurse.

4. **The normal serum sodium level is 135 to 145 mEq/L. This client's level is 125 mEq/L which is low. The nurse should contact the client and make an appointment.**

5. The normal cholesterol is lower than 200 mg/dL. The normal triglyceride value is lower than 150 mg/dL. This client's cholesterol and triglyceride level is within normal range and does not warrant intervention from the clinic nurse.

CLINICAL JUDGMENT GUIDE: This is an alternate type of question included in the NCLEX-RN®. The nurse must be able to select all the options that answer the question correctly. There are no partially correct answers.

33. 1. In some cultures, the husband often speaks for the wife and family, and requesting the husband not to speak may be insulting. This action may cause the wife to leave as well.

2. In some cultures, the husband often is the spokesperson and makes decisions for the wife and family. Asking the husband to leave the room may cause the client to leave as well.

3. **This behavior may be cultural, and the nurse should continue to allow the husband to answer the questions, while the nurse looks at the client. The nurse must be respectful of the client's culture. The nurse can, however, ask whether the client agrees with the husband's answers.**

4. This is disrespectful to the client's culture. Many times, the nurse must honor the client's culture while caring for the client.

CLINICAL JUDGMENT GUIDE: The NCLEX-RN® test plan includes nursing care addressing cultural diversity. The nurse needs to be aware of cultural differences.

34. Correct order is 3, 4, 1, 5, 2.

3. **The nurse needs to determine if the client is unresponsive before taking any action. If the client is unresponsive, then perform compressions.**

4. **The American Heart Association recommends 30 compressions followed by two breaths.**

1. **After completing compressions, open the client's airway to ensure a patent airway.**

5. **The nurse should then administer two breaths with a CPR mask and face shield or bag-valve-mask device.**

2. **The nurse then must determine whether the client's heart is pumping by checking the carotid pulse.**

CLINICAL JUDGMENT GUIDE: This is an alternate type of question included in the NCLEX-RN® test plan. The nurse must be able to perform skills in the correct order.

35. 1. **The client diagnosed with end-stage COPD usually prefers a cool climate, with fans to help ease breathing. A warm area would increase the effort the client would require to breathe. This action would warrant intervention by the nurse.**

2. The client diagnosed with end-stage COPD should be maintained on a low oxygen rate, such as 2 L/min to prevent depression of the hypoxic drive. High levels of oxygen will depress the client's ability to breathe. This action would not warrant intervention by the nurse.

3. The client will usually sit in the orthopneic position, usually slumped over a bedside table, to help ease breathing. This is called the three-point stance. This action would not warrant intervention by the nurse.

4. The client in end-stage COPD has great difficulty breathing; therefore, sleeping in a recliner is sometimes the only way the client can sleep. This action would not warrant intervention by the nurse.

CLINICAL JUDGMENT GUIDE: The nurse only delegates tasks in which the UAP has been trained to perform. Delegation means the nurse is responsible for the UAP's actions; therefore, the nurse must evaluate the UAP's understanding of the procedure the UAP is asked to perform.

36. 1. The UAP cannot perform sterile dressing changes.

2. The UAP cannot perform sterile procedures.

3. The UAP cannot teach the client.

4. **The UAP can transfer the client from the bed to the chair three times a day.**

CLINICAL JUDGMENT GUIDE: The nurse cannot delegate assessment, evaluation, teaching, medications, or an unstable client to a UAP.

37. 1. The staff member is violating HIPAA, and the nurse should take action immediately.

2. **The nurse should first ask the staff member not to discuss the client with a friend. Discussing any information about a client is a violation of HIPAA.**

3. The nurse should address the staff member in the restaurant. The nurse could tell the clinical manager, but the nurse must stop the conversation in the restaurant immediately.

4. The nurse should not tell the client about the breach of confidentiality.

CLINICAL JUDGMENT GUIDE: There will be management questions on the NCLEX-RN®. In many instances, there is no test-taking strategy; the nurse must be knowledgeable regarding management issues. The Health Insurance Portability and Accountability Act (HIPAA) passed into law in 1996 to standardize exchange of information between health-care providers and to ensure client record confidentiality.

38. 1. **This statement warrants intervention because fluids will help prevent dehydration and renal calculi. The nurse should explain the client needs to increase fluids.**

2. ROM exercises help prevent deep vein thrombosis (DVT). This statement does not require intervention by the nurse. The UAP can perform skills if taught and performance is evaluated by the nurse.

3. Keeping the client off the buttocks is an appropriate intervention for a client on strict bedrest. This comment does not require intervention by the nurse.

4. Pulling the client across the sheets will cause skin breakdown. Because the UAP is not doing this, no intervention by the nurse is needed.

CLINICAL JUDGMENT GUIDE: Delegation means the nurse is responsible for the UAP's actions and performance. The nurse must correct the UAP's performance to ensure the client is cared for safely in the hospital or the home.

39. 1. The client's oxygen should always be placed correctly but it is not the priority intervention for difficulty breathing.

2. **Because the client has difficulty breathing while lying in bed, allowing the client to sit in a recliner will help the client; therefore, this is the priority intervention.**

3. Often clients report a fan blowing on the face helps with difficulty breathing but this is not a priority intervention.

4. Slow, deep breaths will not help the client diagnosed with difficulty breathing as much as will sitting in a recliner.

CLINICAL JUDGMENT GUIDE: In questions that ask the test taker to identify a priority intervention, all the options are something a nurse can

implement. The test taker must identify the most important intervention.

40. 1. The body naturally begins to slow down, and clients may not wish to take in liquids or nourishment. This can produce a natural euphoria and make the dying process easier on the client. IV fluids would interfere with this process and would increase secretions the client cannot handle, thus making the client more uncomfortable.

2. A percutaneous endoscopic gastrostomy (PEG) feeding tube would increase the intake of the client and would increase secretions the client cannot handle. This can require suctioning the client and further augmenting the client's discomfort.

3. **Refusal to take in food and liquids produces a natural euphoria and makes the dying process easier on the client. This is an appropriate teaching statement.**

4. This is a therapeutic response, but factual information is needed by the wife to accept the process.

CLINICAL JUDGMENT GUIDE: The NCLEX-RN® addresses questions concerned with end-of-life care. This is included in the Psychosocial Integrity section of the test plan.

41. 1. The home health nurse may be a possibility if a hospice organization is not available, but hospice is the best referral.

2. The nurse would not refer the client to his or her own pastor. The nurse could place a call to notify the pastor at the client's request, but this would not be considered a referral.

3. **One of the guidelines for admission to a hospice agency is a terminal process with a life expectancy of 6 months or fewer. These organizations work to assist the client and family to live life to its fullest while providing for comfort measures and a peaceful, dignified death.**

4. The hospital social worker is not an appropriate referral at this time.

CLINICAL JUDGMENT GUIDE: The nurse must be knowledgeable about appropriate referrals and implement the referral to the most appropriate person or agency.

42. 1. This is advising and crossing professional boundaries. The nurse should not try to influence the client in these types of concerns.

2. This is advising and crossing professional boundaries. The nurse should not try to influence the client in these types of concerns.

3. **This response allows the client to make his or her own decision. It validates that the nurse heard the concern but does not advise the client.**
4. This is advising and crossing professional boundaries. The nurse should not try to influence the client in these types of concerns.

CLINICAL JUDGMENT GUIDE: The nurse must always remember that nurses have positions of authority in a health-care environment. Nurses must maintain professional boundaries at all times and refuse to cross professional boundaries.

43. Correct answers are 1, 2, 3, and 5.
1. **Some nurses see the big picture and seek solutions based on what makes people feel comfortable rather than on logic.**
2. **Some nurses see the world from a logical perspective and focus on a specific intervention.**
3. **Some nurses ask fewer questions than others, especially if they perceive that asking the question will make them look foolish or ignorant.**
4. Different nurses communicate differently. The manager should recognize these differences when attempting to arrive at a common goal.
5. **All nurses should keep an open mind when communicating with others in the workplace. Open-mindedness correlates with flexibility and teamwork.**

CLINICAL JUDGMENT GUIDE: This is an alternate type of question included in the NCLEX-RN®. The nurse must be able to select all the options that answer the question correctly. There are no partially correct answers.

44. 1. The attitude of the staff member changes from one day to the next. The "why" is not important for the manager to know. The important thing for the manager to know is whether the staff member can control the attitude.
2. **The first step is an informal meeting with the staff member to discuss the inappropriate attitude and how it affects the staff. The manager should document the conversation informally with the date and time (the staff member does not need to see this documentation) for future reference. If the situation is not resolved, a formal counseling must take place.**
3. This step would follow the informal discussion if the attitude did not improve.

4. This is a step sometimes used to get the attention of the staff member when formal counseling has not been effective. This step occurs just before termination.

CLINICAL JUDGMENT GUIDE: There will be management questions on the NCLEX-RN®. In many instances, there is no test-taking strategy; the nurse must be knowledgeable regarding management issues.

45. 1. E-mails should be easy to read and concise. Individuals may not take the time to read and understand poorly worded, lengthy e-mails.
2. Some communication is appropriate by e-mail, but when discussing a problem with an individual, it is best to use face-to-face communication in which both parties can give and receive feedback.
3. Capital letters in e-mails may be interpreted as shouting or yelling at the receiver.
4. **E-mail communication should be concise and easy to read. If the e-mail requires a lot of information, then the writer should use bullets to separate information.**

CLINICAL JUDGMENT GUIDE: There will be management questions on the NCLEX-RN®. In many instances, there is no test-taking strategy; the nurse must be knowledgeable regarding management issues.

46. 1. **The problem is not a nursing problem. The HCP should be discussing the problem with an individual from the department that "owns" the problem.**
2. This is not a nursing problem.
3. This is not a nursing problem.
4. This will only make the HCP angrier. The HCP should be directed to discuss the problem with the department that can "fix" the problem.

CLINICAL JUDGMENT GUIDE: There will be management questions on the NCLEX-RN®. In many instances, there is no test-taking strategy; the nurse must be knowledgeable regarding management issues.

47. Correct order is 1, 4, 3, 2, 5.
1. **The nurse should begin the care by assessing the client. Remember the nursing process.**
4. **The nurse should have the client's chest and dressing exposed and should check to make sure the chest tube is securely taped at this time.**

3. The nurse then follows the chest tube to the drainage system and assesses the system.
2. The last part of the chest tube drainage system to assess is the suction system.
5. The nurse should make sure that emergency supplies are at the bedside last.

CLINICAL JUDGMENT GUIDE: This is an alternate type of question included in the NCLEX-RN® test plan. The nurse must be able to perform skills in the correct order. Assessment should always be the first intervention if the client is not in distress.

48. 1. Bronchiectasis is a condition in which the lungs' airways are abnormally stretched and widened. This is caused by mucous blockage, which allows bacteria to grow and leads to infection. Signs and symptoms include coughing, abnormal breath sounds, and clubbing; therefore, the nurse would not assess this client first.
2. Byssinosis (brown lung disease) is a lung disease caused by exposure to dust from cotton processing, hemp, and flax. Signs and symptoms include chest tightness, cough, and wheezing; therefore, this client would not be assessed first.
3. **Cystic fibrosis (CF) is an inherited disease that causes thick, sticky mucus to form in the lungs, pancreas, and other organs. In the lungs, this mucus blocks the airways, causing lung damage and making it hard to breathe. A pulse oximeter reading of 90% equates to approximately a 60% arterial saturation. The nurse should assess this client first.**
4. Pneumoconiosis, known as black lung disease, is an occupational lung disease caused by inhaling coal dust. The signs and symptoms are shortness of breath and chronic cough; therefore, this client would not be assessed first.

CLINICAL JUDGMENT GUIDE: The test taker must determine which sign or symptom is not expected for the disease process. If the sign or symptom is not expected, then the nurse should assess the client first. This type of question is determining if the nurse is knowledgeable regarding signs or symptoms of a variety of disease processes.

49. 1. Activity intolerance is not a priority over gas exchange. If gas exchange does not occur, the client will die.
2. Coping is a psychosocial problem, and physiological problems are the priority.

3. Impaired gas exchange is the priority problem for this client. If the client does not have adequate gas exchange, the client will die. Remember Maslow's Hierarchy of Needs.
4. Self-care deficit is not a priority over gas exchange.

CLINICAL JUDGMENT GUIDE: The NCLEX-RN® integrates the nursing process throughout the Client Needs categories and subcategories. The nursing process is a scientific, clinical reasoning approach to client care that includes assessment, analysis, planning, implementation, and evaluation. The nurse will be responsible for identifying nursing diagnoses for clients.

50. 1. Consolidation indicates fluid or exudates in the lung—pneumonia. This would not indicate the client is improving.
2. **Bilateral breath sounds indicate the left lung has re-expanded and the treatment is effective.**
3. Vigorous bubbling in the suction chamber indicates that there is a leak in the system, but this does not indicate the treatment is effective.
4. Crepitus (subcutaneous emphysema) indicates that oxygen is escaping into the subcutaneous layer of the skin, but this does not indicate the lung has re-expanded, which is the goal of the treatment.

CLINICAL JUDGMENT GUIDE: The nurse should realize a normal finding indicates the medical treatment is effective. If the nurse is vacillating between two options and one option is equipment, the nurse should select the client's body as the correct answer.

51. 1. Jugular vein distention would indicate the client has congestive heart failure (CHF). This is not a complication of a loop diuretic.
2. Rales and rhonchi are symptoms of pulmonary edema, not a complication of a loop diuretic.
3. **Leg cramps may indicate a low serum potassium level, which can occur because of the administration of the loop diuretic, bumetanide (Bumex).**
4. This would indicate the loop diuretic, bumetanide (Bumex), is effective and is not a complication of the medication.

CLINICAL JUDGMENT GUIDE: The nurse must be aware of expected actions of medications. The nurse must be aware of assessment data indicating the medication is effective or the medication is causing a side effect or an adverse effect.

52. 1. **Nonmaleficence means to do no harm. This statement is letting the client know that the concern has been heard but does not give the client bad news before surgery. The nurse is aware that someone having surgery should be of sound mind, and finding out your child is dead would be horrific.**
    2. This is an example of veracity.
    3. This is an example of paternalism, telling the client what he or she should do.
    4. This is a therapeutic response, not an example of nonmaleficence.

CLINICAL JUDGMENT GUIDE: The NCLEX-RN® test plan includes nursing care that addresses ethical principles, including autonomy, beneficence, justice, and veracity, to name a few.

53. 1. **The Joint Commission is an organization that monitors health-care facilities for compliance with standards of care. Accreditation is voluntary, but most third-party payers will not reimburse a facility that is not accredited by some outside organization.**
    2. Accreditation does not guarantee reimbursement, although most third-party payers require some accreditation by an outside organization.
    3. Accreditation does not reduce the hospital's liability.
    4. Medicare or Medicaid will not review a facility routinely if The Joint Commission has accredited the facility, but a representative will review the facility in cases of reported problems.

CLINICAL JUDGMENT GUIDE: The NCLEX-RN® test plan includes nursing care that is ruled by legal requirements as well as The Joint Commission, Medicare and Medicaid Services, Centers for Disease Control and Prevention, and Occupational Safety and Health Administration rules and regulations. The nurse must be knowledgeable regarding these standards.

54. 1. **The nurse should "offer self" to the significant other. Ignoring the needs of the significant other at this time makes the significant other feel that the nurse does not care, and if the nurse does not care for "me," then did the nurse provide adequate care to my loved one? This action is very important to assist in the grieving process.**
    2. The UAP can gather the deceased client's belongings.

3. The UAP can perform post-mortem care.
4. The representative of the organ donation team will make this request. Organ banks think it is best for specially trained individuals to discuss organ donation with the significant others.

CLINICAL JUDGMENT GUIDE: The NCLEX-RN® addresses questions concerned with end-of-life care. This is included in the Psychosocial Integrity section of the test plan. If unsure of the correct option, selecting an option addressing an individual is a better choice.

55. 1. Warfarin (Coumadin) is an oral, not intravenous, medication.
    2. **The therapeutic PTT results should be 1.5 to 2 times the control, or 51 to 68 seconds. The client's value of 53 is within the therapeutic range. The nurse should continue the heparin drip as is.**
    3. The International Normalized Ratio (INR) is not up to therapeutic range yet, so warfarin (Coumadin) should be administered.
    4. These laboratory values do not provide any information about acetylsalicylic acid (Aspirin) administration, but the nurse should ask the HCP whether aspirin (an antiplatelet) should be discontinued because the client is receiving two anticoagulants—heparin and warfarin.

CLINICAL JUDGMENT GUIDE: This is an alternate type of question included in the NCLEX-RN® test plan. The test taker must be able to read an EHR, must be knowledgeable regarding laboratory data, and must be able to make appropriate decisions as to the nurse's most appropriate action.

56. 1. A Rapid Response Team (RRT) is called when the nurse assesses a client whose condition is deteriorating. The purpose of an RRT is to intervene to prevent a code. In the scenario described, the situation has not progressed to an arrest. The nurse should call an RRT, but administering oxygen is the first intervention.
    2. **The first action is to increase the client's oxygen to 100%.**
    3. The nurse could check the ABG results, but the client is in distress and the nurse should implement an intervention to relieve the distress.
    4. A fast-acting inhaler should be used, but not until after the oxygen has been increased and an RRT called.

CLINICAL JUDGMENT GUIDE: The nurse should remember: If a client is in distress and the nurse can do something to relieve the distress, that should be done first, before assessment. The test taker should select an option that directly helps the client's condition.

57. 1. The client may eventually need to be transferred to a facility that accepts long-term ventilator-dependent clients, but the nurse would not anticipate this at this time.
2. The client on a ventilator will have blood gases ordered more often than daily.
3. The stem does not indicate that the client is ready to be removed from the ventilator.
4. **A client who has been intubated for 10 to 14 days and still requires mechanical ventilation should have a surgically placed tracheostomy to prevent permanent vocal cord damage.**

CLINICAL JUDGMENT GUIDE: The nurse must be knowledgeable regarding expected medical treatment for the client. This is a knowledge-based question.

58. 1. The child's skin will normally taste salty, but this is not the priority intervention to teach.
2. The parents should be asked about the client's stools during an assessment because the effectiveness of the pancreatic enzymes is evaluated by the consistency of the stool. This is not the priority intervention because the child must take the enzymes before monitoring the consistency of the stool.
3. **Cystic fibrosis is a genetic condition that results in blockage of the pancreatic ducts. The child needs pancreatic enzymes to be administered with every meal and snack so the enzymes will be available when the food gets to the small intestine.**
4. Cystic fibrosis is one of the few diseases that requires salt replacement, but salt replacement is not more important than taking the pancreatic enzymes.

CLINICAL JUDGMENT GUIDE: The nurse must be knowledgeable regarding expected medical treatment for the client. This is a knowledge-based question.

59. 1. The UAP should be sensitive to the client's preferences and not insist that the client miss the program.
2. The UAP should arrange an acceptable time for the client, and the UAP can return to complete the task at the agreed-on time.

3. **This is the best instruction for the nurse to give to the UAP.**
4. The bath has not been refused. The client does not want the program interrupted.

CLINICAL JUDGMENT GUIDE: Delegation means the nurse is responsible for the UAP's actions and performance. The nurse must provide guidance to the UAP.

60. 1. **Effective group process involves all members of the group.**
2. Unanimous decisions may indicate groupthink, which can be a problem in a group process.
3. Effective group process involves all members of the group, not just two.
4. Not allowing deviation from the agenda is an autocratic style and limits the creativity and involvement of the group.

CLINICAL JUDGMENT GUIDE: There will be management questions on the NCLEX-RN®. In many instances, there is no test-taking strategy; the nurse must be knowledgeable regarding management issues.

61. 1. **The ventilator should be checked to determine which alarm is sounding. This is the first step in assessing the client's problem.**
2. The nurse should assess the ventilator and the client and then notify the respiratory therapist, if needed.
3. The client should be assessed, but the ventilator may require only a simple adjustment to fix the problem and turn off the alarm. This is one instance in which the nurse should assess the machine before assessing the client because the machine is breathing for the client.
4. The client should be manually ventilated if the nurse cannot determine the cause of the ventilator alarm.

CLINICAL JUDGMENT GUIDE: The nurse must determine if the client is in distress. Remember: If in distress, do not assess. The nurse must intervene to help the client. In most situations, the nurse should not select equipment over the client's body; however, when the equipment is breathing for the client the equipment should be assessed first.

62. 1. **Acute respiratory distress syndrome is diagnosed when the client has an arterial blood gas of lower than 50% while receiving oxygen at 10 LPM. The nurse should prepare for the client to be intubated.**

2. The nurse should intervene while the client is breathing by calling the HCP and assisting in the intubation and setup of the mechanical ventilator. If the client has an arrest before this can be arranged, the client would be ventilated with a bag/mask device.

3. If the nurse does not intervene immediately, an arrest situation will occur, at which time a Code Blue would be called and CPR started.

4. If the client does not have a patent IV, the nurse should start one, but not before preparing for intubation.

CLINICAL JUDGMENT GUIDE: The nurse must be knowledgeable regarding expected medical treatment for the client. This is a knowledge-based question.

63. 1. **These blood gases indicate respiratory acidosis that could be caused by ineffective cough, with resulting air trapping. The nurse should encourage the client to turn, cough, and deep breathe.**

2. The Pao_2 level is within normal limits, 80 to 100. Administering oxygen is not the first intervention.

3. The nurse knows the arterial blood gas oxygen level, which is an accurate test. The pulse oximeter only provides an approximate level.

4. This is not the first intervention. The nurse can intervene to treat the client before notifying the HCP.

CLINICAL JUDGMENT GUIDE: The nurse must be knowledgeable regarding expected medical treatment for the client. This is a knowledge-based question.

64. 1. The nurse should first prevent circulatory collapse by starting two IVs and initiating normal saline or Ringer's lactate. The cross-match may be needed if the shock condition is caused by hemorrhage.

2. **The client is exhibiting symptoms of shock. The nurse should start IV lines to prevent the client from progressing to circulatory collapse.**

3. All clients have a history taken and physical examination performed as part of the admission process to the emergency department, but this is not the first intervention.

4. Checking the client's allergies to medications is important, but it is not the first intervention in a client exhibiting signs of shock.

CLINICAL JUDGMENT GUIDE: The nurse should remember if a client is in distress and the nurse

can do something to relieve the distress, that should be done first, before assessment. The test taker should select an option that directly helps the client's condition.

65. **Correct answers are 3 and 5.**
1. This client is nearing discharge status. Postoperative clients are progressed rapidly. A medical-surgical nurse could take care of this client.

2. Chest tubes are frequently cared for on a medical-surgical unit; the medical-surgical nurse can care for this client.

3. **This client's status is uncertain. The ICU nurse would be an appropriate assignment for this client because the client will be moved to the ICU soon.**

4. A medical-surgical nurse can care for this client.

5. **The intensive care nurse should care for this client requiring titration of multiple medications simultaneously.**

CLINICAL JUDGMENT GUIDE: The charge nurse must decide which clients need a higher level of expertise to make this decision. Those clients requiring a higher level of expertise should be assigned to the nurse with the greatest knowledge in certain areas. This is an alternate type of question included in the NCLEX-RN®. The nurse must be able to select all the options that answer the question correctly. There are no partially correct answers.

66. 1. **This position allows for access to the client's back area. The chest tube for a hemothorax is positioned low and posterior to allow for gravity to assist in the removal of fluid from the thoracic area.**

2. This is the position for giving an enema.

3. This is the position used to assist with a lumbar puncture.

4. This is a resting position; it is not preparing for a chest tube placement.

CLINICAL JUDGMENT GUIDE: The nurse must have knowledge of basic anatomy and physiology to answer this question. "Hemo" means blood and "thorax" refers to the thoracic cavity. Blood is in the area where the lung needs to expand. Blood is heavier than air so the client should be positioned to access the area where dependent drainage will occur.

67. 1. Starting an intravenous line must be done before being able to initiate a piggyback medication.

2. **In order to treat the client with the most**

effective medication and not skew the results of a sputum culture, the specimen must be obtained before initiating antibiotics.

3. New orders for intravenous antibiotics must be considered a priority to prevent the client from going into gram-negative sepsis, a potentially lethal situation. However, in order to initiate the ceftriaxone (Rocephin) antibiotic, the nurse must make sure a correct diagnosis is able to be made.

4. Respiratory treatments are important, but not before starting the antibiotics.

CLINICAL JUDGMENT GUIDE: To arrive at the correct priority intervention, the test taker must decide if one option must be accomplished before initiating other options.

68. 1. Shortness of breath after ambulating is expected for a client diagnosed with COPD.

2. **Clients diagnosed with deep vein thrombosis are at risk for pulmonary embolism (PE). Anxiety is a symptom of PE. The nurse must determine if interventions are needed for PE, a life-threatening emergency.**

3. Anyone can take a specimen to the laboratory.

4. An empyema is an abscess in the thoracic cavity. These vital signs would be expected for this client.

CLINICAL JUDGMENT GUIDE: When deciding which client to assess first, there are rules. 1. Is the situation life threatening or life altering? 2. Is the information/data presented abnormal or unexpected? 3. Is the information expected for the disease process? Or is the problem a psychosocial one? 4. Are the data within normal limits? The test taker should choose the correct answer based on 1 first, 2 next, 3 next, and 4 last.

69. **Answer: 2,160 mL intake and 925 mL output. The urinary output is not used in this calculation. The nurse must add up both IV fluids and oral fluids to obtain the total intake for this client;**
    1,500 + 100 = 1,600 IV fluids;
    (1 ounce = 30 mL)
    12 ounces × 30 mL = 360 mL,

6 ounces × 30 mL = 180 mL,
4 ounces × 30 mL = 120 mL;
360 + 180 + 120 = 660 oral fluids. Total intake is 1,600 + 660 = 2,260. The urinary output 800 mL plus chest drainage 125 mL equals 925 mL for shift output.

CLINICAL JUDGMENT GUIDE: The **NCLEX-RN®** test plan includes dosage calculations under **Pharmacological and Parenteral Therapies. This category is included under Physiological Integrity, which promotes physical health and wellness by providing care and comfort, reducing client risk potential, and managing health alterations.**

70. 1. **Bronchiolitis is an inflammation of the bronchioles, which are the small airways in the lungs. Signs and symptoms include wheezy cough, rapid breathing, cyanosis, nasal flaring, muscle retractions, and fever. Because the client is exhibiting expected signs and symptoms, this client should be assigned to the graduate nurse.**

2. Dull percussion and vocal fremitus indicate consolidation. Consolidation is fluid instead of air in the alveolar space. This is a potentially life-threatening situation and should not be assigned to a new graduate.

3. Flail chest describes a situation in which a portion of the rib cage is separated from the rest of the chest wall, usually because of a severe blunt trauma, such as a serious fall or a car accident. This affected portion is unable to contribute to expansion of the lungs. Flail chest is a serious condition that can lead to long-term disability and even death. The charge nurse should assign this client to a more experienced nurse.

4. The client diagnosed with reactive airway disease, asthma, should be asymptomatic; therefore, when the client is wheezing, he or she is having an acute exacerbation and should be assigned to a more experienced nurse.

CLINICAL JUDGMENT GUIDE: When the test taker is deciding which client should be assigned to a new graduate, the most stable client should be assigned to the least experienced nurse.

The correct answer number and rationale for why it is the correct answer are given in **boldface type.** Rationales for why the other possible answer options are incorrect also are given, but they are not in boldface type.

1. 1. The client diagnosed with pneumonia is expected to have bilateral crackles, and an Sao$_2$ of 96% is stable; therefore, this client would not be assigned to the most experienced nurse.
   2. **This client is exhibiting typical signs of adult respiratory distress syndrome (ARDS); therefore, the charge nurse should assign the most experienced nurse to this client.**
   3. The postoperative client diagnosed with purulent drainage could be developing an infection and should be assessed but is not a priority over a client who is experiencing respiratory distress.
   4. The client with a tonsillectomy is expected to have pain on the same day of surgery; any nurse should be able to care for this client.

2. 1. The nurse should administer the prescribed antibiotic, ceftriaxone (Rocephin), as soon as possible but not before obtaining a sputum culture.
   2. The client diagnosed with pneumonia needs more than 2 L oxygen via nasal cannula, which would be appropriate for a client diagnosed with chronic obstructive pulmonary disease.
   3. **The nurse needs to obtain a sputum culture before administering ceftriaxone (Rocephin) antibiotic because the culture and sensitivity will be skewed if the client receives antibiotics. This should be the first HCP implemented.**
   4. The client diagnosed with pneumonia is not placed in respiratory isolation. This HCP order should be questioned.

3. 1. **Placing the client in the orthopneic position will help the client breathe easier. The position assumed by clients diagnosed with orthopnea is one in which they are sitting propped up in bed by several pillows.**
   2. The client diagnosed with COPD must have low oxygen levels of fewer than 3 L/min. COPD clients breathe because of oxygen hunger and high levels of O$_2$ provide so much oxygen that the client loses the stimulus to breathe.
   3. The client is in distress; therefore, the nurse should not assess but instead do something to help the client. The nurse should not treat a machine.
   4. The nurse should implement an intervention first because the client is in distress, then notify the respiratory therapist.

4. 1. **The LPN would be able to care for a client 2 days postoperative; crepitus is air in the subcutaneous tissue but is not life threatening.**
   2. The client who is confused is not stable; therefore, the nurse cannot assign this client to the LPN. The nurse cannot assign assessment, teaching, evaluation, or an unstable client to the LPN.
   3. The nurse cannot assign teaching; therefore, this client cannot be assigned to an LPN.
   4. The client's pulse oximeter reading is lower than 93%; therefore, this client is unstable and cannot be assigned to an LPN.

5. 1. The client diagnosed with active tuberculosis is usually administered rifampin, which causes urine and bodily fluids to turn orange.
   2. The client who is post-op would be expected to have pain, so this client would not need immediate intervention. The client who has signs or symptoms not expected for the disease process or condition would require immediate intervention.
   3. **The client diagnosed with a pneumothorax should not have blood in the collection chamber; the client diagnosed with a hemothorax would be expected to have bloody drainage. This client requires immediate intervention by the charge nurse.**
   4. A client diagnosed with bacterial pneumonia would be expected to have elevated temperature and chills; therefore, this client does not require immediate intervention.

6. 1. Sucralfate (Carafate) coats the stomach and must be administered on an empty stomach; therefore, the nurse would not question administering this medication.
   2. The therapeutic digoxin level is 0.8 to 2.0 mg/dL; therefore, the nurse would not question administering this medication.
   3. The therapeutic PTT for the client receiving heparin is 58 to 78; therefore, the nurse would not question administering this medication.

4. The client on an aminoglycoside antibiotic with an elevated trough level should not receive the medication. The elevation could lead to ototoxicity or nephrotoxicity; therefore, the nurse should question administering this medication.

7. 1. The client needs oxygen to help perfuse the lungs, heart, and body; therefore, this is the first intervention the charge nurse should tell the nurse to implement.
2. The client will need a ventilation/perfusion scan to confirm the diagnosis of pulmonary embolus, but it is not the nurse's first intervention.
3. The nurse will need to notify the client's health-care provider but not before taking care of the client's body.
4. Assessing the client is indicated, but it is not the first intervention in this situation. Remember: If the client is in distress, do not assess; take an action to help the client.

8. 1. The nurse should document the client's reports in the nurse's notes but it is not the first intervention. The nurse should first assess the client.
2. Taking slow deep breaths will not address the client's pain of 6 on the pain scale.
3. The nurse must first determine whether the pain is expected for the client's condition or whether the client is experiencing a complication requiring nursing or medical intervention. This is the nurse's first intervention.
4. The nurse must check the MAR when it is determined the pain is expected and requires pain medication, but it is not the first intervention.

9. Correct answers are 1, 4, and 5.
1. The client should be in a high-Fowler's position to facilitate lung expansion.
2. The system must be patent and intact to function properly but it should be assessed more often than every shift. It should be assessed every 2 to 4 hours.
3. The client can have bathroom privileges, and ambulation facilitates lung ventilation and expansion.
4. The tubing should not have any dependent loops. Looping the tubing prevents direct pressure on the chest tube itself and keeps tubing off the floor, addressing both a safety and an infection control issue.
5. The collection chamber of the chest drainage system (Pleur-evac) should be marked at the end of every shift and is part of the total output for the client.

10. 1. The client suspected of having ARDS is not stable and should not be assigned to an LPN. A more experienced nurse should be assigned to this client.
2. The LPN cannot administer blood; therefore, this client should not be assigned to the LPN.
3. Jugular vein distention and hypotension are signs of a tension pneumothorax, which is a medical emergency, and the client should be assigned to an RN.
4. A client scheduled for a bronchoscopy is stable and should be assigned to the LPN. This client is the most stable and least critical.

Gastrointestinal Management

Let whoever is in charge keep this simple question in her head—NOT how can I always do the right thing myself but how can I provide for this right thing always to be done.

—Florence Nightingale

QUESTIONS

1. The nurse is caring for clients on a medical unit. Which task should the nurse implement **first?**
   1. Change the abdominal surgical dressing for a client who has ambulated in the hall.
   2. Discuss the correct method of placing Montgomery straps on the client with the UAP.
   3. Assess the client who called the desk to say he is nauseated and just vomited.
   4. Place a call to the extended care facility to give the report on a discharged client.

2. The nurse is preparing a client for a barium study of the stomach and esophagus. Which nursing interventions should the nurse perform? **Select all that apply.**
   1. Obtain informed consent from the client for the diagnostic procedure.
   2. Discuss the need to increase oral fluid intake after the procedure.
   3. Explain to the client that he or she will have to drink a white, chalky substance.
   4. Tell the client not to eat or drink anything before the procedure.
   5. Instruct the client to avoid smoking 30 minutes before the procedure.

3. Which client warrants **immediate** intervention from the nurse on the medical unit?
   1. The client diagnosed with dyspepsia who has eructation and bloating
   2. The client diagnosed with pancreatitis who has steatorrhea and pyrexia
   3. The client diagnosed with diverticulitis who has left lower quadrant pain and fever
   4. The client diagnosed with Crohn's disease who has right lower abdominal pain and diarrhea

4. The RN staff nurse and the unlicensed assistive personnel (UAP) are caring for clients on a medical-surgical unit. Which tasks should the RN assign to the UAP? **Select all that apply.**
   1. Instruct the UAP to feed the 69-year-old client who is experiencing dysphagia.
   2. Request the UAP change the linens for the 89-year-old client diagnosed with fecal incontinence.
   3. Tell the UAP to assist the 54-year-old client with a bowel management program.
   4. Ask the UAP to obtain vital signs on the 72-year-old client diagnosed with cirrhosis.
   5. Direct the UAP to apply compression stockings to the 64-year-old client who had abdominal surgery.

5. Which behavior by the unlicensed assistive personnel (UAP) requires **immediate** intervention by the RN staff nurse?
   1. The UAP is refusing to feed the client diagnosed with acute diverticulitis.
   2. The UAP would not place the client who was on bedrest on the bedside commode.
   3. The UAP placed the client with a continuous feeding tube in the supine position.
   4. The UAP placed sequential compression devices on the client who is on strict bedrest.

6. The nurse is concerned about the documentation for blood administration, and other staff members agree the documentation is cumbersome and needs to be revised. Which action is **most** appropriate for the nurse to implement **first?**
   1. Discuss the blood administration documentation with the chief nursing officer.
   2. Contact an individual to help design new blood transfusion documentation.
   3. Learn to adapt to the present documentation and do not take any further action.
   4. Volunteer to be on an ad hoc committee to research alternate documentation.

7. The charge nurse is entering HCP orders for a client scheduled for a barium enema into the EHR. In addition to the radiology department, which department of the hospital should be notified of the procedure?
   1. Cardiac catheterization department
   2. Dietary department
   3. Nuclear medicine department
   4. Hospital laboratory department

8. The RN charge nurse is making assignments on a medical unit. Which client should the charge nurse assign to the new graduate nurse (GN)?
   1. The client who has received three units of packed red blood cells (PRBCs)
   2. The client scheduled for an esophagogastroduodenoscopy (EGD) in the morning
   3. The client diagnosed with short bowel syndrome who has diarrhea and a K+ level of 3.3 mEq/L
   4. The client who has just returned from surgery for a sigmoid colostomy

9. At 0830, the day shift nurse is preparing to administer medications to the client NPO for an endoscopy. Which medication should the nurse **question** administering? **Select all that apply.**

Client's Name: Mr. D. Date: Today	Account Number: 123456 Allergies: Penicillin	
Medication	1901–0700	0701–1900
Digoxin 0.125 mg PO every day		0900
Furosemide 40 mg PO bid		0900
		1600
Ranitidine 150 mg in 250 mL NS IV continuous infusion every 24 hours	0300 NN@11 mL/hr	
Vancomycin 850 mg IVPB every 24 hours	2100	0900
Magnesium hydroxide, simethicone, aluminum hydroxide 30 mL PO PRN heart burn		
Signature/Initials	Night Nurse RN/NN	Day Nurse RN/DN

   1. Digoxin 0.125 mg PO every day
   2. Furosemide 40 mg PO bid
   3. Ranitidine 150 mg in 250 mL NS IV continuous infusion every 24 hours
   4. Vancomycin 850 mg IVPB every 24 hours
   5. Magnesium hydroxide, simethicone, aluminum hydroxide 30 mL PO PRN heartburn

10. Which client should the nurse assess **first** after receiving the p.m. shift assessment?
    1. The client diagnosed with Barrett's esophagus who has dysphagia and pyrosis
    2. The client diagnosed with proctitis who has tenesmus and passage of mucus through the rectum
    3. The client diagnosed with liver failure who is jaundiced and has ascites
    4. The client diagnosed with abdominal pain who has an 8-hour urinary output of 150 mL/hr

11. The nurse is planning the care of a client diagnosed with acute gastroenteritis. Which nursing problem is **priority?**
    1. Altered nutrition
    2. Self-care deficit
    3. Impaired body image
    4. Fluid and electrolyte imbalance

12. The nurse is preparing to administer morning medications to clients on a medical unit. Which medication should the nurse administer **first?**
    1. Methylprednisolone to a client diagnosed with Crohn's disease
    2. Donepezil to a client diagnosed with dementia
    3. Sucralfate to a client diagnosed with ulcer disease
    4. Enoxaparin to a client on bedrest after abdominal surgery

13. The nurse has received the morning shift report on a surgical unit in a community hospital. Which client should the nurse assess **first?**
    1. The client who is 6 hours postoperative small bowel resection who has hypoactive bowel sounds in all four quadrants
    2. The client who is scheduled for an abdominal-peritoneal resection this morning and is crying and upset
    3. The client who is 1 day postoperative for abdominal surgery and has a rigid, hard abdomen
    4. The client who is 2 days postoperative for an emergency appendectomy and is reporting abdominal pain, rating it as an 8 on a pain scale of 1 to 10

14. The charge nurse is reviewing the morning laboratory results. Which data should the charge nurse report to the HCP via telephone?
    1. Ms. B.G., who is 4 hours postoperative for gastric lap banding

Client Name: B.G.	Account Number: 3674960	Allergies: NKDA
Diagnosis:	Height: 61 inches	
Weight in kg: 97.7	Weight in pounds: 215	

Laboratory Report

Laboratory Test	Client Value	Normal Value
WBC	15	4.5–11.1 10^3/microL
RBC	4.5	Male: 4.21–5.81 10^6 cells/microL
		Female: 3.61–5.11 10^6 cells/microL
Hgb	14	Male: 14–17.3 g/dL
		Female: 11.7–15.5 g/dL
Hct	42	Male: 42%–52%
		Female: 36%–48%
Glucose	90	Fasting: Fewer than 100 mg/dL
		Random: Fewer than 200 mg/dL
Potassium	3.5	3.5–5.3 mEq/L or mmol/L

2. Ms. R.M., who is 1 day postoperative total colectomy with creation of an ileal conduit

Client Name: R.M.	Account Number: 5903856	Allergies: Sulfa
Diagnosis:	Height: 62 inches	
Weight in kg: 61.4	Weight in pounds: 135	

Laboratory Report

Laboratory Test	Client Value	Normal Value
WBC	10	4.5–11.1 10^3/microL
RBC	4.0	Male: 4.21–5.81 10^6 cells/microL
		Female: 3.61–5.11 10^6 cells/microL
Hgb	12	Male: 14–17.3 g/dL
		Female: 11.7–15.5 g/dL
Hct	36	Male: 42%–52%
		Female: 36%–48%
Glucose	95	Fasting: Fewer than 100 mg/dL
		Random: Fewer than 200 mg/dL
Potassium	3.5	3.5–5.3 mEq/L or mmol/L

3. Mr. S.P., who is 4 days postoperative for gastric bypass surgery

Client Name: S.P.	Account Number: 2640832	Allergies: PCN
Diagnosis:	Height: 69 inches	
Weight in kg: 61.4	Weight in pounds: 300	

Laboratory Report

Laboratory Test	Client Value	Normal Value
WBC	11	4.5–11.1 10^3/microL
RBC	4.8	Male: 4.21–5.81 10^6 cells/microL
		Female: 3.61–5.11 10^6 cells/microL
Hgb	15	Male: 14–17.3 g/dL
		Female: 11.7–15.5 g/dL
Hct	45	Male: 42%–52%
		Female: 36%–48%
Glucose	180	Fasting: Fewer than 100 mg/dL
		Random: Fewer than 200 mg/dL
Potassium	4.0	3.5–5.3 mEq/L or mmol/L

4. Mr. H.C., who is 8 hours postoperative for exploratory laparotomy

Client Name: H.C.	Account Number: 3721147	Allergies: NKDA
Diagnosis:	Height: 72 inches	
Weight in kg: 86.4	Weight in pounds: 190	

Laboratory Report

Laboratory Test	Client Value	Normal Value
WBC	11	4.5–11.1 10^3/microL
RBC	4.8	Male: 4.21–5.81 10^6 cells/microL
		Female: 3.61–5.11 10^6 cells/microL
Hgb	16	Male: 14–17.3 g/dL
		Female: 11.7–15.5 g/dL
Hct	48	Male: 42%–52%
		Female: 36%–48%
Glucose	95	Fasting: Fewer than 100 mg/dL
		Random: Fewer than 200 mg/dL
Potassium	4.5	3.5–5.3 mEq/L or mmol/L

15. The nurse is preparing clients for surgery. Which client has the **greatest** potential for experiencing complications?
    1. The client scheduled for removal of an abdominal mass who is overweight
    2. The client scheduled for a gastrectomy who has arterial hypertension
    3. The client scheduled for an open cholecystectomy who smokes two packs of cigarettes per day
    4. The client scheduled for an emergency appendectomy who smokes marijuana on a daily basis

16. The nurse is performing ostomy care for a client who had an abdominal-peritoneal resection with a permanent sigmoid colostomy. **Rank in order of performance.**
    1. Cleanse the stomal site with mild soap and water.
    2. Assess the stoma for a pink, moist appearance.
    3. Monitor the drainage in the ostomy drainage bag.
    4. Apply stoma adhesive paste to the skin around the stoma.
    5. Attach the ostomy drainage bag to the abdomen.

17. The nurse is reviewing the HCP's orders for a client who is scheduled for an emergency appendectomy and is being transferred from the emergency department (ED) to the surgical unit. Which order should the nurse implement **first?**
    1. Obtain the client's informed consent.
    2. Administer 2 mg of IV morphine, every 4 hours, PRN.
    3. Shave the lower right abdominal quadrant.
    4. Administer the on-call IVPB antibiotic.

18. The client 1 day postoperative abdominal surgery has an evisceration of the wound. Which intervention should the nurse implement **first?**
    1. Place sterile normal saline gauze on the eviscerated area.
    2. Reinforce the abdominal dressing with an ABD pad.
    3. Assess the client's abdominal bowel sounds.
    4. Place the client in the left lateral position.

19. The medical-surgical nurse has just received the a.m. shift report. Which client should the nurse assess **first?**
1. The client diagnosed with a paralytic ileus who has absent bowel sounds
2. The client who is 2 days post-op abdominal surgery and has a soft, tender abdomen
3. The client who is 6 hours postoperative and has an abdominal wound dehiscence
4. The client who had a liver transplant and is being transferred to the rehabilitation unit

20. The client is being prepared for a colonoscopy in the day surgery center. The RN charge nurse observes the RN primary nurse instructing the unlicensed assistive personnel (UAP) to assist the client to the bathroom. Which action should the charge nurse implement?
1. Take no action because this is appropriate delegation.
2. Tell the UAP to obtain a bedside commode for the client.
3. Discuss the inappropriate delegation of the nursing task.
4. Document the situation in an adverse occurrence report.

21. The nurse is caring for clients on a surgical unit. Which client should the nurse assess **first?**
1. The client who has been vomiting for 2 days and has an ABG of pH 7.47, Pao_2 95, $Paco_2$ 44, Hco_3 30
2. The client who is 8 hours postoperative for splenectomy and who is reporting abdominal pain, rating it as a 9 on a pain scale of 1 to 10
3. The client who is 12 hours postoperative abdominal surgery and has dark green bile draining in the nasogastric tube
4. The client who is 2 days postoperative for hiatal hernia repair and is reporting feeling constipated

22. The unlicensed assistive personnel (UAP) tells the RN primary nurse angrily, "You are the worst nurse I have ever worked with and I really hate working with you." Which action should the RN primary nurse implement **first?**
1. Don't respond to the comment and appraise the situation.
2. Tell the UAP to leave the unit immediately.
3. Report this comment and behavior to the RN charge nurse.
4. Explain to the UAP that he or she cannot talk to the RN primary nurse in this manner.

23. The client is admitted to the critical care unit after a motor vehicle accident. The client asks the nurse, "Do you know if the person in the other car is all right?" The nurse knows the person died. Which statement supports the ethical principle of veracity?
1. "I am not sure how the other person is doing."
2. "I will try to find out how the other person is doing."
3. "You should rest now and try not to worry about it."
4. "I am sorry to have to tell you, but the person died."

24. The client admitted to the critical care unit tells the nurse, "I have an advance directive (AD) and I do not want to have cardiopulmonary resuscitation (CPR)." Which intervention should the nurse implement **first?**
1. Ask the client for a copy of the AD so that it can be entered into the EHR.
2. Inform the health-care provider of the client's request as soon as possible.
3. Determine whether the client has a durable power of attorney for health care.
4. Request the hospital chaplain to come and talk to the client about this request.

25. The client is diagnosed with esophageal bleeding. Which assessment data warrants **immediate** intervention by the nurse?
1. The client's hemoglobin/hematocrit is 11.4/32.
2. The client's abdomen is soft to touch and nontender.
3. The client's vital signs are T 99, AP 114, RR 18, BP 88/60.
4. The client's nasogastric tube has coffee ground drainage.

26. Which task should the RN staff nurse in the long-term care facility delegate to the unlicensed assistive personnel (UAP)?
    1. Assist the resident up in a wheelchair for meals.
    2. Assess the incontinent client's perianal area.
    3. Discuss requirements with the client for going out on a pass.
    4. Explain how to care for the client's colostomy to the family.

27. The RN primary nurse and the unlicensed assistive personnel (UAP) are caring for a client on a medical unit who has difficulty swallowing and is incontinent of urine and feces. Which task should the RN delegate to the unlicensed assistive personnel (UAP)?
    1. Check the client's gastrostomy feeding tube for patency.
    2. Place hydrocolloid wound dressing on the client's coccyx.
    3. Apply nonmedicated ointment to the client's perineum.
    4. Suction the client during feeding to prevent aspiration.

28. Which behavior by the unlicensed assistive personnel (UAP) **warrants** intervention by the long-term care RN staff nurse?
    1. The UAP is giving the client with a gastrostomy tube a glass of water.
    2. The UAP is ambulating the client outside using a safety belt.
    3. The UAP is assisting the client with putting a jigsaw puzzle together.
    4. The UAP is giving a back rub to the client who is on bedrest.

29. The nurse is preparing to teach the client how to irrigate his sigmoid colostomy. Which intervention should the nurse implement **first?**
    1. Demonstrate the procedure on a model.
    2. Provide the client with written instructions.
    3. Ask the client whether he has any questions.
    4. Show the client all the equipment needed.

30. The LPN tells the RN primary nurse the client diagnosed with liver failure is getting more confused. Which intervention should the RN implement **first?**
    1. Assess the client's neurological status.
    2. Notify the client's health-care provider.
    3. Request a STAT ammonia serum level.
    4. Tell the LPN to obtain the client's vital signs.

31. The nurse is changing the client's colostomy bag. Which interventions should the nurse implement? **Rank in order of priority.**
    1. Remove the client's colostomy bag.
    2. Apply the client's new colostomy bag.
    3. Don nonsterile gloves.
    4. Assess the client's stoma site.
    5. Cleanse the area around the client's stoma.

32. Which task is **most** appropriate for the RN home health-care nurse to delegate to the unlicensed assistive personnel (UAP)?
    1. Instruct the UAP to give ginkgo biloba to the client diagnosed with Alzheimer's.
    2. Ask the UAP to perform the tube feedings for a client with a gastrostomy tube.
    3. Request the UAP to perform the daily colostomy irrigation for the client.
    4. Tell the UAP to wash and dry the client's hair.

33. Which behavior by the UAP **warrants** intervention by the RN home health (HH) nurse?
    1. The UAP does not accept a birthday gift from the client.
    2. The UAP gives the client a vase of flowers from the UAP's garden.
    3. The UAP picked up the client's prescriptions from the pharmacy.
    4. The UAP cleaned the client's bathroom, including scrubbing the commode.

34. The client, diagnosed with diverticulosis, called the home health-care agency and told the nurse, "I am having really bad pain in my left lower stomach and I think I have a fever." Which action should the nurse take?
    1. Recommend the client take an antacid and lie flat in the bed.
    2. Instruct one of the nurses to visit the client immediately.
    3. Tell the client to have someone drive him or her to the emergency room.
    4. Ask the client what she has had to eat in the last 8 hours.

35. The client with a sigmoid colostomy has an excoriated area around the stoma that has not improved for more than 2 weeks. Which intervention is **most** appropriate for the home health nurse to implement?
    1. Refer the client to the wound care nurse.
    2. Notify the client's health-care provider.
    3. Continue to monitor the stoma site.
    4. Place hydrocolloid paste over the excoriated area.

36. The client, who is terminally ill, tells the nurse, "I just want to live to see my grandson graduate in 2 months." Which stage of grief is the client experiencing?
    1. Anger
    2. Bargaining
    3. Depression
    4. Acceptance

37. The nurse is discussing end-of-life (EOL) care with the client diagnosed with pancreatic cancer. Which statements are the goals for end-of-life care? **Select all that apply.**
    1. To provide comfort and supportive care during the dying process
    2. To plan and arrange the funeral for the client
    3. To improve the client's quality of life for the remaining time
    4. To help ensure a dignified death for the client and family
    5. To assist with the financial cost of the dying process

38. The client, who is terminally ill, refuses hospice services because he says it is "giving up" and would prefer his family to take care of him. Which is the **most** appropriate action by the nurse?
    1. Discuss the philosophy and services of hospice care with the client.
    2. Take no other action and support the client's decision.
    3. Contact the client's health-care provider to discuss the prognosis.
    4. Talk to the client's family members about his choice to refuse hospice.

39. The nurse is discussing end-of-life issues with a client. The nurse is explaining about a document used for listing the person the client will allow to make health-care decisions for the client should he or she become unable to make informed health-care decisions. Which document is the nurse discussing with the client?
    1. Advance directive
    2. Directive to physicians
    3. Living will
    4. Durable power of attorney for health care

40. The significant other of a client diagnosed with liver cancer and who is dying asks the nurse, "What is bereavement counseling?" Which statement is the nurse's **best** response?
    1. "Bereavement counseling helps the client accept the terminal illness."
    2. "It provides support to you and your family in the transition to a life without your loved one."
    3. "We provide counseling to you and your loved one during the dying process."
    4. "It is group counseling for family members whose loved ones have died."

41. The nurse is working in a digestive disease disorder clinic. Which nursing action is an example of evidence-based practice (EBP)?
    1. Turn on the tap water to help a client urinate.
    2. Use two identifiers to identify a client before a procedure.
    3. Educate a client based on current published information.
    4. Read nursing journals about the latest procedures.

42. The RN charge nurse notices an RN staff nurse recapping a needle in a client's room. Which action should the charge nurse take **first?**
    1. Tell the staff nurse not to recap the needle.
    2. Quietly ask the staff nurse to step into the hall.
    3. Reprimand the staff nurse for not following procedure.
    4. Notify the house supervisor of the staff nurse's behavior.

43. The administrative supervisor is staffing the hospital's medical-surgical units during an ice storm and has received many calls from staff members who are unable to get to the hospital. Which action should the supervisor implement **first?**
    1. Inform the chief nursing officer.
    2. Notify the on-duty staff to stay.
    3. Call staff members who live close to the facility.
    4. Implement the emergency disaster protocol.

44. The RN clinic nurse is working in a community health clinic. Which nursing tasks should the RN clinic nurse delegate to the unlicensed assistive personnel (UAP)? **Select all that apply.**
    1. Instruct the UAP to take the client's history.
    2. Request the UAP to document the client's symptoms.
    3. Ask the UAP to obtain the client's weight and height.
    4. Tell the UAP to complete the client's follow-up care.
    5. Have the UAP take the client's temperature.

45. The staff nurse is working with a colleague who begins to act erratically and is loud and argumentative. Which action should be taken by the nurse?
    1. Ask the supervisor to come to the unit.
    2. Determine what is bothering the nurse.
    3. Suggest the nurse go home.
    4. Smell the nurse's breath for alcohol.

46. The charge nurse is making assignments on a medical-surgical unit. Which client should be assigned to the **most** experienced nurse?
    1. The client diagnosed with lower esophageal dysfunction who is experiencing regurgitation
    2. The client diagnosed with Barrett's esophagitis who is scheduled for an endoscopy
    3. The client diagnosed with gastroesophageal reflux disease who has bilateral wheezes
    4. The client who is 1 day post-op hiatal hernia repair and has pain rated a 4 on a pain scale of 1 to 10

47. The client is experiencing severe diarrhea and has a serum potassium level of 3.3 mEq/L. Which intervention should the nurse implement **first?**
    1. Notify the client's health-care provider.
    2. Assess the client for leg cramps.
    3. Place the client on cardiac telemetry.
    4. Prepare to administer intravenous potassium.

48. The unlicensed assistive personnel (UAP) notifies the RN charge nurse that the client is angry with the care he is receiving and is packing to leave the hospital. Which intervention should the RN charge nurse implement **first?**
    1. Ask the client's nurse why the client is upset.
    2. Discuss the problem with the client.
    3. Notify the health-care provider (HCP).
    4. Have the client sign the against medical advice (AMA) form.

49. The RN primary nurse is caring for a 14-year-old female client diagnosed with bulimia. Which intervention should the RN primary nurse delegate to the unlicensed assistive personnel (UAP)?
    1. Talk with the parents about setting goals for the client.
    2. Stay with the client for 15 to 20 minutes after each meal.
    3. Encourage the client to verbalize low self-esteem.
    4. List for the dietitian the amount of food the client consumed.

50. The client tells the nurse in the bariatric clinic, "I have tried to lose weight on just about every diet out there but nothing works." Which statement is the nurse's **best** response?
    1. "Which diets and modifications have you tried?"
    2. "How much weight are you trying to lose?"
    3. "This must be difficult. Do you want to talk?"
    4. "You may need to get used to being overweight."

51. The client 2 days postoperative from a laparoscopic cholecystectomy tells the office nurse, "My right shoulder hurts so bad I can't stand it." Which statement is the nurse's **best** response?
    1. "This is a result of the carbon dioxide gas used in surgery."
    2. "Call 911 and go to the emergency department immediately."
    3. "Increase the pain medication the surgeon ordered."
    4. "You need to ambulate in the hall to walk off the gas pains."

52. The nurse is administering medications. At 1400, the client diagnosed with gastroenteritis is reporting being nauseated and has had a formed brown stool. Which intervention should the nurse implement?

Client Name: T.R. Height: 5'8" Date: Today	Account Number: 5948726 Weight in pounds: 202		Allergies: Milk Date of Birth: 07/22/1948
Medication	1901–0700		0701–1900
Diphenoxylate and atropine 1 or 2 tablets after each stool up to 8 in 24 hours	0400		0900
Ondansetron 4–8 mg IVP every 4 hours PRN for nausea	0030 (4 mg)		0630 (4 mg) 1230 (4 mg)
Signature/Initials	Night Nurse RN/NN		Day Nurse RN/DN

    1. Administer ondansetron 4 mg IVP.
    2. Administer diphenoxylate and atropine 2 tabs PO.
    3. Notify the client's health-care provider.
    4. Tell the client nothing can be administered for the nausea.

53. The nurse is caring for a client who is hemorrhaging from a duodenal ulcer. Which **collaborative** interventions should the nurse implement? **Select all that apply.**
   1. Prepare to administer a Sengstaken-Blakemore tube.
   2. Assess the client's vital signs.
   3. Administer a proton-pump intravenously.
   4. Obtain a type and crossmatch for four units of blood.
   5. Monitor the client's intake and output.

54. The nurse is caring for a client diagnosed with peptic ulcer disease. Which assessment data would cause the client to require an **immediate** intervention by the nurse?
   1. The client has hypoactive bowel sounds.
   2. The client's output is 480 mL for 12-hour shift.
   3. The client has T 98.6, AP 98, RR 22, BP 102/78.
   4. The client has coffee ground emesis.

55. The nurse is caring for a client 1 day postoperative sigmoid resection. There is a large amount of bright red blood on the dressing. Which intervention should the nurse implement **first?**
   1. Assess the client's apical pulse and blood pressure.
   2. Auscultate the client's bowel sounds.
   3. Notify the health-care provider immediately.
   4. Reinforce the dressing with a sterile gauze pad.

56. The nurse is preparing to hang a new bag of total parenteral nutrition on a client who has had an abdominal perineal resection. The bag has 2,000 mL of 50% dextrose, 10 mL of trace elements, 20 mL of multivitamins, 20 mL of potassium chloride, and 500 mL of lipids. The bag is to infuse over the next 24 hours. At what rate should the nurse set the pump?

   [   ]

57. The unlicensed assistive personnel (UAP) tells the RN staff nurse a client, who had a laparoscopic cholecystectomy, is reporting abdominal pain. Which intervention should the RN implement **first?**
   1. Check the medication administration record for the last pain medication the client received.
   2. Instruct the UAP to ask the client to rate her pain on a 1 to 10 pain scale.
   3. Assess the client to rule out any postoperative surgical complications.
   4. Tell the UAP to obtain the client's vital signs and pulse oximeter reading.

58. The male client is 30 minutes post-procedure liver biopsy. Which action by the unlicensed assistive personnel (UAP) requires the RN primary nurse to intervene?
   1. The UAP offered the client a urinal to void.
   2. The UAP gave the client a glass of water.
   3. The UAP turned the client on the left side.
   4. The UAP took the client's vital signs.

59. The client diagnosed with liver failure is experiencing pruritus secondary to severe jaundice and is scratching the upper extremities. Which intervention should the RN primary nurse implement **first?**
   1. Request the UAP to assist the client to take a hot, soapy shower.
   2. Apply an emollient to the client's upper extremities.
   3. Place mittens on both hands of the client.
   4. Administer diphenhydramine 25 mg PO to the client.

60. The client diagnosed with hepatitis asks the nurse, "Is there any herb I can take to help my liver get better?" Which statement is the nurse's **best** response?
   1. "You should ask your health-care provider about taking herbs."
   2. "Milk thistle is an antioxidant and may improve liver function."
   3. "You should not take any medication that is not prescribed."
   4. "Why would you want to take any herbs?"

61. Which task would be **most** appropriate for the RN staff nurse on the GI unit to delegate to the unlicensed assistive personnel (UAP)?
    1. Request the UAP to draw the serum liver function test.
    2. Ask the UAP to remove the nasogastric tube.
    3. Tell the UAP to empty the client's colostomy bag.
    4. Instruct the UAP to enter HCP orders into the EHR.

62. The client is diagnosed with gastroenteritis. Which laboratory data warrants **immediate** intervention by the nurse?
    1. A serum sodium level of 152 mEq/L
    2. An arterial blood gas of pH 7.37, Pao_2 95, $Paco_2$ 43, Hco_3 24
    3. A serum potassium level of 4.8 mEq/L
    4. A stool sample that is positive for fecal leukocytes

63. Which nursing problem is the highest **priority** for the client diagnosed with gastroenteritis from staphylococcal food poisoning?
    1. Fluid and electrolyte imbalance
    2. Alteration in bowel elimination
    3. Nutrition, altered: less than body requirements
    4. Oral mucous membrane, altered

64. The nurse has received the a.m. shift report. Which client should the nurse assess **first**?
    1. The client diagnosed with peptic ulcer disease who is reporting acute epigastric pain
    2. The client diagnosed with acute gastroenteritis who is upset and wants to go home
    3. The client diagnosed with inflammatory bowel disease who is receiving total parenteral nutrition
    4. The client diagnosed with hepatitis B who is uncomfortable, jaundiced, and anorexic

65. The client who has had abdominal surgery is reporting pain and tells the nurse, "I felt something pop in my stomach." Which intervention should the nurse implement **first**?
    1. Check the client's apical pulse and blood pressure.
    2. Determine the client's pain on a 1 to 10 pain scale.
    3. Assess the client's surgical wound site.
    4. Administer pain medication intravenously.

66. The client who is 2 days postoperative abdominal surgery has a Jackson-Pratt (JP) drain. Which assessment data indicates the JP drain is functioning appropriately?
    1. The bulb is round and has 40 mL of fluid.
    2. The drainage tube is pinned to the dressing.
    3. The drainage tube insertion site is pink and has no foul drainage.
    4. The bulb has suction and is compressed.

67. The nurse is caring for the following clients on a surgical unit. Which client should the nurse assess **first**?
    1. The client with an inguinal hernia repair who has a urine output of 160 mL in 4 hours
    2. The client with an emergency appendectomy who was transferred from PACU
    3. The client who is 4 hours postoperative abdominal surgery who has flatulence
    4. The client who is 6 hours post-procedure colonoscopy and is being discharged

68. The client who is morbidly obese is 8 hours postoperative gastric bypass surgery. Which nursing intervention is of the greatest **priority**?
    1. Instruct the client to use the incentive spirometer.
    2. Weigh the client daily in the same clothes and at the same time.
    3. Apply sequential compression devices to the client's lower extremities.
    4. Assist the client to sit in the bedside chair.

69. The charge nurse has completed the report. Which client should be seen **first?**
1. The client diagnosed with ulcerative colitis who had five loose stools the previous shift
2. The elderly client admitted from another facility who is refusing to be seen by the nurse
3. The client diagnosed with intractable vomiting who has tented skin turgor and dry mucous membranes
4. The client diagnosed with hemorrhoids who had spotting of bright red blood on the toilet tissue

70. The RN staff nurse, a licensed practical nurse (LPN), and a unlicensed assistive personnel (UAP) are caring for clients on a medical floor. Which nursing tasks can the RN assign or delegate? **Select all that apply.**
1. Instruct the UAP to discontinue the client's total parenteral nutrition.
2. Ask the UAP to give the client 30 mL of magnesium hydroxide, aluminum hydroxide for heartburn.
3. Tell the LPN to administer a bulk laxative to a client diagnosed with constipation.
4. Request the LPN to assess the abdomen of a client who has had reports of pain.
5. Have the UAP assist the 1 day postoperative cholecystectomy client to the bathroom.

GASTROINTESTINAL CLINICAL SCENARIO

The RN charge nurse is monitoring a 36-bed unit which admits demographically diverse clients diagnosed with gastrointestinal disorders and clients for pre- or post-gastrointestinal surgery. The large regional hospital's gastrointestinal disorder unit is staffed with four RNs, two LPNs, and two UAPs as well as a unit secretary.

1. The RN charge nurse is making assignments. Which client should be assigned to the graduate nurse (GN) who has been on the unit for 1 month?
   1. The 39-year-old client diagnosed with gastroesophageal reflux disease who is reporting pyrosis
   2. The elderly client who had an endoscopy this morning and has absent bowel sounds
   3. The middle age client diagnosed with gastroesophageal reflux disease who has bilateral wheezing
   4. The obese client who is 1-day post-op cholecystectomy and refuses to deep breathe

2. The middle age client diagnosed with inflammatory bowel disease has a serum potassium level of 4.4 mEq/L. Which intervention should the nurse implement **first?**
   1. Notify the health-care provider.
   2. Continue to monitor the client.
   3. Request telemetry for the client.
   4. Prepare to administer potassium IV.

3. The 59-year-old client has been admitted to the hospital diagnosed with hemorrhaging from a duodenal ulcer. Which independent interventions should the RN charge nurse instruct the primary nurse to implement? **Select all that apply.**
   1. Complete the admission assessment.
   2. Evaluate BP lying, sitting, and standing.
   3. Administer antibiotics intravenously.
   4. Administer blood products.
   5. Obtain a hemoglobin and hematocrit.

4. The RN charge nurse is discharging an elderly client with a new sigmoid colostomy. Which statement made by the client indicates to the charge nurse the client needs **more** teaching?
   1. "If my stoma becomes a purple color I will notify my HCP."
   2. "I can eat the foods I used to eat when I go home."
   3. "I should wear a colostomy pouch over my stoma."
   4. "I will irrigate my colostomy every week with 750 mL of tap water."

5. The nurse is preparing to hang a new bag of total parenteral nutrition on a 47-year-old client who has had an abdominal perineal resection. The bag has 2,000 mL of 50% dextrose, 15 mL of trace elements, 30 mL of multivitamins, 20 mL of potassium chloride, and 200 mL of lipids. The bag is to infuse over the next 24 hours. At what rate should the nurse set the pump?

   [   ]

6. The elderly client is admitted to the medical unit with a diagnosis of acute diverticulitis. Which order should the RN charge nurse clarify with the health-care provider?
   1. Insert a nasogastric tube.
   2. Start IV D$_5$W at 125 mL/hr.
   3. Schedule the client for a sigmoidoscopy.
   4. Place the client on bedrest with bathroom privileges.

7. The RN charge nurse observes the unlicensed assistive personnel (UAP) turning the jaundiced client who has just had a liver biopsy to the supine position. Which action should the charge nurse implement **first**?
   1. Tell the UAP to keep the client on bedrest for 2 hours.
   2. Praise the UAP for placing the client in the supine position.
   3. Instruct the UAP to place the client on the right side.
   4. Complete an incident report on the UAP's behavior.

8. One of the primary nurses tells the RN charge nurse she stuck herself in the finger with a "used" needle and cleaned the site with soap and water. Which intervention should the charge nurse implement **first**?
   1. Notify the infection control nurse.
   2. Complete an adverse occurrence report.
   3. Request post-exposure prophylaxis.
   4. Check the hepatitis status of the client.

9. Which nursing task is **most** appropriate for the RN charge nurse to delegate to the unlicensed assistive personnel (UAP)?
   1. Bathe the middle age client diagnosed with liver failure who has a Sengstaken-Blakemore tube inflated.
   2. Teach the client with an abdominal incision to splint the incision when coughing.
   3. Assist the jaundiced client diagnosed with pruritus to the bathroom for a shower and a.m. care.
   4. Tell the UAP to assist the RN staff nurse performing a paracentesis on the obese client diagnosed with liver failure.

10. The charge nurse is making rounds on the unit. Which client should the charge nurse assess **first**?
    1. The 67-year-old client diagnosed with peptic ulcer disease who is receiving blood and has a hemoglobin of 10.1 and hematocrit 35
    2. The middle age client diagnosed with ulcerative colitis who has had 10 loose stools and has a potassium level of 3.5 mEq/L
    3. The malnourished client who is 1-day post-op abdominal surgery with a hard, rigid abdomen and elevated temperature
    4. The elderly client diagnosed with acute diverticulitis whose nasogastric tube is draining green bile

The correct answer number and rationale for why it is the correct answer are given in **boldface type**. Rationales for why the other possible answer options are incorrect also are given, but they are not in boldface type.

1. 1. This client should be seen in a timely manner, but not before the client who is vomiting.
2. This can take some time and should not be hastily completed because the nurse must know the task is being done correctly before delegating it to a UAP. This should be done at a time arranged between the UAP and the nurse.
3. **This client has experienced a physiological problem and the nurse must assess the client and the emesis to decide on possible interventions.**
4. The nurse could call the extended care facility after assessing the client who has vomited and after dressing the client's leg.

CLINICAL JUDGMENT GUIDE: The test taker should use some tool as a reference to guide in the decision-making process. In this situation, Maslow's Hierarchy of Needs should be applied. Physiological needs have priority over psychosocial ones.

2. Correct answers are 1, 3, and 4.
1. **A barium study of the upper GI system is an x-ray procedure and requires the client to sign an informed consent form.**
2. The barium can cause constipation after the procedure; therefore, the client should increase fluid intake.
3. **The client will have to drink a white, chalky substance that creates a lining on the inner wall of the gastrointestinal tract.**
4. **The test is a barium study of the upper GI system and requires the client's upper GI system to be empty. This client should be NPO for at least 8 to 10 hours before the test.**
5. The client should not smoke for several hours before the procedure as this causes secretions to build and obstruct the diagnostic image.

CLINICAL JUDGMENT GUIDE: The nurse must be knowledgeable regarding diagnostic tests. The nurse must know pre-procedure and post-procedure interventions, as well as which ones require informed consent.

3. 1. The nurse would expect the client diagnosed with dyspepsia (upset stomach) to have eructation (belching) and bloating; therefore, this client does not warrant immediate intervention.
2. The nurse would expect the client diagnosed with pancreatitis to have steatorrhea (fat, frothy stools) and pyrexia (fever); therefore, this client does not warrant immediate intervention.
3. The nurse would expect the client diagnosed with diverticulitis to have left lower quadrant pain and fever; therefore, this client does not warrant immediate intervention.
4. **The client diagnosed with Crohn's disease should be asymptomatic, so pain and diarrhea warrant intervention by the nurse. Pain could indicate a complication.**

CLINICAL JUDGMENT GUIDE: "Warrants immediate intervention" means the nurse must determine which client is the priority to assess. The nurse would assess a client in pain if all the other options had clients with expected signs or symptoms.

4. Correct answers are 2, 3, 4, and 5.
1. The nurse should not delegate to the UAP the task of feeding a client who is not stable and at risk for complications during feeding, because of dysphagia. This requires judgment that the UAP is not expected to possess.
2. **UAPs can change linens for clients who are incontinent; therefore, this task could be delegated to a UAP.**
3. **The UAP can assist the client to the bathroom and document the results of the attempt.**
4. **The UAP can obtain the vital signs on a stable client.**
5. **The UAP can apply compression stockings to the client who had abdominal surgery.**

CLINICAL JUDGMENT GUIDE: This is an alternate type of question included in the NCLEX-RN®. The nurse must be able to select all the options that answer the question correctly. There are no partially correct answers. An RN cannot delegate assessment, teaching, evaluation, medications, or an unstable client to a UAP. Tasks that cannot be delegated are nursing interventions requiring nursing judgment.

5. 1. The client diagnosed with acute diverticulitis should be NPO; therefore, the UAP should not feed a client. This action does not warrant immediate intervention.
   2. The UAP should not allow the client on bedrest to use the bedside commode; therefore, this does not warrant immediate intervention by the nurse.
   3. **A client with a continuous feeding tube should be in the Fowler's or high-Fowler's position to prevent aspiration pneumonia. This action requires immediate intervention by the nurse.**
   4. The UAP can place sequential compression devices on a client; therefore, this does not warrant immediate intervention.

CLINICAL JUDGMENT GUIDE: Delegation means the nurse is responsible for the UAP's actions and performance. The nurse must correct the UAP's performance to ensure the client is cared for safely in the hospital or the home.

6. 1. The nurse should go through the chain of command when attempting to make a change.
   2. This may be an appropriate action at some point, but this would not be implemented until after assessing the old documentation and identifying areas to be changed.
   3. The nurse should be a change agent.
   4. **The staff nurse should be a part of the solution to a problem; volunteering to be on a committee of peers is the best action to effect a change.**

CLINICAL JUDGMENT GUIDE: There will be management questions on the NCLEX-RN®. Concepts of Management is included under the category Safe and Effective Environment and subcategory Management of Care. This is a knowledge-based question.

7. 1. Because this procedure is performed in the radiology department and is testing the gastrointestinal system, the cardiac catheter laboratory does not need to be informed of the procedure.
   2. **The client must be NPO for 8 to 10 hours before the procedure. Therefore, the dietary department should be notified to hold the meal trays.**
   3. The procedure is performed using barium or Gastrografin, neither of which contains any nuclear material. The nuclear medicine department does not need to be informed of the procedure.

   4. The procedure does not involve the clinical laboratory; therefore, this department does not need to be notified.

CLINICAL JUDGMENT GUIDE: The test taker must be knowledgeable regarding the role of all members of the multidisciplinary health-care team. Referrals are included under the category Safe and Effective Care Environment and subcategory Management of Care.

8. 1. This client is unstable and should not be assigned to a new graduate nurse.
   2. **This client is being prepared for a test in the morning and is the least acute of the clients listed. The new graduate should be assigned to this client.**
   3. This client is hypokalemic secondary to diarrhea and is at risk for cardiac dysrhythmias. This client should be assigned to a more experienced nurse. Short bowel syndrome is a malabsorption disorder caused by the surgical removal of the small intestine or rarely because of the complete dysfunction of a large segment of bowel.
   4. A client returning from surgery with a sigmoid colostomy is at risk for postoperative complications and should be assigned to a more experienced nurse.

CLINICAL JUDGMENT GUIDE: The test taker must determine which client is the most stable; therefore, this is an "except" question. Three clients are either unstable or have potentially life-threatening conditions.

9. Correct answers are 1, 2, and 5.
   1. **The nurse should not administer any PO medications such as digoxin (Lanoxin) because the client is NPO.**
   2. **This medication is PO; therefore, furosemide (Lasix) should not be administered until after the endoscopy.**
   3. Ranitidine (Zantac) is an intravenous medication, so it can be administered even though the client is NPO.
   4. Vancomycin is an intravenous medication, so it can be administered even though the client is NPO.
   5. **Magnesium hydroxide, simethicone, aluminum hydroxide (Mylanta) is a PRN medication and it is PO; therefore, it should not be administered until after the procedure.**

CLINICAL JUDGMENT GUIDE: This is an alternate type of question included in the NCLEX-RN® test plan. The test taker must be able to read

a medication administration record (MAR), be knowledgeable regarding medications, and be able to make a decision as to the nurse's most appropriate intervention.

10. 1. The client diagnosed with Barrett's esophagus is expected to have dysphagia (difficulty swallowing) and pyrosis (heartburn); therefore, this client would not be assessed first.
2. Proctitis is an inflammation of the anus and the lining of the rectum, affecting only the last 6 inches of the rectum. Symptoms are ineffectual straining to empty the bowels (tenesmus), diarrhea, rectal bleeding and possible discharge, involuntary spasms and cramping during bowel movements, left-sided abdominal pain, passage of mucus through the rectum, and anorectal pain. Because the signs and symptoms are expected, this client would not be assessed first.
3. Jaundice and ascites are expected in a client diagnosed with liver failure; therefore, the nurse should not assess this client first.
4. **The client has a urinary output of fewer than 30 mL/hr; therefore, this client may be going into renal failure and should be assessed first.**

CLINICAL JUDGMENT GUIDE: The test taker should ask, "Is it normal or expected for the disease process?" If it is normal or expected, then do not assess this client first. If more than one option is not expected or normal, then the test taker should ask which client is in a more life-threatening situation, needs more assessment, or may need the nurse to notify the health-care provider.

11. 1. Altered nutrition is a concern, but a client can live for several weeks on minimal intake.
2. Self-care deficit is a psychosocial problem; physiological problems have priority.
3. Impaired body image is a psychosocial problem; physiological problems have priority.
4. **Fluid and electrolyte imbalance can cause cardiac dysrhythmias. This is the priority problem.**

CLINICAL JUDGMENT GUIDE: The NCLEX-RN® integrates the nursing process throughout the Client Needs categories and subcategories. The nursing process is a scientific, clinical reasoning approach to client care that includes assessment, analysis, planning, implementation, and evaluation. The nurse will be responsible for identifying nursing diagnoses for clients.

12. 1. This is a routine medication that has a timeframe of 30 minutes before and after the scheduled time to be administered. Methylprednisolone (Solu-Medrol), a steroid, does not need to be the first medication administered.
2. Donepezil (Aricept), an acetylcholinesterase inhibitor, can be administered within a 30-minute timeframe. This medication does not need to be the first medication administered.
3. **Sucralfate (Carafate), a mucosal barrier agent, must be administered before the client eats in order for the medication to coat the gastric mucosa. This medication should be administered first.**
4. Enoxaparin (Lovenox), an anticoagulant, can be administered within the 30-minute timeframe. This medication does not need to be the first medication administered.

CLINICAL JUDGMENT GUIDE: The test taker should know medications that are priority medications, such as life-sustaining medications, insulin, and mucolytics (Carafate). These medications should be administered first by the nurse.

13. 1. A client who is 6 hours postoperative abdominal surgery would be expected to have decreased bowel sounds; therefore, this client would not be assessed first.
2. Surgery is scary, and the client who is crying and upset should be assessed, but not before a potentially life-threatening surgical emergency. Psychosocial problems do not take priority over physiological problems.
3. **A hard, rigid abdomen indicates peritonitis, which is a life-threatening emergency. This client should be assessed first.**
4. The client who is 2 days postoperative and who is reporting and rating pain as an 8 should be assessed, but the pain is not life threatening and, therefore, does not take priority over the client diagnosed with probable peritonitis.

CLINICAL JUDGMENT GUIDE: When deciding which client to assess first, the nurse should determine whether the signs or symptoms the client is exhibiting are normal or expected for the client's situation. After eliminating the expected options, the test taker should determine which situation is more life threatening.

14. 1. **Because a client undergoing an elective procedure such as gastric lap banding is usually healthy preoperatively, an elevated postoperative WBC may indicate infection requiring notification of the HCP.**
    2. The H&H of 12/36 is within normal limits; therefore, this laboratory result does not warrant intervention.
    3. The glucose level is elevated but it does not indicate if this is a fasting or random sample. Many clients who are obese have diabetes and must be at least 50 pounds overweight to have gastric bypass surgery.
    4. A serum potassium level of 4.5 mEq/L is within normal limits; therefore, this does not warrant notifying the health-care provider.

CLINICAL JUDGMENT GUIDE: The nurse must be knowledgeable regarding normal laboratory values. These values must be memorized and the nurse must be able to determine if a laboratory value is normal for the client's disease process or medications the client is taking, or if the health-care provider should be notified.

15. 1. A client who is overweight and having abdominal surgery is not at a higher risk for postoperative complications than any other client.
    2. The client's high blood pressure should be monitored closely and medications administered to decrease the hypertension, but this would not cause the client to have a higher risk for postoperative complications.
    3. **The location of the incision for an open cholecystectomy, the general anesthesia needed, and a heavy smoking history make this client high risk for pulmonary complications. Most cholecystectomies are performed laparoscopically; however, an open cholecystectomy could be indicated for clients with suspected gallbladder cancer, cholecystobiliary fistulas, and severe cardiopulmonary disease.**
    4. Use of marijuana daily does not increase the risk of pulmonary complications for a client having gastric surgery.

CLINICAL JUDGMENT GUIDE: This is an "except" question, but it does not say all the options are correct "except." Only one option would cause the nurse to suspect high risk of postoperative complications. Remember: Smoking cigarettes puts clients at risk for multiple problems, so it would be a good choice.

16. Correct order is 3, 2, 1, 4, 5.
    3. **The nurse must first assess the drainage in the bag for color, consistency, and amount.**
    2. **After removing the bag, the nurse should assess the site to ensure circulation to the stoma. A pink, moist appearance indicates adequate circulation.**
    1. **The nurse should cleanse the area with mild soap and water to ensure that the skin is prepared for the adhesive paste.**
    4. **The nurse should then apply adhesive paste to the clean, dry skin.**
    5. **The ostomy drainage bag is attached last.**

CLINICAL JUDGMENT GUIDE: This is an alternate type of question included in the NCLEX-RN® test plan. The nurse must be able to perform skills in the correct order. Obtaining informed consent and performing an assessment should always be the first interventions.

17. 1. **The nurse must first obtain the operative permit, or determine whether it has been signed by the client, before implementing any other orders.**
    2. The client cannot give informed consent after receiving pain medication; therefore, administration of morphine cannot be implemented first.
    3. The operating room staff usually performs shave preps, but the nurse would not implement this before medicating the client.
    4. The on-call IVPB is not administered until the operating room (OR) is prepared for the client. New standards recommend that the prophylactic IVPB antibiotic be administered within 1 hour of opening the skin during a surgical procedure.

CLINICAL JUDGMENT GUIDE: The NCLEX-RN® test plan includes perioperative nursing care. The nurse must be knowledgeable regarding preoperative and postoperative care, which is generic for all clients undergoing surgery. Obtaining informed consent is a priority intervention.

18. 1. **Evisceration is the removal of viscera (internal organs, especially those in the abdominal cavity). If the bowels protrude from the abdominal incision, the nurse must apply sterile normal saline gauze and then notify the client's surgeon.**
    2. The nurse can place an ADB pad on the normal sterile saline gauze.

3. The nurse can assess the bowel sounds, but not before applying sterile normal saline gauze.

4. The client should be placed in the supine position; the left lateral position will not affect the client's abdominal evisceration.

CLINICAL JUDGMENT GUIDE: The test taker should apply the nursing process in questions that ask, "Which intervention should the nurse implement first?" If the client is in distress, do not assess. The nurse should do something directly to help the client's situation.

19. 1. This client diagnosed with a paralytic ileus would be expected to have absent bowel sounds; therefore, this client should not be assessed first.

2. The client who is postoperative abdominal surgery should have a soft, tender abdomen; therefore, this client should not be assessed first.

3. **Wound dehiscence is the premature "bursting" open of a wound along surgical sutures, and is an emergency that would require the nurse to assess this client first.**

4. This client should be prepared for transfer to the rehabilitation unit, but not before assessing a client diagnosed with a complication of surgery.

CLINICAL JUDGMENT GUIDE: The nurse must determine which client is experiencing an unexpected or abnormal situation for the surgery or condition. All the clients should be assessed and cared for, but the nurse must determine which one should be assessed first.

20. 1. **The primary nurse's instruction to the UAP to assist the client to the bathroom is an appropriate delegation that ensures the safety of the client. It requires no action by the charge nurse.**

2. There is no information in the stem that indicates the client needs a bedside commode; therefore, this is not an appropriate action.

3. The UAP can assist a client who is stable to ambulate; therefore, this is not inappropriate delegation.

4. An adverse occurrence report is completed whenever potential or actual harm has come to the client. Ambulating the client with assistance is not harmful.

CLINICAL JUDGMENT GUIDE: The nurse must ensure the UAP can perform any delegated

nursing tasks. It is the nurse's responsibility to evaluate the task, and demonstrate or teach the UAP how to perform the task.

21. 1. The ABGs reflect metabolic alkalosis, which is expected in a client who has excessive vomiting; therefore, this client would not be assessed first.

2. **Pain is a priority because the nurse must determine if this is expected postoperative pain or a complication of the surgery. This client should be assessed first.**

3. Dark green bile should be draining from the client's nasogastric tube; therefore, this client should not be assessed first.

4. The client who is reporting being constipated would not be a priority over a client with surgical pain.

CLINICAL JUDGMENT GUIDE: When deciding which client to assess first, the nurse should determine whether the signs and symptoms the client is exhibiting are normal or expected for the client situation. After eliminating the expected option, the test taker should determine which situation is more life threatening.

22. 1. **The nurse should first appraise the situation and not do anything. This is the pivotal point at which the nurse can return the anger or appraise the situation. The most important action to take is to empathize with the UAP and determine the provocation for the behavior.**

2. The primary nurse could tell the UAP to leave the unit, but this is responding to the anger and not the reason for the anger.

3. The comment may need to be reported to the charge nurse, but not until the primary nurse can determine what caused the comment. The UAP may be upset about something else entirely.

4. This is not the first action when dealing with someone who is angry. This comment may cause further angry behavior by the UAP and will not diffuse the situation. The nurse is the professional person and should control the situation.

CLINICAL JUDGMENT GUIDE: There will be management questions on the NCLEX-RN®. In many instances, there is no test-taking strategy for these questions. The nurse must be knowledgeable regarding management issues addressing how to deal with conflict and personnel issues.

23. 1. Beneficence is the ethical principle to do good actively for the client. Because the client is in the ICU, the client is critically ill and does not need any type of news that will further upset him or her. This statement supports the ethical principle of beneficence.
   2. The statement supports beneficence, which is to do good.
   3. This statement avoids directly telling the client the other individual is dead.
   4. **This statement supports the ethical principle of veracity, which is the duty to tell the truth. This statement will probably further upset the client and cause psychological distress, which may hinder the recovery period.**

CLINICAL JUDGMENT GUIDE: The NCLEX-RN® test plan includes nursing care that addresses ethical principles including autonomy, beneficence, justice, and veracity, to name a few.

24. 1. A copy of the advance directive should be placed in the client's electronic health record (EHR), but it is not the nurse's first intervention.
   2. **The nurse should first inform the HCP so the order can be documented in the client's EHR. The HCP must write the do not resuscitate (DNR) order before the client's wishes can be honored.**
   3. The person with the durable power of attorney for health care can make health-care choices for the client if the client is unable to verbalize his or her wishes, but the first intervention is to have the HCP write a DNR order.
   4. The client has a right to make this request, and the chaplain does not need to talk to the client about the advance directive.

CLINICAL JUDGMENT GUIDE: There will be management questions on the NCLEX-RN®. Advance directives are included under the category Safe and Effective Environment and subcategory Management of Care.

25. 1. The client's H&H is not within normal limits, but remember: "Hemoglobin 9 think about transfusion time." This laboratory information does not warrant immediate intervention.
   2. A soft, nontender abdomen is expected and does not warrant immediate intervention by the nurse.
   3. **The client's apical pulse (AP) is above normal and the BP is low, which are signs**

of hypovolemic shock, which warrants immediate intervention by the nurse.
   4. Coffee ground drainage indicates "old blood," which would not be unexpected in the client who has esophageal bleeding.

CLINICAL JUDGMENT GUIDE: The test taker should ask, "Is the assessment data normal for the disease process?" If it is normal for the disease process, then the nurse would not need to intervene; if it is not normal for the disease process, then this warrants intervention by the nurse.

26. 1. **Getting a client up in a wheelchair for meals is an appropriate delegation to an unlicensed assistive personnel (UAP). This task does not require nursing judgment.**
   2. Assessing an incontinent client's perianal area requires nursing judgment and cannot be delegated to the UAP.
   3. Discussing requirements with a client for going out on a pass should be done by the nurse responsible for completing the required documentation and providing any medication that the resident should take along.
   4. Explaining colostomy care is teaching, and the RN cannot ask the UAP to teach.

CLINICAL JUDGMENT GUIDE: The nurse cannot delegate assessment, evaluation, teaching, administering medications, or the care of an unstable client to a UAP.

27. 1. Checking the patency of a percutaneous endoscopic gastrostomy (PEG) feeding tube requires nursing judgment, and feeding the client through the tube is based on this judgment. The unlicensed assistive personnel (UAP) should not be asked to perform this task.
   2. The nurse should assess the coccyx and the area where the hydrocolloid dressing (DuoDERM) should be placed. The UAP should not be asked to perform this task.
   3. **The UAP can apply nonmedicated ointment to protect the client's perineum when bathing and changing the client's incontinence pads. This will protect the client from skin breakdown.**
   4. The nurse should not delegate suctioning during feeding to a UAP. This indicates the client is unstable.

CLINICAL JUDGMENT GUIDE: When the test taker is deciding which option is the most appropriate task to delegate or assign, the test taker should choose the task that allows each member of the staff to function within his or her full scope of practice. Do not assign a task to a staff member that requires a higher level of expertise than that staff member has; similarly, do not assign a task to a staff member that could be assigned to a staff member with a lower level of expertise.

28. 1. **The client with a gastrostomy tube cannot eat or drink oral fluids; therefore, this behavior warrants intervention by the nurse.**
    2. At the long-term care center, the clients are allowed to go outside and the unlicensed assistive personnel (UAP) ambulating the client with a safety belt is appropriate behavior.
    3. Assisting the client with an activity is an appropriate behavior by the UAP in a long-term care center.
    4. Giving a back rub to a client on bedrest is a wonderful thing for the UAP to do for the client.

CLINICAL JUDGMENT GUIDE: The nurse must ensure the UAP can perform any delegated nursing tasks. It is the nurse's responsibility to evaluate the task and demonstrate or teach the UAP how to perform the task. It is also the nurse's responsibility to intervene if the UAP is exhibiting an unsafe behavior.

29. 1. The nurse should demonstrate the procedure on a model, but the first intervention should be to assess, to determine whether the client has any questions.
    2. The nurse should provide the client with written instructions, but the first intervention should be to assess, to determine whether the client has any questions.
    3. **The client cannot learn if he has any questions or concerns. Therefore, the first intervention is to ask the client whether he has any questions. The nurse must allay any of the client's concerns or fears before beginning to teach the client.**
    4. The nurse should show the client all the equipment, but the first intervention should be to assess, to determine whether the client has any questions.

CLINICAL JUDGMENT GUIDE: The nurse should always apply the nursing process when answering

a question requiring the nurse to "determine which intervention to implement first." The first part of the nursing process is to assess.

30. 1. **The nurse should first assess the client's neurological status to determine the status of the client.**
    2. The nurse may need to contact the client's HCP, but the nurse should assess the client first, before contacting the HCP.
    3. Increasing confusion is a symptom of hepatic encephalopathy and checking the client's ammonia level would be appropriate, but not before assessing the client.
    4. The nurse should assess the client first, before the LPN obtaining further data.

CLINICAL JUDGMENT GUIDE: Any time the nurse receives information about a client (who may be experiencing a complication) from another staff member, the nurse must assess the client. The nurse should not make decisions about the client's needs based on another staff member's information.

31. Correct order is 3, 1, 4, 5, 2.
    3. **The nurse should first put on nonsterile gloves, because of body fluid contamination.**
    1. **The nurse should remove the bag carefully and ensure no drainage in the bag gets on the client's skin.**
    4. **The nurse should ensure the stoma site is moist and pink.**
    5. **The area around the stoma should be cleansed with soap and water and allowed to dry thoroughly.**
    2. **Lastly, the nurse should apply the new colostomy bag.**

CLINICAL JUDGMENT GUIDE: The nurse must rank the interventions in order of priority. This is an alternate type of question included in the NCLEX-RN® test plan. Remember, Standard Precautions are always a priority.

32. 1. Even if the client is prescribed the herb ginkgo biloba by the health-care provider, the nurse cannot delegate any type of medication administration to the unlicensed assistive personnel (UAP).
    2. In some situations, the UAP may be able to perform tube feedings in the home, but the nurse should assign the least invasive procedure to the UAP.
    3. In some situations, the UAP may be able to do colostomy irrigations in the home, but the nurse should assign the least invasive procedure to the UAP.

4. **The UAP can wash and dry the client's hair, as this is the least invasive task, so this would be the most appropriate task for the nurse to delegate to the UAP.**

CLINICAL JUDGMENT GUIDE: The nurse cannot delegate assessment, teaching, evaluation, medications, or an unstable client to the UAP. The nurse should always assign the least invasive task or the task that requires the least educated employee.

33. 1. Because the UAP cannot accept gifts or money from the client, this would not warrant an intervention.
2. The UAP can bring flowers to the client. This does not violate any rules.
3. **The UAP should not take money from the client to pick up prescriptions and the UAP is not responsible for doing errands for the client. If money is missing or medications are missing, this could result in a difficult situation. The home health (HH) nurse should tell the UAP not to do this type of activity for the client.**
4. Cleaning the house is not part of the UAP's job description, but this would not warrant intervention by the HH nurse.

CLINICAL JUDGMENT GUIDE: The nurse is responsible for knowing the scope of practice for health-care team member subordinates.

34. 1. The client is having signs and symptoms of diverticulitis, which can be potentially life threatening; therefore, the client should get medical assistance immediately.
2. The client needs to be seen by a health-care provider to be prescribed antibiotics; therefore, there is no reason for an HH nurse to visit the client.
3. **The nurse must have knowledge of disease processes. The client is verbalizing signs of acute diverticulitis, which requires the client to be NPO and prescribed antibiotics. The client needs to receive immediate medical attention.**
4. The client is verbalizing signs and symptoms of acute diverticulitis, which requires medical attention. It does not matter what the client has had to eat.

CLINICAL JUDGMENT GUIDE: The nurse must be knowledgeable in expected medical treatments for the client. This is a knowledge-based question.

35. 1. According to the NCLEX-RN® test plan under management of care, the nurse should be knowledgeable regarding referrals. The wound care nurse is trained to care for a client with a colostomy and is knowledgeable in treating complications.
2. The most appropriate intervention is to refer the client to a member of the multidisciplinary team who has expertise in the area in which the client is having the problem. In this case, the wound care nurse has the expertise to care for the stoma site.
3. After 2 weeks, the nurse should obtain further assistance in treating the stoma site.
4. Hydrocolloid (Karaya) paste will not be effective in treating the excoriated area; therefore, this is not an appropriate intervention.

CLINICAL JUDGMENT GUIDE: The test taker must be knowledgeable regarding the role of all members of the multidisciplinary health-care team as well as HIPAA rules and regulations. These will be tested on the NCLEX-RN® examination.

36. 1. Denial is the first stage of grief. Anger is the second stage of grief: "Why me? It's not fair!" The individual recognizes that denial cannot continue. Because of anger, the person is very difficult to care for because of misplaced feelings of rage and envy.
2. **Bargaining: "I'll do anything for a few more years." The third stage involves the hope that the individual can somehow postpone or delay death. The client's comments indicate bargaining.**
3. Depression: "I am so sad, why bother with anything?" During the fourth stage, the dying person begins to understand the certainty of death. Because of this, the individual may become silent, refuse visitors, and spend much of the time crying and grieving.
4. Acceptance: "It's going to be okay." In this last stage, the individual begins to come to terms with his or her mortality or the mortality of a loved one.

CLINICAL JUDGMENT GUIDE: The nurse caring for clients who are dying needs to know the stages of death. Each stage of death requires the nurse to address the psychosocial needs of the client in a different way.

37. Correct answers are 1, 3, and 4.
   1. This is a goal for EOL care.
   2. This will need to be done during the client's dying process, but it is not a goal for EOL care.
   3. This is a goal for EOL care.
   4. This is a goal for EOL care.
   5. Addressing the financial cost of the dying process is not a goal for EOL care.

CLINICAL JUDGMENT GUIDE: This is an alternate type of question included in the NCLEX-RN®. The nurse must be able to select all the options that answer the question correctly. There are no partially correct answers. The nurse must know the role of the other areas of nursing so that the nurse can refer the client and family to the appropriate resource.

38. 1. Some families are close-knit and often prefer to care for their own family members; therefore, they would not seek hospice or palliative care. The nurse should attempt to help the client understand the philosophy, the benefits, and the help hospice can give the client and family.
   2. The nurse should attempt to help the client and family understand hospice so the client can make an informed decision.
   3. The health-care provider does not need to be contacted to reaffirm the client is dying.
   4. The nurse should first talk to the client and then to the family.

CLINICAL JUDGMENT GUIDE: The client has a right to refuse any health care, but the nurse first must ensure the client fully understands the focus of the care. When the client fully understands and then refuses the care, the nurse must respect the client's rights.

39. 1. "Advance directive" is a general term used to describe documents that give instructions about future medical care and treatments and who should make them in the event the client is unable to communicate.
   2. A directive to health-care providers is a written document specifying the client's wish to be allowed to die without heroic or extraordinary measures.
   3. "Living will" is a lay term used frequently to describe any number of documents giving instructions about future medical care and treatments.
   4. The nurse is specifically describing the term "durable power of attorney for

health care." It is a document included in an advance directive.

CLINICAL JUDGMENT GUIDE: The nurse must be aware of documents clients use when addressing end-of-life issues. This is a knowledge-based question, but nurses must be able to ensure the client's last requests are honored.

40. 1. Bereavement counseling is for the survivors, not the client.
   2. This is the definition of bereavement counseling.
   3. Bereavement counseling is for the survivors, not the client.
   4. Bereavement counseling may include group counseling, but it could also be individual counseling. This is not the nurse's best response.

CLINICAL JUDGMENT GUIDE: The nurse must be able to explain the support provided by hospice. Losing a loved one is a huge loss to most people, and the nurse's responsibility is to help the survivors work through the stages of grief.

41. 1. Many nurses follow this practice, but no research has been completed to support this practice.
   2. This is part of The Joint Commission's Patient Safety Goals, not evidence-based practice.
   3. Evidence-based practice (EBP) is the conscientious use of current best evidence in making decisions about nursing care. Using the "evidence," or research, to teach a client is evidence-based practice.
   4. Reading the journal is a step in EBP, but EBP requires using the information in practice.

CLINICAL JUDGMENT GUIDE: The NCLEX-RN® test plan includes nursing care based on evidence-based practice. The nurse must be knowledgeable regarding nursing research.

42. 1. The charge nurse should stop the nurse from recapping the needle, but not in front of the client.
   2. The charge nurse should not reprimand the nurse in front of the client or client's family. The charge nurse should ask the nurse to step into the hall, where the client cannot hear.
   3. Reprimanding the nurse is not the first action.
   4. Notifying the house supervisor is not the first action.

CLINICAL JUDGMENT GUIDE: In any business, including a health-care facility, correcting a fellow staff member's behavior should not occur in front of a customer or, in this instance, the client.

43. 1. The chief nursing officer should be informed, but this is not the first action.
   2. **The first action for the administrative supervisor is to make sure the clients receive care. The supervisor cannot allow the on-duty staff to leave until replacement staff members have been arranged.**
   3. The supervisor should call any staff that can get to the hospital in an attempt to staff the hospital, but this is not the first action to implement.
   4. An emergency disaster protocol may be implemented, but the first intervention is to ensure the clients have a nurse on duty.

CLINICAL JUDGMENT GUIDE: The nurse must be knowledgeable regarding emergency preparedness. Employees receive this information in employee orientation and are responsible for implementing procedures correctly. The NCSBN NCLEX-RN® test plan includes questions on a safe and effective care environment.

44. **Correct answers are 3 and 5.**
   1. The nurse cannot delegate any task requiring nursing judgment. Taking a client's history requires knowing which questions need to be asked to assess the client's problems.
   2. Documenting the client's symptoms is a nursing responsibility that the nurse must perform. It cannot be delegated to the unlicensed assistive personnel (UAP).
   3. **The UAP can obtain the client's height and weight. This is a task the nurse should delegate.**
   4. The client's follow-up care may require teaching, judgment, or further assessment; therefore, the nurse should not delegate this action to a UAP. When delegating to a UAP, the nurse must provide clear, concise, and specific instructions. The nurse cannot delegate teaching.
   5. **The UAP can take the client's temperature. This is a task the nurse should delegate.**

CLINICAL JUDGMENT GUIDE: This is an alternate type of question included in the NCLEX-RN®. The nurse must be able to select all the options

that answer the question correctly. There are no partially correct answers. An RN cannot delegate assessment, teaching, evaluation, medications, or an unstable client to a UAP. Tasks that cannot be delegated are nursing interventions requiring nursing judgment.

45. 1. **The actions of the colleague indicate possible drug or alcohol impairment. The staff nurse is not in a position of authority to require the potentially impaired nurse to submit to a drug test. The administrative supervisor should assess the situation and initiate the appropriate follow-up. The nurse must make sure an impaired nurse is not allowed to care for clients.**
   2. The nurse is not a counselor, and a staff nurse should not attempt to confront an impaired colleague.
   3. The administrative supervisor and the charge nurse are the only staff members who have the authority to send a nurse home.
   4. The nurse should not attempt to determine the cause of the behavior. This is outside the nurse's authority.

CLINICAL JUDGMENT GUIDE: There will be management questions on the NCLEX-RN®. Concepts of Management is included under the category Safe and Effective Environment and subcategory Management of Care.

46. 1. Regurgitation (effortless return of food or gastric contents from the stomach into the esophagus or mouth) is a common manifestation of GERD; therefore, this client would not be assigned to the most experienced nurse.
   2. Barrett's esophagitis is a complication of GERD; new graduates can prepare a client for a diagnostic procedure.
   3. **This client is exhibiting symptoms of asthma, a complication of GERD; therefore, the client should be assigned to the most experienced nurse.**
   4. Pain is expected with a surgical procedure and a less experienced nurse could administer pain medication.

CLINICAL JUDGMENT GUIDE: The test taker must determine which client is the most unstable and would require the most experienced nurse, thus making this an "except" type of question. Three clients are either stable or have non–life-threatening conditions.

47. 1. The nurse should notify the HCP, but it is not the first intervention.
2. The nurse should assess the client for leg cramps, indicating hypokalemia, but the nurse should first ensure the client's cardiac status is stable.
3. **The client is at high risk for cardiac dysrhythmias, because of hypokalemia. The nurse should first assess the cardiac status, then implement other interventions. Remember Maslow's Hierarchy of Needs.**
4. The client will need IV potassium, but this requires an HCP order; therefore, this intervention is not implemented first.

CLINICAL JUDGMENT GUIDE: Before selecting "notify the HCP" as the correct answer, the test taker must examine the other three options. If information in any of the other options contains data that will relieve the client's distress, prevent a life-threatening situation, or provide information the HCP will need to make an informed decision, then the test taker should eliminate the "notify the HCP" option.

48. 1. The charge nurse should discuss the client's anger with the client immediately because the client is preparing to leave the hospital. The charge nurse can talk with the primary nurse after talking with the client.
2. **This is the first action for the charge nurse. The client is preparing to leave, and a delay in going to the client's room could result in the client leaving before the situation can be resolved.**
3. The HCP should be notified, but the charge nurse should assess the situation first.
4. The client will be asked to sign the against medical advice form if he insists on leaving, but the charge nurse should attempt to resolve the situation successfully first.

CLINICAL JUDGMENT GUIDE: The nurse should always apply the nursing process when answering a question requiring the nurse to "determine which intervention to implement first." The first part of the nursing process is to assess.

49. 1. Planning the care of the client cannot be delegated to an unlicensed assistive personnel (UAP), and the client, not the parents, should set the goals.
2. The UAP should stay with the client for an hour after a meal. Leaving the client after 20 minutes would allow the client time to induce vomiting.

3. This requires the nurse to utilize therapeutic conversation and nursing judgment. The nurse cannot delegate this intervention to a UAP.
4. **The UAP can document the amount of food consumed on a calorie-count form for the dietitian to evaluate.**

CLINICAL JUDGMENT GUIDE: An RN cannot delegate assessment, teaching, evaluation, medications, or an unstable client to a UAP. Tasks that cannot be delegated are nursing interventions requiring nursing judgment.

50. 1. **This is an assessment question and should be asked to determine if what the client has attempted has been unsuccessful.**
2. The amount of weight loss desired is not as important as assessment of previous unsuccessful strategies.
3. This is a therapeutic statement, but the nurse should assess the client.
4. This statement is not helpful, and the nurse working in a bariatric clinic should know that there are many options for weight loss, including surgery.

CLINICAL JUDGMENT GUIDE: Assessment is the first step of the nursing process, and the test taker should use the nursing process or some other systematic process to assist in determining priorities.

51. 1. **During a laparoscopic cholecystectomy, carbon dioxide is instilled into the client's abdomen. Postoperatively, the gas migrates to the shoulder by gravity and causes shoulder pain.**
2. This is not an emergency situation, and the nurse should explain this to the client.
3. The nurse should not tell the client to increase the pain medication. This is prescribing.
4. These pains are "gas" pains, but they are not intestinal gas pains that can be relieved by ambulation.

CLINICAL JUDGMENT GUIDE: The nurse must be knowledgeable regarding expected medical treatment for the client. This is a knowledge-based question.

52. 1. The medication is ordered every 4 hours and it has been fewer than 4 hours since ondansetron (Zofran) was last administered. The nurse cannot administer the PRN medication.

2. Diphenoxylate and atropine (Lomotil) is for diarrhea and the client has a soft, brown, formed stool; therefore, the nurse would not administer this medication.
3. **The nurse should call the health-care provider to discuss the situation. The client is nauseated and needs something, but there is nothing ordered that has not been given.**
4. The nurse should not tell the client there is nothing that can be done. The nurse needs to call the health-care provider.

CLINICAL JUDGMENT GUIDE: Before selecting "notify the HCP" as the correct answer, the test taker must examine the other three options. If information in any of the other options contains data that will relieve the client's distress, prevent a life-threatening situation, or provide information the HCP will need to make an informed decision, then the test taker should eliminate the "notify the HCP" option.

53. Correct answers are 1, 3, and 4.
    1. **The HCP must order the insertion of a Sengstaken-Blakemore tube, so this is a collaborative nursing intervention.**
    2. Assessing the client's vital signs does not require an HCP's order, so this is an independent nursing intervention, not a collaborative intervention.
    3. **This is a collaborative intervention that the nurse should implement. It requires an order from the HCP.**
    4. **Obtaining laboratory data requires an HCP's order, so this is a collaborative intervention.**
    5. Monitoring the client's intake and output does not require an HCP's order, so this is an independent nursing intervention, not a collaborative intervention.

CLINICAL JUDGMENT GUIDE: This is an alternate type of question included in the NCLEX-RN®. The nurse must be able to select all the options that answer the question correctly. There are no partially correct answers.

54. 1. Hypoactive bowel sounds are not normal, but it would not warrant immediate intervention. As long as the bowels are moving, it is not an emergency.
    2. The client should have 30 mL of urine output an hour; therefore, this information is normal and does not warrant immediate intervention.

3. These vital signs are normal; therefore, they do not warrant immediate intervention.
4. **Coffee ground emesis indicates bleeding and old blood, and warrants intervention by the nurse. Further assessment is needed to determine if the client is hypovolemic and the HCP should be notified.**

CLINICAL JUDGMENT GUIDE: The test taker should ask, "Is the assessment data normal for the disease process?" If it is normal for the disease process, then the nurse would not need to intervene; if it is not normal for the disease process, then this warrants intervention by the nurse.

55. 1. **The nurse should first determine if the client is hypovolemic before taking any other action. This will determine the nurse's next action.**
    2. The nurse should auscultate the client's bowel sounds to determine if they are present, but not before taking the client's pulse and blood pressure.
    3. The nurse should assess the situation before notifying the HCP.
    4. The nurse may need to reinforce the dressing if the dressing becomes too saturated, but this would occur only after a thorough assessment is completed.

CLINICAL JUDGMENT GUIDE: Before selecting "notify the HCP" as the correct answer, the test taker must examine the other three options. If information in any of the other options contains data that will relieve the client's distress, prevent a life-threatening situation, or provide information the HCP will need to make an informed decision, then the test taker should eliminate the "notify the HCP" option.

56. Answer: 106 gtts per minute.
    The nurse must divide the total amount to be infused by 24 hours to determine the IV rate. 2,550 mL divided by 24 = 106.25

CLINICAL JUDGMENT GUIDE: The NCLEX-RN® test plan includes dosage calculations under Pharmacological and Parenteral Therapies. This category is included under Physiological Integrity, which promotes physical health and wellness by providing care and comfort, reducing client risk potential, and managing health alterations.

57. 1. The nurse must check the medication administration record (MAR) to determine the last time the client received any pain medication, but not before assessing the

client first. Remember: Assessment is the first step of the nursing process.

2. The nurse must assess the client's pain, not the unlicensed assistive personnel (UAP). The nurse cannot delegate assessment.

3. **The first part of the nursing process is assessment. The nurse must first assess the client's pain to determine if the pain indicates a complication requiring medical intervention, or if this is routine postoperative pain, which is expected.**

4. The nurse should not delegate obtaining the vital signs of a client who may be unstable. The nurse must assess the client.

CLINICAL JUDGMENT GUIDE: Any time the nurse receives information about a client (who may be experiencing a complication) from another staff member, the nurse must assess the client. The nurse should not make decisions about the client's needs based on another staff member's information.

58. 1. The client should stay on his right side for at least 2 hours post-procedure, so giving the client a urinal to void in is an appropriate action and does not warrant intervention.

2. The client is not NPO after the procedure, so giving the client water is an appropriate action and does not warrant intervention.

3. **Direct pressure is applied to the site and then the client is placed on the right side to maintain site pressure for at least 2 hours. Turning the client to the left side warrants intervention by the nurse so the client will not hemorrhage.**

4. The unlicensed assistive personnel (UAP) can take the vital signs for the client who is stable; therefore, this action would not warrant intervention.

CLINICAL JUDGMENT GUIDE: Delegation means the nurse is responsible for the UAP's actions and performance. The nurse must correct the UAP's performance to ensure the client is cared for safely in the hospital or the home.

59. 1. Hot water increases pruritus, and soap will cause dry skin, which increases pruritus; therefore, the nurse should discuss this with the UAP.

2. This will help prevent dry skin, which will help decrease pruritus, but this is not the client's first intervention. The nurse should first directly protect the client's skin.

3. **Mittens will help prevent the client from scratching the skin and causing skin**

breakdown, which is a priority for the client diagnosed with liver failure. The client has decreased vitamin K, which will lead to bleeding. The client is also immunosuppressed, which will lead to infection.

4. Diphenhydramine (Benadryl) will help decrease the pruritus, but it will take at least 30 minutes to work. Protecting the client's skin integrity is the priority.

CLINICAL JUDGMENT GUIDE: The nurse should remember that if a client is in distress and the nurse can do something to relieve the distress, then it should be done first, before assessment. The test taker should select an option that directly helps the client's condition.

60. 1. This is "passing the buck," and this is not the best option to select. The nurse should answer the client's question.

2. **Milk thistle has an active ingredient, silymarin, which has been used to treat liver disease for more than 2,000 years. It is both an antioxidant and anti-inflammatory and may improve liver function. This response gives the client factual information.**

3. The nurse should not discourage complementary therapies.

4. This is a judgmental statement and the nurse should encourage the client to ask questions.

CLINICAL JUDGMENT GUIDE: The nurse must be knowledgeable regarding complementary alternative medicine, which includes herbs used to treat medical conditions.

61. 1. The laboratory technician draws serum blood studies, not the unlicensed assistive personnel (UAP).

2. The nurse should not request the UAP to remove the NG tube. This is an invasive tube and judgment is required to remove it.

3. **The UAP can empty feces from a colostomy bag; this is not changing the colostomy bag, just emptying the feces.**

4. The UAP cannot enter HCP orders into the EHR. The UAP assists the nurse with direct client care.

CLINICAL JUDGMENT GUIDE: An RN cannot delegate assessment, teaching, evaluation, medications, or an unstable client to a UAP. Tasks that cannot be delegated are nursing interventions requiring nursing judgment. The test taker must be knowledgeable regarding the role of all members of the multidisciplinary health-care team.

62. 1. **The normal serum sodium level is 135 to 145 mEq/L; this sodium level is elevated, indicating the client is dehydrated, which warrants intervention by the nurse.**

    2. These are normal arterial blood gas results; therefore, the nurse would not need to intervene.

    3. The normal serum potassium level is 3.5 to 5.3 mEq/L; therefore, this laboratory information does not warrant intervention by the nurse.

    4. A stool specimen showing fecal leukocytes would support the diagnosis of gastroenteritis and not warrant immediate intervention by the nurse.

CLINICAL JUDGMENT GUIDE: The nurse must be knowledgeable regarding normal laboratory values. These values must be memorized and the nurse must be able to determine if a laboratory value is normal for the client's disease process or medications the client is taking.

63. 1. **Fluid and electrolyte imbalance is a priority because of the potential for metabolic acidosis and hypokalemia, which are both life threatening, especially in the elderly.**

    2. The client will have diarrhea, but it is not a priority over fluid and electrolyte imbalance.

    3. The client will probably be NPO and will not want to eat, but this diagnosis is not a priority over fluid and electrolyte imbalance.

    4. The client's oral mucous membranes may be dry because of vomiting and diarrhea, but it is not a priority over fluid and electrolyte imbalance.

CLINICAL JUDGMENT GUIDE: The NCLEX-RN® integrates the nursing process throughout the Client Needs categories and subcategories. The nursing process is a scientific, clinical reasoning approach to client care that includes assessment, analysis, planning, implementation, and evaluation. The nurse will be responsible for identifying nursing diagnosis for clients.

64. 1. **Pain should be assessed, even if it is expected for the client's diagnosis, if the other clients are stable.**

    2. The nurse needs to talk to this client, but should assess the client with pain first.

    3. The client diagnosed with IBD who is receiving total parenteral nutrition is stable and would not be assessed first.

    4. The client diagnosed with hepatitis B would be expected to be jaundiced and anorexic, so this client would not be assessed first.

CLINICAL JUDGMENT GUIDE: The test taker should use some tool as a reference to guide in the decision-making process. In this situation, Maslow's Hierarchy of Needs should be applied. Physiological needs have priority over psychosocial ones.

65. 1. The nurse should assess the client for hypovolemia, but the first intervention is to assess the client's surgical wound to determine if wound dehiscence has occurred.

    2. The nurse should determine the client's pain, but not before determining the cause of the pain.

    3. **Assessing the surgical incision is the first intervention because this may indicate the client has wound dehiscence.**

    4. The nurse should not administer pain medication without assessing for potential complications first.

CLINICAL JUDGMENT GUIDE: Assessment is the first step of the nursing process, and the test taker should use the nursing process or some other systematic process to assist in determining priorities.

66. 1. The Jackson-Pratt (JP) drain bulb should be depressed, which indicates suction is being applied. The drain needs to be emptied and suction reapplied, which indicates the drain is not functioning appropriately.

    2. The tube should be pinned to the dressing to prevent the client drain from accidentally being pulled out of the insertion site, but this does not indicate the drain is functioning appropriately.

    3. The insertion site should be pink and without any signs of infection, which include drainage, warmth, and redness, but it does not indicate the drain is functioning appropriately.

    4. **The Jackson-Pratt (JP) drain should be sunken in or depressed, indicating that suction is being applied, which indicates the drain is functioning appropriately.**

CLINICAL JUDGMENT GUIDE: The NCLEX-RN® includes Safe Use of Equipment as a subcategory under Safety and Infection Control, which addresses content on protecting clients, family or significant others, and health-care personnel from health and environmental hazards.

67. 1. The client should urinate 30 mL/hour, so 160 mL in 4 hours is appropriate; the nurse should not assess this client first.

2. **This client was just transferred from the post anesthesia care unit (PACU); therefore, the nurse should assess this client first to perform a baseline assessment and ensure the client is stable.**
3. Flatulence, "gas," indicates the bowels are working, which is normal for a client with abdominal surgery, so this client should not be seen first.
4. The client being discharged would be stable and not a priority for the nurse.

CLINICAL JUDGMENT GUIDE: The test taker must determine which sign or symptom is expected for the surgical procedure. Clients being transferred from more intensive nursing areas to less intensive areas should be assessed upon arrival to the unit.

68. 1. **The client that is morbidly obese will have a large abdomen that prevents the lungs from expanding, and predisposes the client to respiratory complications. Having the client use an incentive spirometer will help prevent respiratory complications.**
2. The client may be weighed daily, but this is not a priority over respiratory complications.
3. Preventing deep vein thrombosis (DVT) is an important intervention, but oxygenation is a priority.
4. The nurse should get the client out of bed as soon as possible to help prevent deep vein thrombosis, but this is not a priority over oxygenation.

CLINICAL JUDGMENT GUIDE: The test taker should use some tool as a reference to guide in the decision-making process. In this situation, Maslow's Hierarchy of Needs should be applied. Oxygenation is a priority.

69. 1. The client diagnosed with ulcerative colitis can have 10 to 12 loose stools a day; therefore, this client should not be seen first.
2. This client should be assessed, but is not a priority over a client diagnosed with a physiological problem.
3. **This client has signs of dehydration, which is not expected when a client is vomiting. The client should remain hydrated even when the client is vomiting.**
4. This is not normal, but it is expected for a client diagnosed with hemorrhoids.

CLINICAL JUDGMENT GUIDE: The test taker must determine which sign or symptom is not expected for the disease process. If the sign or symptom is not expected, then the nurse should assess that client first. This type of question is determining if the nurse is knowledgeable regarding signs or symptoms of a variety of disease processes.

70. **Correct answers are 3 and 5.**
1. Total parenteral nutrition is an intravenous medication; the nurse cannot delegate medication administration to the UAP.
2. The nurse cannot delegate medication administration to the UAP.
3. **The LPN can administer medications to a client.**
4. The RN cannot assign assessment to the LPN.
5. **The UAP can assist the stable postoperative client to the bathroom.**

CLINICAL JUDGMENT GUIDE: The nurse cannot assign assessment, teaching, evaluation, or an unstable client to an LPN. The nurse cannot delegate assessment, teaching, evaluation, medications, or an unstable client to the UAP.

CLINICAL SCENARIO ANSWERS AND RATIONALES

The correct answer number and rationale for why it is the correct answer are given in **boldface type.** Rationales for why the other possible answer options are incorrect also are given, but they are not in boldface type.

1. 1. **Pyrosis is heartburn and is expected in a client diagnosed with GERD. The new graduate can care for this client and administer an antacid.**

2. An endoscopy is a diagnostic test and the client should have bowel sounds; therefore, if the client has no bowel sounds, then this is an unexpected complication and requires a more experienced nurse.
3. This client is exhibiting symptoms of asthma, a complication of GERD; therefore, the client should be assigned to the more experienced nurse.

4. A postoperative cholecystectomy client who is obese and, because of the pain, refuses to deep breathe is at risk of developing pneumonia. This client should have a more experienced nurse to ensure the client takes deep breaths.

2. 1. The HCP would not need to be notified because the potassium level is within the normal limits of 3.5 to 5.5 mEq/L.
   2. **The client's potassium level is within normal limits, so the nurse should continue to monitor the client. The normal level is 3.5 to 5.3 mEq/L or mmol/L.**
   3. Hypokalemia can lead to cardiac dysrhythmias, but the client's potassium level is within normal limits.
   4. The client will need potassium to correct the hypokalemia, but the client's potassium level is within normal limits.

3. **Correct answers are 1 and 2.**
   1. **An admission assessment is an independent intervention that the nurse should implement.**
   2. **Evaluating blood pressure is an independent intervention that the nurse should implement. If the client is able, BPs should be taken lying down, sitting, and standing to assess for orthostatic hypotension.**
   3. This is a collaborative intervention that the nurse should implement. It requires an order from the HCP.
   4. Administering blood products is collaborative, requiring an order from the HCP.
   5. The HCP must order any laboratory work, so this is not an independent nursing intervention.

4. 1. A purple stoma indicates necrosis and requires immediate intervention, so the client should notify the HCP; therefore, the client understands the teaching.
   2. The client should be on a regular diet, and the colostomy will have been working for several days before discharge. The client's statement indicates an understanding of the teaching.
   3. The client should wear a colostomy pouch over the stoma, so it will collect the feces coming from the stoma.
   4. **A sigmoid colostomy must be irrigated daily, so the client will have a bowel movement daily. This statement indicates the client needs more teaching.**

5. **Answer: 94 mL/hour.**
   First determine the total amount to be infused during 24 hours.

6. 1. The client will have a nasogastric tube because the client will be NPO, which will decompress the bowel and help remove hydrochloric acid.
   2. Preventing dehydration is a priority with the client who is NPO.
   3. **The charge nurse should question a sigmoidoscopy. Invasive tests are not completed during an acute exacerbation of diverticulosis.**
   4. The client is in severe pain and should be on bedrest, which will help rest the bowel.

7. 1. The client should be on bedrest for 2 hours, but must be on the right side to prevent hemorrhaging.
   2. The client must be on the right side for 2 hours to prevent hemorrhaging.
   3. **The client should be placed on the right side, same side as liver, to prevent hemorrhaging after the liver biopsy.**
   4. An incident report may need to be completed, but not before taking care of the client by placing the client on the right side.

8. 1. The nurse must notify the infection control nurse as soon as possible so that treatment can start if needed, but this is not the first intervention.
   2. **The charge nurse must first have the nurse complete the adverse occurrence report, so there is written documentation concerning the situation. Then the charge nurse should notify the infection control nurse, who will arrange for post-exposure prophylaxis and then determine if the client has hepatitis.**
   3. Post-exposure prophylaxis may be needed, but this is not the first action.
   4. The infection control nurse will check the status of the client whom the needle was used on before the nurse stuck herself.

9. 1. The client with an inflated Sengstaken-Blakemore tube has acute esophageal varices bleeding and is not stable; therefore, this nursing task cannot be delegated.
   2. The nurse cannot delegate assessment, teaching, evaluation, medications, or an unstable client.
   3. **The client diagnosed with pruritus (itching) is stable and the unlicensed assistive personnel (UAP) can assist with**

showering and a.m. care; therefore, this task can be delegated by the charge nurse.
4. The nurse cannot perform a paracentesis; only an HCP can perform this procedure. Therefore, the UAP cannot assist the nurse.

10. 1. This client's hemoglobin and hematocrit is low, but the client is receiving blood; therefore, this client is stable and does not need to be assessed first.
2. The client diagnosed with ulcerative colitis would be expected to have 10 loose stools

and the potassium level is within normal limits; therefore, this client does not need to be assessed first.
3. **A hard, rigid abdomen and elevated temperature is indicative of peritonitis, which is an acute postoperative complication of abdominal surgery and requires immediate intervention. The charge nurse should assess this client first.**
4. Green bile draining from the NG tube is expected and does not require assessment by the charge nurse.

Renal and Genitourinary Management 6

You are the people who are shaping a better world. One of the secrets of inner peace is the practice of compassion.

—Dalai Lama

QUESTIONS

1. The nurse is caring for the following clients on a medical unit. Which client should the nurse assess **first?**
   1. The client diagnosed with acute glomerulonephritis who has oliguria and periorbital edema
   2. The client diagnosed with benign prostatic hypertrophy who has blood oozing from the intravenous site
   3. The client diagnosed with renal calculi who is complaining of flank pain rated as a 5 on a scale of 1 to 10
   4. The client diagnosed with nephrotic syndrome who has proteinuria and hypoalbuminemia

2. The nurse is inserting an indwelling catheter into a male elderly client. Which intervention should the nurse implement **first?**
   1. Ask the client if he has any prostate problems.
   2. Determine if the client has a povidone iodine allergy.
   3. Lubricate the end of the indwelling catheter.
   4. Ensure urine is obtained in the indwelling catheter.

3. The nurse is preparing to administer intravenous narcotic medication to the client who has renal calculi and is reporting pain rated as 8 on a 1 to 10 pain scale. The client's vital signs are stable. Which intervention should the nurse implement **first?**
   1. Clamp the IV tubing proximal to the port of medication administration.
   2. Administer the narcotic medication slowly over 2 minutes.
   3. Check the medication administration record (MAR) against the hospital identification band.
   4. Determine if the client's intravenous site is patent.

4. The nurse is administering medications to clients on a surgical unit. Which medication should the nurse administer **first?**
   1. Morphine IV infusion to the client who is 8 hours postoperative and is reporting pain, rating it as a 7 on a 1 to 10 pain scale
   2. Vancomycin intravenous piggyback (IVPB) to the client diagnosed with an infected abdominal wound
   3. Pantoprazole IVPB to the client who is at risk for developing a stress ulcer
   4. Furosemide intravenous push (IVP) to the client who has undergone surgical debridement of the right lower limb

5. The RN staff nurse and unlicensed assistive personnel (UAP) are caring for clients on a surgical unit. Which action by the UAP warrants **immediate** intervention?
   1. The UAP empties the indwelling catheter bag for the client with transurethral resection of the prostate (TURP).
   2. The UAP assists a client who received an IV narcotic analgesic 30 minutes ago to ambulate in the hall.
   3. The UAP provides apple juice to the client with a nephrectomy who has just been advanced to a clear liquid diet.
   4. The UAP applies moisture barrier cream to the elderly client diagnosed with urinary incontinence who has an excoriated perianal area.

6. The RN charge nurse is making shift assignments to the surgical staff, which consists of two RNs, two licensed practical nurses (LPNs), and two unlicensed assistive personnel (UAP). Which assignment would be **most** appropriate for the RN charge nurse to make?
   1. Instruct the RN staff nurse to administer all PRN medications.
   2. Instruct the UAP to clean the recently vacated room.
   3. Assign the LPN to change the client's ileal conduit bag.
   4. Request the LPN to complete the admission for a new client.

7. The charge nurse is making assignments in the day surgery center. Which client should be assigned to the **most** experienced nurse?
   1. The 24-year-old client who had a circumcision and is being prepared for discharge
   2. The client scheduled for a cystectomy who is crying and upset about the surgery
   3. The client diagnosed with kidney cancer who is receiving two units of blood
   4. The client who has end-stage renal disease and had an arteriovenous fistula created

8. The nurse is completing the admission assessment on the client scheduled for cystectomy with creation of an ileal conduit. The client tells the nurse, "I am taking saw palmetto for my enlarged prostate." Which intervention should the nurse implement **first**?
   1. Notify the client's HCP to write an order for the herbal supplement.
   2. Ask the client why he is taking an herb for his enlarged prostate.
   3. Consult with the pharmacist to determine any potential drug interactions.
   4. Look up saw palmetto in the *Physicians' Desk Reference* (PDR).

9. The client is upset because the HCP told her she has syphilis. The client asks the nurse, "This is so embarrassing. Do you have to tell anyone about this?" Which statement is the nurse's **best** response?
   1. "This must be reported to the Public Health Department and your sexual partners."
   2. "According to HIPAA, I cannot report this to anyone without your permission."
   3. "You really should tell your sexual partners, so they can be treated for syphilis."
   4. "I realize you are embarrassed. Would you want to talk about the situation?"

10. The RN primary nurse is caring for clients on the renal unit. Which task is **most** appropriate for the RN to delegate to the unlicensed assistive personnel (UAP)?
    1. Instruct the UAP to calculate the clients' urinary intake and output.
    2. Request the UAP to double-check a unit of blood that is being administered.
    3. Tell the UAP to change the surgical dressing on the client with a kidney transplant.
    4. Ask the UAP to transfer the client from the renal unit to the intensive care unit.

11. The nurse is caring for clients on a renal unit and making assignments for the day shift. Which client should the nurse assess **first**?
    1. The client diagnosed with interstitial cystitis who has urinary urgency and pain in the bladder
    2. The client diagnosed with acute post–streptococcal glomerulonephritis who has hematuria with a smoky appearance
    3. The client diagnosed with Goodpasture syndrome who has pallor, anemia, and renal failure
    4. The client diagnosed with nephrolithiasis who has hematuria and is complaining of pain, rating it as a 9 on a 1 to 10 pain scale

12. Which action by the licensed practical nurse (LPN) requires intervention by the critical care RN charge nurse?
1. The LPN has the trough drawn after hanging the aminoglycoside.
2. The LPN changes out a "sharps" container that is over the fill line.
3. The LPN asks another nurse to observe wastage of a narcotic.
4. The LPN inserts an indwelling urinary catheter into the client.

13. The unlicensed assistive personnel (UAP) reports to the RN primary nurse that the client's urine output has bright red blood. Which intervention should the RN implement **first**?
1. Instruct the UAP to take a urine specimen to the laboratory.
2. Document the findings in the client's nursing notes.
3. Assess the client's urine specimen and complete a renal assessment.
4. Ask the UAP to take the client's vital signs.

14. The RN charge nurse is making client assignments. Which client should the charge nurse assign to the graduate nurse (GN) who has just finished orientation?
1. The client with a cystectomy who had a creation of an ileal conduit
2. The client on continuous hemodialysis who is awaiting a kidney transplant
3. The client diagnosed with renal trauma secondary to a motor vehicle accident
4. The client who has had abdominal surgery and whose wound has eviscerated

15. The charge nurse on the intensive care unit (ICU) is notified of a bus accident with multiple injuries and clients are being brought to the emergency department (ED). The hospital is implementing the disaster policy. Which action should the nurse take **first**?
1. Determine which clients could be discharged home immediately.
2. Call any off-duty nurses to notify them to come in to work.
3. Assess the staffing to determine which staff could be sent to the ED.
4. Request all visitors to leave the hospital as soon as possible.

16. The 18-year-old client diagnosed with renal trauma is admitted to the critical care unit after a serious motor vehicle accident resulting from driving under the influence. The mother comes to the unit and starts yelling at her son about "driving drunk." Which action should the nurse implement?
1. Allow the mother to continue talking to her son.
2. Notify the hospital security to remove the mother.
3. Escort the mother to a private area and talk to her.
4. Tell the mother if she wants to stay, she must be quiet.

17. The nurse is caring for an 84-year-old male client diagnosed with benign prostatic hypertrophy. The client has undergone a transurethral resection of the prostate (TURP) and is reporting bladder spasms. Which intervention should the nurse implement **first**?
1. Administer an antispasmodic medication for bladder spasms.
2. Calculate the client's urinary output.
3. Palpate the client's abdomen for bladder distention.
4. Assess the client's three-way urinary catheter for patency.

18. The nurse is caring for clients on a surgical unit. Which client should the nurse assess **first** after shift report?
1. The client diagnosed with polycystic kidney disease who has a BP of 170/100.
2. The client diagnosed with bladder cancer who has gross painless hematuria.
3. The client diagnosed with renal calculi who thinks he passed a stone.
4. The client diagnosed with acute pyelonephritis who has nausea/vomiting and is dehydrated.

19. The 78-year-old client diagnosed with Alport syndrome asks the clinic nurse, "What should I do so I won't get sick this winter?" Which statements should the nurse include in the teaching? **Select all that apply.**
    1. "You should not be around any crowds during the winter months."
    2. "It is recommended you get a flu vaccine yearly."
    3. "You need to eat well-balanced meals each day."
    4. "Dress warmly when it is colder than 40 degrees Fahrenheit outside."
    5. "Wash your hands frequently throughout the day."

20. The elderly female client tells the nurse, "I have vaginal dryness and it hurts when my husband and I make love." Which **priority** intervention should the nurse discuss with the client?
    1. Tell the client to discuss hormone replacement therapy with her HCP.
    2. Encourage the client to refrain from having sexual intercourse.
    3. Recommend the client use a vaginal lubricant before intercourse.
    4. Explain to the client that vaginal dryness is not uncommon in the elderly.

21. The elderly female client diagnosed with osteoporosis is prescribed alendronate. Which intervention is the **priority** when administering this medication?
    1. Administer the medication first thing in the morning.
    2. Ask the client whether she has a history of peptic ulcer disease.
    3. Encourage the client to walk for at least 30 minutes a day.
    4. Have the client remain upright for 30 minutes after administering the medication.

22. Which nursing task should the RN staff nurse on the renal unit assign to the licensed practical nurse (LPN)?
    1. Insert an indwelling urinary catheter before surgery.
    2. Turn and reposition the client every 2 hours.
    3. Measure and record the urine in the bedside commode.
    4. Feed the client who choked on food during the last meal.

23. The nurse on a medical unit has just received the evening shift report. Which client should the nurse assess **first?**
    1. The client diagnosed with renal vein thrombosis who has a heparin drip infusion and a PTT of 92
    2. The client on peritoneal dialysis who has a clear dialysate draining from the abdomen
    3. The client on hemodialysis whose right upper arm fistula has an audible bruit
    4. The client diagnosed with cystitis who is reporting burning on urination

24. The nurse is preparing to administer medications. Which medication should the nurse administer **first?**
    1. Digoxin due at 0900
    2. Furosemide due at 0800
    3. Propoxyphene due in 2 hours
    4. Acetaminophen due in 5 minutes

25. Which intervention should the nurse implement **first** when assisting a client diagnosed with a flaccid bladder to urinate?
    1. Perform the Credé's maneuver on the client.
    2. Perform intermittent catheterization on the client.
    3. Place the client on the bedside commode.
    4. Request the client to drink a full glass of water.

26. The nurse is caring for clients in a family practice clinic. Which client should the nurse assess **first?**
    1. The male client diagnosed with chronic pyelonephritis who has costovertebral tenderness
    2. The female client who is having burning and pain on urination
    3. The female client diagnosed with urethritis who reports dysuria, urgency, and frequent urination
    4. The male client who has hesitancy, terminal dribbling, and intermittency

27. The RN clinic nurse and unlicensed assistive personnel (UAP) are working in a family practice clinic. Which task should the RN delegate to the UAP?
    1. Give the client sample medications for a urinary tract infection (UTI).
    2. Show the client how to use a self-monitoring blood glucometer.
    3. Answer the telephone triage line and take messages from clients.
    4. Take the vital signs of a client scheduled for a physical examination.

28. Which task is **most** appropriate for the RN staff nurse on the renal unit to delegate to the unlicensed assistive personnel (UAP)?
    1. Escort the client diagnosed with acute pyelonephritis to the radiology department for a CT scan.
    2. Obtain a sterile urine specimen for the client to evaluate for a urinary tract infection.
    3. Hang the bag of D_5W for the client diagnosed with post–streptococcal glomerulonephritis.
    4. Provide discharge instructions for the client diagnosed for nephrotic syndrome.

29. Which task should the RN employee health nurse delegate to the unlicensed assistive personnel (UAP)?
    1. Request the UAP read the PPD result administered to the client 72 hours ago.
    2. Ask the UAP to obtain a urine specimen for the client having a urine drug screening.
    3. Tell the UAP to apply an ice pack to the client who slipped and has a sprained right ankle.
    4. Instruct the UAP to complete the incident report for the RN who had a "dirty needle stick."

30. The RN clinic nurse manager in the medical-surgical outpatient clinic is making assignments. Which task is **most** appropriate to delegate/assign to the UAP/LPN?
    1. Ask the LPN to administer the flu vaccine to the client.
    2. Tell the UAP to call the pharmacist to refill a prescription.
    3. Request the LPN to obtain the height and weight of the client.
    4. Instruct the UAP to empty the trashcans in the clients' rooms.

31. Which behavior **warrants** intervention by the clinical manager in the medical-surgical outpatient clinic?
    1. The UAP is discussing a client's condition in the waiting room.
    2. The LPN is talking to a client over the phone about laboratory tests.
    3. The RN is triaging phone messages during his or her lunch break.
    4. The UAP is taking vital signs for the client being placed in a room.

32. The UAP in the school nurse's office is listening to a female student who is pregnant and scared to tell her parents. Which action should the RN school nurse implement?
    1. Tell the UAP she cannot talk to the female student.
    2. Call the student's parents and tell them their daughter is pregnant.
    3. Do not take any action and allow the UAP to listen to the student.
    4. Ask the UAP to leave and continue to talk to the student.

33. The RN clinic nurse observes an LPN discussing an intravenous pyelogram, a diagnostic test, with a client in the waiting room of the outpatient clinic. Which action should the RN implement?
    1. Praise the LPN for talking to the client about the diagnostic test.
    2. Tell the LPN the RN needs to talk to her in the office area.
    3. Go to the waiting room and tell the LPN not to discuss this there.
    4. Inform the HCP that the LPN was talking to the client in the waiting room.

34. The charge nurse in a large outpatient clinic notices the staff members are arguing and irritable with one another and the atmosphere has been very tense for the past week. Which action should the charge nurse take?
    1. Wait for another week to see whether the situation resolves itself.
    2. Write a memo telling all staff members to stop arguing.
    3. Schedule a meeting with the staff to discuss the situation.
    4. Tell the staff to stop arguing or they will be terminated.

35. The employee health nurse is obtaining a urine specimen for a pre-employment drug screen. Which action should the nurse implement **first?**
    1. Obtain informed consent for the procedure.
    2. Maintain the chain of custody for the specimen.
    3. Allow the client to go to any bathroom in the clinic.
    4. Take and record the client's tympanic temperature.

36. The client comes to the clinic reporting pain and burning on urination. Which action should the nurse implement **first?**
    1. Assess and document the client's vital signs.
    2. Determine whether the client has seen any blood in the urine.
    3. Request the client give a midstream urine specimen.
    4. Ask the client whether she wipes front to back after a bowel movement.

37. The nurse is working at the emergency health clinic in a disaster shelter. Which intervention is the **priority** when initially assessing the client?
    1. Find out how long the client will be in the shelter.
    2. Determine whether the client has his or her routine medications.
    3. Document the client's health history in writing.
    4. Assess the client's vital signs, height, and weight.

38. The HCP orders an intravenous pyelogram for the 27-year-old male client diagnosed with a possible renal calculi. The client is diagnosed with schizophrenia and is delusional. Which action should the clinic nurse implement?
    1. Ask the client whether he is allergic to yeast.
    2. Request the client to sign a permit for the procedure.
    3. Obtain informed consent from the client's significant other.
    4. Discuss the local hospital's day surgery procedure with the client.

39. The home health (HH) aide tells the RN home health nurse one of the older male clients is taking saw palmetto every day. Which statement is the RN's **best** response?
    1. "Herbal supplements are dangerous and I will talk to the client."
    2. "Saw palmetto is used to treat benign prostatic hypertrophy. Let him take it."
    3. "I will notify the client's health-care provider as soon as possible."
    4. "Many clients use herbal supplements. He has a right to take it."

40. The home health (HH) aide caring for the client who is postoperative kidney transplant asks the RN home health nurse, "Why is the physical therapist coming to visit the client?" Which statement is the home health RN's **best** response?
    1. "The physical therapist will evaluate the client's swallowing difficulty."
    2. "The physical therapist will assist the client with fine motor coordination."
    3. "The physical therapist will assist with caregiver concerns and making referrals."
    4. "The physical therapist will work with the client on strengthening and endurance."

41. The home health (HH) nurse is admitting a female client diagnosed with end-stage renal disease who refuses to be placed on hemodialysis. The client is ready to die, but verbalizes having so many regrets in her life. Which intervention would be **most** appropriate for the nurse?
    1. Contact the agency chaplain to come talk to the client.
    2. Call her church pastor and discuss the client's concerns.
    3. Ask the client whether or not she would want to pray with the nurse.
    4. Determine whether or not the client has an advance directive.

42. The nurse is preparing to perform a dressing change on a female client who has end-stage renal disease. The nurse notes the client's husband is silently holding the client's hand and praying. Which action should the nurse implement **first?**
    1. Continue to prepare for the dressing change in the room.
    2. Call the chaplain to help the client and spouse pray.
    3. Quietly leave the room and come back later for the dressing change.
    4. Ask the husband whether or not he would want the nurse to join in the prayer.

43. The unit manager on the renal unit is evaluating the staff nurse. Which data should be included in the nurse's yearly evaluation? **Select all that apply.**
    1. The fact that the nurse clocked in late to work twice in the last year
    2. The client's complaint stating the nurse did not answer a call light during a code
    3. The number of times the nurse switched shifts with another nurse
    4. The appropriateness of the nurse's written documentation in the EHR
    5. The nurse's membership in the American Nephrology Nurses Association

44. The hospice nurse is providing follow-up care with the family member of a client who died with chronic renal disease. Which intervention is the **priority?**
    1. Attend the client's funeral service or visitation.
    2. Check on the family member 1 to 2 months after the death of the client.
    3. Make sure the arrangements are what the client wanted.
    4. Help the family member dispose of the client's belongings as soon as possible.

45. The nurse is attempting to start an intravenous (IV) line in an elderly client who is dehydrated. After two unsuccessful attempts, which interventions should the nurse implement? **Select all that apply.**
    1. Keep trying to get a patent IV access.
    2. Ask the HCP to order oral fluid replacement.
    3. Ask a second nurse to attempt to start the IV.
    4. Place cold packs on the client's arms for comfort.
    5. Obtain the portable vein finder device to assist the IV start.

46. The client diagnosed with chronic kidney disease (CKD), and who has a left forearm graft, is assigned to the RN primary nurse and unlicensed assistive personnel (UAP). Which action by the UAP requires **immediate** intervention by the RN?
    1. The UAP avoids using soap while bathing the client.
    2. The UAP takes the BP on the client's left arm.
    3. The UAP tells the client she should not eat chips.
    4. The UAP measures a scant amount of urine in the BSC.

47. The nurse is on the day shift in a long-term care facility. Which medication should the nurse **question** administering to the elderly client diagnosed with chronic pyelonephritis and heart failure?

Client Name: Mr. C.D. Height: 65 inches Date of Birth: 02/10/1942	Account Number: 245869 Weight in pounds: 165 Date: Today	Allergies: NKDA Weight in kg: 75
Medication	0701-1900	1901-0700
Digoxin 0.125 mg PO daily	0900	
Furosemide 40 mg PO daily	0900	
Potassium 20 mEq PO daily	0900	
	1800	
Biscacodyl 5mg PO daily	0900	
Signature/Initials	Day Nurse RN/DN	Night Nurse RN/NN

1. Digoxin
2. Furosemide
3. Potassium
4. Bisacodyl

48. The elderly client diagnosed with heart failure is scheduled to receive a unit of packed red blood cells (PRBCs). The PRBCs are prepared in 350 mL of solution. At what rate should the nurse set the pump?

[   ]

49. Which interventions should the RN staff nurse delegate to the unlicensed assistive personnel (UAP) when caring for the client who is 2 days postoperative open surgery of the kidney? **Select all that apply.**
1. Explain the procedure for using the patient-controlled analgesia (PCA) pump.
2. Check the client's flank surgical dressing for drainage.
3. Take and record the client's vital signs and pulse oximeter reading.
4. Empty the client's indwelling catheter bag at the end of the shift.
5. Assist the client to ambulate in the hallway three to four times a day.

50. The client with open surgery of the kidney has an apical pulse of 118 and BP of 88/58. Which intervention should the nurse implement **first?**
1. Obtain the client's pulse oximeter reading.
2. Check the client's last hemoglobin and hematocrit.
3. Notify the client's surgeon immediately.
4. Monitor the client's urine output.

51. The 88-year-old female client is reporting urinary frequency and dribbling. Which nursing interventions should be implemented? **Rank in order of performance.**
1. Have the UAP make rounds on the client every 2 hours.
2. Give the client perineal pads to place inside her underwear.
3. Place an absorbent pad on the client's bed.
4. Put a bedside commode at the client's bedside.
5. Instruct the client in providing a clean-catch urine specimen.

52. The nurse in the dialysis center is initiating the morning dialysis run. Which client should the nurse assess **first?**
1. The client who has a hemoglobin of 9.0 mg/dL and hematocrit of 26%
2. The client who does not have a palpable thrill or auscultated bruit
3. The client who is reporting a 3.6 kg weight gain and is refusing dialysis
4. The client on peritoneal dialysis who is reporting a hard, rigid abdomen

53. The male client diagnosed with chronic kidney disease has received the initial dose of erythropoietin 1 week ago. Which data **warrants** the nurse to notify the health-care provider?
    1. The client has a pulse oximeter reading of 95%.
    2. The client has a platelet count of 155,000.
    3. The client has a blood pressure reading of 184/102.
    4. The client has a tympanic temperature of 99.8°F.

54. The nurse is developing a nursing care plan for the client diagnosed with chronic kidney disease. Which nursing problem should be addressed **first?**
    1. Self-care deficit
    2. Knowledge deficit
    3. Chronic pain
    4. Excess fluid volume

55. The client diagnosed with chronic kidney disease is placed on a fluid restriction of 1,500 milliliters per day. On the 7 a.m. to 7 p.m. shift the client drank an 8-ounce cup of coffee, 8 ounces of juice, 16 ounces of tea, and 8 ounces of water with medications. What amount of fluid can the 7 p.m. to 7 a.m. nurse give to the client?

    [   ]

56. The client receiving dialysis is reporting feeling dizzy and light-headed. Which **priority** intervention should the nurse implement?
    1. Place the client in the reverse Trendelenburg position.
    2. Decrease the volume of blood being removed from the client.
    3. Bolus the client 300 mL of 0.9% saline solution.
    4. Notify the health-care provider as soon as possible.

57. The client is NPO and is receiving total parenteral nutrition (TPN) via a subclavian line. Which precautions should the nurse implement? **Select all that apply.**
    1. Place the client's TPN on a gravity intravenous line.
    2. Monitor the client's blood glucose every 24 hours.
    3. Weigh the client daily, first thing in the morning.
    4. Change the client's IV tubing with every TPN bag administered.
    5. Monitor the client's intake and output every shift.

58. The client has received IV solutions for 3 days through a 20-gauge IV catheter placed in the left cephalic vein. On morning rounds the nurse notes the IV site is tender to palpation, it is edematous, and a red streak has formed. Which interventions should the nurse implement? **Rank in order of performance.**
    1. Start a new IV in the right hand.
    2. Discontinue the intravenous line.
    3. Complete an incident report.
    4. Place a warm washcloth over the old IV site.
    5. Document the situation in the client's EHR.

59. The RN staff nurse and unlicensed assistive personnel (UAP) are caring for a group of clients. Which nursing intervention should the RN perform?
    1. Measure the client's output from the indwelling catheter.
    2. Record the client's intake and output on the I&O sheet.
    3. Instruct the client on appropriate fluid restrictions.
    4. Provide water for a client diagnosed with acute pyelonephritis.

60. The nurse emptied 2,340 mL from the drainage bag of a continuous irrigation of a client who had a transurethral resection of the prostate (TURP). The amount of irrigation in the hanging bag was 3,000 mL at the beginning of the shift. There was 1,550 mL left in the bag 8 hours later. What is the correct urine output at the end of the 8 hours?

    [   ]

61. Which nursing diagnosis is the **priority** for the client who has undergone a transurethral resection of the prostate (TURP)?
    1. Potential for sexual dysfunction
    2. Potential for altered urinary elimination
    3. Potential for infection
    4. Potential for hemorrhage

62. The client is 1-day postoperative transurethral resection of the prostate (TURP). Which action by the unlicensed assistive personnel (UAP) **warrants** intervention by the RN staff nurse?
    1. The UAP increased the client's irrigation fluid to clear clots from the tubing.
    2. The UAP elevated the client's scrotum on a towel roll for support.
    3. The UAP emptied the client's indwelling urinary catheter bag.
    4. The UAP brought ice water to the client's bedside.

63. The male client diagnosed with renal calculi is admitted to the medical unit. Which intervention should the nurse implement **first?**
    1. Request the client to urinate in a urinal.
    2. Assess the client's pain.
    3. Increase the client's oral fluid intake.
    4. Strain the client's urine.

64. The female client diagnosed with renal calculi is scheduled for a STAT kidney, ureter, bladder (KUB). Which statement by the client **warrants** intervention by the nurse?
    1. "I am allergic to shellfish and iodine."
    2. "I just had my lunch tray and ate all of it."
    3. "I have not had my period for 3 months."
    4. "I am having pain in my lower back."

65. The client diagnosed with renal calculi is scheduled for a 24-hour urine specimen collection. Which interventions should the nurse implement? **Select all that apply.**
    1. Keep the client NPO during the time the urine is being collected.
    2. Instruct the client to urinate, and include this urine when starting collection.
    3. Place the client's urine in an appropriate specimen container for 24 hours.
    4. Insert an indwelling catheter in the client after having the client empty his or her bladder.
    5. Post signs on the client's door alerting staff to save all the client's urine output.

66. The client diagnosed with renal calculi is 1-hour post-procedure lithotripsy. Which task is **most** appropriate for the RN primary nurse to delegate to the unlicensed assistive personnel (UAP)?
    1. Tell the UAP to check the amount, color, and consistency of the client's urine output.
    2. Request the UAP to transcribe the client's health-care provider's orders.
    3. Instruct the UAP to strain the client's urine and place any sediment in a sterile container.
    4. Ask the UAP to take the client's post-procedural vital signs.

67. The client had surgery to remove a kidney stone. Which laboratory assessment data **warrants** intervention by the nurse?
    1. A serum potassium level of 5.2 mEq/L
    2. A urinalysis showing blood in the urine
    3. A creatinine level of 1.1 mg/dL
    4. A white blood cell count of 9.510^3/microL

68. Which intervention should the nurse implement **first** for the client diagnosed with urinary incontinence?
    1. Palpate the bladder after an incontinent episode.
    2. Administer oxybutynin.
    3. Ensure the client does not sit or lie in the urine.
    4. Instruct the client to go to the bathroom every 2 hours.

69. The nurse is caring for an elderly female client who has an indwelling catheter. Which data **warrants** notifying the health-care provider?
    1. The client's vital signs are T 98, AP 90, RR 16, BP 142/88.
    2. The client has had a change in her mental status.
    3. The client's urine is cloudy with sediment.
    4. The client has no discomfort or pain.

70. The RN primary nurse is observing the unlicensed assistive personnel (UAP) provide care to a client with an indwelling catheter. Which action by the UAP warrants **immediate** intervention by the RN?
    1. The UAP does not secure the tubing to the client's leg.
    2. The UAP wears gloves when providing catheter care to the client.
    3. The UAP positions the collection bag on the side of the client's bed.
    4. The UAP cares for the client's catheter after washing his or her hands.

RENAL AND GENITOURINARY CLINICAL SCENARIO

The clinical manager on a 20-bed renal unit in a large county hospital is the RN charge nurse for the 7 p.m. to 7 a.m. shift today because the regular charge nurse is on emergency family leave. The client population is primarily socioeconomically disadvantaged. Staff for the shift includes two RNs, one LPN, and two unlicensed assistive personnel (UAPs).

1. The RN and the UAP are caring for clients on the unit. Which nursing task would be **most** appropriate for the RN to delegate to the UAP?
    1. Assist the radiology technician with a portable chest x-ray on an obese client.
    2. Evaluate the elderly client's 8-hour intake and output.
    3. Perform in and out catheterization on an adolescent client for a sterile urine specimen.
    4. Administer a cation-exchange resin enema on a 51-year-old female client.

2. The RN is preparing to perform hemodialysis on the depressed middle age client diagnosed with end-stage renal disease. Which data warrants **immediate** intervention from the RN?
    1. A hemoglobin of 9.8 mg/dL and hematocrit of 30%
    2. Inability to palpate thrill or auscultate a bruit
    3. Reports being exhausted and unable to sleep
    4. No urine output in the past 12 hours

3. The client diagnosed with renal cell carcinoma who is 1-day postoperative cystectomy has a nasogastric tube (NGT) in place and an IV running at 150 mL/hr via an IV pump. Which data should the RN report to the health-care provider?
    1. The client's peripheral intravenous access is infiltrated.
    2. The client has hypoactive bowel sounds.
    3. The client has crackles bilaterally in the lower lobes.
    4. The client has 2+ bilateral pedal pulses.

4. The elderly male client is diagnosed with chronic glomerulonephritis. Which lab value indicates the condition has worsened?
    1. The BUN is 18 mg/dL.
    2. The creatinine level is 1.0 mg/dL.
    3. The glomerular filtration rate (GFR) is 60 mL/minute.
    4. The 24-hour creatinine clearance is 120 mL/minute.

5. The UAP emptied 3,000 mL from the drainage bag of a continuous bladder irrigation (CBI) of a 75-year-old client who had a transurethral resection of the prostate (TURP). The amount of irrigation in the bag hanging was 4,000 mL at the beginning of the shift. There was 2,000 mL left in the bag at 0700. What is the corrected urine volume output for the shift?

[   ]

6. The elderly client returned from surgery after having a TURP and has a P 96, R 20, BP 110/70, and light pink urine draining in the indwelling urinary catheter bag. Which interventions should the RN implement? **Select all that apply.**
   1. Assess the urine in the continuous irrigation drainage bag.
   2. Increase the irrigation fluid in the continuous irrigation catheter.
   3. Lower the head of the bed while raising the foot of the bed (Trendelenburg).
   4. Contact the surgeon to give an update on the client's condition.
   5. Monitor the client's postoperative hematocrit and hemoglobin.

7. The young female client diagnosed with renal calculi is admitted to the unit. Which intervention should the RN implement **first?**
   1. Complete the admission assessment documentation.
   2. Assess the client's pain and rule out complications.
   3. Increase the client's oral fluid intake.
   4. Enter into the EHR the health-care provider's orders.

8. The obese client with constant left flank pain diagnosed with renal calculi is scheduled for a lithotripsy procedure. Which post-procedure client-care task is **most** appropriate for the RN to delegate to the UAP?
   1. Assess the amount, color, and consistency of urine output.
   2. Teach the client about care of the indwelling urinary catheter.
   3. Instruct the UAP to strain the client's urine.
   4. Assess the client for burning on urination.

9. The charge nurse is making rounds on clients in the renal unit. Which client should the charge nurse assess **first?**
   1. The depressed client diagnosed with end-stage renal disease on hemodialysis who has a palpable thrill
   2. The young female client diagnosed with acute glomerulonephritis who has hematuria and proteinuria
   3. The elderly client diagnosed with bladder cancer who has painless urination with bright red urine
   4. The malnourished male client with an ileal conduit who has not had any drainage in the drainage bag

10. The RN staff nurse and the LPN are caring for clients on the renal unit. Which intervention should the RN assign to the LPN?
    1. Teach the elderly client about home care of the suprapubic catheter.
    2. Monitor the obese post-op client with a WBC of 22,000 mm/dL.
    3. Administer antineoplastic medications to the client diagnosed with bladder cancer.
    4. Administer a narcotic analgesic to the client diagnosed with renal calculi.

ANSWERS AND RATIONALES

The correct answer number and rationale for why it is the correct answer are given in **boldface type.** Rationales for why the other possible answer options are incorrect also are given, but they are not in boldface type.

1. 1. The nurse would expect the client diagnosed with acute glomerulonephritis to have oliguria and periorbital edema. Acute glomerulonephritis is a disorder of the glomeruli (glomerulonephritis), or small blood vessels in the kidneys.
   2. **The nurse would not expect the client diagnosed with BPH to have oozing blood from the intravenous site. This may indicate disseminated intravascular coagulation (DIC), which is a potentially life-threatening complication and requires immediate intervention.**
   3. The nurse would expect the client diagnosed with renal calculi to have pain, but a level 5 indicates the pain is under control; therefore, this client does not need to be seen first.
   4. The nurse would expect the client diagnosed with nephrotic syndrome to have proteinuria (protein in the urine) and hypoalbuminemia (decreased protein in the blood). Nephrotic syndrome is a nonspecific disorder in which the kidneys are damaged, causing them to leak large amounts of protein into the urine.

CLINICAL JUDGMENT GUIDE: The nurse must determine which sign or symptom is not expected for the disease process. If the sign or symptom is not expected, or if it is an emergency situation, the nurse should assess the client first. This type of question is determining if the nurse is knowledgeable regarding signs or symptoms of a variety of disease processes.

2. 1. This is an appropriate question, but even clients diagnosed with prostate problems can have an indwelling catheter if inserted carefully.
   2. **Povidone iodine (Betadine) is included in the indwelling catheter kit; therefore, another form of cleaning agent must be used when inserting the catheter. Therefore, this is the first intervention.**
   3. This is appropriate, but not the first intervention.
   4. Urine should be obtained in the catheter, but it is not the first intervention.

CLINICAL JUDGMENT GUIDE: When the question asks, "Which intervention should be implemented first?" it means all the options are things a nurse could implement, but only one should be implemented first. The nurse should use the nursing process and remember: If the client is in distress, do not assess; if the client is not in distress, the nurse should assess.

3. 1. The nurse should clamp the tubing to ensure the medication goes directly into the client and not retrograde up the tubing, but it is not the first administration.
   2. The medication should be administered over 2 minutes, but it is not the first intervention.
   3. The nurse should always ensure the medication is being administered to the correct client, but the nurse should first make sure the route of administration is safe.
   4. **Ensuring the site is patent is the first intervention because even if it is the correct client, the medication should not be administered if the IV site is infiltrated.**

CLINICAL JUDGMENT GUIDE: When the question asks, "Which intervention should be implemented first?" it means all the options are things a nurse could implement, but only one should be implemented first. The nurse should use the nursing process and remember: If the client is in distress, do not assess; if the client is not in distress, the nurse should assess.

4. 1. **The client who is in pain is the priority. None of the other clients have a life-threatening condition. Pain is considered the fifth vital sign.**
   2. Routine antibiotics are not a priority over a client who has postoperative pain.
   3. Risk for a stress ulcer is a potential, not an actual problem, and proton-pump inhibitors are administered routinely to help prevent stress ulcers.
   4. The loop diuretic is a routine medication prescribed for a medical comorbid condition, not for surgical debridement.

CLINICAL JUDGMENT GUIDE: When the nurse is making a decision about prioritizing medication administration, client comfort takes priority over regularly scheduled medications.

5. 1. The unlicensed assistive personnel (UAP) can empty an indwelling catheter drainage bag because this does not require judgment.
   2. The client who received a narcotic analgesic 30 minutes ago is at risk for falling because of the effects of the medication; therefore, the UAP should not ambulate this client. The nurse should intervene.
   3. The UAP can provide juice to the client, and apple juice is part of the client's liquid diet.
   4. Moisture barrier cream is not a medication; therefore, the UAP can apply such creams to an intact perianal area.

CLINICAL JUDGMENT GUIDE: The nurse cannot delegate assessment, evaluation, teaching, administration of medications, or an unstable client to an unlicensed assistive personnel (UAP).

6. 1. The LPN can administer routine as well as some PRN medications; assigning the LPN to administer all PRN medications is not appropriate.
   2. The housekeeping department, not the UAP, is assigned to clean recently vacated rooms.
   3. It is within an LPN's scope of practice to change an ileal conduit drainage bag; therefore, this would be the most appropriate assignment for the LPN.
   4. The nurse would be the most appropriate staff member to complete the admission assessment.

CLINICAL JUDGMENT GUIDE: When the nurse is deciding which option is the most appropriate task to delegate or assign, the nurse should choose the task that allows each staff member to function within his or her scope of practice. Remember, the nurse cannot delegate assessment, teaching, evaluation, medications, or an unstable client to the UAP and cannot assign assessment, teaching, evaluation, or an unstable client to the LPN.

7. **1. The most experienced nurse should be assigned to the client who requires teaching before being discharged. Postoperative complications can occur, so the client must be knowledgeable regarding when to call the health-care provider and how to take care of the surgical site.**
   2. A less experienced nurse can talk to the client who is crying and upset. The most experienced nurse should care for a client who requires more knowledge.
   3. A less experienced nurse can administer and monitor blood transfusion to the client.

4. Although the creation of an arteriovenous fistula requires assessment and teaching on the part of the most experienced nurse, this client is not being discharged home at this time.

CLINICAL JUDGMENT GUIDE: The nurse must determine which client is the most unstable or requires extensive teaching. This client requires the most experienced nurse, thus making this type of question an "except" question. Three clients are either stable or have non–life-threatening conditions.

8. 1. If the HCP deems that the client can continue to take the herbal supplement, then an order must be written; however, this is not the first intervention.
   2. The nurse could ask for clarification of the reason he is taking the herbal supplement, but this is not the first intervention. Many clients use herbal supplements for a variety of health-care needs.
   3. According to the NCSBN NCLEX-RN® test plan, collaboration with interdisciplinary team members is part of the management of care. The nurse should first consult with the pharmacist to determine whether the client is taking any medications that could interact with the saw palmetto.
   4. The PDR is available to research medications, not herbal supplements.

CLINICAL JUDGMENT GUIDE: The nurse must be knowledgeable regarding interventions when administering medications to clients undergoing surgery, such as: the client should not receive any PO medications, the client should not receive any medications that could increase bleeding, or determining if the client is taking any complementary alternative medications, such as herbs.

9. **1. HIPAA does not apply in some situations, including the reporting of sexually transmitted diseases to the Public Health Department. The Public Health Department will attempt to notify any sexual partners the client reports.**
   2. This is a false statement. HIPAA does not apply in certain situations, and the nurse must be knowledgeable regarding HIPAA guidelines.
   3. The client should notify her sexual partners so they can be treated; however, in response to the client asking, "Does anyone have to

know?" the nurse's best response is to provide facts.

4. This is a therapeutic response aimed at encouraging the client to verbalize feelings, but the nurse should provide factual information in this situation.

CLINICAL JUDGMENT GUIDE: There will be management questions on the NCLEX-RN®. In many instances, there is no test-taking strategy for these questions; the nurse must be knowledgeable of management issues. The Health Insurance Portability and Accountability Act (HIPAA) passed into law in 1996 to standardize exchange of information between healthcare providers and to ensure patient record confidentiality.

10. 1. **The unlicensed assistive personnel (UAP) can calculate intake and output for clients. The UAP cannot evaluate the numbers to determine if the treatment is effective, but the UAP can obtain the numbers.**

    2. Two nurses must double-check a unit of blood before infusing the blood; therefore, this task cannot be delegated.

    3. The surgeon or the nurse must change the surgical dressing for a kidney transplant. This task cannot be delegated to personnel with a lower level of expertise.

    4. The UAP cannot transfer the unstable client from the renal unit to the intensive care unit.

CLINICAL JUDGMENT GUIDE: An RN cannot delegate assessment, teaching, evaluation, medications, or an unstable client to a UAP. Tasks that cannot be delegated are nursing interventions requiring nursing judgment.

11. 1. Interstitial cystitis is a chronic, painful inflammatory disease of the bladder characterized by urgency or frequency, as well as pain in the bladder or pelvis. Because the signs and symptoms are expected, the nurse would not assess this client first.

    2. The clinical manifestations of acute post–streptococcal glomerulonephritis are varied, including generalized body edema, hypertension, oliguria, hematuria with a smoky or rusty appearance, and proteinuria. Because the signs and symptoms are expected, the nurse would not assess this client first.

    3. Goodpasture syndrome is a rare autoimmune disease seen primarily in young male smokers characterized by hematuria, weakness, pallor,

anemia, and renal failure. Because the signs and symptoms are expected, the nurse would not assess this client first.

4. **Nephrolithiasis, kidney stones, is characterized by pain and hematuria, but the nurse must assess the pain to determine whether a complication has occurred or it is the expected routine pain. Pain is the common priority of these four clients.**

CLINICAL JUDGMENT GUIDE: The nurse can use Maslow's Hierarchy of Needs to determine which client to assess first. Pain is a physiological need.

12. 1. **The trough should be drawn before the aminoglycoside, vancomycin, antibiotic is hung. This requires intervention by the critical care charge nurse.**

    2. The LPN should change out a "sharps" container that is full; if not changed, then this constitutes an OSHA violation.

    3. The LPN must have a narcotic wastage observed by another nurse.

    4. The LPN can insert an indwelling urinary catheter in his or her scope of practice.

CLINICAL JUDGMENT GUIDE: The nurse must know the scope of practice for the LPN. The nurse must know the correct procedure for administering medications to the client and OSHA standards.

13. 1. The unlicensed assistive personnel (UAP) can take a specimen to the laboratory, but this is not the first intervention.

    2. The findings should be documented in the nurse's notes, but it is not the first intervention.

    3. **The nurse must first assess the UAP's findings and the client before taking any further action.**

    4. The UAP can take the client's vital signs, but it is not the first intervention for the nurse.

CLINICAL JUDGMENT GUIDE: A rule of thumb when answering test questions is this: If anyone gives the nurse information about a client, the nurse's first intervention is to assess the client. The nurse should always make decisions based on his or her assessment of the client.

14. 1. **Although cystectomy is a major surgical procedure, it has a predictable course, and no complications were identified. After removing the bladder, the client must have an ileal conduit. This is expected with this type of surgery and the**

new graduate nurse could be assigned this client.

2. A client on continuous hemodialysis would require a nurse trained in this area of nursing; therefore, this client should be assigned to a more experienced nurse.

3. Renal trauma is unpredictable and requires continuous assessment. A more experienced nurse should be assigned to this client.

4. An eviscerated wound indicates the client's incision has opened and the bowels are out of the abdomen. This client is critically ill and should not be assigned to an inexperienced nurse.

CLINICAL JUDGMENT GUIDE: When the test taker is deciding which client should be assigned to a new graduate, the most stable client should be assigned to the least experienced nurse.

15. 1. The charge nurse should have as many beds as possible available for any clients who must be transferred to the unit. The charge nurse should send a nurse to the ED and then assess the bed situation.

2. This may need to be done, but it is not the first intervention, and the charge nurse could assign this to a staff member who is not providing direct client care.

3. **Most disaster policies require one nurse to be sent immediately from each area; therefore, this intervention should be implemented first. The charge nurse must determine which staff nurse would be most helpful in the ED without compromising the staffing in the ICU.**

4. The charge nurse should not request anyone to leave the hospital. This is not typical protocol for a disaster.

CLINICAL JUDGMENT GUIDE: The nurse must be knowledgeable regarding emergency preparedness. Employees receive this information in employee orientation and are responsible for implementing procedures correctly. The NCSBN NCLEX-RN® test plan includes questions on a safe and effective care environment.

16. 1. The nurse must diffuse the situation and remove the mother from the client's room because a seriously ill client does not need to be yelled at.

2. Hospital security does not need to be called unless the mother refuses to leave the client's room in the critical care unit.

3. **The nurse should remove the mother from the room and allow her to vent her feelings about the accident her son sustained while he was under the influence.**

4. The nurse should remove the mother because she is upset and let her vent. Telling the mother she must be quiet is condescending, and when someone is upset, telling the person to be quiet is not helpful.

CLINICAL JUDGMENT GUIDE: The NCLEX-RN® test plan includes Therapeutic Communication as a subcategory in Psychosocial Integrity. The nurse should allow clients and family to vent feelings.

17. 1. The nurse may need to administer an antispasmodic medication, but not before assessment of the client. Bladder spasms in a client who has had a TURP are usually caused by clots remaining in the bladder. A three-way indwelling catheter that is working properly will flush the clots from the bladder.

2. The nurse should calculate the client's urine output, but that is not the first intervention and will not address the client's pain.

3. The nurse could palpate the client's bladder for distention, but this will not help decrease the client's pain.

4. **The three-way indwelling catheter is placed during surgery to keep blood clots from remaining in the bladder and causing bladder spasms and increasing bleeding. The nurse should first assess the drainage system to make sure that it has not become obstructed with a clot.**

CLINICAL JUDGMENT GUIDE: The test taker should use a systematic guide when deciding on a priority intervention. The nursing process is an excellent tool for the test taker to use in this question. Assessment is the first step of the nursing process.

18. 1. The client diagnosed with polycystic kidney disease, the most common life-threatening genetic disease in the world, is expected to have hypertension along with hematuria and a feeling of heaviness in the back, side, or abdomen. The nurse should not assess this client first because the clinical manifestations are expected.

2. The clinical manifestation of bladder cancer is painless gross hematuria; therefore, the nurse would not assess this client first.

3. The nurse should check to determine whether the client has passed a stone, but this is a desired outcome and could wait until the client with an emergency has been assessed and appropriate interventions initiated.

4. **The client diagnosed with acute pyelonephritis, an inflammation of the renal parenchyma and collecting system, is not expected to get dehydrated; therefore, this client should be assessed first.**

CLINICAL JUDGMENT GUIDE: The test taker must read all the options to determine whether an option contains a life-threatening situation. If an option contains information that is expected or within normal limits, that client does not have priority.

19. **Correct answers are 2, 3, 4, and 5.**
    1. Avoiding all crowds may help the elderly client avoid getting a cold or the flu, but it is not usually possible and can be detrimental mentally and physically to the client.
    2. **The yearly flu shot helps to prevent getting sick during the winter months, because the flu can cause serious illness, and even death, in the elderly. Alport syndrome is also known as hereditary nephritis.**
    3. **Eating a well-balanced diet is important to maintain health and support a healthy immune system.**
    4. **Dressing appropriately in the winter months is important as poor circulation can cause distress and impact immunity in the elderly.**
    5. **Frequent hand washing can help avoid illness and prevent spreading germs to others.**

CLINICAL JUDGMENT GUIDE: This is an alternate type of question included in the NCLEX-RN®. The nurse must be able to select all the options that answer the question correctly. There are no partially correct answers. The nurse must be able to teach health promotion to clients. Immunizations are a priority for children and the elderly.

20. 1. Hormone replacement therapy may be needed, but not because of vaginal dryness. The client should discuss this with her HCP, but it does not address the client's statement.
    2. Many elderly people are sexually active and sexual activity should be encouraged, not discouraged, by the nurse.
    3. **Vaginal lubricant will help with the vaginal dryness and help decrease pain during sexual intercourse.**

4. Vaginal dryness is common in the elderly, but the nurse should discuss ways to address the dryness, not explain that it is normal.

CLINICAL JUDGMENT GUIDE: When the question asks for the priority intervention, it means one or more of the options could be something a nurse might discuss with the client. The test taker should select the option that answers the client's statement directly.

21. 1. The bisphosphonate medication alendronate (Fosamax) should be administered in the morning on an empty stomach to increase absorption, but it is not a priority over the client's sitting up for 30 minutes. The client should remain upright for at least 30 minutes to prevent regurgitation into the esophagus and esophageal erosion.
    2. The client diagnosed with peptic ulcer disease may be more at risk for esophageal erosion, but the HCP should have assessed this before prescribing this medication for the client.
    3. The client diagnosed with osteoporosis should be encouraged to walk to increase bone density, but this is not pertinent when administering the medication.
    4. **The bisphosphonate medication alendronate (Fosamax) should be administered on an empty stomach with a full glass of water to promote absorption of the medication. The client should remain upright for at least 30 minutes to prevent regurgitation into the esophagus and esophageal erosion.**

CLINICAL JUDGMENT GUIDE: The nurse must be aware of interventions that need to be implemented when administering medications. The nurse must know which interventions will help prevent untoward complications when administering medications.

22. 1. **The LPN is qualified to perform a sterile procedure, such as inserting an indwelling catheter before surgery. This is an appropriate assignment.**
    2. Turning and repositioning a client can be delegated to an unlicensed assistive personnel (UAP).
    3. Emptying a client's bedside commode and recording the amount of urine can be delegated to a UAP.
    4. The nurse should feed the client who choked during the last meal to assess the client's

ability to swallow. This client is unstable and cannot be assigned or delegated.

CLINICAL JUDGMENT GUIDE: The nurse cannot delegate or assign assessment, teaching, evaluation, or an unstable client to an LPN. The LPN can transcribe HCP orders, can call HCPs on the phone to obtain orders for a client, and can perform sterile procedures.

23. 1. **The therapeutic PTT level should be 1.5 to 2 times the normal PTT of 39 seconds. The therapeutic levels of heparin are 58 and 78. With a PTT of 92, the client is at risk for bleeding, and the heparin drip should be held. The nurse should assess this client first.**
    2. The client on peritoneal dialysis should have clear dialysate, so this client does not have to be assessed first.
    3. The client on hemodialysis should have an audible bruit over the fistula, which indicates the fistula is patent.
    4. Cystitis is inflammation of the urinary bladder, and burning on urination is an expected symptom.

CLINICAL JUDGMENT GUIDE: The test taker must determine if any of the assessment data are normal or abnormal for the client's diagnosis. If the data are abnormal, then this client should be seen first.

24. 1. Digoxin (Lanoxin), a cardiac glycoside, can be administered later because it is a routine medication.
    2. Furosemide (Lasix), a loop diuretic, can be administered within the 1-hour leeway (30 minutes before and after); it does not need to be administered first.
    3. Propoxyphene (Darvon), an analgesic, is not due yet; the nurse should assess the client and determine whether nonpharmacological interventions to relieve pain can be implemented, but this medication cannot be administered for 2 hours.
    4. **Acetaminophen (Tylenol), an analgesic, is administered for mild-to-moderate pain. By the time the nurse obtains the medication and performs all the steps to administer a medication correctly, it will be time for the client to receive the Tylenol. This medication should be administered first.**

CLINICAL JUDGMENT GUIDE: The nurse must be knowledgeable regarding how and when to administer medications.

25. 1. **Credé's maneuver is a method used for expressing urine by pressing the hand on the bladder, especially a paralyzed bladder. It is a noninvasive procedure and should be implemented first before catheterization, which is an invasive procedure.**
    2. Intermittent catheterization is an invasive procedure, which may lead to possible infection when done every 3 to 4 hours.
    3. The nurse could place the client on the bedside commode, but this is used for clients diagnosed with an uninhibited bladder pattern.
    4. Drinking water before attempting to urinate will not help the client.

CLINICAL JUDGMENT GUIDE: If the nurse is undecided between an invasive and a noninvasive procedure, the nurse should select the noninvasive procedure first.

26. 1. The client diagnosed with pyelonephritis typically presents with costovertebral tenderness over the affected side; therefore, this is expected and the nurse would not assess this client first.
    2. **More than likely this client has a urinary tract infection, which requires a midstream urinalysis. Of these four clients, this client should be seen first to have the test ordered.**
    3. The client diagnosed with urethritis would present with these symptoms; therefore, the clinic nurse would not need to see this client first.
    4. Hesitancy, terminal dribbling, and intermittency are signs and symptoms of benign prostatic hypertrophy, which may require surgery; therefore, this client should not be seen before a client diagnosed with a possible urinary tract infection.

CLINICAL JUDGMENT GUIDE: When deciding which client to assess first, the test taker should determine whether the signs and symptoms the client is exhibiting are normal for the client situation. After eliminating the expected options, the test taker should determine which situation can be cured and which is more life threatening.

27. 1. The nurse should not delegate medication administration, including giving the client boxes of sample medications, to an unlicensed assistive personnel (UAP).
    2. Showing the client how to use a glucometer is teaching the client, and the nurse cannot delegate teaching.

3. Triaging calls requires nursing judgment; this responsibility cannot be delegated to the UAP.

4. **The UAP is trained to take vital signs on a client who is stable. This task could safely be delegated by the nurse.**

CLINICAL JUDGMENT GUIDE: The nurse cannot delegate assessment, evaluation, teaching, administration of medications, or care of an unstable client to a UAP.

28. 1. **The unlicensed assistive personnel (UAP) can escort a client who is stable to the radiology department; therefore, this is the most appropriate task to delegate to the UAP.**

2. The UAP cannot obtain a sterile specimen; therefore, this task cannot be delegated.

3. The UAP cannot hang intravenous bags because they are medications, and medication administration cannot be delegated to a UAP.

4. Discharge instructions are teaching, and teaching cannot be delegated to a UAP.

CLINICAL JUDGMENT GUIDE: An RN cannot delegate assessment, teaching, evaluation, medications, or an unstable client to a UAP. Tasks that cannot be delegated are nursing interventions requiring nursing judgment.

29. 1. The unlicensed assistive personnel (UAP) cannot administer medication or evaluate the effectiveness of medication; therefore, this task cannot be delegated.

2. This is a legal issue and should not be delegated to the UAP.

3. **The UAP can apply ice to the right ankle because the client is stable.**

4. The nurse should complete the incident report, not the UAP.

CLINICAL JUDGMENT GUIDE: The nurse cannot delegate assessment, teaching, evaluation, medications, or an unstable client to the UAP. Remember, most forms should be completed by the individual whom the form is about, not completed by someone who is not aware of the situation.

30. 1. **The LPN can administer medication to the client; therefore, this is an appropriate assignment.**

2. The unlicensed assistive personnel (UAP) cannot call in prescription refills to the pharmacist.

3. The LPN can obtain the weight and height of a client, but the UAP can do this task, so it is more appropriate to delegate it to the UAP.

4. The UAP can empty the trashcans, but the custodian or housekeeper would be a more appropriate delegation of this task.

CLINICAL JUDGMENT GUIDE: The nurse cannot delegate assessment, teaching, evaluation, medications, or an unstable client to the UAP. The nurse cannot assign assessment, teaching, evaluation, or an unstable client to the LPN. Remember to delegate or assign the task to the least educated person who can safely do the task.

31. 1. **The unlicensed assistive personnel (UAP) is violating HIPAA rules concerning confidentiality, so the clinical manager should intervene.**

2. The LPN can talk to the client over the phone about laboratory tests so this does not warrant intervention.

3. The RN can triage phone messages, so this does not warrant intervention.

4. The UAP can take vital signs on a client who is stable, and clients in an outpatient clinic are considered stable unless otherwise specified.

CLINICAL JUDGMENT GUIDE: The nurse is responsible for the actions and behavior of UAPs and LPNs working in the unit. The nurse must correct behavior as needed.

32. 1. The unlicensed assistive personnel (UAP) is a member of the health-care team and should be able to listen to a student's concerns.

2. The nurse cannot violate the student's rights, even in the school nurse setting.

3. **The nurse should allow the UAP to continue to talk to the female student, and then the nurse can talk to the student after the UAP and student finish talking.**

4. The UAP has established a relationship with the student and should be allowed to talk to the student. If the student wanted to talk to the school nurse, he would have done so.

CLINICAL JUDGMENT GUIDE: The nurse is responsible for the actions and behavior of UAPs in any health-care setting. The nurse should know when to intervene and when not to intervene.

33. 1. This is a breach of confidentiality. The LPN should not discuss the client's health problem in the waiting room area where everyone can hear.

2. **The nurse should remove the LPN from the situation without embarrassing the LPN. Asking the LPN to come to the of-**

fice area is the appropriate action for the nurse to take. The LPN's action is a violation of HIPAA.

3. The nurse should not correct the LPN's behavior in front of the client. This is embarrassing to both the LPN and the client.

4. The nurse does not have to report this to the HCP. The nurse can talk to the LPN concerning this breach of confidentiality.

CLINICAL JUDGMENT GUIDE: The nurse is responsible for knowing and complying with local, state, and federal standards of care. The LPN's discussion of a confidential matter in a public area is a violation of HIPAA.

34. 1. The charge nurse must address this situation because it has been going on for more than a week.

2. Writing a memo does nothing to discover the cause of the tense atmosphere.

3. **The charge nurse should call a meeting and attempt to determine what is causing the staff's behavior and the tense atmosphere. The charge nurse could then problem-solve, with the goal being to have a more relaxed atmosphere in which to work.**

4. This is threatening, which is not an appropriate way to resolve a staff problem.

CLINICAL JUDGMENT GUIDE: In any business, including a health-care facility, arguing should not occur among staff of any level where the customers—in this case, the clients—can hear it or see it. The nurse should address the situation directly with the staff members.

35. 1. Obtaining a urine sample is not an invasive procedure and does not require informed consent.

2. **The urine specimen must adhere to a chain of custody, so the client cannot dispute the results.**

3. The bathroom for drug testing should not have access to any water via a sink, so that the client cannot dilute the urine specimen.

4. The tympanic temperature is taken in the client's ear and is not required for a urine drug sample.

CLINICAL JUDGMENT GUIDE: There are management questions on the NCLEX-RN®. In many instances, there is no test-taking strategy for these questions. The nurse must be knowledgeable regarding management issues, and know

what must comply with local, state, and federal requirements.

36. 1. Any client seen in the clinic should have the vital signs taken, but given the signs and symptoms of the client, the nurse should first obtain a urinalysis.

2. The nurse should determine whether there has been blood in the urine, but it is not the nurse's first intervention. The HCP needs a urinalysis to confirm the probable diagnosis.

3. **The client is verbalizing the classic signs and symptoms of a urinary tract infection, but it must be confirmed with a urinalysis. The nurse should first obtain the specimen so the results will be available by the time the HCP sees the client.**

4. The nurse should always teach the client and asking this question is appropriate, but it is not the clinic nurse's first intervention.

CLINICAL JUDGMENT GUIDE: The client's signs and symptoms often provide the nurse with the most likely problem, and the nurse should confirm the condition with a laboratory test, if possible. Clinic and emergency department nurses obtain tests so the HCP will have the results when seen.

37. 1. The nurse may need to know how long the client will be in the shelter, but this is not a priority during the initial assessment of the client.

2. **During a disaster, the priority is to determine whether the client has routine medications that can be taken while in the shelter. If clients have life-sustaining medications, then obtaining the medications becomes a priority. Remember, psychiatric medications are life sustaining.**

3. The client's health history is important, but no matter what the history is, if the client does not have life-sustaining medications, the client will end up in the hospital.

4. The client should be assessed but unless the client has verbalized a specific symptom in this situation, assessment of vital signs, height, and weight is not a priority.

CLINICAL JUDGMENT GUIDE: The nurse must be knowledgeable regarding emergency preparedness. This is part of hospital requirements since 9/11. The NCSBN NCLEX-RN® test plan includes questions on a safe and effective care environment.

38. 1. The nurse should ask whether the client is allergic to iodine or shellfish.
2. An incompetent client cannot sign the consent form. Because the client is diagnosed with schizophrenia, asking him to sign a permit form is not an appropriate intervention.
3. **An incompetent client is an individual who is not autonomous and cannot give or withhold consent—for example, individuals who are cognitively impaired, mentally ill, neurologically incapacitated, or under the influence of mind-altering drugs. This client is diagnosed with schizophrenia, a mental illness, and is delusional; therefore, the client's significant other must sign for the procedure.**
4. This procedure is performed in the radiology department, not in a day surgery department.

CLINICAL JUDGMENT GUIDE: The NCLEX-RN® test plan includes questions on nursing care ruled by legal requirements. The nurse must be knowledgeable regarding these issues.

39. 1. Some herbal supplements can interact with prescribed medications and become dangerous, but saw palmetto is not one of them.
2. **The herbal supplement, saw palmetto, is recommended by many urologists and used to treat BPH; therefore, this is the most appropriate statement.**
3. The nurse should notify the client's HCP, but the best response is to support the client's use of saw palmetto for BPH.
4. This is a true statement, but the nurse should address the client taking the saw palmetto, not make a general statement.

CLINICAL JUDGMENT GUIDE: The NCLEX-RN® tests complementary alternative medicine (CAM), so the nurse must be familiar with the common herbs used to treat disease processes.

40. 1. This is the role of the speech therapist, a member of the home care team.
2. This is the role of the occupational therapist, a member of the home care team.
3. This is the role of the social worker, a member of the home care team.
4. **This is the role of the physical therapist, a member of the home care team.**

CLINICAL JUDGMENT GUIDE: The home health (HH) nurse must know the roles of the members of the home care team. The HH nurse must be able to make appropriate referrals.

41. 1. **The NCSBN NCLEX-RN® test plan includes referrals under Management of Care. The client is in spiritual distress, and the chaplain is the member of the team who addresses spiritual needs.**
2. The nurse should not discuss the client's concerns with the client's pastor. The nurse should contact the agency chaplain; then, if needed, the agency chaplain could talk to the client's pastor.
3. This is crossing professional boundaries. The nurse should not impose his or her religious beliefs on the client. If the client asks the nurse to pray, then the nurse could—but the nurse should not ask the client to pray.
4. The client is verbalizing thoughts about dying, not asking questions about living wills. This would not be an appropriate intervention.

CLINICAL JUDGMENT GUIDE: The test taker must be knowledgeable regarding the roles of all members of the multidisciplinary health-care team.

42. 1. This is a private moment between the client and spouse; the nurse should not impose on the situation.
2. The client and spouse did not ask for help; the nurse should not assume that help is needed.
3. **This is a private moment and should be respected by the nurse. The nurse should allow the client and spouse quiet time together.**
4. This is a private moment between the client and spouse; the nurse should not impose on the situation.

CLINICAL JUDGMENT GUIDE: The nurse must be aware of spiritual needs and help to support the client's needs whenever possible.

43. Correct answers are 4 and 5.
1. Clocking in late twice in a year's time is not a pattern of behavior.
2. The nurse involved in a code would not be able to leave the code to answer a call light.
3. The nurse has covered himself or herself, or may be changing to cover someone else. This action is assuming responsibility for the client care on the unit and does not require a mention in the evaluation, unless the nurse is changing at the request of management.

4. The nurse's care is being evaluated, including the nurse's documentation. The completeness of documentation should be included in the evaluation.
5. The nurse's membership in the American Nephrology Nurses Association helps the nurse remain up-to-date on current trends, which impacts the care provided. This information should be included in the evaluation.

CLINICAL JUDGMENT GUIDE: This is an alternate type of question included in the NCLEX-RN®. The nurse must be able to select all the options that answer the question correctly. There are no partially correct answers. There will be management questions on the NCLEX-RN®. In many instances, there is no test-taking strategy for these questions; the nurse must be knowledgeable regarding management issues.

44. 1. This is a nice gesture, but the priority is to provide support when the family and friends have returned to their own lives.
2. **The family and friends will have returned to their own lives 1 to 2 months after a family member has died. This is when the next of kin needs support from the hospice nurse. Hospice will follow up with the significant other for up to 13 months.**
3. This is the family's responsibility, not that of the hospice nurse.
4. This is not the nurse's responsibility and should be discouraged for a short period of time. In the immediate grieving period, the significant other may get rid of possessions that later he or she may wish had been kept.

CLINICAL JUDGMENT GUIDE: The test taker must be knowledgeable regarding the roles of all members of the multidisciplinary health-care team. This knowledge will be tested on the NCLEX-RN® examination.

45. **Correct answers are 3 and 5.**
1. The nurse should not continue to attempt IV access if there is another nurse available who may be able to insert the IV line successfully.
2. The client needs IV replacement at this time.
3. **After two attempts, the nurse should arrange for a second nurse to attempt the placement.**
4. Cold packs would cause the circulatory system to contract and make it more difficult to

start an IV line. Hot packs dilate the blood vessels.
5. **With a portable vein finder device, infrared light is absorbed by hemoglobin in the blood and makes the veins appear darker in contrast to the surrounding tissue facilitating IV starts.**

CLINICAL JUDGMENT GUIDE: The nurse must be able to perform skills safely. The nurse should not continue to inflict pain on the client after attempting invasive procedures more than twice.

46. 1. The unlicensed assistive personnel (UAP) should not use soap when bathing a client diagnosed with CKD. Soap is drying and the client diagnosed with CKD has altered skin integrity.
2. **The nurse should stop the UAP from using the arm with the graft. Pressure on the graft could occlude the graft.**
3. The UAP can tell the client not to eat contraband food. This is not teaching.
4. This is an appropriate action for the UAP; the nurse would not need to intervene.

CLINICAL JUDGMENT GUIDE: "Delegation" means that the nurse is responsible for the UAP's actions and performance. The nurse must correct the UAP's performance to ensure the client is cared for safely, in the hospital or the home.

47. 1. Digoxin (Lanoxin) is frequently ordered for elderly clients with a history of heart failure. The nurse should take an apical heart rate and hold the medication if the apical pulse is lower than 60. This is a maintenance dose of the medication.
2. Furosemide (Lasix), a loop diuretic, is frequently prescribed for clients with a history of heart failure. The nurse should determine if the client is having muscle cramping, which is a sign of potassium deficiency. The nurse would not question administering this medication without an indication of potassium deficiency.
3. Potassium (K Dur) is given to prevent potassium depletion when administering a diuretic.
4. **Bisacodyl (Dulcolax) is a stimulant laxative. Overuse of stimulant laxatives can cause laxative dependency and colon obstruction. The nurse should contact the HCP and arrange for a bulk laxative if the client requires a daily laxative.**

CLINICAL JUDGMENT GUIDE: This is an alternate type of question included in the NCLEX-RN® test plan. The test taker must be able to read a medication administration record (MAR), be knowledgeable regarding medications, and be able to make an appropriate decision as to the nurse's most appropriate intervention.

48. **Answer: 88 mL per hour (350 divided by 4 hours = 87.5 mL per hour).**
   The client is diagnosed with heart failure, which indicates the client is at high risk for fluid volume overload when administering any type of fluids. Blood must be administered within 4 hours.

CLINICAL JUDGMENT GUIDE: The NCLEX-RN® test plan includes dosage calculations under Pharmacological and Parenteral Therapies. This category is included under Physiological Integrity, which promotes physical health and wellness by providing care and comfort, reducing client risk potential, and managing health alterations.

49. **Correct answers are 3, 4, and 5.**
    1. Teaching is the responsibility of the nurse and cannot be delegated to an unlicensed assistive personnel (UAP).
    2. The word "check" indicates a step in the assessment process, and the nurse cannot delegate assessing to a UAP.
    3. **The client is 2 days postoperative and vital signs should be stable so the UAP can take vital signs. The nurse must make sure the UAP knows when to immediately notify him or her of vital signs not within the guidelines the nurse provides to the UAP.**
    4. **This action does not require judging, assessing, teaching, or evaluating on the part of the UAP. This task can be delegated to the UAP.**
    5. **A client who is 2 days postoperative should be ambulating frequently. The UAP can perform this task.**

CLINICAL JUDGMENT GUIDE: This is an alternate type of question included in the NCLEX-RN®. The nurse must be able to select all the options that answer the question correctly. There are no partially correct answers.

50. 1. The nurse could obtain the client's pulse oximeter reading, but this client is hemor-

rhaging and the surgeon should be notified immediately.
    2. Checking the client's last H&H could be done, but this client's AP and BP are indicating hemorrhaging; therefore, the first intervention is to notify the client's surgeon.
    3. **The client's apical pulse (AP) and blood pressure (BP) indicate the client is hemorrhaging; therefore, the nurse should first notify the client's surgeon.**
    4. The nurse could monitor the client's urine output, but it will not help the client's hemorrhaging; therefore, this is not the nurse's first intervention.

CLINICAL JUDGMENT GUIDE: The test taker needs to read all the options carefully before choosing the option that says, "Notify the HCP." If any of the options will provide information the HCP needs to know in order to make a decision, the test taker should choose that option. If, however, the HCP does not need any additional information to make a decision and the nurse suspects the condition is serious or life threatening, the priority intervention is to call the HCP.

51. **Correct order is 4, 5, 2, 3, 1.**
    4. **Safety should be the primary concern of the nurse. A bedside commode will provide the client with an option that is easier to get to than walking to the bathroom and prevent the client from slipping on urine that may be dribbled.**
    5. **The nurse needs to obtain a urine culture so antibiotic therapy can be initiated.**
    2. **This will help the client stay dry and not soil clothes, as well as allowing some independence in ambulation in the room and hallways.**
    3. **This will protect the bed and the client from soiling.**
    1. **Providing frequent assistance with toileting will prevent the client from having incontinence.**

CLINICAL JUDGMENT GUIDE: This is an alternate type of question included in the NCLEX-RN® test plan. The nurse must be able to implement interventions in the correct order.

52. 1. These laboratory findings are low, but would not require a blood transfusion. These laboratory findings are often expected in a client who is anemic secondary to chronic kidney disease.

2. This client's dialysis access is compromised and should be assessed, but this is not life threatening.

3. This client should be seen, but not before a potentially life-threatening situation.

4. **The client on peritoneal dialysis who has a hard, rigid abdomen has a potentially life-threatening complication; this client should be assessed first and then sent to the hospital.**

CLINICAL JUDGMENT GUIDE: The test taker must determine if any of the assessment data are normal or abnormal for the client's diagnosis. If the data are abnormal, then this client should be seen first. If the data are normal, then a client diagnosed with a physiological problem is the client the nurse should assess first.

53. 1. This pulse oximeter reading is above 93%; therefore, this information does not warrant notifying the health-care provider.

2. The client's platelet count is within normal limits; therefore, this information does not warrant notifying the health-care provider.

3. **After the initial administration of erythropoietin, a biological response modifier, a client's antihypertensive medications may need to be adjusted. Therefore, this elevated blood pressure warrants notifying the health-care provider. Erythropoietin therapy is contraindicated in clients diagnosed with hypertension that cannot be controlled.**

4. The client's tympanic temperature is within normal limits; therefore, this does not warrant notifying the health-care provider.

CLINICAL JUDGMENT GUIDE: The test taker should select the option that is potentially life threatening, or a complaint that would require the medication to be adjusted or discontinued. The nurse should notify the HCP if the medication is causing an adverse effect, not an expected side effect.

54. 1. The stem of the question does not provide any information indicating the client has a self-care deficit, and it is not automatically suspected with a client diagnosed with chronic kidney disease.

2. Teaching is always an important part of the care plan, but it is not a priority over a physiological problem.

3. Chronic pain may occur with a client diagnosed with chronic kidney disease, but would not be a priority over excess fluid volume.

4. **Excess fluid volume is a priority because of the stress placed on the heart and vessels, which could lead to heart failure, pulmonary edema, and death.**

CLINICAL JUDGMENT GUIDE: The NCLEX-RN® integrates the nursing process throughout the Client Needs categories and subcategories. The nursing process is a scientific, clinical reasoning approach to client care that includes assessment, analysis, planning, implementation, and evaluation. The nurse will be responsible for identifying a nursing diagnosis for clients.

55. **Answer: 300 mL.**
The nurse must add up how many milliliters of fluid the client drank on the 7 a.m. to 7 p.m. shift, then subtract that number from 1,500 mL to determine how much fluid the client can receive on the 7 p.m. to 7 a.m. shift. One ounce is equal to 30 mL. The client drank 40 ounces (8 + 8 + 16 + 8) of fluid, or 1,200 mL (40 × 30) of fluid. Therefore, the client can have 300 mL (1,500 − 1,200) of fluid on the 7 p.m. to 7 a.m. shift.

CLINICAL JUDGMENT GUIDE: The NCLEX-RN® test plan includes dosage calculations under Pharmacological and Parenteral Therapies. This category is included under Physiological Integrity, which promotes physical health and wellness by providing care and comfort, reducing client risk potential, and managing health alterations.

56. 1. Reverse Trendelenburg position has the nurse elevating the client's chair, which will not help the client's dizziness and light-headedness.

2. Decreasing the volume of blood being removed is an appropriate intervention, but it will not help the client's dizziness and light-headedness as fast as will infusing normal saline.

3. **Normal saline infusion increases the amount of volume in the bloodstream, which will decrease the client's light-headedness and dizziness.**

4. Hypotension is an expected occurrence in clients receiving dialysis; therefore, the HCP does not need to be notified.

CLINICAL JUDGMENT GUIDE: When the question asks, "Which intervention should be implemented first?" it means all the options are things a nurse could implement, but only one should be implemented first. The nurse should use the nursing process and remember: If the client is in distress, do not assess; if the client is not in distress, the nurse should assess.

57. **Correct answers are 3, 4, and 5.**
    1. TPN is a hypertonic solution that has enough calories, proteins, lipids, electrolytes, and trace elements to sustain life. It is administered via a pump to prevent a too rapid infusion. It should not be administered without a pump or via a gravity intravenous line.
    2. TPN contains 50% dextrose solution; therefore, the client is monitored to ensure that the pancreas is adapting to the high glucose levels. The glucose level is checked every 6 hours, not every 24 hours.
    3. **The client is weighed daily in the same clothes and at the same time to monitor for fluid overload and evaluate daily weight.**
    4. **The IV tubing is changed with every bag because the high glucose level can cause bacterial growth.**
    5. **Intake and output are monitored to observe for fluid balance.**

CLINICAL JUDGMENT GUIDE: This is an alternate type of question included in the NCLEX-RN®. The nurse must be able to select all the options that answer the question correctly. There are no partially correct answers.

58. **Correct order is 2, 1, 4, 5, 3.**
    2. **The client has signs of phlebitis and the IV must be removed to prevent further complications.**
    1. **A new IV will be started in the right hand after the IV is discontinued.**
    4. **A warm washcloth placed on an IV site sometimes provides comfort to the client. If this is done, it should be done for 20 minutes, four times a day.**
    5. **All pertinent situations should be documented in the client's EHR.**
    3. **Depending on the health-care facility, this may or may not be done, but client care comes before documentation.**

CLINICAL JUDGMENT GUIDE: This is an alternate type of question included in the NCLEX-RN® test plan. The nurse must be able to perform skills in the correct order. Documentation is always completed after direct client care.

59. 1. An unlicensed assistive personnel (UAP) can empty the catheter and measure the amount.

2. The UAP can record intake and output on the I&O sheet.
3. **The nurse cannot delegate teaching to the UAP.**
4. The client has a disease, but all the UAP is being asked to do is take water to the client.

CLINICAL JUDGMENT GUIDE: This is an "except" question. The nurse could determine which task is appropriate to delegate to the UAP; three options would be appropriate to delegate. The nurse should implement the task that is not appropriate to delegate. Remember, the nurse cannot delegate assessment, teaching, evaluation, medications, or an unstable client to the UAP.

60. **Answer: 890 mL.**
    First, determine the amount of irrigation fluid: 3,000 − 1,550 = 1,450 mL of irrigation fluid. Then, subtract 1,450 irrigation fluid from the drainage of 2,340 to determine the urine output: 2,340 − 1,450 = 890 mL of urine output.

CLINICAL JUDGMENT GUIDE: The NCLEX-RN® test plan includes dosage calculations under Pharmacological and Parenteral Therapies. This category is included under Physiological Integrity, which promotes physical health and wellness by providing care and comfort, reducing client risk potential, and managing health alterations.

61. 1. TURPs may cause sexual dysfunction, but if there were a sexual dysfunction, it is not a priority over a physiological problem, such as hemorrhaging.
    2. This may be a possible nursing diagnosis, but is not a priority over hemorrhaging, which is the priority nursing diagnosis.
    3. All postoperative clients have the risk of infection, but the client with a TURP priority nursing concern is hemorrhaging because of the surgical procedure.
    4. **This is a potential life-threatening nursing diagnosis and is the client's priority. This is the reason for the three-way continuous bladder irrigation.**

CLINICAL JUDGMENT GUIDE: The NCLEX-RN® integrates the nursing process throughout the Client Needs categories and subcategories. The nursing process is a scientific, clinical reasoning approach to client care that includes assessment, analysis, planning, implementation, and evaluation. The nurse will be responsible for identifying nursing diagnoses for clients.

ANSWERS

62. 1. **The unlicensed assistive personnel (UAP) cannot increase the irrigation fluid because this requires assessment and judgment. This behavior warrants intervention by the nurse.**
    2. Elevating the scrotum on a towel for support is an intervention a UAP can implement. It does not require judgment and the client is stable; therefore, action does not warrant intervention by the nurse.
    3. The UAP can empty catheter bags, because this does not require any judgment. This action does not warrant intervention by the nurse.
    4. The client can bring ice water to the client's bedside, because the client is not NPO.

CLINICAL JUDGMENT GUIDE: "Delegation" means the nurse is responsible for the UAP's actions and performance. The nurse must correct the UAP's performance to ensure the client is cared for safely, in the hospital or the home.

63. 1. The client should use a urinal, so the nurse can strain the urine before placing it in the commode.
    2. **Assessment is the first part of the nursing process and is always the priority. The intensity of the renal colic pain can be so intense it can cause a vasovagal response, with resulting hypotension and syncope.**
    3. Increased fluid increases urinary output, which will facilitate movement of the renal stone through the ureter and help decrease pain, but it is not the first intervention.
    4. The nurse should strain the client's urine to determine if the renal calculi have been passed via the urine.

CLINICAL JUDGMENT GUIDE: When the question asks, "Which intervention should be implemented first?" it means that all the options are things a nurse could implement, but only one should be implemented first. The nurse should use the nursing process and remember: If the client is in distress, do not assess; if the client is not in distress, the nurse should assess.

64. 1. A KUB is an x-ray and does not include administering any type of contrast dye.
    2. Food, fluids, and ordered medication are not restricted before a KUB.
    3. **An x-ray should not be completed on a client who may be pregnant. The x-rays could harm the fetus.**
    4. The client diagnosed with renal calculi is expected to have pain, depending on where the calculi are located, but this statement would not warrant intervention for the KUB.

CLINICAL JUDGMENT GUIDE: This question asks the nurse to identify which statement warrants intervention, which indicates three of the options are appropriate for the disease process or disorder but one is incorrect. This is an "except" question, but it does not say all the options are correct "except."

65. **Correct answers are 3 and 5.**
    1. The health-care provider may order certain foods and medications when obtaining a 24-hour urine collection to evaluate for calcium oxalate or uric acid, but the client will not be NPO.
    2. When the collection begins, the client should completely empty the bladder and discard that urine. The first urine specimen should not be included.
    3. **All urine for 24 hours should be saved and put in a container with a preservative, refrigerated, or put on ice, as indicated. Not following specific instructions will result in an inaccurate test result.**
    4. The urine is obtained in some type of urine collection device such as a bedpan, bedside commode, or commode hat. The client is not catheterized.
    5. **Posting signs will help ensure that all the urine is saved during the 24-hour period. If any urine is discarded, the test may result in inaccurate information or the need to start the test over.**

CLINICAL JUDGMENT GUIDE: This is an alternate type of question included in the NCLEX-RN®. The nurse must be able to select all the options that answer the question correctly. There are no partially correct answers.

66. 1. The urine must be assessed for bleeding and cloudiness. Initially, the urine is bright red, but the color soon diminishes, and cloudiness may indicate an infection. This assessment should not be delegated to an unlicensed assistive personnel (UAP).
    2. The UAP cannot transcribe a health-care provider's orders.
    3. **The UAP can strain the client's urine. This task does not require judgment or evaluation. Any sediment should be placed in a sterile container and sent to the laboratory for analysis.**

4. The kidney is highly vascular. Hemorrhaging and the resulting shock are potential complications of lithotripsy, so the nurse should not delegate vital signs post-procedure.

CLINICAL JUDGMENT GUIDE: The nurse cannot delegate assessment, teaching, evaluation, medications, or an unstable client to a UAP. Tasks that cannot be delegated are nursing interventions requiring nursing judgment.

67. 1. This potassium level is within normal limits, 3.5 to 5.5 mEq/L.
    2. **Hematuria is not uncommon after removal of a kidney stone, but cause for further assessment by the nurse. It may indicate hemorrhaging, which is life threatening.**
    3. A creatinine level of 1.1 mg/dL is normal for a male or a female client.
    4. This white blood cell count is within the normal limits of 4.5 to 11.1 10³/microL.

CLINICAL JUDGMENT GUIDE: The nurse must be knowledgeable regarding normal laboratory values. These values must be memorized, and the nurse must be able to determine if the laboratory value is normal for the client's disease process or for medications the client is taking.

68. 1. **The nurse should assess first to determine the etiology of the incontinence before the treatment plan can be formulated. By palpating the bladder after voiding, the nurse can determine if the incontinence was the result of overdistention of the bladder.**
    2. Medications—for instance, anticholinergic agents such as oxybutynin—can cause adverse effects. Nonpharmacological methods of treatment are preferred before medications are administered.
    3. The nurse should ensure the client does not have skin breakdown secondary to urinary incontinence, but the first intervention is assessment.
    4. The nurse should instruct the client to go to the bathroom every 2 hours to attempt to urinate, which may decrease the number of incontinent episodes.

CLINICAL JUDGMENT GUIDE: When the question asks, "Which intervention should be implemented first?" it means that all the options are things a nurse could implement, but only one should be implemented first.

The nurse should use the nursing process and remember: If the client is in distress, do not assess; if the client is not in distress, the nurse should assess.

69. 1. These vital signs are within normal limits and would not require further investigation.
    2. **When an elderly client's mental status changes, the nurse should notify the HCP because it is not normal or expected. This could indicate a urinary tract infection secondary to an indwelling catheter. Elderly clients often do not present with classic signs and symptoms of infection.**
    3. The client's urine should be clear and light yellow, but cloudy urine with sediment is not life threatening. The nurse would not need to notify the client's HCP.
    4. The client should have no discomfort and pain; therefore, this would not warrant further investigation.

CLINICAL JUDGMENT GUIDE: When the question asks, "Which data set warrants notifying the HCP?" it is an "except" question. Three of the data sets are expected with the client's disease process or condition, whereas one is not expected and warrants notifying the HCP.

70. 1. **The client's catheter should be secured on the leg to prevent manipulation, which increases the risk for a urinary tract infection. This warrants immediate intervention by the nurse.**
    2. The unlicensed assistive personnel (UAP) must adhere to Standard Precautions when providing care to the client; therefore, this doesn't warrant immediate intervention by the nurse.
    3. The drainage bag should be kept below the level of the bladder to prevent reflux of urine into the renal system; therefore, this does not warrant intervention by the nurse.
    4. Hand hygiene is important before and after handling any portion of the drainage system; therefore, this does not warrant intervention by the nurse.

CLINICAL JUDGMENT GUIDE: When the question asks, "Which intervention warrants immediate intervention?" it is an "except" question. Three of the interventions indicate the UAP understands the appropriate care for the client, and one indicates the UAP does not understand the appropriate care.

CLINICAL SCENARIO ANSWERS AND RATIONALES

The correct answer number and rationale for why it is the correct answer are given in **boldface type**. Rationales for why the other possible answer options are incorrect also are given, but they are not in boldface type.

1. 1. **The UAP can assist the radiology technician with the portable chest x-ray. The RN cannot delegate assessment, teaching, evaluation, medications, or an unstable client. If the UAP is pregnant, then the nurse should not delegate this task.**
   2. The UAP can obtain the client's intake and output, but the nurse must evaluate the data to determine if interventions are needed or if interventions are effective.
   3. In some units, UAPs can perform urinary catheterization, but of the four options, the nurse should delegate the least invasive task.
   4. This is a medication enema, and the UAP cannot administer medications. Also, for this to be ordered, the client must be unstable with an excessively high serum potassium level.

2. 1. The laboratory findings are low, but would not require a blood transfusion. These laboratory findings are often expected in a client who is anemic secondary to ESRD.
   2. **The dialysis access is compromised; therefore, this client warrants intervention by the RN because the hemodialysis cannot be performed.**
   3. It is not uncommon for a client undergoing dialysis to be exhausted and sleep through the treatment; therefore, this does not warrant intervention.
   4. The client in end-stage renal disease would not have urinary output; therefore, this does not warrant intervention from the RN.

3. 1. The RN can restart the client's IV access without notifying the health-care provider.
   2. Hypoactive bowel sounds may be abnormal, but airway problems take priority over gastrointestinal distress. Remember Maslow's Hierarchy of Needs.
   3. **The client may be developing pneumonia or acute respiratory distress syndrome; therefore, the RN should notify the health-care provider. This is a complication of surgery.**
   4. A 2+ pedal pulse is expected data; therefore, the RN does not need to notify the health-care provider.

4. 1. Normal blood urea nitrogen levels are 8 to 21 mg/dL or 10 to 31 mg/dL for clients older than age 90 years.
   2. Normal creatinine levels are 0.61 to 1.21 mg/dL for male clients.
   3. **Glomerular filtration rate (GFR) is approximately 120 mL per minute. If the GFR is decreased to 60 mL per minute, the kidneys are functioning at about one-half filtration capacity.**
   4. Normal creatinine clearance is 85 to 125 mL per minute for males and 75 to 115 mL per minute for females.

5. **Answer: 1,000 mL.**
   First, determine the amount of irrigation fluid: 4,000 − 2,000 = 2,000 mL of irrigation fluid. Then, subtract 2,000 of irrigation fluid from the drainage of 3,000 to determine the urine output: 3,000 − 2,000 = 1,000 mL of urine output.

6. Correct answers are 1 and 5.
   1. **The client is stable, but the RN should assess the drainage. The drainage should be light pink for a client who had a TURP.**
   2. The client is stable; therefore, the RN should not increase the irrigation fluid, unless the drainage is dark red.
   3. If the client is hypovolemic, the head of the bed should be lowered and the foot should be elevated to protect the brain. This client is stable.
   4. The surgeon needs to be notified if the client is unstable or experiencing a complication of surgery. This client is stable; therefore, the RN should not notify the surgeon.
   5. **The RN should monitor the client's laboratory values for bleeding or infection.**

7. 1. The RN needs to complete the admission assessment, but the priority should always be the client's body; therefore, assessing pain is priority.
   2. **Assessment is the first part of the nursing process and is always a priority. The intensity of the renal colic pain can be so intense it can cause a vasovagal response, with resulting hypotension and syncope.**
   3. Increased fluid increases urinary output, which will facilitate movement of the renal stone through the ureter and help decrease pain, but it is not the first intervention.

4. The nurse should transcribe the client's HCP order, but this is not a priority over the client's body pain. The charge nurse can check the HCP orders to determine if there is any priority order.

8. 1. The urine must be assessed for bleeding and cloudiness. Initially, the urine is bright red, but the color soon diminishes, and cloudiness may indicate an infection. This assessment should not be delegated to the UAP.
   2. Teaching cannot be delegated to the UAP, and the client diagnosed with renal calculi should not have an indwelling urinary catheter.
   3. **The client's urine must be strained to determine if the renal stone was dissolved and is being passed out of the body. Straining the urine is not assessment, teaching, evaluation, medications, or an unstable client; therefore, this can be delegated to the UAP.**
   4. The client may experience burning on urination after lithotripsy; however, assessment should not be delegated to the UAP.

9. 1. The client with a palpable thrill is stable; therefore, the charge nurse would not need to see this client first.

2. The client diagnosed with acute glomerulonephritis is expected to have hematuria and proteinuria; therefore, the charge nurse should not assess this client first.
3. The sign or symptom of bladder cancer is painless hematuria; therefore, the charge nurse would not need to see this client first.
4. **An ileal conduit is a procedure that diverts urine from the bladder and provides an alternate cutaneous pathway for urine to exit the body. Urinary output should always be at least 30 mL per hour. This client should be assessed to make sure that the stents placed in the ureters have not become dislodged, or to ensure that edema of the ureters is not occurring.**

10. 1. Teaching cannot be assigned to an LPN, no matter how knowledgeable the LPN.
    2. This client has the laboratory symptoms of an infection; therefore, the RN cannot assign an unstable client to the LPN.
    3. Antineoplastic medication can only be administered by a qualified registered nurse.
    4. **The LPN can administer narcotic analgesics to a client; therefore, this would be an appropriate assignment.**

Neurological Management

Let us never consider ourselves finished nurses . . . we must be learning all our lives.

—Florence Nightingale

QUESTIONS

1. The charge nurse has received laboratory data for clients in the medical department. Which client would require intervention by the charge nurse?
   1. The client diagnosed with a stroke who has a platelet level of 250 x 10³/microL
   2. The client diagnosed with a seizure disorder who has a valproic acid level of 75 mcg/mL
   3. The client diagnosed with multiple sclerosis on prednisone who has a glucose level of 208 mg/dL
   4. The client receiving phenytoin who has serum levels of 24 mcg/dL

2. The nurse is administering medications for clients on a neurological unit. Which medication should the nurse administer **first?**
   1. A pain medication to a client reporting a headache rated an 8 on a 1 to 10 pain scale
   2. A steroid to the client experiencing an acute exacerbation of multiple sclerosis
   3. An anticholinesterase medication to a client diagnosed with myasthenia gravis
   4. An antacid to a client diagnosed with pyrosis who has called several times over the intercom

3. The nurse has just received the shift report. Which client should the nurse assess **first?**
   1. The client diagnosed with Guillain-Barré syndrome who has ascending paralysis to the knees
   2. The client diagnosed with a C-6 spinal cord injury who has autonomic dysreflexia
   3. The client diagnosed with Parkinson's disease who is experiencing a "pill rolling" tremor
   4. The client diagnosed with Huntington's disease who has writhing, twisting movements of the face

4. The RN primary nurse and unlicensed assistive personnel (UAP) are caring for a client diagnosed with right-sided paralysis. Which action by the UAP **requires** the RN to intervene?
   1. The UAP places the gait belt around the client's waist before ambulating.
   2. The UAP places the client on the abdomen with the client's head to the side.
   3. The UAP places her hand under the client's right axilla to help the client move up in bed.
   4. The UAP praises the client for performing activities of daily living independently.

5. The charge nurse is making client assignments for a neurological medical floor. Which client should be assigned to the **most** experienced nurse?
   1. The elderly client who is experiencing a stroke-in-evolution
   2. The client diagnosed with a transient ischemic attack 48 hours ago
   3. The client diagnosed with Guillain-Barré syndrome who reports leg pain
   4. The client diagnosed with Alzheimer's disease who is wandering in the halls

6. The client diagnosed with a cerebrovascular accident (CVA) has residual right-sided hemiparesis and difficulty swallowing, but is scheduled for discharge. Which referral is **most** appropriate for the case manager to make at this time?
   1. Inpatient rehabilitation unit
   2. Home health-care agency
   3. Long-term care facility
   4. Outpatient therapy center

7. The RN primary nurse and LPN are caring for a client diagnosed with a stroke. Which intervention should the RN assign to the LPN?
   1. Feed the client who is being allowed to eat for the first time.
   2. Administer the client's anticoagulant subcutaneously.
   3. Check the client's neurological signs and limb movement.
   4. Teach the client to turn the head and tuck the chin to swallow.

8. The RN staff nurse is caring for a client diagnosed with Alzheimer's disease. Which nursing tasks can the RN staff nurse delegate to the unlicensed assistive personnel (UAP)? **Select all that apply.**
   1. Check the client's skin under the restraints.
   2. Administer the client's antipsychotic medication.
   3. Perform the client's morning hygiene care.
   4. Ambulate the client to the bathroom.
   5. Obtain the client's routine vital signs.

9. The RN primary nurse on the surgical unit is working with an unlicensed assistive personnel (UAP). Which task is **most** appropriate for the RN to delegate to the UAP?
   1. Change an abdominal dressing on a client who is 2 days postoperative.
   2. Check the client's IV insertion site on the right arm.
   3. Monitor vital signs on a client who has just returned from surgery.
   4. Escort a client who has been discharged to the client's vehicle.

10. Which client diagnosed with a spinal cord injury (SCI) should the charge nurse assess **first** after receiving the change-of-shift report?
    1. The client diagnosed with a C-6 SCI who is describing dyspnea symptoms and has a respiratory rate of 12 breaths/minute
    2. The client diagnosed with an L-4 SCI who is frightened about being transferred to the rehabilitation unit
    3. The client diagnosed with an L-2 SCI who is reporting a headache and feeling very hot all of a sudden
    4. The client diagnosed with a C-4 SCI who is on a ventilator and has a pulse oximeter reading of 98%

11. The client diagnosed with a C-6 spinal cord injury (SCI) comes to the emergency department reporting a throbbing headache and has a BP of 200/120. Which intervention should the nurse implement **first?**
    1. Place the client on a telemetry unit.
    2. Complete a neurological assessment.
    3. Insert an indwelling urinary catheter.
    4. Request a STAT CT scan on the head.

12. The RN ICU nurse and unlicensed assistive personnel (UAP) are caring for a client diagnosed with right-sided paralysis secondary to a cerebrovascular accident. Which action by the UAP **requires** the RN to intervene?
1. The UAP performs passive range-of-motion (ROM) exercises for the client.
2. The UAP places the client on the abdomen with the head to the side.
3. The UAP uses a lift sheet when moving the client up in bed.
4. The UAP praises the client for attempting to feed him- or herself.

13. The critical care RN charge nurse is making client assignments for the shift. Which client should the charge nurse assign to the graduate nurse (GN) who just completed orientation?
1. The client diagnosed with amyotrophic lateral sclerosis on a ventilator who is dying and whose family is at the bedside
2. The client diagnosed with a closed head injury and increasing intracranial pressure receiving IV mannitol
3. The client diagnosed with a C-5 spinal cord injury who is experiencing spinal shock and is on dopamine
4. The client diagnosed with a seizure disorder who has been experiencing status epilepticus for the past 24 hours

14. The critical care nurse is caring for a client diagnosed with a head injury secondary to a motorcycle accident who, on morning rounds, is responsive to painful stimuli and assumes decorticate posturing. Two hours later, which data would warrant **immediate** intervention by the nurse?
1. The client has purposeful movement when the nurse rubs the sternum.
2. The client extends the upper and lower extremities in response to painful stimuli.
3. The client is aimlessly thrashing in the bed when a noxious stimulus is applied.
4. The client is able to squeeze the nurse's hand on a verbal request.

15. The RN charge nurse is making rounds and notices that the sharps container in the client's room is above the fill line. Which action should the charge nurse implement?
1. Complete an adverse occurrence report.
2. Discuss the situation with the primary nurse.
3. Instruct the UAP to change the sharps container.
4. Notify the infection control nurse immediately.

16. The wife of a client diagnosed with a brain tumor tells the nurse, "I don't know how I will make it if something happens to my husband. I love him so much." Which statement is **most** appropriate for the nurse?
1. "I will call the chaplain to come and talk to you."
2. "Do you have any family support to be with you?"
3. "You don't know how you will make it if something happens."
4. "Do not worry, everything will be all right. You are a strong woman."

17. Which **priority** client problem should be included in the care plan for the client diagnosed with Guillain-Barré syndrome who is admitted to the critical care unit?
1. Decreased cardiac output
2. Fear and anxiety
3. Complications of immobility
4. Ineffective breathing pattern

18. To which collaborative health-care team member should the RN critical care nurse refer the client in the late stages of myasthenia gravis (MG)?
1. Occupational therapist
2. Physical therapist
3. Social worker
4. Speech therapist

19. The nurse caring for a client is accidentally stuck with the stylet used to start an IV infusion. Which actions should the nurse implement next? **Rank in order of performance.**
    1. Have the laboratory draw the client's and the nurse's blood.
    2. Notify the charge nurse and follow hospital protocol.
    3. Contact the infection control nurse to start post-exposure prophylactic medication.
    4. Follow up with the employee health nurse to have laboratory work drawn.
    5. Flush the skin with water and attempt to get the area to bleed.

20. The nurse is caring for clients in a long-term care facility. Which client should the nurse assess **first** after receiving the morning report?
    1. The client diagnosed with Parkinson's disease who began to hallucinate during the night
    2. The client diagnosed with congestive heart failure who has 3+ pitting edema of both feet
    3. The client diagnosed with Alzheimer's disease who was found wandering in the hall at 0200
    4. The client diagnosed with terminal cancer who has lost 8 pounds since the last weight taken 4 weeks ago

21. The nurse in a long-term care facility is administering medications to a group of clients. Which medication should the nurse administer **first?**
    1. Acetylsalicylic acid to a client diagnosed with cerebrovascular disease
    2. Neostigmine to a client diagnosed with myasthenia gravis
    3. Cephalexin to a client diagnosed with an acute urinary tract infection
    4. Acyclovir to a client diagnosed with Bell's palsy

22. The nurse in a long-term care facility is developing the plan of care for a client diagnosed with end-stage Alzheimer's disease. Which client problem is **priority** for this client?
    1. Inability to do activities of daily living
    2. Increased risk for injury
    3. Potential for constipation
    4. Ineffective family coping

23. The clinic nurse is providing discharge instructions to an elderly client diagnosed with cataracts. Which interventions are important for the nurse to implement? **Select all that apply.**
    1. Teach the client to increase the light in the home.
    2. Encourage the client to wear dark glasses outside.
    3. Discuss the need to have the cataracts removed.
    4. Tell the family to avoid rearranging the furniture in the home.
    5. Provide instructions with visual aids or large print.

24. A wife tells the clinic nurse her husband had been fine and is now confused, doesn't know where he is, and is **not** acting the way he usually does. Which intervention should the nurse implement **first?**
    1. Perform a neurological assessment.
    2. Notify the client's health-care provider.
    3. Ask the wife to explain more about the behavior.
    4. Determine when the client last had something to eat.

25. The RN charge nurse observes the client's RN primary nurse telling the unlicensed assistive personnel (UAP) to feed an elderly client diagnosed with a cerebrovascular accident (CVA). Which question should the charge nurse ask the client's nurse?
    1. "How does the client swallow the medications?"
    2. "Did you complete your head-to-toe assessment?"
    3. "Does the client have some thickener in the room?"
    4. "Why would you delegate feeding to a UAP?"

26. The client diagnosed with a cerebrovascular accident (CVA) is confined to a wheelchair for most of the waking hours. Which intervention is **priority** for the nurse to implement?
    1. Encourage the client to move the buttocks every 2 hours.
    2. Order a high-protein diet to prevent skin breakdown.
    3. Get a pressure-relieving cushion to place in the wheelchair.
    4. Refer the client to physical therapy for transfer teaching.

27. As the nurse enters the room of a newly admitted client, the client begins to have a tonic-clonic seizure. Which actions should the nurse implement? **Select all that apply.**
    1. Identify the first area that began seizing.
    2. Note the time the client's seizure began.
    3. Begin to pad the client's bed rails.
    4. Provide the client with privacy during the seizure.
    5. Immediately insert an oral airway.

28. The RN rehabilitation unit nurse tells the unlicensed assistive personnel (UAP) to assist the client recovering from Guillain-Barré syndrome with a.m. care. Which action by the UAP warrants **immediate** intervention?
    1. The UAP closes the door and cubicle curtain.
    2. The UAP massages the client's back with lotion.
    3. The UAP checks the temperature of the bathing water.
    4. The UAP puts the side rails up when bathing the client.

29. The client diagnosed with a right-sided cerebral vascular accident (CVA), or stroke, is admitted to the rehabilitation unit. Which interventions should be included in the nursing care plan? **Select all that apply.**
    1. Position the client to prevent shoulder adduction.
    2. Refer the client to occupational therapy daily.
    3. Encourage the client to move the affected side.
    4. Perform quadriceps exercises five times a day.
    5. Instruct the client to hold the fingers in a fist.

30. The nurse is the **first** person on the scene of a motor vehicle accident. The driver is in the driver's seat unconscious. Which action should the nurse implement **first**?
    1. Stabilize the driver's cervical spine.
    2. Do not move the client from the accident.
    3. Ensure the driver has a patent airway.
    4. Control any external bleeding.

31. The clinic nurse is making assignments for the large family practice clinic. Which task should be assigned to a staff nurse who is 4 months pregnant?
    1. Have the staff nurse answer the telephone calls from clients.
    2. Instruct the staff nurse to work in the radiology department.
    3. Tell the staff nurse to work in the front desk triage area.
    4. Assign the staff nurse to work in the oncology clinic.

32. Which task is **most** appropriate for the RN clinic nurse to delegate to the unlicensed assistive personnel (UAP)?
    1. Request the UAP to ride in the ambulance with a client.
    2. Ask the UAP to escort the client in a wheelchair to the car.
    3. Instruct the UAP to show the client how to use crutches.
    4. Tell the UAP to call the pharmacy to refill a prescription.

33. The employee health nurse is caring for an employee who fell off a ladder and is describing low back pain radiating down both legs. Which intervention should the nurse implement **first?**
    1. Refer the client to an HCP for further evaluation.
    2. Complete the workers' compensation documentation.
    3. Investigate the cause of the fall off the ladder.
    4. Notify the employee's supervisor of the incident.

34. The employee health nurse is caring for an employee who reports tripping and is describing right knee pain. There is no visible injury, and the client has a normal neurovascular assessment. Which intervention should the nurse implement?
    1. Request the employee to return to work.
    2. Obtain a urine specimen for a drug screen.
    3. Send the client to the emergency department.
    4. Place a sequential compression device on the leg.

35. The rural emergency department nurse is triaging victims at the site of a disaster. The victims are tagged using a color code system. Which client should be evacuated first? **Rank in order of priority.**
    1. The client assigned a red tag who is alert and diagnosed with a sucking chest wound
    2. The client assigned a green tag who cannot stop crying and can't answer questions
    3. The client assigned a yellow tag whose abdomen is hard and tender to the touch
    4. The client assigned a black tag with full-thickness burns on more than 60% of the body
    5. The client assigned a white tag who has no injuries and is comforting the victims

36. The home health (HH) nurse enters the home of an 80-year-old female client who had a cerebrovascular accident (CVA), or stroke, 2 months ago. The client is reporting a severe headache. Which intervention should the nurse implement **first?**
    1. Determine what medication the client has taken.
    2. Assess the client's pain on a pain scale of 1 to 10.
    3. Ask whether the client has any acetaminophen.
    4. Tell the client to sit down, and take her blood pressure.

37. A client is suspected of having bacterial meningitis and the nurse is assisting the health-care provider with a lumbar puncture. Which intervention should the nurse implement **first?**
    1. Have the client lie in the lateral recumbent position.
    2. Tell the client to empty the bladder.
    3. Encourage the client to complete an advance directive.
    4. Keep the client NPO before the procedure.

38. The home health (HH) nurse is scheduling visits for the day. Which client should the nurse visit **first?**
    1. The client diagnosed with an L-4 SCI who is describing a severe, pounding headache
    2. The client diagnosed with amyotrophic lateral sclerosis (ALS) who is depressed and wants to die
    3. The client diagnosed with Parkinson's disease who is walking with a short, shuffling gait
    4. The client diagnosed with a C-5 SCI who reports redness and drainage at the halo vest sites

39. The clinic nurse is triaging client telephone calls. Which client should the nurse call **first?**
    1. The client diagnosed with AIDS who has developed Kaposi's sarcoma
    2. The client diagnosed with dementia who is having difficulty dressing himself
    3. The client diagnosed with trigeminal neuralgia who is having lightning-like shock to the cheeks
    4. The client who has vomiting and abdominal cramping pain and a friend with botulism

40. The home health (HH) nurse is caring for a 22-year-old female client who sustained an L-5 spinal cord injury 2 months ago. The client says, "I will never be happy again. I can't walk, I can't drive, and I had to quit college." Which intervention should the nurse implement **first?**
    1. Allow the client to express her feelings of powerlessness.
    2. Refer the client to the home health-care agency social worker.
    3. Recommend contacting the American Spinal Cord Association.
    4. Ask the client whether she has any friends who come and visit.

41. The client being admitted with transient ischemic attack (TIA) is reporting a headache. The client is allergic to morphine, iodine, and codeine. Which health-care provider order should the nurse **question?**
    1. Schedule for CT scan with contrast in a.m.
    2. Administer acetaminophen 650 mg PO for headache.
    3. Take client's vital signs per protocol.
    4. Provide the client with a low-fat, low-cholesterol diet.

42. The home health (HH) nurse is admitting a female client diagnosed with myasthenia gravis. The client tells the nurse, "Even with my medication I get exhausted when I do anything." Which intervention should the nurse implement?
    1. Talk to the client's spouse about helping around the house more.
    2. Contact the HH occupational therapist to discuss the client's concern.
    3. Allow the client to verbalize her feelings of being exhausted.
    4. Recommend the client make an appointment with her HCP.

43. The nurse is caring for clients in the emergency department. Which client should the nurse assess **first?**
    1. The client diagnosed with an epidural hematoma
    2. The client who had a seizure who is in the postictal state
    3. The client diagnosed with encephalitis who has a headache
    4. The client diagnosed with multiple sclerosis who has scanning speech

44. The nurse in the neurological clinic is triaging phone calls. Which client should the nurse contact **first?**
    1. The client diagnosed with a tension headache who is reporting nausea and vomiting
    2. The client diagnosed with a migraine headache who is reporting bilateral throbbing pain
    3. The client diagnosed with a cluster headache who is reporting unilateral sharp pain
    4. The client diagnosed with hypertension who is reporting pressure-type pain in the back of the head

45. A client sustained a severe head injury, and his wife is concerned about what to do if he has a seizure when they go home. Which statement indicates the wife understands the **most** important action to take if her husband has a seizure?
    1. "I should check to see if my husband urinates on himself."
    2. "I will move the furniture out of his way."
    3. "I will call 911 as soon as the seizure begins."
    4. "I will make sure he rests after the seizure is over."

46. The multidisciplinary team is meeting to discuss a client diagnosed with right-sided weakness who has developed a stage 2 pressure ulcer over the sacral area that is **not** healing. Which **priority** intervention should the client's home health (HH) nurse recommend?
    1. Recommend the client get a hospital bed with a trapeze bar.
    2. Recommend a home health aide provide care 7 days a week for the client.
    3. Recommend the client be transferred to a skilled nursing unit.
    4. Recommend a referral to the home health-care agency wound care nurse.

47. The home health (HH) aide tells the RN home health nurse the client diagnosed with multiple sclerosis is having problems getting out of the bed to the chair, and is now having problems getting into the shower. Which intervention should the RN implement?
    1. Ask the HH aide whether the bathroom has grab bars.
    2. Assess the client's ability to transfer in the home.
    3. Instruct the HH aide to give the client a bed bath.
    4. Contact the agency physical therapist about the situation.

48. The nurse is teaching the client diagnosed with tension-type headaches. Which statement indicates the client needs **more** teaching?
    1. "I will do some type of exercise every day."
    2. "I am going to do yoga techniques when I get a headache."
    3. "Cold packs to the back of my neck will help my headache."
    4. "Foods containing amines such as cheese and chocolate can cause headaches."

49. The client in a multiple car crash dies in the emergency department. Which **priority** intervention should the emergency department nurse implement when addressing the needs of the client's family?
    1. Ask if the client wanted to be an organ donor.
    2. Give the family the client's personal belongings.
    3. Escort the family to a private room to grieve.
    4. Determine which funeral home should be contacted.

50. The neurologist has explained to the family of a 22-year-old client diagnosed with a traumatic brain injury placed on a ventilator after a motor vehicle accident that the client has **no** brain function. Which referral is appropriate at this time?
    1. Local funeral director
    2. Hospice agency
    3. Home health nurse
    4. Organ procurement organization

51. The nurse is caring for clients in an ophthalmology clinic. Which client **warrants** intervention by the nurse?
    1. The client diagnosed with cataracts who reports decreased vision and abnormal color perception
    2. The client diagnosed with a retinal detachment who reports a painless loss of peripheral vision
    3. The client diagnosed with an external hordeolum who reports reddened tender area under eye
    4. The client diagnosed with primary open-angle glaucoma who reports excruciating eye pain

52. The nurse is at a park and observes a person fall and a stick become impaled into the right eye. Which intervention should the nurse implement **first**?
    1. Tell someone to call 911 immediately.
    2. Stabilize the stick in the accident victim's eye.
    3. Apply direct pressure to the right eye.
    4. Use a non-toxic liquid and irrigate the eye.

53. The RN staff nurse and unlicensed assistive personnel (UAP) are caring for a minimally responsive client diagnosed with multiple sclerosis who weighs more than 400 pounds. Which action is **priority** when moving the client in the bed?
    1. Obtain a lifting device made for lifting heavy clients.
    2. Do not attempt to move the client because of the weight.
    3. Get another UAP to help move the client in the bed.
    4. Tell the family that the client must assist in moving in the bed.

54. The terminally ill client diagnosed with amyotrophic lateral sclerosis (ALS), also known as Lou Gehrig's disease, has a DNR order in place and is currently reporting "pain all over." The nurse notes the client has shallow breathing and a P 67, R 8, BP 104/62. Which intervention should the nurse implement?
    1. Administer the narcotic pain medication IVP.
    2. Turn and reposition the client for comfort.
    3. Refuse to administer pain medication.
    4. Notify the HCP of the client's vital signs.

55. The nurse in a rehabilitation facility is evaluating the progress of a female client who sustained a C-6–C-7 spinal cord injury. Which outcome indicates the client is **improving?**
    1. The client can maneuver the automatic wheelchair into the hallway.
    2. The client states she will be able to return to work in a few weeks.
    3. The client uses eye blinks to communicate yes and no responses.
    4. The client's spouse built a wheelchair ramp onto their house.

56. The nurse is triaging phone calls in a neurosensory clinic. Which client should the nurse contact **first?**
    1. The client diagnosed with Méniére's disease who is reporting vertigo and tinnitus
    2. The client diagnosed with otitis media with effusion describing a feeling of fullness in the ear
    3. The client diagnosed with external otitis who has serosanguineous drainage and otalgia
    4. The client diagnosed with otosclerosis who has bilateral hearing loss

57. The nurse is planning care for the client diagnosed with Parkinson's disease (PD). Which client problem is **priority?**
    1. Altered nutrition
    2. Altered mobility
    3. Altered elimination
    4. Altered body image

58. A client comes to the emergency department after having bleach splash in the eyes. Which intervention should the nurse implement **first?**
    1. Cover both the eyes with sterile patches.
    2. Assess the client's visual acuity.
    3. Irrigate the eyes with sterile solution.
    4. Elevate head of bed 45 degrees.

59. The 24-year-old client diagnosed with a traumatic brain injury is being transferred to a rehabilitation unit. Which health-care provider order should the nurse **question?**
    1. Physical therapy to work on lower extremity strength daily
    2. Occupational therapy to work on cognitive functioning bid
    3. A soft diet with mechanically ground meats and thickening agent in fluids
    4. Methylprednisolone IVP q 6 hours

60. The rehabilitation nurse is planning the discharge of a 68-year-old client whose status post–subarachnoid hemorrhage includes residual speech and balance deficits. Which referral should the nurse initiate at this time?
    1. Hospice organization
    2. Speech therapist
    3. Physical therapist
    4. Home health agency

61. The client is postoperative right eye enucleation. Which statement indicates the client needs **more** discharge teaching?
    1. "It will be approximately 2 weeks before I can get a prosthetic eye."
    2. "I can show you how I insert the conformer in the socket in case it falls out."
    3. "I should insert the eye drops into the lower conjunctiva of my eye."
    4. "If I develop an increased temperature I should call my health-care provider."

62. The nurse is caring for a client newly diagnosed with multiple sclerosis. Which referral is appropriate at this time?
1. Social worker to apply for disability
2. Dietitian for a nutritional consult
3. Psychological counselor for therapy
4. Chaplain to discuss spiritual issues

63. The RN staff nurse, LPN, and UAP have been assigned to care for clients on a neurology unit. Which nursing task is **most** appropriate to assign to the LPN?
1. Administer adrenocorticotropic hormone to the client diagnosed with multiple sclerosis.
2. Take the vital signs for the client who is experiencing status epilepticus.
3. Assist the client diagnosed with Parkinson's disease to ambulate to the bathroom.
4. Assess the newly admitted client diagnosed with pneumonia and restless legs syndrome.

64. The nurse is administering medications on a neurological unit. Which medication should the nurse administer **first?**
1. The osmotic diuretic to the client diagnosed with a closed head injury
2. The morning medications to the client scheduled for physical therapy
3. The narcotic pain medication to a client diagnosed with increased intracranial pressure
4. Gabapentin to the client diagnosed with restless leg syndrome

65. The RN charge nurse observes the new graduate nurse (GN) delegating tasks to the unlicensed assistive personnel (UAP) and the UAP appears to be ignoring the graduate nurse. Which action should the charge nurse implement **first?**
1. Wait and observe how the graduate nurse handles the situation.
2. Tell the UAP to get busy and complete the assigned tasks.
3. Discuss learning to assert authority with the new graduate.
4. Informally counsel the UAP about the response to the new nurse.

66. The nurse is on the day shift of a rehabilitation unit. Given the following medication administration record (MAR), which medication should the nurse administer **first?**

Client Name: D. F. Height: 69 inches Date of Birth: 05/07/1955	Account Number: 9251645 Weight in Pounds: 178 Date: Today	Allergies: Penicillin Weight in kg: 80.9
Medication	**1901–0700**	**0701–1900**
Levothyroxine 0.75 mcg PO daily		
Morphine sulfate 30 mg PO bid		
Fleets enema per rectum Q day		
Metformin 850 mg PO bid		
Signature/Initials	Night Nurse RN/NN	Day Nurse RN/DN

1. Administer the levothyroxine.
2. Administer the morphine sulfate.
3. Administer the Fleets enema.
4. Administer the metformin.

67. The client on the rehabilitation unit post–motor vehicle accident has been prescribed 50 mg of baclofen per dose orally for muscle spasms. Baclofen comes in 10-mg, 20-mg, and 75-mg tablets. How many tablets should the nurse administer and in which quantity?

----

68. The 19-year-old client is in the rehabilitation unit following a traumatic brain injury. Which intervention should the RN staff nurse delegate to the unlicensed assistive personnel (UAP)? **Select all that apply.**
1. Make safety rounds hourly.
2. Refer the client to a college and career counselor.
3. Assist the client with meals.
4. Clamp and unclamp the indwelling catheter every 2 hours.
5. Discuss discharge placement with the parents.

69. The 69-year-old client post–right cerebral vascular accident (CVA) is on the rehab unit diagnosed with left-sided weakness. Where should the nurse place the quad cane when assisting the client to ambulate?

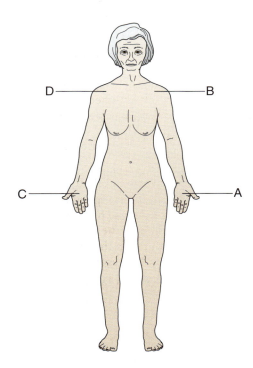

1. A
2. B
3. C
4. D

70. The male client is in the emergency department after a fall, resulting in a closed head injury. The admitting nurse notes the client responds by opening his eyes and pushing the nurse's arm away when painful stimuli is applied but the client does **not** make any verbal response. Which rating on the Glasgow Coma Scale should be documented by the nurse?

Glasgow Coma Scale

Appropriate Stimulus	Response	Score
Eyes Open		
*Approach to bedside	Spontaneous response	4
*Verbal command	Opens eyes to name on command	3
*Pain	Lack of opening of eyes to previous stimuli but opens to pain	2
	Lack of opening of eyes to any stimulus	1
	Untestable	0
Best Verbal Response		
Verbal questioning with maximum arousal	Oriented to person, place, time, and events	5
	Confusion, conversant but disoriented	4
	Disorganized use of words	3
	Incomprehensible words, groaning	2
	Lack of sound even with painful stimuli	1
	Untestable	0
Best Motor Response		
Verbal command	Follows verbal command	6
Pain (pressure on proximal nail bed)	Localizes pain, attempts to remove offending stimulus	5
	Flexion withdrawal of arm in response to pain without abnormal posturing	4
	Abnormal flexion, flexing of arm at elbow and pronation, making a fist	3
	Abnormal extension, extension of arm at elbow with adduction, and internal rotation of arm at shoulder	2
	Lack of response	1
	Untestable	0

1. Client scored a 12 on the Glasgow Coma Scale.
2. Client scored a 10 on the Glasgow Coma Scale.
3. Client scored an 8 on the Glasgow Coma Scale.
4. Client scored a 6 on the Glasgow Coma Scale.

NEUROLOGICAL CLINICAL SCENARIO

The RN charge nurse is on the 10-bed neurological intensive care unit and 20-bed neurological step-down unit in a large research hospital with level I adult and level II pediatric trauma classifications. The charge nurse supervises 15 RNs in the ICU, 30 RNs in the step-down unit, one new graduate nurse (GN), and 15 UAPs.

1. The day shift RN staff nurse and the UAP are caring for an elderly client diagnosed with a right-sided cerebrovascular accident (CVA) with hemi-paralysis. Which action by the UAP **requires** the RN to intervene?
   1. The UAP places the call light on the client's left side.
   2. The UAP assists the client to eat the breakfast meal.
   3. The UAP uses the draw sheet to move the client up in bed.
   4. The UAP places a small pillow under the client's left shoulder.

2. The 45-year-old hypertensive client diagnosed with a right-sided cerebrovascular accident (CVA) is reporting a severe headache. Which intervention should the nurse implement **first?**
   1. Administer acetaminophen.
   2. Prepare for a STAT computed tomography (CT) scan.
   3. Notify the client's health-care provider.
   4. Assess the client's neurological status.

3. The nurse is caring for clients on the neurological intensive care unit. Which client should the nurse assess **first?**
   1. The client diagnosed with a C-6 SCI who is reporting dyspnea and has crackles in the lungs
   2. The young adult client diagnosed with Guillain-Barré syndrome who is reporting ascending paralysis
   3. The client diagnosed with traumatic brain injury who has a Glasgow Coma Scale score of 6
   4. The obese client diagnosed with a cerebrovascular accident (CVA) who has expressive aphasia

4. The ICU unit is very busy and the charge nurse is entering the health-care provider's admission orders for an elderly client diagnosed with a closed head injury into the EHR. Which medication order should the charge nurse **question?**
   1. An SQ anticoagulant
   2. An IV osmotic diuretic
   3. An IV anticonvulsant
   4. An IV proton-pump inhibitor

5. The nurse is caring for a quadriplegic client who had a C-6 SCI 2 years ago and is admitted for stage IV pressure ulcers in the coccyx area. The client is reporting a severe headache and the BP is 190/110. Which intervention should the nurse implement **first?**
   1. Insert a urinary catheter into the client.
   2. Complete a neurological assessment.
   3. Put the client in the Trendelenburg position.
   4. Palpate the client's bladder.

6. The charge nurse is making rounds and enters the room as the pediatric client is having a tonic-clonic seizure. Which **priority** intervention should the charge nurse implement?
   1. Place the client on the side.
   2. Call the Rapid Response Team.
   3. Determine if the client is incontinent of urine.
   4. Provide the client with privacy during the seizure.

7. The UAP is attempting to put an oral airway in the mouth of a client having a tonic-clonic seizure. Which intervention should the RN charge nurse take **first?**
   1. Complete an adverse occurrence report.
   2. Instruct the UAP to stop inserting the oral airway.
   3. Assist the UAP to insert the oral airway.
   4. Note the time of the seizure and observe the seizure.

8. The charge nurse is telling the graduate nurse the correct procedure for assisting the health-care provider with a lumbar puncture to R/O meningitis on a young adult. Which interventions should the charge nurse discuss with the graduate nurse? **Select all that apply.**
   1. Obtain an informed consent from the client or spouse.
   2. Determine if the client is allergic to iodine or shellfish.
   3. Place the client in the supine position with the foot of the bed elevated.
   4. Instruct the client to relax and breathe normally.
   5. Explain to the client what to expect during the procedure.

9. The charge nurse is making shift assignments. Which client should be assigned to the **most** experienced nurse?
   1. The malnourished client diagnosed with bacterial meningitis who is experiencing photophobia
   2. The paraplegic client diagnosed with an L-4 SCI who has spastic muscle spasms of the lower extremities
   3. The elderly client diagnosed with Parkinson's who has a mask-like face and has pill rolling
   4. The client diagnosed with amyotrophic lateral sclerosis (ALS) who is having respiratory distress

10. The nurse is caring for clients on a neurological intensive care unit. Which client should be assessed **first?**
    1. The client recovering from an MVA diagnosed with increased intracranial pressure whose Glasgow Coma Scale went from 11 to 14
    2. The quadriplegic client diagnosed with a C-6 SCI who has bradycardia, hypotension, and hyperflexia
    3. The client with a brainstem herniation whose big toe moves toward the top surface of the foot and the other toes fan out after the sole of the foot has been firmly stroked
    4. The 20-year-old client diagnosed with West Nile virus who has a temperature of 101.2°F and generalized body aches

The correct answer number and rationale for why it is the correct answer are given in **boldface type.** Rationales for why the other possible answer options are incorrect also are given, but they are not in boldface type.

1. 1. The serum platelet level is within the normal range of 140 to 400 x 10^3/ microL; therefore, this client does not warrant intervention by the charge nurse.
2. A therapeutic valproic acid (Depakote) level is 50 to 125 mcg/mL; therefore, this laboratory result does not warrant action by the nurse.
3. Steroids, such as prednisone, elevate a client's blood glucose level; therefore, this does not warrant intervention by the nurse.
4. **The therapeutic range for the anticonvulsant phenytoin (Dilantin) is 10–20 mcg/mL. This client's higher level warrants intervention because the serum level is above the therapeutic range.**

CLINICAL JUDGMENT GUIDE: The nurse must be knowledgeable of normal laboratory values. These values must be memorized and the nurse must be able to determine if the laboratory value is normal for the client's disease process or medications the client is taking.

2. 1. A pain medication is important to administer in a timely manner, but its administration is not a priority over a medication that must be administered on time to prevent respiratory complications.
2. A steroid medication is not a priority over a client who may experience respiratory difficulty. Steroids must be given to prevent adrenal sufficiency but it does not have to be administered first.
3. **Anticholinesterase medications administered for myasthenia gravis must be administered on time to preserve muscle functioning, especially the functioning of the muscles of the upper respiratory tract. This is the priority medication.**
4. Clients who have called for medications should be attended to, but this client would not receive an antacid for heartburn before the client diagnosed with myasthenia gravis or the client in pain.

CLINICAL JUDGMENT GUIDE: The nurse must be aware of expected actions of medications, and assess data indicating whether the medication is effective or the medication is causing a side effect or an adverse effect.

3. 1. The nurse would expect the client diagnosed with Guillain-Barré syndrome to have ascending paralysis and the problem has just reached the knees, so the nurse should not need to assess this client first.
2. **The client diagnosed with a C-6 SCI is expected to have autonomic dysreflexia but it is an emergency situation; therefore, the nurse should assess this client first.**
3. "Pill rolling," a hand tremor wherein the thumb and forefinger appear to move in a rotary fashion as if rolling a pill, is an expected clinical manifestation of Parkinson's; therefore, the nurse would not assess this client first.
4. The client diagnosed with Huntington's disease has chorea, which includes abnormal and excessive involuntary movements; therefore, this client would not be assessed first.

CLINICAL JUDGMENT GUIDE: The nurse must determine which sign or symptom is not expected for the disease process. If the sign or symptom is not expected or it is an emergency situation, then the nurse should assess the client first. This type of question determines if the nurse is knowledgeable of signs or symptoms of a variety of disease processes.

4. 1. Placing a gait belt on a client before ambulating is an appropriate action for safety and would not require the nurse to intervene.
2. Placing the client in a prone position helps promote hyperextension of the hip joints, which is essential for normal gait and helps prevent knee and hip flexion contractures; therefore, this would not require the nurse to intervene.
3. **This action is inappropriate and would require intervention by the nurse because pulling on a flaccid shoulder joint could cause shoulder dislocation; the client should be pulled up by placing the arm underneath the client's back or using a lift sheet.**
4. The client should be encouraged and praised for attempting to perform any activities independently, such as combing hair or brushing teeth.

CLINICAL JUDGMENT GUIDE: The nurse must ensure the UAP can perform any tasks that are delegated. It is the nurse's responsibility to demonstrate to or teach the UAP how to perform the task, and evaluate the task.

5. **1. With an evolving stroke, the client experiences a worsening of signs or symptoms over several minutes to hours; thus, the client is at risk for dying and should be cared for by the most experienced nurse.**
   2. A transient ischemic attack by definition lasts fewer than 24 hours; thus, this client should be stable at this time.
   3. Pain is expected in clients diagnosed with Guillain-Barré syndrome, and symptoms typically occur on the lower half of the body, which wouldn't affect the airway. Therefore, a less experienced nurse could care for this client.
   4. The charge nurse could assign this client to an unlicensed assistive personnel (UAP).

CLINICAL JUDGMENT GUIDE: When the nurse is deciding which client should be assigned to the most experienced nurse, the most critical and unstable client should be assigned to the most experienced nurse.

6. **1. This client should be referred to an inpatient rehabilitation facility for intensive therapy before deciding on long-term placement (home with home health care or a long-term care facility). The initial rehabilitation a client receives can set the tone for all further recuperation. This is the appropriate referral at this time.**
   2. A home health-care agency may be needed when the client returns home, but the most appropriate referral is to a rehabilitation center where intensive therapy can take place.
   3. A long-term care facility may be needed at some point, but the client should be given the opportunity to regain as much lost ability as possible at this time.
   4. The outpatient center would be utilized when the client is ready for discharge from the inpatient center.

CLINICAL JUDGMENT GUIDE: The nurse must be knowledgeable of the role of all members of the multidisciplinary health-care team, as well as HIPAA rules and regulations. These will be tested on the NCLEX-RN® examination.

7. 1. The nurse should be the first one to feed the client in order for the nurse to evaluate the client's ability to swallow and not aspirate.
   2. **The LPN could administer routine parenteral medications. This is the best task to assign to the LPN.**

3. This involves assessing the client; therefore, the nurse should not delegate this assignment to the LPN.
   4. Teaching is the responsibility of the RN.

CLINICAL JUDGMENT GUIDE: The nurse cannot assign assessment, teaching, evaluation, or an unstable client to a LPN. The LPN calls HCPs on the phone to obtain orders for a client.

8. **Correct answers are 3, 4, and 5.**
   1. Checking the client's skin involves assessment; therefore, the nurse cannot delegate this assignment to the UAP.
   2. The nurse cannot delegate medication administration to a UAP.
   3. **The UAP can perform routine hygiene care. The nurse must then make the time to assess the client's skin.**
   4. **The UAP can ambulate a client to the bathroom.**
   5. **The UAP can take routine vital signs.**

CLINICAL JUDGMENT GUIDE: This is a type of alternate question included in the NCLEX-RN® examination. The nurse must be able to select all the options that answer the question correctly. There are no partial correct answers.

9. 1. The UAP cannot change abdominal dressings because the incision must be assessed for healing.
   2. The UAP cannot check the client's IV site. Remember, "check" is assessment.
   3. The nurse must monitor the vital signs on a client recently returned from surgery to determine whether the client is stable; the UAP can take vital signs and report results to the nurse.
   4. **The UAP can escort the client to the vehicle after discharge.**

CLINICAL JUDGMENT GUIDE: A nurse cannot delegate assessment, teaching, evaluation, medications, or an unstable client to a UAP. Tasks that cannot be delegated are nursing interventions requiring nursing judgment.

10. **1. This client diagnosed with dyspnea and a respiration rate of 12 has signs and symptoms of a respiratory complication and should be assessed first because ascending paralysis at the C-6 level could cause the client to stop breathing.**
   2. This is a psychosocial need and should be addressed, but it is not a priority over a physiological problem.
   3. A client diagnosed with a lower SCI would not be at risk for autonomic dysreflexia; therefore,

a report of headache and feeling hot would not be a priority over an airway problem.

4. The client with a pulse oximeter reading greater than 93% is receiving adequate oxygenation.

CLINICAL JUDGMENT GUIDE: When deciding which client to assess first, the test taker should determine whether the signs and symptoms the client is exhibiting are normal or expected for the situation. After eliminating the expected options, the test taker should determine which situation is more life threatening.

11. 1. The client is experiencing autonomic dysreflexia, a complication of SCI above the T6, and the most common cause is a full bladder. Placing the client on telemetry is not the nurse's first intervention.

2. Completing a neurological assessment is an intervention a nurse could implement, but it should not be the first for a client experiencing autonomic dysreflexia.

3. **Autonomic dysreflexia is a life-threatening condition and can be considered a medical emergency requiring immediate attention. The nurse should not assess but should intervene, and the most common cause is a full bladder.**

4. A CT scan of the head would be appropriate if the elevated BP was secondary to a CVA, not because of a complication of a SCI.

CLINICAL JUDGMENT GUIDE: When the test question asks the test taker to determine which intervention should be implemented first, it means that all the options are something a nurse could implement. The test taker should apply the nursing process: If the client is in distress then do not assess; the nurse should do something to help the client.

12. 1. It would be appropriate for the UAP to perform ROM exercises to help prevent contractures; therefore, this action would not require the nurse to intervene.

2. **This is not an appropriate intervention because the client is at risk for increased intracranial pressure (ICP); therefore, the client should not be placed on the stomach. The prone position helps promote hyperextension of the hip joints, which is essential for normal gait and helps prevent knee and hip flexion contractures, and is done in rehabilitation.**

3. The client should be pulled up in bed by placing the arm underneath the back or using

a lift sheet; therefore, the nurse would not need to intervene.

4. The client should be encouraged and praised for attempting to perform any activities independently, such as combing hair, brushing teeth, or feeding him- or herself. The nurse would not need to intervene.

CLINICAL JUDGMENT GUIDE: The nurse must ensure the UAP can perform any tasks that are delegated. It is the nurse's responsibility to demonstrate to or teach the UAP how to perform the task, and evaluate the task.

13. 1. **The less experienced nurse could care for the client on a ventilator and console the family as needed.**

2. A client diagnosed with increased intracranial pressure requires a more experienced critical care nurse.

3. This client is unstable and requires a more experienced critical care nurse.

4. Status epilepticus is a state of continuous seizure activity and is the most serious complication of epilepsy. This is a neurological emergency. This client should be assigned to a more experienced nurse.

CLINICAL JUDGMENT GUIDE: The most stable client should be assigned to the graduate nurse. The more critical clients should be assigned to the more experienced nurses.

14. 1. Purposeful movement following painful stimuli would indicate an improvement in the client's condition and would not warrant intervention by the nurse.

2. **Extension of the upper and lower extremities is assuming a decerebrate posture, which indicates the client's intracranial pressure (ICP) is increasing. This would warrant immediate intervention by the nurse.**

3. Aimless thrashing would indicate an improvement in the client's condition and would not warrant intervention by the nurse.

4. If the client is able to follow simple commands, then the client's condition is improving and would not warrant intervention by the nurse.

CLINICAL JUDGMENT GUIDE: The test taker should ask, "Are the assessment data normal?" for the disease process. If the data are normal for the disease process, then the nurse would not need to intervene; if they are not normal for the disease process, then this warrants intervention by the nurse.

ANSWERS

15. 1. An adverse occurrence report is completed for incidents occurring to clients.
2. The nurse should talk to the primary nurse, but the sharps container should be changed immediately.
3. **The UAP can change a sharps container. This must be done because a sharps container above the fill line is a violation of Occupational Safety and Health Administration (OSHA) rules and can result in a financial fine.**
4. The infection control nurse does not need to be notified of this situation.

CLINICAL JUDGMENT GUIDE: The nurse is responsible for knowing and complying with local, state, and federal standards of care.

16. 1. The nurse should address the client's comment and not "pass the buck" to someone else.
2. The nurse should address the client's statement and not attempt to problem-solve at this point in the conversation.
3. **The nurse is reflecting the client's comments, which will encourage the client to ventilate her feelings. This is the most appropriate response.**
4. This is false reassurance and an inappropriate response to the client's statement.

CLINICAL JUDGMENT GUIDE: The NCLEX-RN® test plan includes Therapeutic Communication as a subcategory of Psychosocial Integrity. The nurse should allow clients and family to express feelings.

17. 1. The client diagnosed with Guillain-Barré syndrome is at risk for airway compromise resulting from the ascending paralysis. Cardiac output is not a priority.
2. The client's psychological needs are important, but psychosocial problems are not a priority.
3. Complications of immobility are pertinent but do not take priority over the airway.
4. **Guillain-Barré syndrome produces ascending paralysis that will cause respiratory failure; therefore, the breathing pattern is the priority.**

CLINICAL JUDGMENT GUIDE: The NCLEX-RN® integrates the nursing process throughout the Client Needs categories and subcategories. The nursing process is a scientific, clinical reasoning approach to client care that includes assessment, analysis, planning, implementation, and evaluation. The nurse will be responsible for identifying nursing problems for clients.

18. 1. The occupational therapist addresses assisting the client diagnosed with ADLs, but with MG the client will have no problems with ADLs if the client takes the medication correctly, 30 minutes before performing ADLs.
2. A physical therapist addresses transfer and movement issues with the client, but this would not be a priority in the critical care unit.
3. The social worker assists the client with discharge issues or financial issues, but this would not be appropriate for the client in the critical care unit.
4. **Speech therapists address swallowing problems, and clients diagnosed with myasthenia gravis (MG) are dysphagic and are at risk for aspiration; the speech therapist can help match food consistency to the client's ability to swallow and thus help enhance client safety. This referral would be appropriate in the critical care unit.**

CLINICAL JUDGMENT GUIDE: The NCLEX-RN® integrates the nursing process throughout the Client Needs categories and subcategories. The nursing process is a scientific, clinical reasoning approach to client care that includes assessment, analysis, planning, implementation, and evaluation. The nurse will be responsible for identifying nursing diagnoses for clients.

19. Correct order is 5, 2, 1, 3, 4.
5. **The nurse should flush the area with soap and water and attempt to get the site to bleed.**
2. **The nurse should notify the charge nurse immediately after cleaning the area to avoid any delays in treatment and to initiate hospital protocol.**
1. **The laboratory should draw the client's and the nurse's baseline laboratory blood work.**
3. **Post-exposure prophylaxis should be started, if applicable, within 4 hours of the stick.**
4. **Follow up with the employee health nurse is done at 3 months and 6 months.**

CLINICAL JUDGMENT GUIDE: The NCLEX-RN® test plan includes nursing care that is ruled by legal requirements as well as The Joint Commission, Centers for Medicare & Medicaid Services, the Centers for Disease Control and

Prevention, and Occupational Safety and Health Administration rules and regulations. The nurse must be knowledgeable of these standards.

20. **1. The client diagnosed with Parkinson's disease who has begun to hallucinate may be experiencing an adverse reaction to one of the medications used to treat the disease. The nurse should assess this client first.**
   2. Peripheral edema is expected in a client diagnosed with heart failure. This client does not need to be assessed first.
   3. Wandering and lack of sleeping are expected in a client diagnosed with Alzheimer's disease. This client does not need to be assessed first.
   4. Weight loss in a client diagnosed with terminal cancer is expected. The nurse should review the client's intake, food preferences, and pain control before making an intervention. Weight loss does not occur in a matter of minutes to hours, and this client's needs do not merit assessment before the client diagnosed with a new problem.

CLINICAL JUDGMENT GUIDE: The nurse should determine whether a new problem is occurring or whether the problem is expected for the disease process. If the symptom is expected for the disease process and it is not life threatening, then that client does not have priority.

21. 1. A daily acetylsalicylic acid (aspirin) is not a priority medication. This medication can be administered within 30 minutes before or 30 minutes after the scheduled time.
   2. Neostigmine (Prostigmin) promotes muscle function in clients diagnosed with myasthenia gravis. This medication should always be administered on time to prevent loss of muscle tone, especially the muscles of the upper respiratory tract. This is the priority medication to administer at this time.
   3. Cephalexin (Keflex), an oral antibiotic, can be administered within 30 minutes before or after the scheduled timeframe.
   4. Acyclovir (Zovirax) alone or in combination with prednisone may be used to treat Bell's palsy but this medication is not a priority medication.

CLINICAL JUDGMENT GUIDE: When the nurse is deciding on a priority medication, the test taker must first decide on the expected response of the client. If the expected response prevents or treats

an emergency situation, then that medication becomes the priority medication to administer.

22. 1. Clients diagnosed with Alzheimer's disease may have problems with completing activities of daily living, but this is not the client's priority problem.
   2. Safety is the highest priority for clients diagnosed with end-stage Alzheimer's disease because the client is unaware of his or her own surroundings and can easily wander from an area of safety.
   3. The client in end-stage disease may have an increased risk for constipation, but this is not a priority over safety of the client.
   4. The client's family is often distraught over seeing their loved one deteriorate because of Alzheimer's, but it is not a priority over the safety of the client.

CLINICAL JUDGMENT GUIDE: The test taker can use Maslow's Hierarchy of Needs to determine the correct answer. On the pyramid of needs, beginning at the bottom, physiological needs have priority, followed by safety.

23. Correct answers are 1, 2, 4, and 5.
   1. Cataracts cause less light to be filtered through an opaque lens to the retina. The client should have as much light as possible in the home to prevent falls.
   2. Dark glasses protect the eyes from the sun's rays when outside, as they do for anyone, so they should be encouraged in this client.
   3. This is the responsibility of the HCP, not the nurse.
   4. The furniture in the client's house should not be moved. If the furniture is left in its usual position, the client will be less likely to fall or stumble.
   5. Discharge instructions should be provided with visual aids or large print. This allows the client to review the materials with less difficulty.

CLINICAL JUDGMENT GUIDE: This question requires the test taker to use knowledge of the disease process and Maslow's Hierarchy of Needs. Cataracts cause opacity of the lens of the eye. The test taker should address nursing interventions that promote client safety and independence.

24. **1. The nurse should first assess the client's neurological status. It is not normal for an elderly person to have a change in behavior; this is cause for assessment.**

2. The nurse may need to notify the HCP but not before completing a neurological assessment.

3. The nurse should first assess the client before further interviewing the client's wife.

4. The nurse could determine the last time the client ate, because the confusion could be caused by hypoglycemia, but the first intervention is to complete a neurological assessment.

CLINICAL JUDGMENT GUIDE: Any time the nurse receives information about a client who may be experiencing a complication, the nurse must assess the client. The nurse should not make decisions about the client's needs based on another staff member's information.

25. 1. **This question will determine whether the nurse has assessed the client's ability to swallow. The nurse cannot delegate unstable clients, and a client newly diagnosed with a CVA may be unstable and have difficulty swallowing.**

2. This question does not address the client's ability to swallow.

3. Thickener (Thick-It) might be needed if the client has difficulty swallowing, but the charge nurse has not established that the client has swallowing difficulty.

4. A UAP can feed clients who are stable and do not require nursing judgment during the process.

CLINICAL JUDGMENT GUIDE: The nurse cannot delegate assessment, evaluation, teaching, administering medications, or the care of an unstable client to a UAP.

26. 1. The client should be encouraged to move the buttocks to increase blood circulation to the area, but a wheelchair cushion used every time the client is in the wheelchair will help prevent pressure ulcers.

2. A high-protein diet will assist with maintaining a positive nitrogen balance that will support wound healing, but it will not prevent pressure from causing a breakdown of the skin.

3. **All clients remaining in a wheelchair for extended periods of time should have a wheelchair cushion that relieves pressure to prevent skin breakdown.**

4. The more the client can move from the wheelchair to a chair to the bed, the more it will help decrease the possibility of a pressure ulcer, but a wheelchair cushion helps relieve pressure continuously.

CLINICAL JUDGMENT GUIDE: The nurse must be knowledgeable of expected medical treatment for the client. This is a knowledge-based, or comprehension, question.

27. Correct answers are 1, 2, and 4.
1. **Identifying the first area that began seizing will provide information and clues as to the origin of the seizure in the brain.**

2. **The nurse should first look at his or her watch and time the seizure.**

3. The client's bed rails should be padded, but this intervention should not be performed when a client is beginning to have a seizure. The nurse should protect the client and assess the seizure. The seizure may be over by the time the nurse can pad the side rails.

4. **The client should be protected from onlookers as much as possible.**

5. The nurse should never attempt to insert anything into the mouth of a client during a seizure. Doing so can cause injury to the client's mouth or obstruction of the client's airway.

CLINICAL JUDGMENT GUIDE: This is an alternate type of question included in the NCLEX-RN® examination. The nurse must be able to select all the correct options. There are no partially correct answers.

28. 1. Closing the door and cubicle curtain protects the client's privacy and would not warrant immediate intervention from the nurse.

2. Providing a back massage is a wonderful action to take and would not warrant intervention by the nurse.

3. Checking the temperature of the bathwater prevents scalding the client with water that is too hot or making the client uncomfortable with water that is too cold. This action would not warrant immediate intervention.

4. **The client is recovering from a potentially debilitating disease, and in the rehabilitation unit the client should be out of the bed as much as possible. Bathing the client in bed would warrant intervention by the nurse.**

CLINICAL JUDGMENT GUIDE: Delegation means the nurse is responsible for the UAP's actions and performance. The nurse must correct the UAP's performance to ensure the client is cared for safely in the hospital, the rehabilitation unit, or the home.

29. Correct answers are 1, 2, 3, and 4.

   1. Placing a small pillow under the shoulder will prevent the shoulder from adducting toward the chest and developing a contracture.

   2. The client should be referred to occupational therapy for assistance with performing activities of daily living (ADLs).

   3. The client should not ignore the paralyzed side, and the nurse must encourage the client to move it as much as possible; a written schedule may assist the client in exercising.

   4. These exercises should be done at least five times a day for 10 minutes at a time to help strengthen the muscles used for walking.

   5. The fingers should be positioned so that they are barely flexed, to prevent contracture.

CLINICAL JUDGMENT GUIDE: This is an alternate type of question included in the NCLEX-RN®. The nurse must be able to select all the options that answer the question correctly. There are no partially correct answers.

30. 1. The nurse should stabilize the client's cervical spine to help prevent a spinal cord injury or the client's spine can sustain irreparable damage during movement.

   2. Unless the driver is in danger (car on fire or in water) the nurse should not move the driver.

   3. The nurse should first ensure a patent airway. According to Maslow's Hierarchy of Needs, airway is always the priority.

   4. The nurse should control external bleeding but the first intervention is the airway.

CLINICAL JUDGMENT GUIDE: The test taker should use some tool as a reference to guide in the decision-making process. In this situation, Maslow's Hierarchy of Needs should be applied.

31. **1. This would be the most appropriate assignment because the nurse would not be exposed to any contagious diseases or dangerous radiological procedures.**

   2. The pregnant nurse should not be exposed to x-rays, which could endanger the fetus.

   3. Working in the front desk triage area would allow the pregnant nurse to be exposed to any type of contagious or infectious disease. This is not an appropriate assignment.

   4. The oncology clinic will have clients receiving chemotherapeutic agents that may endanger the fetus; this would not be the most appropriate assignment. Even if the nurse is not administering the medication, the most appropriate assignment is to assign the nurse to an area that poses no danger to the fetus.

CLINICAL JUDGMENT GUIDE: Pregnant nurses can refuse and should not be assigned duties that could harm the fetus. Most medications and many diagnostic tests and treatments can harm the fetus.

32. 1. If the client must be transferred from the clinic to the hospital, then the client is unstable and therefore should not be assigned to a UAP.

   2. The client is stable because he or she is being sent home; therefore, the UAP could safely complete this task.

   3. Showing the client how to walk with crutches is teaching, and the nurse cannot delegate teaching to the UAP.

   4. The UAP should not be calling a pharmacy because this is not within the scope of practice of unlicensed personnel. The HCP is responsible for delegating this task.

CLINICAL JUDGMENT GUIDE: A nurse cannot delegate assessment, teaching, evaluation, medications, or an unstable client to a UAP. Tasks that cannot be delegated are nursing interventions requiring nursing judgment.

33. **1. The nurse should first care for the client and refer the client to an HCP for possible x-rays, pain medication, and further treatment. The employee health nurse's responsibility is to ensure the employee is safe to work, and this client is not.**

   2. This information should be completed because any injury on the job must be covered by workers' compensation insurance so that all costs will be covered for the client. Documentation is never a priority over caring for the client.

   3. The employee health nurse should determine whether there are unsafe areas in the workplace or whether the employee was negligent, but this is not the nurse's first intervention.

   4. The employee's supervisor does need to be notified, but this is not the nurse's first intervention. The safety of the client is always first.

CLINICAL JUDGMENT GUIDE: When the question asks which intervention should be implemented first, it means all the options are something a nurse could implement, but only one should be implemented first. The test taker should use the nursing process to determine the appropriate action: If the client is in distress, do not assess; if the client is not in distress, then the nurse should assess.

34. 1. If a client is reporting pain, the nurse should not ask the client to return to work. If nothing else, the client should be allowed to stay in the clinic until the pain subsides.
   2. **The employee must submit to a urine drug screen anytime there is an injury. This is standard practice by many employers to help determine whether the employee was under the influence during the time of the accident. Workers' compensation will not be responsible if the employee is under the influence of alcohol or drugs.**
   3. Because there are no visible injuries and the neurovascular assessment is normal, a referral to the emergency department is not warranted. The employee health nurse could send the employee home with further instructions. None of the symptoms warrant the employee needing an x-ray.
   4. A sequential compression device is used to help prevent deep vein thrombosis for clients on bedrest. This is not an appropriate intervention.

CLINICAL JUDGMENT GUIDE: The NCLEX-RN® test plan includes nursing care that is ruled by legal requirements as well as The Joint Commission, Centers for Medicare & Medicaid Services, Centers for Disease Control and Prevention, and Occupational Safety and Health Administration rules and regulations. The nurse must be knowledgeable of these standards.

35. **Correct order is 1, 3, 2, 4, 5.**
   1. **An alert client diagnosed with a sucking chest wound and categorized as red should be evacuated first. A red tag means the injury is life threatening but survivable with minimal intervention. These clients can deteriorate rapidly without treatment.**
   3. **A client whose abdomen is hard and tender and categorized as a yellow should be evacuated second. A yellow tag means the injury is significant and requires medical care but is stable at the moment.**
   2. **A client who cannot stop crying, cannot answer questions, and is categorized as green should be evacuated third.**

A green tag means the injury is minor and treatment can be delayed hours to days. These clients should be moved away from the main triage area. Clients diagnosed with behavioral and psychological problems are included in this category.
   4. **This client who is categorized as black should be evacuated fourth. A black tag means the injury is extensive and chances of survival are unlikely even with definitive care. Clients should receive comfort measures and be separated from other casualties, but not abandoned.**
   5. **The client who is categorized as white does not need to be evacuated until last. A white tag means no care is required.**

CLINICAL JUDGMENT GUIDE: The NCLEX-RN® test plan includes questions on disaster management. The nurse needs to be aware of triaging clients, nursing care, and procedures and protocols during disasters.

36. 1. The nurse should determine what medication the client has taken, but the nurse should first attempt to determine whether the headache is secondary to high blood pressure.
   2. No matter what number the client identifies on the pain scale in the home setting, the nurse must attempt to determine the cause. One way to try to determine the cause or to eliminate a possible cause is to take the client's blood pressure.
   3. If the client's blood pressure is not elevated, the client could take the non-narcotic analgesic acetaminophen (Tylenol), but if the client's blood pressure is elevated, the Tylenol will not help.
   4. **The number 1 risk factor for a CVA is arterial hypertension. Because the client has a history of a CVA and is reporting a severe headache, which is a symptom of hypertension, the nurse should first take the client's blood pressure. If it is elevated, the client needs to be taken to the emergency department. In the home setting, asking about the pain scale would not affect the care the nurse provides.**

CLINICAL JUDGMENT GUIDE: When the question asks which intervention should be implemented first, it means that all the options are something a nurse could implement, but only one should be implemented first. The test taker should use the nursing process to determine the appropriate action: **If the client is in distress, do not assess; if the client is not in distress, then the nurse should assess.**

37. 1. The nurse should assist the client to lie in the "C" position with the back as near as possible to the edge of the bed, but it is not the first intervention.
2. **The first intervention is to empty the client's bladder before the procedure.**
3. All clients should have an advance directive, but it is not mandated by law, and clients can decide not to have one.
4. The client does not have to be NPO for this procedure.

CLINICAL JUDGMENT GUIDE: The nurse must be knowledgeable of normal diagnostic tests pre- and post-procedure. These interventions must be memorized and the nurse must be able to determine if the client is able to have the diagnostic procedure and post-procedure care to ensure the client is safe.

38. 1. A severe, pounding headache would be the priority for a client diagnosed with a T-6 or above spinal cord injury (SCI) because it could be autonomic dysreflexia, but not in a client diagnosed with a lower-level lesion.
2. The client's psychosocial need is not a priority over clients diagnosed with physiological problems. This client should not be visited first.
3. The client diagnosed with Parkinson's disease is expected to have a short, shuffling gait; therefore, this client does not need to be seen first.
4. **The client is reporting an infection at the insertion sites into the bone, which can lead to osteomyelitis. This client is exhibiting a potentially life-threatening condition and should be seen first.**

CLINICAL JUDGMENT GUIDE: When deciding which client to assess first, the test taker should determine whether the signs or symptoms the client is exhibiting are normal or expected for the client situation. After eliminating the expected option, the test taker should determine which situation is more life threatening.

39. 1. A client diagnosed with AIDS would be expected to have Kaposi's sarcoma; therefore, this client would not need to be visited first.
2. A client diagnosed with dementia would be expected to have difficulty dressing; therefore, this client would not need to be visited first.

3. The classic feature of trigeminal neuralgia is excruciating pain described as a burning, knife-like, or lightning-like shock in the lips, upper or lower gums, cheek, forehead, or side of the nose. The nurse would not return this call first because the client is experiencing the normal signs and symptoms for the disease process.
4. **Botulism is the most serious type of food poisoning and the client is exhibiting signs and symptoms of it; therefore, the nurse should return this phone call first.**

CLINICAL JUDGMENT GUIDE: When deciding which client to assess first, the nurse should determine whether the signs and symptoms the client is exhibiting are normal or expected for the client situation. After eliminating the expected options, the test taker should determine which situation is more dangerous for the client.

40. 1. **Therapeutic communication addresses the client's feelings and attempts to allow the client to verbalize feelings. The client is still grieving over her loss, and the nurse should let her vent those feelings.**
2. The social worker may be able to help the client with driving and going back to college, but this is not the nurse's first intervention.
3. The American Spinal Cord Association is an excellent resource for clients diagnosed with spinal cord injuries, but the client is still grieving, and the nurse should allow the client to express her feelings.
4. Attempting to help identify a support system for the client is an appropriate intervention, but the first intervention is to allow the client to vent her feelings.

CLINICAL JUDGMENT GUIDE: The NCLEX-RN® test plan includes Therapeutic Communication as a subcategory of Psychosocial Integrity. The nurse should allow clients and family to vent their feelings.

41. 1. **The client is allergic to iodine; therefore, the client cannot have the CT scan with contrast because it is iodine. The nurse should question this HCP order.**
2. The client is not allergic to Tylenol; therefore, this order should not be questioned.
3. The client should have vital signs taken; therefore, this order should not be questioned.
4. A low-fat, low-cholesterol diet would be appropriate for this client.

CLINICAL JUDGMENT GUIDE: When the stem asks the nurse to determine which health-care provider's order to question, the test taker should realize this is an "except" question. Three of the options are appropriate for the HCP to prescribe and one is not appropriate for the client's disease process or procedure.

42. 1. The client has a chronic illness. The nurse should empower the client to deal with her disease process, not put more responsibility on her spouse.
    2. **The occupational therapist could assist the client in identifying ways to save energy when performing activities of daily living. Myasthenia gravis is a neurological condition that causes skeletal muscle weakness.**
    3. The HH nurse should realize that exhaustion is a symptom of her disease process and should utilize any member of the home health-care team who could help the client. Allowing the client to verbalize her feelings about exhaustion is an appropriate therapeutic intervention, but this client needs specific advice on how to handle her exhaustion.
    4. If the client is taking her medication, she does not need to be referred to her HCP. Myasthenia gravis is a chronic illness, and muscle weakness is the primary symptom.

CLINICAL JUDGMENT GUIDE: The test taker must be knowledgeable of the role of all members of the multidisciplinary health-care team as well as HIPAA rules and regulations. These will be tested on the NCLEX-RN® examination.

43. 1. **An epidural hematoma results from bleeding between the dura and the inner surface of the skull, and is a medical emergency. This client should be seen first.**
    2. Postictal state is a sleepy state the client has after having a seizure. This client is stable; therefore, this client does not have to be assessed first.
    3. The client diagnosed with encephalitis may have fever, headache, nausea, and vomiting. The client needs to be assessed but not before a head injury with active arterial bleeding.
    4. The client diagnosed with multiple sclerosis is expected to have scanning speech; therefore, the nurse should not assess this client first.

CLINICAL JUDGMENT GUIDE: The test taker should use some tool as a reference to guide in the decision-making process. In this situation, Maslow's Hierarchy of Needs should be applied.

44. 1. **The tension headache does not involve nausea or vomiting but may involve photophobia or phonophobia. Because the nausea and vomiting are not expected, the nurse should return this phone call first.**
    2. The migraine headache is a recurring headache characterized by unilateral or bilateral throbbing pain; therefore, this client should not be contacted first.
    3. The pain of cluster headaches is sharp and stabbing on one side of the head, often near the eye. It is not similar to the pulsing pain of a migraine headache. This client does not need to be contacted first.
    4. This is the typical type of pain clients diagnosed with hypertension experience; therefore, this client does not need to be contacted first.

CLINICAL JUDGMENT GUIDE: The test taker must determine which sign or symptom is not expected for the disease process. If the sign or symptom is not expected, then the nurse should assess the client first. This type of question is determining if the nurse is knowledgeable of signs and symptoms of a variety of disease processes.

45. 1. The wife should check to determine whether the client is incontinent of urine, but the client's safety is the priority.
    2. **The most important action the wife can take if her husband has a seizure is to make sure he does not get injured during the seizure. Moving all the furniture out of the way will help ensure the client's safety.**
    3. Seizures are not life threatening. If the wife calls 911, the ambulance will probably arrive after the client's seizure has ended. Seizures lasting longer than 4 to 5 minutes warrant calling 911.
    4. The client should be allowed to rest after the seizure when he is in the postictal state, but it is not the most important action to take. Safety of the client during the seizure is the priority.

CLINICAL JUDGMENT GUIDE: The nurse must be knowledgeable of the expected medical treatment for the client's condition. Safety is the priority for the client, especially when the client is at home.

46. 1. The client may benefit from a hospital bed, but this is not the priority intervention to address the client's non-healing pressure ulcer.
2. HH care agencies do not provide care 7 days a week. Even if the client could have an HH aide 7 days a week, it is not the priority intervention to address the client's non-healing pressure ulcer.
3. The client does not need to be transferred to a skilled nursing unit. The wound care nurse should attempt to heal the pressure ulcer in the home first.
4. **The wound care nurse's primary role is to address non-healing pressure ulcers. This referral is the priority intervention.**

CLINICAL JUDGMENT GUIDE: The test taker must be knowledgeable of the role of all members of the multidisciplinary health-care team as well as HIPAA rules and regulations. These will be tested on the NCLEX-RN® examination.

47. 1. Grab bars address safety issues, but the client is having transfer difficulty, which requires the help of the physical therapist.
2. In most situations, the nurse should assess the client before taking action, but the HH aide has the ability and knowledge to determine if the client is having problems getting out of the bed and into the shower. The nurse should allow the physical therapist to assess the client's transfer ability.
3. The goal of HH nursing is to keep the client as independent as possible, and having the client receive a bed bath is increasing the client's dependency on the HH aide.
4. **The physical therapist is the member of the health-care team who is responsible for helping the client diagnosed with mobility issues.**

CLINICAL JUDGMENT GUIDE: The test taker must be knowledgeable of the role of all members of the multidisciplinary health-care team as well as HIPAA rules and regulations. These will be tested on the NCLEX-RN® examination.

48. 1. Daily exercise, relaxation periods, and socializing are encouraged because each can help decrease the occurrence of headaches. This statement indicates the client understands the teaching.
2. Alternative ways of handling the pain of a headache include techniques such as relaxation, meditation, yoga, and self-hypnosis. This statement indicates the client understands the teaching.

3. **Massage and moist hot packs to the neck and head can help a client diagnosed with tension-type headaches. This statement indicates the client needs more teaching.**
4. Foods containing amines (cheese, chocolate), nitrites (hot dogs), vinegar, onions, caffeine, and alcohol (especially red wine) can trigger a headache. The statement indicates the client understands the teaching.

CLINICAL JUDGMENT GUIDE: This question asks the nurse to identify which statement indicates the client understands the teaching, indicating that three of the options are appropriate for the teaching, but one is incorrect. This is an "except" question, even though it does not say all the options are correct "except."

49. 1. Most organ procurement organizations prefer to ask the family if the client wished to be an organ or tissue donor. The priority intervention for the nurse is to address the family's grieving.
2. The nurse should give the client's personal belongings to the family but the priority intervention is to address the family's grieving.
3. **The nurse's priority intervention should be to address the grieving process of the family.**
4. The client's body will have to be sent to a funeral home but it is not the nurse's priority intervention.

CLINICAL JUDGMENT GUIDE: The nurse must address all areas of the client's death, but the priority intervention is to address the client's family. Helping the client's family initially after the death with the grieving process should be the nurse's priority.

50. 1. The family should designate a funeral home of their choice. The nurse does not make this referral.
2. Hospice is for clients who are dying, but this client is considered brain dead.
3. A home health nurse cannot help this client or family.
4. **A 22-year-old client who experienced a traumatic brain death may be a good candidate for organ donation. Most organ procurement organizations prefer to be the ones to approach the family. This is the best referral.**

CLINICAL JUDGMENT GUIDE: The NCLEX-RN® test plan includes nursing care that is ruled by legal requirements as well as The

Joint Commission, Centers for Medicare & Medicaid Services, Centers for Disease Control and Prevention, and Occupational Safety and Health Administration rules and regulations. The nurse must be knowledgeable of these standards.

51. 1. The client diagnosed with cataracts is expected to have decreased vision and abnormal color perception, and will need surgery but it is elective surgery. Therefore, this client does not warrant intervention.
    2. Loss of peripheral vision is an expected symptom of a retinal detachment and should be seen because the client needs surgery; without surgery, the condition could lead to blindness. But this does not warrant intervention over the client having pain.
    3. A hordeolum is a "sty," which is an infection of the sebaceous glands in the lid margin. It is not an emergency and is treated with warm, moist compresses to the eye four times a day.
    4. **The client diagnosed with primary open-angle glaucoma reports no symptom of pain or pressure, so a client reporting eye pain warrants intervention by the nurse.**

CLINICAL JUDGMENT GUIDE: The test taker must determine which sign or symptom is not expected for the disease process. If the sign or symptom is not expected, then the nurse should assess the client first. This type of question is determining if the nurse is knowledgeable of signs or symptoms of a variety of disease processes.

52. 1. Someone should call 911 because the client needs to go to the emergency department, but the nurse should first take care of the client.
    2. **The nurse should first stabilize the foreign object to help prevent further damage. The stick should not be removed because it will cause more damage and possibly enucleate the eye.**
    3. The nurse should not apply direct pressure to the eye. The nurse should stabilize the foreign object and not apply pressure, which could cause further damage.
    4. The eye should be irrigated for a chemical exposure, not an impaled object.

CLINICAL JUDGMENT GUIDE: The nurse should remember that if a client is in distress and the nurse can do something to relieve the distress,

that action should be done first, before assessment. The nurse should select an intervention that directly helps the client's condition or prevents further damage.

53. 1. **The nurse and the UAP should protect themselves from injury. A lifting device should be used before attempting to move the client.**
    2. The nurse and the UAP should provide the best care possible, including turning the client every 2 hours.
    3. One other person may not be enough to turn or move the client adequately without injuring the staff.
    4. The client is not responsive enough to assist in movement.

CLINICAL JUDGMENT GUIDE: The NCLEX-RN® test plan includes nursing care that is ruled by legal requirements as well as The Joint Commission, Centers for Medicare & Medicaid Services, Centers for Disease Control and Prevention, and Occupational Safety and Health Administration rules and regulations. The nurse must be knowledgeable of these standards.

54. 1. **The nurse should administer the IVP narcotic pain medication even if the client has shallow breathing, with respirations of 8. A nurse should never administer a medication with the intent of hastening the client's death, but medicating a dying client to achieve a peaceful death is an appropriate intervention.**
    2. Repositioning the client would not be effective for "pain all over."
    3. This is cruel to do to a client who is dying and has made himself or herself a DNR.
    4. The HCP has all the orders needed in place. There is no reason to notify the HCP.

CLINICAL JUDGMENT GUIDE: The NCLEX-RN® addresses questions concerned with end-of-life care. This is included in the Psychosocial Integrity section of the test plan. If unsure of the correct option, selecting an intervention addressing an individual is a better choice.

55. 1. **The client's ability to maneuver a wheelchair indicates that the client has progressed in therapy.**
    2. This statement indicates the client is in denial about the prognosis of the injury.
    3. Eye blinks may be used for communication in a client with a higher-level injury.

4. The building of a wheelchair ramp indicates the husband is preparing for the client's return home, not that the client is progressing in therapy.

CLINICAL JUDGMENT GUIDE: The NCLEX-RN® integrates the nursing process throughout the Client Needs categories and subcategories. The nursing process is a scientific, clinical reasoning approach to client care that includes assessment, analysis, planning, implementation, and evaluation. The nurse will be responsible for determining if goals are being met or are not met.

56. 1. Méniére's disease, an excessive accumulation of endolymph in the membranous labyrinth, is characterized by episodic vertigo, tinnitus, fluctuating sensorineural hearing loss, and aural fullness. This client does not need to be contacted first.
2. Otitis media with effusion is an inflammation of the middle ear in which a collection of fluid is present in the middle ear space, resulting in a feeling of fullness of the ear and decreased hearing. This is expected; therefore, the nurse does not need to contact this client first.
3. **This client needs to be contacted so culture and sensitivity (C&S) can be done and mild analgesics prescribed. The ear canal has to be cleansed and antibiotic eardrops administered to the ear. Otalgia is ear pain. This client should be contacted for treatment.**
4. Otosclerosis is an autosomal disease, the fixation of the footplate of the stapes of the oval window, and results in conductive hearing loss; therefore, this client does not need to be notified.

CLINICAL JUDGMENT GUIDE: The test taker must determine which sign or symptom is not expected for the disease process. If the sign or symptom is not expected, then the nurse should assess the client first. This type of question is determining if the nurse is knowledgeable of signs or symptoms of a variety of disease processes.

57. 1. Altered nutrition is a physiological problem but is not a priority over safety.
2. **Altered mobility is a problem experienced by clients diagnosed with Parkinson's disease. It leads to many other concerns, including the risk for falls resulting from the client's shuffling gait. This is the priority problem.**

3. Altered elimination is a problem that the client's altered mobility can cause. This is not, however, the priority problem.
4. Altered body image is a psychological problem and is not a priority.

CLINICAL JUDGMENT GUIDE: The NCLEX-RN® integrates the nursing process throughout the Client Needs categories and subcategories. The nursing process is a scientific, clinical reasoning approach to client care that includes assessment, analysis, planning, implementation, and evaluation. The nurse will be responsible for identifying nursing diagnoses for clients.

58. 1. The nurse must irrigate the eyes, not patch the eyes.
2. The client is in distress and the nurse needs to flush the client's eyes, not assess the visual acuity.
3. **For chemical injuries, the nurse should begin ocular irrigation with sterile, pH-balanced, physiological solution.**
4. The nurse should elevate the head of the bed, but it is not the nurse's first intervention.

CLINICAL JUDGMENT GUIDE: The nurse should remember that if a client is in distress, and the nurse can do something to relieve the distress, it should be done first, before assessment. The nurse should select an option that directly helps the client's condition.

59. 1. The client admitted to a rehabilitation unit is expected to participate in therapy for at least 3 hours each day. The nurse would not question this order.
2. The client admitted to a rehabilitation unit is expected to participate in therapy for at least 3 hours each day. The nurse would not question this order.
3. Clients diagnosed with neurological deficits may have trouble swallowing. The nurse would not question this order.
4. **A client in a rehabilitation unit for a brain injury should not require IV medications. The nurse should question this order.**

CLINICAL JUDGMENT GUIDE: When the stem asks the nurse to determine which health-care provider's order to question, the test taker needs to realize this is an "except" question. Three of the options are appropriate for the HCP to prescribe, and one is not appropriate for the client's disease process or procedure.

60. 1. A hospice organization is designed for terminally ill clients. The client is not terminally ill.

2. The speech therapist helps clients regain speech and swallowing abilities. This therapy should have been occurring while the client was in the rehab facility.

3. The physical therapist assists the client with gait and muscle strengthening. This therapy should have been occurring while the client was in the rehab facility.

4. **The client is being discharged. The nurse should plan for continuity of care by arranging for a home health agency to follow the client at home.**

CLINICAL JUDGMENT GUIDE: The test taker must be knowledgeable of the role of all members of the multidisciplinary health-care team as well as HIPAA rules and regulations. These will be tested on the NCLEX-RN® examination.

61. 1. **It will take approximately 6 weeks for the wound to sufficiently heal before being fitted for a prosthetic eye.**

2. The nurse should ensure the client can insert the conformer in the eye socket and the client should be able to demonstrate this to the nurse. The client does not need more teaching.

3. Eye drops must be placed in the lower conjunctiva; therefore, the client does not need more discharge teaching.

4. The client is at risk for infection and should call the HCP if an elevation in temperature occurs. The client does not need more discharge teaching.

CLINICAL JUDGMENT GUIDE: This question asks the nurse to identify which statement supports the notion that the client needs more teaching, indicating three of the statements are appropriate for the disease process or disorder, but one is incorrect. This is an "except" question even though it does not say all the options are correct "except."

62. 1. The client may be able to maintain the ability to work for several years before needing to apply for disability. The stem does not suggest the client is disabled.

2. The client is newly diagnosed; nutrition would not be a problem at this time.

3. **The client should be referred to a psychological counselor to develop skills for coping with the long-term chronic illness.**

4. The chaplain may need to see the client, but the stem did not indicate the client was having a problem with spiritual distress.

CLINICAL JUDGMENT GUIDE: The test taker must be knowledgeable of the role of all members of the multidisciplinary health-care team as well as HIPAA rules and regulations. These will be tested on the NCLEX-RN® examination.

63. 1. **The LPN can administer medications to clients; therefore, this task is appropriate for the nurse to assign to the LPN.**

2. The client experiencing status epilepticus is an unstable client and the nurse should not assign this task to the LPN.

3. The UAP could assist the client to the bathroom. Remember to assign/delegate tasks based on his or her education and job description.

4. The nurse cannot assign assessment to the LPN.

CLINICAL JUDGMENT GUIDE: When the test taker is deciding which option is the most appropriate task to delegate or assign, the test taker should choose the task that allows each staff member to function within his or her full scope of practice. Do not assign a task to a staff member that falls outside the staff member's or volunteer's expertise. Remember: The nurse cannot delegate assessment, teaching, evaluation, or the care of an unstable client to the LPN.

64. 1. **The client diagnosed with a closed head injury is at risk for increased intracranial pressure and the osmotic diuretic is a priority medication.**

2. The nurse should administer the medications to the client before leaving the unit, but the client diagnosed with a physiological, potentially life-threatening complication is a priority.

3. Before administering a narcotic, the nurse must first assess the client to make sure that administering the medication is not going to mask symptoms.

4. The anticonvulsant gabapentin (Neurontin) is a routine medication and can be administered 30 minutes before or after the routine scheduled time. This is not a priority medication.

CLINICAL JUDGMENT GUIDE: The test taker should know which medications are priority medications such as those indicated in life-threatening situations. These must be administered first.

65. 1. **The charge nurse will not always be available to intercede for the new graduate. The charge nurse should wait and see whether the new graduate is capable of handling the situation before intervening.**

2. The charge nurse should wait to allow the new graduate to deal with the UAP.
3. The charge nurse should wait to allow the new graduate to deal with the UAP.
4. The charge nurse should wait to allow the new graduate to deal with the UAP.

CLINICAL JUDGMENT GUIDE: There will be management questions on the NCLEX-RN®. In many instances, there is no test-taking strategy; the nurse must be knowledgeable of management issues.

66. 1. Levothyroxine (Synthroid) is a daily medication.
    2. **Morphine sulfate (MS Contin) is a narcotic analgesic in sustained-release form. Clients experiencing pain are unlikely to be able to participate fully in the treatment program. The client should be medicated to ensure the ability to comply with the treatment regimen.**
    3. The Fleets enema is utilized daily to assist the client in regaining control of the bowels. This should be administered sometime during the evening hours because administering it during the day would interfere with other therapies such as physical or occupational therapy. Most therapy is completed during the daytime hours.
    4. Metformin (Glucophage) should be administered with meals to prevent nausea and could be the second medication administered.

CLINICAL JUDGMENT GUIDE: This is an alternate type of question included in the NCLEX-RN® test plan. The test taker must be able to read a medication administration record (MAR), be knowledgeable of medications, and be able to make an appropriate decision as to the nurse's most appropriate intervention.

67. **Answer: Two 20-mg tablets and one 10-mg tablet.**
    20 + 20 + 10 = 50 mg
    The nurse cannot split a 75-mg tablet into 2/3 of a tablet, so the client must receive multiple tablets.

CLINICAL JUDGMENT GUIDE: This is an alternate type of question included in the NCLEX-RN®. The nurse must know how to solve math questions.

68. **Correct answers are 1, 3, and 4.**
    1. **The UAP can make hourly rounds on the client, taking the client to the bathroom,** giving the client a drink of water, checking to make sure the client is not climbing out of bed, and so on.
    2. This is the responsibility of the registered nurse or the social worker.
    3. **This client is in rehab and should be stable so that the UAP can set up the tray or feed the client.**
    4. **The UAP can clamp and unclamp an indwelling catheter in a rehab area. This is a noninvasive skill that can be taught to the UAP. It does not require judgment.**
    5. This is the responsibility of the registered nurse or the social worker.

CLINICAL JUDGMENT GUIDE: This is an alternate type of question included in the NCLEX-RN®. The nurse must be able to select all the options that answer the question correctly. There are no partially correct answers.

69. 1. The left hand is weak and cannot be depended on to hold a cane.
    2. The shoulder is not appropriate for a cane.
    3. **The right hand is the strongest hand and should be the one holding the cane. A right-sided CVA results in damage to the left side of the body.**
    4. The shoulder is not appropriate for a cane.

CLINICAL JUDGMENT GUIDE: This is an alternate type of question on the NCLEX-RN® called "hot spot," which asks the nurse to identify the area with the computer arrow.

70. 1. The client has a much lower score than 12 on the Glasgow Coma Scale.
    2. The client has a lower score than 10 on the scale.
    3. **The client received 2 points for lack of opening of eyes to previous stimuli but opens to pain; the client receives 1 point for lack of sound even with painful stimuli; and the client receives 5 points for localizing pain and attempts to remove offending stimulus. This is a total of 8 points.**
    4. The client has a higher score than 6.

CLINICAL JUDGMENT GUIDE: This is an alternate type of question included in the NCLEX-RN® test plan. The test taker must be able to read an EHR, be able to assess the client, and be able to make a decision as to the nurse's most appropriate action.

CLINICAL SCENARIO ANSWERS AND RATIONALES

The correct answer number and rationale for why it is the correct answer are given in **boldface type.** Rationales for why the other possible answer options are incorrect also are given, but they are not in boldface type.

1. 1. **The client diagnosed with a right-sided CVA has left-sided paralysis, so placing the call light on the left side is inappropriate. The client would not be able to use the call light because the left side is paralyzed; the nurse should intervene.**
   2. The UAP should assist the client with meals because the client is unable to use the left arm.
   3. Using a draw sheet is an appropriate way to move the client up in bed.
   4. Placing a small pillow under the shoulder will prevent the shoulder from adducting toward the chest and developing a contracture, so this action does not require the nurse to intervene.

2. 1. The client may need acetaminophen, a nonopioid analgesic, for the pain but the nurse should first assess the client to determine whether this is a headache or whether the client has an evolving CVA, which would require notifying the health-care provider.
   2. The client may need a CT scan but that cannot be determined until the nurse assesses the client to determine if the headache is indicative of an evolving stroke.
   3. The nurse must assess the client to obtain data that will be needed when notifying the health-care provider; therefore, this is not the nurse's first intervention.
   4. **The nurse must first assess the client to determine whether the client's neurological status is deteriorating, which requires notifying the HCP; or if the headache is expected, then it would require an analgesic.**

3. 1. The client may be developing pneumonia and needs to be assessed but not before a client with a Glasgow Coma Scale of 6, which is life threatening.
   2. Ascending paralysis is a symptom of Guillain-Barré syndrome; therefore, the nurse would not need to assess this client first.

3. **A 15 on the Glasgow Coma Scale indicates the client is neurologically intact, and a 6 indicates the client is not neurologically intact; therefore, the nurse should see this client first.**
   4. The nurse should expect a client diagnosed with a CVA (stroke) to have some sequelae of the problem, including the inability to speak.

4. 1. **This medication could possibly cause bleeding; therefore, this medication should be questioned by the charge nurse.**
   2. An osmotic diuretic is the medication of choice used to treat increased intracranial pressure which can occur with a closed head injury.
   3. Any client diagnosed with a head injury will be on prophylactic anticonvulsants to prevent seizure activity, so the nurse would not question this order.
   4. Clients in the ICU are administered proton-pump inhibitors to help prevent stress ulcers; therefore, the nurse would not question this order.

5. 1. If the client's bladder is full, the nurse needs to insert a urinary catheter, which will relieve the headache. The client may be experiencing autonomic dysreflexia, but the nurse will need to palpate the bladder first.
   2. The client is in distress; therefore, the nurse should not assess the client first.
   3. The client should be put in the Trendelenburg position for hypovolemia, not for autonomic dysreflexia.
   4. **The nurse should first palpate the client's bladder to determine if the client is experiencing autonomic dysreflexia, which is what the nurse should consider first with the client's signs and symptoms.**

6. 1. **Placing the client on the side to maintain a patent airway is the charge nurse's priority intervention.**
   2. The Rapid Response Team is called when the client is alive but the nurse thinks the client is in a potentially life-threatening situation. This is a possible intervention but it is not a priority as the nurse walks in the room.

3. The nurse should determine if the client is incontinent of urine or stool and assess the client's seizure for type of activity, but it is not a priority over maintaining a patent airway.
4. The client should have privacy but it is not a priority over maintaining a patent airway.

7. 1. An adverse occurrence report may need to be completed, but it is not the nurse's first intervention.
   2. **The charge nurse's first intervention is to stop the UAP from inserting the oral airway. Once the seizure has started, there should be no attempts to insert anything in the mouth. At times an oral airway could be inserted if the client has an aura and before the seizure, but not once the seizure has started.**
   3. Once a seizure has started nothing should be inserted in the client's mouth.
   4. The nurse should observe the time the seizure started and the seizure activity but it is not the first intervention.

8. Correct answers are 1, 4, and 5.
   1. **A lumbar puncture is an invasive procedure; therefore, an informed consent is required.**
   2. A lumbar puncture does not insert dye into the client; therefore, this is not an appropriate intervention.
   3. The client should be in the side-lying position with the back arched. This position increases the space between the vertebrae, which allows the HCP easier entry into the spinal column.
   4. **The client is encouraged to relax and breathe normally; the client should feel some pressure in the back but there should be no pain.**

5. **The nurse should always explain to the client what is happening before and during a procedure.**

9. 1. The client diagnosed with bacterial meningitis would be expected to have photophobia, so the most experienced nurse would not need to be assigned to this client.
   2. The client diagnosed with an L-4 SCI could have spastic muscle spasms and is not a complication; therefore, a less experienced nurse could care for this client.
   3. A less experienced nurse would be assigned the client diagnosed with Parkinson's disease because these symptoms are expected for this client.
   4. **The client diagnosed with ALS has deteriorating respiratory distress, which is expected, but with these four clients the most experienced nurse should be assigned to the client who has respiratory distress. Maslow's Hierarchy of Needs identifies airway as a priority.**

10. 1. A Glasgow Coma Scale of 15 indicates intact neurological status, so an increase from 11 to 14 is good and the nurse would not need to see this client first.
    2. **These signs and symptoms indicate spinal shock; therefore, this client should be assessed first and appropriate medications administered.**
    3. This is the sign of a positive Babinski, which is expected in a client diagnosed with a brainstem herniation, so this client would not need to be assessed first.
    4. These are expected signs and symptoms of West Nile virus; therefore, the nurse would not need to assess this client first.

SCENARIO ANSWERS

Endocrine Management 8

Intuition will tell the thinking mind where to look next.

—John Salk

QUESTIONS

1. After receiving the shift report, the 7:00 p.m. to 7:00 a.m. nurse is reviewing the medication administration record (MAR) of the client diagnosed with type 2 diabetes. Which intervention should the nurse implement?

Client's Name: M.P. Height: 70 inches	Account Number: 1234567 Weight: 265 lb	Allergies: NKDA Date:
Medication	1901–0700	0701–1900
Regular insulin by bedside glucose subcu ac & hs		
Lower than 60 notify HCP 150 0 units 151–200 2 units		0730 DN BG 420 units
201–250 4 units 251–300 6 units		1130 DN BG 245 4 units
301–350 8 units 351–400 10 units Greater than 400 notify HCP		1630 DN BG 398 10 units
Insulin isophane 48 units bid subcu ac		0730 DN 1630 DN
Signature/Initials	Night Nurse RN/NN	Day Nurse RN/DN

1. Make sure the client receives a snack at bedtime.
2. Check the client's blood glucose level immediately.
3. Have the unlicensed assistive personnel (UAP) give the client some orange juice.
4. Teach the client about the symptoms of diabetic ketoacidosis (DKA).

2. Which task is **most** appropriate for the RN staff nurse to delegate to the unlicensed assistive personnel (UAP)?
   1. Request the UAP to take the diabetic client's HS snack to the client.
   2. Ask the UAP to silence the alarm on the client's PCA pump.
   3. Tell the UAP to witness the client's advance directive.
   4. Ask the UAP to show the client how to take the client's radial pulse.

3. Which task is **most** appropriate for the RN charge nurse to assign to the licensed practical nurse (LPN)?
   1. Tell the LPN to change the client's subclavian dressing.
   2. Request the LPN to obtain the client's daily weight.
   3. Assign the LPN to care for the client in myxedema coma.
   4. Ask the LPN to complete discharge teaching to the client.

4. The new graduate nurse on the endocrine unit is having difficulty completing the workload in a timely manner. Which suggestion could the RN preceptor make to help the new graduate become **more** organized?
   1. Suggest the new nurse take a break whenever the nurse feels overwhelmed with tasks.
   2. Tell the new nurse to start the shift with a work organization sheet for the assigned clients.
   3. Instruct the new nurse to take five deep breaths at the beginning of the shift, and then begin.
   4. Review each day's assignments for the new nurse and organize the work for the new nurse.

5. The rehabilitation nurse is caring for a client diagnosed with type 2 diabetes who is 1 week postoperative for left carotid endarterectomy. The client's 11:30 a.m. bedside glucometer reading is 408 mg/dL. Based on the medication administration record (MAR), which intervention should the nurse implement **first**?

Client's Name: P. S. Height: 69 inches	Account Number: 1234569 Weight: 165 pounds		Allergies: NKDA Date:
Medication		1901–0700	0701–1900
Regular insulin by bedside glucose subcu ac & hs			
Lower than 60 notify HCP 150 0 units			0730 DN BG 142 0 units
151–200 2 units			
201–250 4 units			
251–300 6 units			
301–350 8 units			
351–400 10 units			
Greater than 400 notify HCP			
Signature/Initials		Night Nurse RN/NN	Day Nurse RN/DN

   1. Notify the health-care provider.
   2. Administer 10 units regular insulin.
   3. Notify the laboratory to draw a serum glucose level.
   4. Recheck the bedside glucometer reading.

6. The RN charge nurse on the endocrine surgical unit is making assignments. Which task should be delegated or assigned to the team members?
    1. Request the licensed practical nurse (LPN) assess the client who is hypoglycemic.
    2. Ask the unlicensed assistive personnel (UAP) to assist feeding the client with an adrenalectomy who has a paralytic ileus.
    3. Instruct the UAP to insert a nasogastric (N/G) tube into the client who has had a thyroidectomy.
    4. Tell the LPN to perform an intermittent urinary catheterization for the client diagnosed with acromegaly.

7. Which task is **most** appropriate for the RN staff nurse to delegate or assign when caring for clients on a surgical unit?
    1. Instruct the licensed practical nurse (LPN) to feed the client who is 1-day postoperative unilateral thyroidectomy.
    2. Ask another nurse to administer an IVP pain medication to a postoperative client in severe pain.
    3. Request the unlicensed assistive personnel (UAP) to check the client whose vital signs are AP 112, RR 26, BP 92/58.
    4. Instruct the licensed practical nurse (LPN) to obtain the pretransfusion assessment on a postoperative client.

8. The client diagnosed with Addison's disease is being prepared for emergency surgery and is asking to complete an advance directive. Which type of advance directive should the nurse recommend the client complete at this time?
    1. Power of attorney
    2. Living will
    3. Do not resuscitate (DNR) order
    4. Durable power of attorney for health care

9. The nurse is caring for clients in the post-anesthesia care unit (PACU). Which client requires **immediate** intervention by the PACU nurse?
    1. The client who had a bilateral adrenalectomy who is exhibiting masseter rigidity
    2. The client who had a subtotal thyroidectomy who has not urinated since surgery
    3. The client who had general anesthesia who is sleepy but arouses easily to verbal stimuli
    4. The client who had a pituitary tumor removed and has hypoactive bowel sounds

10. The RN charge nurse on a busy 20-bed endocrinology unit must send one staff member to the nursery. Which staff member is **most** appropriate to send to the nursery?
    1. The nurse who has worked on the endocrinology unit for 4 years
    2. The graduate nurse who has been on the endocrinology unit for 6 months
    3. The licensed practical nurse (LPN) who has worked in a newborn nursery at another facility
    4. The unlicensed assistive personnel (UAP) who has six small children of her own

11. The nurse is working in an endocrinology unit. Which client warrants **immediate** intervention by the nurse?
    1. The client diagnosed with acromegaly who has club-like fingertips and large feet
    2. The client diagnosed with syndrome of inappropriate antidiuretic hormone who has decreased urine output
    3. The client diagnosed with Cushing's syndrome who has truncal obesity and thin, fragile skin
    4. The client diagnosed with pheochromocytoma who has a severe pounding headache and chest pain

12. The night nurse enters the client's room and finds the client crying. The client asks the nurse, "Am I dying? I think something is terribly wrong with me, but no one is telling me." The nurse knows the client has pancreatic cancer and has less than 6 months to live. Which response is an example of the ethical principle of veracity?
    1. "You are concerned no one is telling you something is wrong."
    2. "Your diagnosis is pancreatic cancer."
    3. "If you feel something is wrong you should speak with your doctor in the morning."
    4. "What makes you think there is something wrong and you are dying?"

13. The critical care nurse has just received the a.m. shift report on a client diagnosed with heart failure and who has pre-existing type 2 diabetes. After reviewing the client's medication administration record (MAR), which medication should the nurse administer **first?**

Client's Name: A. R. Height: 67 inches	Account Number: 1234560 Weight: 148 pounds		Allergies: Penicillin Date:
Medication	**1901–0700**		**0701–1900**
Metformin 100 mg PO bid	2000		0800
70/30 insulin 24 units subcu			0730
Digoxin 0.125 mg IVP qd			0800
Ceftriaxone 100 mg IVPB	0700		
Signature/Initials	Night Nurse RN/NN		Day Nurse RN/DN

    1. Administer metformin 100 mg PO.
    2. Administer digoxin 0.125 mg IVP.
    3. Administer ceftriaxone 100 mg IVPB.
    4. Administer 70/30 insulin subcutaneously.

14. Which client should the charge nurse on a medical unit assign to a nurse who is 5 months pregnant?
    1. The client who completed chemotherapy treatment and who is immunosuppressed
    2. The client diagnosed with postoperative hyperparathyroidism who has shingles (herpes zoster)
    3. The client diagnosed with hyperthyroidism who is receiving radioactive iodine I-131
    4. The client diagnosed with AIDS who has a cytomegalovirus infection

15. The client diagnosed with hypothyroidism and a diagnosis of myxedema coma is admitted to the critical care unit. Which assessment data warrants **immediate** intervention by the nurse?
    1. The client's blood glucose level is 74 mg/dL.
    2. The client's temperature is 96.2°F; AP, 54; R, 12; and BP, 90/58.
    3. The client's ABG values are pH, 7.33; Pao_2, 78; $Paco_2$, 48; Hco_3, 25.
    4. The client is lethargic and sleeps all the time.

16. The nurse is preparing to administer morning medications. Which medication should the nurse administer **first?**
    1. The levothyroxine to a client diagnosed with hypothyroidism
    2. The insulin isophane to a client diagnosed with type 2 diabetes
    3. The prednisone to a client diagnosed with Addison's disease
    4. The tiotropium inhaler to a client diagnosed with chronic asthma

17. The nurse is working on an endocrinology unit. Which client should the nurse assess **first?**
    1. The client diagnosed with diabetes insipidus who has polyuria and polydipsia
    2. The client who is 1-day postoperative thyroidectomy who has neck edema
    3. The client who has hypoparathyroidism who has painful muscle cramps and irritability
    4. The client diagnosed with Addison's disease who has weakness, fatigue, and anorexia

18. The client is admitted to the endocrinology unit newly diagnosed with an acute exacerbation of central diabetes insipidus (DI). Which intervention is the **priority** nursing intervention?
    1. Obtain the client's baseline weight.
    2. Administer desmopressin acetate intranasally.
    3. Administer intravenous hypotonic saline.
    4. Monitor the client's intake and output.

19. The unlicensed assistive personnel (UAP) tells the nurse the client who had a thyroidectomy has a T 104°F, P 128, RR 26, BP 164/88. Which intervention should the nurse implement **first?**
    1. Prepare to administer propranolol.
    2. Notify the health-care provider immediately.
    3. Assess the client's vital signs and surgical dressing.
    4. Administer acetaminophen PO STAT.

20. The unlicensed assistive personnel (UAP) tells the RN primary nurse that a client is crying and upset because she has been told her husband has just died. Which intervention should the nurse implement?
    1. Tell the UAP to go and sit with the client.
    2. Make a referral for the chaplain to see the client.
    3. Ask the HCP to prescribe a mild sedative.
    4. Leave the client alone in the room to grieve.

21. At 1000, the client diagnosed with type 1 diabetes is reporting being jittery, having a headache, and feeling dizzy. Which intervention should the nurse implement **first?**
    1. Give the client glucose tablets.
    2. Provide the client with the lunch meal.
    3. Request the laboratory to draw a serum glucose level.
    4. Determine the last time the client received insulin.

22. An elderly client diagnosed with thyroid cancer frequently makes statements that are inappropriate for the situation, and is not oriented to place, time, or date. The HCP has ordered a magnetic resonance imaging (MRI) scan of the client's brain. Which intervention should the nurse implement?
    1. Administer a mild sedative to prevent claustrophobia.
    2. Order a vest restraint for use by the client during the MRI.
    3. Make sure the client does not have a pacemaker.
    4. Ask a family member to stay with the client while the test is performed.

23. An elderly female client is admitted from the long-term care facility diagnosed with hyperglycemic hyperosmolar nonketotic coma. The client does not have any family or friends present. Which resource(s) should the admission nurse utilize to obtain information about the client?
    1. Having the nurse wait until a significant other can be contacted
    2. The verbal report from the ambulance workers and STAT laboratory work
    3. The transfer form from the nursing home and old hospital records
    4. The health-care provider's telephone orders about care needed

24. The nurse administering medications to clients on a medical unit discovers the wrong medication was administered to a client, Mrs. Jones. Mrs. Jones had replied she was Mrs. Smith when the nurse asked her name from the MAR. Which step in medication administration did the nurse violate when administering the medication?
    1. Asking the client to repeat her name
    2. Verifying the client's armband with the MAR
    3. Checking the medication against the MAR
    4. Documenting the medication on the MAR

25. The female client diagnosed with type 2 diabetes and a urinary tract infection (UTI) describes frequent UTIs. Which interventions should the nurse implement? **Select all that apply.**
    1. Encourage the client to empty her bladder regularly and completely.
    2. Instruct the client to drink 8 ounces of cranberry or lingonberry juice a day.
    3. Explain the importance of taking oral hypoglycemic medications.
    4. Discuss the importance of taking all the antibiotics.
    5. Teach the client to measure her urine output with each voiding.

26. Which laboratory data should the nurse monitor for the client receiving intravenous methylprednisolone?
    1. Potassium level
    2. Sodium level
    3. Liver enzymes
    4. Glucose level

27. The nurse is working in an outpatient clinic triaging phone calls. Which client **warrants** notifying the health-care provider?
    1. The client diagnosed with type 2 diabetes receiving hemodialysis who has gained 6 pounds since the last dialysis treatment
    2. The client diagnosed with type 1 diabetes who has early stage chronic renal disease and reports having to go to the bathroom several times at night
    3. The client diagnosed with syndrome of inappropriate antidiuretic hormone who is very upset because no one has returned the previous phone call
    4. The client diagnosed with type 1 diabetes who had a kidney transplant and reports decreased urine output and flu-like symptoms

28. Which client should the endocrinology nurse assess **first** after receiving the shift report?
    1. The client who is 1-day postoperative transsphenoidal hypophysectomy who has clear drainage from the nose
    2. The client diagnosed with Graves' disease who has exophthalmos and bruits over the thyroid gland
    3. The client diagnosed with hyperparathyroidism who is reporting weakness, loss of appetite, and constipation
    4. The client diagnosed with Addison's disease who has orthostatic hypotension, nausea, and vomiting

29. Which client is the **priority** to be assigned to a case manager in the outpatient clinic so that care can be achieved?
    1. The client diagnosed with renal calculi who is 2 weeks post–lithotripsy procedure
    2. The client diagnosed with type 2 diabetes and coronary artery disease (CAD)
    3. The client who is diagnosed with hypothyroidism receiving radiation treatment
    4. The client diagnosed with Addison's disease who is on corticosteroid therapy

30. Which client is **most** appropriate for the parish nurse to care for?
    1. The post-gestational diabetic client who had triplets and is a single parent
    2. The Catholic client who is confined to the home because of severe arthritis
    3. The obese client diagnosed with Cushing's syndrome who is requesting help with losing weight
    4. The client diagnosed with chronic renal disease who is being cared for in the home by the wife

31. Which task should the RN ambulatory care nurse delegate to the unlicensed assistive personnel (UAP)?
    1. Ask the UAP to remove the trash from the room of the client who received radioactive iodine diagnosed with hyperthyroidism.
    2. Instruct the UAP to escort the client outside who is asking to smoke a cigar.
    3. Request the UAP check the surgical dressing on the client with an ileal conduit.
    4. Tell the UAP to take the glucometer reading on the client about to go to surgery.

32. The nurse is hanging 1,000 mL of IV fluids to run for 8 hours. The IV tubing is a microdrip. At how many gtt/min should the IV rate be set?

    [   ]

33. The clinic nurse is caring for clients using complementary alternative medicine (CAM). Which intervention is an example of CAM? **Select all that apply.**
    1. The client diagnosed with hypothyroidism who takes *Centella asiatica*
    2. The client diagnosed with type 2 diabetes who takes cinnamon daily
    3. The client diagnosed with coronary artery disease (CAD) who takes a daily low-dose aspirin
    4. The client who uses acupuncture to help quit smoking cigarettes
    5. The client who uses hypnosis to improve memory function

34. Which statement is an example of community-oriented, population-focused nursing?
    1. The nurse cares for an elderly client living in the community who has had a kidney transplant.
    2. The nurse develops an educational program for the type 2 diabetics in the local area.
    3. The nurse refers a client diagnosed with Cushing's syndrome to the registered dietitian.
    4. The nurse provides pamphlets to the client diagnosed with chronic renal disease.

35. Which **priority** intervention should the nurse implement when teaching the client diagnosed with type 2 diabetes about glucometer testing?
    1. Instruct the client to keep a written record of the glucometer readings.
    2. Recommend the client check the glucometer reading in the morning.
    3. Have the client demonstrate how to correctly perform the blood sugar test.
    4. Tell the client to dispose of the lancets and strips appropriately.

36. Which client would **most** benefit from acupressure, a traditional Chinese medicine, which is considered complementary alternative medicine (CAM)?
    1. The client diagnosed with thyroid cancer who has chemotherapy-induced nausea
    2. The client diagnosed with type 2 diabetes and chronic renal disease
    3. The postpartum client who is diagnosed with Sheehan syndrome
    4. The client diagnosed with arterial hypertension

37. The home health director of nurses hears a nurse and the occupational therapist loudly disagreeing about the care of a newly admitted client while they are sitting in an area that is accessible to anyone coming into the office. Which action should the director of nurses implement **first?**
    1. Ask the staff members to move the argument to another room.
    2. Request both individuals to come into the director's office.
    3. Call the secretary with instructions for the staff to quit arguing.
    4. Tell the staff members that arguing is not allowed in the office.

38. Which client should the nurse on the endocrinology unit assess **first?**
    1. The client diagnosed with hypothyroidism whose vital signs are T 94.2, AP 48, RR 14, BP 90/68
    2. The client diagnosed with hypoparathyroidism who has a positive Chvostek's sign
    3. The client who is 1-day postoperative thyroidectomy who is hoarse
    4. The client diagnosed with diabetes insipidus who is drinking large amounts of water

39. Which activities are examples of home health-care nurse responsibilities when caring for clients diagnosed with endocrine disorders? **Select all that apply.**
    1. Complete nutritional counseling and teaching for a client on a high-fiber diet.
    2. Discuss preoperative teaching for the client having a total right hip replacement.
    3. Manage oxygen therapy for a client diagnosed with chronic obstructive pulmonary disease (COPD).
    4. Teach the client and family about administration and side effects of medications.
    5. Draw blood for studies related to monitoring disease processes and therapy.

40. The unlicensed assistive personnel (UAP) has just taken the blood pressure of a client who had a thyroidectomy. The UAP tells the RN primary nurse that the client's hand turned into a claw when the blood pressure was taken. Which intervention should the nurse implement **first?**
    1. Prepare to administer intravenous calcium gluconate.
    2. Assess the client for signs or symptoms of hypoparathyroidism.
    3. Request the UAP to elevate the client's head of the bed.
    4. Notify the client's health-care provider immediately.

41. The client diagnosed with type 2 diabetes who has chronic renal disease asks the nurse, "How can I qualify for home health care when I go home?" Which statement is the nurse's **best** response?
    1. "You must need constant skilled care by the nurse."
    2. "You must have a family member living with you."
    3. "You must be homebound to receive home health care."
    4. "You must be referred by the hospital social worker."

42. The nurse is providing complementary alternative medicine (CAM) by teaching the client diagnosed with hyperthyroidism to focus attention, increase self-awareness, and increase concentration on an object. Which type of mind-body intervention is the nurse teaching?
    1. Meditation
    2. Imagery
    3. Aromatherapy
    4. Acupressure

43. Which **priority** intervention should the nurse implement for the client diagnosed with syndrome of inappropriate antidiuretic hormone (SIADH)?
    1. Maintain the prescribed daily fluid restriction.
    2. Position the client's head of bed with no more than 10 degrees of elevation.
    3. Turn and reposition the client every 2 hours while on bedrest.
    4. Provide frequent oral hygiene every 2 hours for the client.

44. The home health (HH) agency chief nursing officer (CNO) is making assignments for the nurses. Which client should be assigned to the new graduate nurse who just completed orientation?
    1. The client diagnosed with Cushing's syndrome who is dyspneic and confused
    2. The client who does not have the money to get prescriptions filled
    3. The client diagnosed with full-thickness burns on the arm who needs a dressing change
    4. The client reporting pain who is diagnosed with diabetic neuropathy

45. The RN staff nurse on the endocrinology unit is caring for clients, assisted by an unlicensed assistive personnel (UAP). Which task is **most** appropriate to delegate to the UAP?
    1. Feed the client who is 1-day postoperative transsphenoidal hypophysectomy.
    2. Obtain a urine specimen for the client diagnosed with diabetes insipidus.
    3. Take the vital signs for the client diagnosed with myxedema coma.
    4. Assess the pulse oximeter reading of the client diagnosed with an Addisonian crisis.

46. The clinical nurse manager on the endocrine unit overhears the staff nurses who are upset and arguing over how the clients are being assigned by the charge nurse. Which statement indicates a democratic leadership style by the clinical nurse manager?
1. "My charge nurse makes the assignments and I support how she does it."
2. "As long as there are no reports from the clients I will not interfere."
3. "I appreciate you telling me about the situation and I will handle it."
4. "I will schedule a meeting and we will all sit down and discuss the situation."

47. The hospice nurse is writing a care plan for a client diagnosed with type 2 diabetes mellitus who has peripheral neuropathy. Which client problem has **priority** for the client?
1. Altered glucose metabolism
2. Anticipatory grieving
3. Alteration in comfort
4. Spiritual distress

48. The unlicensed assistive personnel (UAP) tells the RN staff nurse the client diagnosed with thyroid cancer who is terminally ill is having deep-rapid breathing, but then doesn't breathe for about a minute. Which intervention should the nurse implement **first?**
1. Explain the client is having Cheyne-Stokes respirations.
2. Notify the hospital chaplain to come to the client's room.
3. Go to the client's room immediately and assess the client.
4. Contact the client's family that the client's death is near.

49. Which interventions should the RN primary nurse implement for the client diagnosed with hyperthyroidism? **Select all that apply.**
1. Establish a supportive and trusting relationship to help the client cope.
2. Assist with exercises involving large muscle groups.
3. Instruct the unlicensed assistive personnel (UAP) to apply multiple blankets to the bed.
4. Explain that the caregiver should not leave the client alone.
5. Place the client in a cool room away from high-traffic areas.

50. Which statement by the client experiencing exophthalmos indicates the client needs **more** teaching by the endocrinology nurse?
1. "I will use artificial tears to moisten my eyes."
2. "I need to wear dark glasses to prevent irritation."
3. "I should not move my eyes unless absolutely necessary."
4. "I should lightly tape my eyes shut when I sleep."

51. Which action by the unlicensed assistive personnel (UAP) **warrants** intervention by the RN primary nurse caring for the client diagnosed with type 2 diabetes and chronic renal disease who is on hemodialysis?
1. The UAP times the client's activities to help conserve energy.
2. The UAP applies a lubricant to the lips and oral mucous membranes.
3. The UAP ties a sheet around the client sitting in the chair.
4. The UAP uses a fan to facilitate movement of cool air.

52. The RN nurse supervisor in the home health (HH) office is assigning tasks for the day. Which task is **most** appropriate for the nurse supervisor to assign to the licensed practical nurse (LPN)?
1. Tell the LPN to complete the admission assessment for the client diagnosed with Cushing's disease.
2. Request the LPN to evaluate the client's response to the new pain medication regimen.
3. Request the LPN perform the wound care for the client diagnosed with a stage 4 pressure ulcer.
4. Instruct the LPN to visit the client diagnosed with type 2 diabetes who is stable and needs a hospital bed.

53. The charge nurse is reviewing the morning laboratory results for the clients. Which laboratory results require notifying the client's health-care provider?
    1. The client diagnosed with hypoparathyroidism who has a decreased serum calcium level
    2. The client diagnosed with Cushing's disease who has a decreased urine cortisol level
    3. The client diagnosed with diabetes insipidus who has a low urine specific gravity
    4. The client diagnosed with hyperthyroidism who has an increased TSH level

54. The nurse on the medical unit is preparing to administer 0900 medications. Which medication should the nurse **question** administering?
    1. Levothyroxine to the client diagnosed with hypothyroidism
    2. Metformin to the type 2 diabetic who just had a CT scan with dye
    3. Insulin (human recombinant) to the client diagnosed with type 1 diabetes who is no longer NPO
    4. Prednisone to a client diagnosed with Addison's disease

55. The RN staff nurse and unlicensed assistive personnel (UAP) are caring for clients on an endocrinology unit. Which tasks should the RN delegate to the UAP? **Select all that apply.**
    1. Ambulate the client who had a unilateral adrenalectomy.
    2. Change the linens on the client diagnosed with acute thyrotoxicosis who is diaphoretic.
    3. Bring ice-cold water to the client diagnosed with diabetes insipidus.
    4. Take the vital signs of a client who has just returned from the post-anesthesia care unit (PACU).
    5. Deliver the lunch tray to the client receiving regular insulin on a sliding scale.

56. The unit manager of an endocrinology unit is overbudget for the year and must transfer one staff member to another unit. Which option is the **best** action for the unit manager to take before deciding which staff member to transfer?
    1. Assess each staff member's abilities.
    2. Choose the last staff member hired.
    3. Ask for input from the staff members.
    4. Request the transfer documentation form.

57. The clinic nurse is caring for a 10-year-old client diagnosed with type 2 diabetes mellitus. Which client problem is the **priority?**
    1. Altered nutrition, excessive intake
    2. Risk for low self-esteem
    3. Hypoglycemia
    4. Risk for loss of body part

58. The overhead page has just announced a Code Red, actual fire, on a unit two floors below the unit where the RN staff nurse is working. Which action should the nurse implement **first?**
    1. Turn off the oxygen supply to the rooms.
    2. Evacuate the clients to a lower floor.
    3. Close all of the doors to the clients' rooms.
    4. Make a list of clients to discharge.

59. The nurse is preparing to administer medications for clients on a medical unit. The client diagnosed with hypothyroidism is describing being hot all the time, feeling palpitations, and being jittery. Which intervention should the nurse implement **first?**
    1. Check the client's serum thyroid levels.
    2. Assess the client for diarrhea.
    3. Document the finding in the EHR.
    4. Hold the client's thyroid medication.

60. The nurse is administering medications on an endocrinology unit. Which medication should the nurse **question** administering?
    1. The propylthiouracil to the client diagnosed with hyperthyroidism
    2. The desmopressin acetate to the client diagnosed with diabetes insipidus
    3. The somatropin to the client diagnosed with hypopituitarism
    4. The propranolol to the client diagnosed with hypothyroidism

61. The hospice nurse caring for a client diagnosed with diabetes mellitus type 2 observes the client eating a bowl of ice cream. Which intervention should the nurse implement **first?**
    1. Allow the client to enjoy the ice cream.
    2. Check the client's blood glucose.
    3. Remind the client not to eat ice cream.
    4. Suggest the client eat low-fat sweets.

62. The RN staff nurse is caring for the client who is 1-day postoperative transsphenoidal hypophysectomy. Which action by the unlicensed assistive personnel (UAP) **warrants** intervention by the nurse?
    1. The UAP places the client with the HOB 30 degrees elevated.
    2. The UAP tells the client not to cough vigorously.
    3. The UAP is helping the client splint the incision.
    4. The UAP is taking the client's vital signs.

63. The charge nurse of a surgical unit has been notified of an external disaster with multiple casualties. Which client should the charge nurse request to be discharged from the hospital to make room for clients from the disaster?
    1. The client scheduled for a bilateral adrenalectomy in the morning whose preoperative teaching has not been started
    2. The client who had a total abdominal hysterectomy 2 days ago and PCA machine has been discontinued
    3. The client who is postoperative bilateral thyroidectomy who has a hemoglobin of 7 mg/dL and a hematocrit of 22.1%
    4. The client diagnosed with type 2 diabetes who has just had a kidney transplant and is experiencing fever and pain at the surgical site

64. For which client's laboratory data should the charge nurse notify the HCP?
    1. The potassium level of 3.6 mEq/L in a client diagnosed with heart failure who is taking furosemide
    2. The PTT level of 78 in the client diagnosed with pulmonary embolism who is receiving IV heparin
    3. The blood urea nitrogen (BUN) of 84 mg/dL in a client diagnosed with end-stage renal disease (ESRD) and peripheral edema
    4. The blood glucose level of 543 mg/dL in a client diagnosed with uncontrolled diabetes mellitus type 1

65. Which nursing intervention is the **priority** for the intensive care nurse to implement when caring for a client diagnosed with diabetic ketoacidosis (DKA)?
    1. Assess for a fruity breath odor.
    2. Check blood glucose levels ac and hs.
    3. Monitor the client's pulse oximeter readings.
    4. Maintain the regular insulin IV rate on an infusion pump.

66. The client diagnosed with type 2 diabetes mellitus has a hemoglobin A1C of 11 mg/dL. Which intervention should the nurse implement **first?**
    1. Check the client's current blood glucose level.
    2. Assess the client for neuropathy and retinopathy.
    3. Teach the client about the effects of uncontrolled hyperglycemia.
    4. Monitor the client's BUN and creatinine levels.

67. The nurse is working in a primary health-care clinic reviewing laboratory data. Which laboratory data should the nurse report to the HCP **first?**

1. Mr. F.G., who was seen for his annual physical examination

Laboratory Report

Laboratory Test	Client Value	Normal Value
WBC	16.3	4.5 to 11.1 10³/microL
RBC	4.3	Male: 4.21 to 5.81 10⁶ cells/microL
		Female: 3.61 to 5.11 10⁶ cells/microL
Hgb	13.3	Male: 14 to 17.3 g/dL
		Female: 11.7 to 15.5 g/dL
Hct	42	Male: 42% to 52%
		Female: 36% to 48%
Platelets	149	150 to 450 (10³ mm)

2. Ms. J.K., who reported a runny nose and cough

Laboratory Report

Laboratory Test	Client Value	Normal Value
WBC	5.3	4.5 to 11.1 10³/microL
RBC	3.9	Male: 4.21 to 5.81 10⁶ cells/microL
		Female: 3.61 to 5.11 10⁶ cells/microL
Hgb	12	Male: 14 to 17.3 g/dL
		Female: 11.7 to 15.5 g/dL
Hct	36.9	Male: 42% to 52%
		Female: 36% to 48%
Platelets	150	150 to 450 (10³ mm)

3. Ms. L.M., who received an influenza vaccination

Laboratory Report

Laboratory Test	Client Value	Normal Value
Glucose	125	Fasting: Less than 100 mg/dL
		Random: Less than 200 mg/dL
Potassium	4.9	3.5 to 5.3 mEq/L or mmol/L
Sodium	140	135 to 145 mEq/L or mmol/L

4. Mr. O.R., who reported insomnia and work stress

Laboratory Report

Laboratory Test	Client Value	Normal Value
Glucose	100	Fasting: Less than 100 mg/dL
		Random: Less than 200 mg/dL
Potassium	5.1	3.5 to 5.3 mEq/L or mmol/L
Sodium	136	135 to 145 mEq/L or mmol/L

68. The client diagnosed with type 1 diabetes is receiving regular insulin by sliding scale. The client's glucometer reading is 249. The order reads blood glucose level:
Fewer than 150 0 units
151–200 5 units
201–250 8 units
251–300 12 units
More than 301 Contact health-care provider
How much insulin should the nurse administer to the client?

[ ]

69. The RN clinic nurse in the outpatient clinic is working with an unlicensed assistive personnel (UAP). Which tasks are **most** appropriate for the nurse to delegate to the UAP? **Select all that apply.**
    1. Take the client to the examination room and take the vital signs.
    2. Weigh the client and document the weight in the client's EHR.
    3. Prepare the examination room for the next client.
    4. Discuss the prescriptions prescribed by the health-care provider.
    5. Call the pharmacy to authorize a refill on a client's prescription.

70. The nurse in an outpatient clinic is triaging telephone calls. **Rank in order of priority.**
    1. The call from a husband who states his wife started on an antidepressant and now will not wake up
    2. The call from a client who states the medication that was prescribed for her type 2 diabetes mellitus is too expensive
    3. The client diagnosed with hypothyroidism who is reporting feeling hot, having hand tremors, and having diarrhea
    4. The call from the pharmacist wanting an authorization to change a medication from a brand name to a generic name drug
    5. The call from the client who had a magnetic resonance imaging (MRI) scan 2 days ago and has not received the results

CLINICAL SCENARIO

ENDOCRINE CLINICAL SCENARIO

The RN charge nurse is overseeing an endocrine unit in a large medical center located in the metropolitan, rapidly expanding inner city. She is working with five additional RNs, three LPNs, two UAPs, and a unit secretary. They are working on a Monday from 0700 to 1900. There are 10 culturally diverse clients of all ages on the 15-bed endocrine intensive care and dialysis unit.

1. The 24-year-old client diagnosed with type 1 diabetes mellitus is reporting nausea and vomiting. Which interventions should the nurse implement? **Select all that apply.**
    1. Ask the client about vomiting and, if so, how many times.
    2. Determine the client's blood glucose level.
    3. Find out what medications the client has taken for the nausea.
    4. Tell the client to drink diet sodas to keep from being dehydrated.
    5. Make sure the client does not take insulin during the illness.

2. The 19-year-old client newly diagnosed with type 1 diabetes mellitus asks the nurse about "sick day rules." Which instructions should the nurse include in the teaching? **Select all that apply.**
   1. Tell the client to monitor urine ketones when sick.
   2. Instruct the client to go immediately to the emergency department when feeling sick.
   3. Teach the client to take over-the-counter medications that are sugar-free.
   4. Have the client call the health-care provider if showing ketones in the urine.
   5. Discuss trying to intake carbohydrates equal to usual caloric intake.

3. The nurse is caring for an obese client who reported to the ED with nausea and vomiting. The client is diagnosed with diabetes ketoacidosis (DKA) and admitted to the intensive care unit (ICU). Which interventions should the ICU nurse implement at this time? **Select all that apply.**
   1. Assess the client for dehydration and electrolyte imbalance.
   2. Perform bedside glucose monitoring hourly.
   3. Initiate an intravenous drip of NS and regular insulin.
   4. Perform oral care.
   5. Monitor potassium and sodium levels frequently.

4. The RN ICU nurse and the UAP are caring for an elderly client diagnosed with diabetes ketoacidosis (DKA). The UAP is performing foot care on the client. Which action by the UAP requires the nurse to intervene?
   1. The UAP cleans the feet with warm water and soap.
   2. The UAP thoroughly dries the feet, patting gently.
   3. The UAP applies lotion to the feet between the toes.
   4. The UAP places cotton socks on the client's feet.

5. The young adult client diagnosed with type 1 diabetes recovers from the DKA and is being discharged from the hospital. The nurse is preparing the discharge information. Which information should the nurse include in the discharge instructions? **Select all that apply.**
   1. Discuss "sick day rules" with the client.
   2. Review self-monitoring of blood glucose.
   3. Perform an inspection of the feet daily.
   4. Encourage weight loss.
   5. Teach to have regular eye examinations.

6. The 22-year-old client newly diagnosed with type 1 diabetes is being discharged from the hospital after recovering from diabetes ketoacidosis (DKA). Which referral should the nurse initiate at this time?
   1. Referral to the physical therapist
   2. Referral to a hospice organization
   3. Referral to a diabetes educator
   4. Referral to a fitness trainer

7. The middle-age client diagnosed with type 1 diabetes asks the nurse, "What are the benefits of continuous glucose monitoring (CGM)?" Which statement is the nurse's **best** response?
   1. "You will never have to perform a fingerstick blood glucose check again."
   2. "The CGM system is much cheaper than performing fingerstick checks."
   3. "The CGM system adjusts your insulin dosage to the blood sugar results automatically."
   4. "You will be able to see the trends in your blood glucose levels."

8. The nurse is teaching the 76-year-old client with an insulin pump. Which statement indicates the client **needs more** teaching?
   1. "When I sleep, I will clip my insulin pump to my pajamas."
   2. "My insulin pump will help stabilize my blood sugar levels."
   3. "I will need to monitor my blood glucose frequently."
   4. "I can perform any type of exercise wearing my insulin pump."

9. The obese client diagnosed with lipohypertrophy uses an insulin pump to control blood sugar. The client asks the nurse, "How can I prevent lipohypertrophy?" Which **priority** intervention should the nurse discuss with the client?
   1. "Rotate the catheter insertion site frequently."
   2. "Wash your hands before adjusting your insulin pump."
   3. "Avoid insertion of the catheter in the inner thigh."
   4. "Take all oral antibiotics as prescribed."

10. The nurse is performing a triple preparation procedure for insertion of an insulin pump catheter into a diabetic client. Which interventions should the nurse implement? **Rank in order of performance.**
    1. Apply an antiseptic and adhesive wipe to the area and let dry.
    2. Insert the infusion catheter set in a continuous motion.
    3. Wash the insertion area with antibacterial soap and let dry.
    4. Wash hands and don nonsterile gloves.
    5. Cleanse the area with antibacterial solution and let dry.

The correct answer number and rationale for why it is the correct answer are given in **boldface type.** Rationales for why the other possible answer options are incorrect also are given, but they are not in boldface type.

1. 1. **The client received an intermediate-acting insulin at 1630 plus the sliding-scale insulin dose to lower the client's blood glucose level. This client should receive a bedtime snack to make sure the client does not experience a hypoglycemic reaction during the night. Intermediate insulin generally peaks 6 to 8 hours after administration, 2230 to 0030 for this client.**
   2. The nurse should check the client's blood glucose at 2100 hours, not at the current time.
   3. Nothing indicates the client needs an intervention for hypoglycemia at this time.
   4. The client diagnosed with type 2 diabetes would experience hyperglycemic hyperosmolar nonketotic coma (HHNC) syndrome, not DKA.

CLINICAL JUDGMENT GUIDE: This is an alternate type of question included in the NCLEX-RN® test plan. The test taker must be able to read a medication administration record (MAR), be knowledgeable of medications, and be able to make a decision as to the nurse's most appropriate intervention.

2. 1. **The UAP can take food to the client because this is not a medication and the client is stable.**
   2. The RN staff nurse should not have the UAP silence the alarm on the client's PCA pump. The nurse should assess the client and the pump to determine the reason for the PCA alarm.
   3. None of the hospital employees should witness the client's advance directive.
   4. The RN cannot delegate teaching to the UAP.

CLINICAL JUDGMENT GUIDE: The nurse should not delegate assessment, teaching, evaluation, medications, or an unstable client to the UAP.

3. 1. **The LPN can change sterile dressings according to his or her scope of practice.**
   2. The UAP can obtain the client's weight; therefore, it should not be assigned to the LPN.
   3. The client in myxedema coma is not a stable client and should be assigned to the RN, not the LPN.

4. Teaching should not be assigned to the LPN, only to the RN.

CLINICAL JUDGMENT GUIDE: The RN should not assign assessment, teaching, evaluation, or the care of an unstable client to an LPN. If any task can be assigned to a UAP, then it should not be assigned to an LPN.

4. 1. The new graduate cannot take a break whenever he or she becomes overwhelmed because the work may never get done. The new graduate should schedule breaks throughout the shift, not when he or she wants to take them.
   2. **The preceptor should recommend that the new graduate use some tool to organize the work so important tasks, such as medication administration and taking vital signs, are not missed.**
   3. Encouraging the new graduate to calm down (five deep breaths) before beginning work is good, but it will not help the new graduate with time management.
   4. The new graduate must find the best way to organize. Doing the organizing for the new graduate will not help.

CLINICAL JUDGMENT GUIDE: There will be management questions on the NCLEX-RN®. Concepts of Management is included under the category Safe and Effective Care Environment and the subcategory Management of Care.

5. 1. The HCP should be notified when the glucose level is verified by the laboratory.
   2. The sliding scale indicates that a blood glucose level of 351 to 400 mg/dL requires 10 units of regular insulin. There is no insulin dosage administered for 408 mg/dL.
   3. This should be done, but not until the nurse rechecks the blood glucose level at the bedside.
   4. **The nurse should first recheck the blood glucose level at the bedside before taking any further action.**

CLINICAL JUDGMENT GUIDE: The test taker needs to read all of the options carefully before choosing the option that says, "Notify the HCP." If any of the options will provide information the HCP needs to know in order to make a decision, the test taker should choose that option. Assessment is the first step in the nursing process.

6. 1. The LPN is not licensed to assess the client who is hypoglycemic, nor should the RN

assign or delegate an unstable client. This client is unstable and requires the RN's assessment skills.

2. The client diagnosed with a paralytic ileus is NPO and should not have any food.

3. The UAP does not have the skill or training to insert a nasogastric tube.

4. **The LPN can perform a sterile procedure such as completing an intermittent urinary catheterization.**

CLINICAL JUDGMENT GUIDE: The test taker must not only know which tasks should be delegated or assigned to the UAP and LPN, but the RN must also know which interventions are appropriate for the client's condition.

7. 1. This would be an inappropriate assignment because the UAP, not the LPN, could feed this stable client.

2. **The RN could request that another nurse administer pain medication so that the client obtains immediate pain relief.**

3. This client's vital signs indicate that the client is unstable; therefore, the RN should check on this client and not delegate the assessment to a UAP.

4. The client who requires a blood transfusion is unstable. The RN should complete the pretransfusion assessment. The RN, not the LPN, assesses.

CLINICAL JUDGMENT GUIDE: The RN cannot delegate assessment, teaching, evaluation, medications, or an unstable client to a UAP. The RN cannot assign assessment, teaching, evaluation, or an unstable client to an LPN. The nurse can assign a task to another nurse.

8. 1. A power of attorney is a legal document authorizing an individual to conduct business for the client. The nurse should not recommend this type of document for a health-care situation.

2. The living will usually requests the client's refusal of life-sustaining treatment. General anesthesia requires the client to be intubated and placed on a ventilator; therefore, the client's request to deny this type of life-sustaining effort will not be honored in the OR. The nurse should not recommend this type of advance directive.

3. A DNR order must be written in the client's EHR by the HCP and may reflect the client's wishes, but it is not an advance directive.

4. **This document would be most appropriate for the nurse to recommend because it names an individual to be responsible in the event the client cannot make health-care decisions for him- or herself.**

CLINICAL JUDGMENT GUIDE: Questions on advance directives are included in the NCLEX-RN®. This content is included under the category Safe and Effective Care Environment and the subcategory Management of Care.

9. 1. **Masseter rigidity is a sign of malignant hyperthermia, which is a life-threatening complication of surgery. The client will also exhibit tachycardia (a heart rate greater than 150 beats/min), hypotension, decreased cardiac output, and oliguria. It is a rare muscle disorder chemically induced by anesthesia.**

2. The client was NPO after midnight and during surgery; therefore, not urinating since surgery does not warrant immediate intervention.

3. The client who received general anesthesia is expected to be sleepy after surgery and easy to arouse; therefore, this client does not warrant immediate intervention.

4. As long as the client has bowel sounds after surgery, hypoactive or hyperactive, then this client does not warrant immediate intervention.

CLINICAL JUDGMENT GUIDE: When deciding which client to assess first, the test taker should determine whether the signs and symptoms the client is exhibiting are normal or expected for the client situation. After eliminating the expected option, the test taker should determine which situation is more life threatening.

10. 1. The nurse who has worked on the unit for 4 years should not be sent because the nurse's expertise is needed on the unit.

2. The graduate nurse, although knowledgeable of the endocrinology unit with 6 months of experience, would not be sent because of lack of experience in the maternal child area.

3. **The LPN with maternal child area experience would be most helpful to the nursery.**

4. The charge nurse should not make assignments based on a staff member's personal life.

CLINICAL JUDGMENT GUIDE: There will be management questions on the NCLEX-RN®. Charge

nurse responsibilities are included under the category Safe and Effective Care Environment.

11. 1. Acromegaly, an excessive secretion of growth hormone, results in overgrowth of the bones and soft tissues. Clubbed fingertips and large feet are expected; therefore, this client doesn't warrant intervention.

2. The client diagnosed with SIADH, because of sustained secretion of antidiuretic hormone (ADH), would be expected to have a low urinary output. This client does not warrant intervention by the nurse.

3. The client diagnosed with Cushing's syndrome would have truncal obesity and thin, fragile skin; therefore, this client does not warrant intervention by the nurse. Cushing's syndrome is caused by excess secretion of glucocorticoids by the adrenal gland.

4. **The client diagnosed with pheochromo-cytoma, a tumor of the adrenal medulla that produces excessive catecholamine, is expected to have a severe pounding headache and chest pain; but of these four clients, this client is having pain, which is a priority. This client warrants intervention by the nurse.**

CLINICAL JUDGMENT GUIDE: The test taker should use some tool as a reference to guide in the decision-making process. In this situation, Maslow's Hierarchy of Needs should be applied. Pain is a priority even if it is expected.

12. 1. This statement is a therapeutic response, but it is not telling the client the truth.

2. **The ethical principle of veracity is the duty to tell the truth.**

3. This statement is "passing the buck," which the nurse should not do if at all possible.

4. This is attempting to obtain more information about the situation, but it is not telling the truth.

CLINICAL JUDGMENT GUIDE: The NCLEX-RN® test plan includes nursing care addressing ethical principles, including autonomy, beneficence, justice, and veracity, to name a few.

13. 1. After the a.m. shift report, the priority medication should be the insulin before the breakfast meal, not metformin (Glucophage).

2. After the a.m. shift report, the priority medication should be the insulin before the breakfast meal, not digoxin.

3. Ceftriaxone (Rocephin), an antibiotic, IVPB is a routine, scheduled medication and should have been administered by the night nurse; there's also a 1-hour leeway when administering this medication. The nurse would have to see whether the IVPB apparatus was hanging at the client's bedside or contact the night nurse before administering this medication.

4. **Insulin is a medication that must be administered before the meal; therefore, this medication is a priority.**

CLINICAL JUDGMENT GUIDE: The test taker should know which medications are priority medications such as life-threatening medications, insulin, and medications that have specific requirements for effectiveness, such as mucosal barrier agents (Carafate). These medications should be administered first by the nurse.

14. 1. **The pregnant nurse can care for clients who have received antineoplastic medications. The nurse should not be exposed to antineoplastic agents outside of the administration bags and tubing. The pregnant nurse can care for a client who is immunosuppressed.**

2. Shingles (herpes zoster) is a painful, blistering skin rash caused by the varicella-zoster virus, the virus that causes chickenpox. The pregnant nurse should not be assigned this client.

3. The client receiving radioactive iodine should not be around pregnant women or young children; therefore, the nurse who is pregnant should not care for this client.

4. The client has cytomegalovirus, which crosses the placental barrier. Therefore, a pregnant nurse should not be assigned this client. Any client diagnosed with a communicable disease that crosses the placental barrier should not be assigned to a nurse who is pregnant.

CLINICAL JUDGMENT GUIDE: There will be management questions on the NCLEX-RN®. Charge nurse responsibilities are included under the category Safe and Effective Care Environment.

15. 1. This is less than the normal fasting range of 100 mg/dL. Hypoglycemia is expected in a client diagnosed with myxedema; therefore, a 74 mg/dL blood glucose level would be expected.

2. The client's metabolism is slowed in myxedema coma, which would result in these vital signs.

3. **These ABGs indicate respiratory acidosis (pH lower than 7.35, $PaCO_2$ higher than 45) and hypoxemia (O_2 lower than 80); therefore, this client would warrant immediate intervention by the nurse. Untreated respiratory acidosis can result in death if not treated immediately.**

4. Lethargy is an expected symptom in a client diagnosed with myxedema; therefore, this would not warrant immediate intervention.

CLINICAL JUDGMENT GUIDE: The nurse must be knowledgeable of expected medical treatment for the client. This is a knowledge-based question. The nurse must be knowledgeable of normal laboratory values. These values must be memorized and the nurse must be able to determine if the laboratory value is normal for the client's disease process or medications the client is taking.

16. 1. Levothyroxine (Synthroid), a thyroid hormone, is a daily medication and can be administered within the 1-hour timeframe (30 minutes before and 30 minutes after the dosing time).

2. **Insulin isophane (Humulin N), a pancreatic hormone, should be administered before a meal for best effects. This medication should be administered first.**

3. Prednisone, a glucocorticoid, is a routine medication and can be administered within the 1-hour timeframe (30 minutes before and 30 minutes after the dosing time).

4. Tiotropium (Spiriva) inhaler, a bronchodilator, is a routine daily medication and can be administered within the 1-hour timeframe (30 minutes before and 30 minutes after the dosing time).

CLINICAL JUDGMENT GUIDE: The test taker should know what medications are priority medications such as life-sustaining medications, insulin, and medications with specific requirements for effectiveness, such as mucosal barrier agents (Carafate). These medications should be administered first by the nurse.

17. 1. The client diagnosed with diabetes insipidus, a deficiency in the production of the antidiuretic hormone, will have an increase in thirst and urination. The nurse should not assess this client first.

2. **The nurse should assess the client with a thyroidectomy for hemorrhaging every 2 hours. Neck edema, irregular breathing, and frequent swelling are signs of hemorrhaging; therefore, the nurse should assess this client first.**

3. The client diagnosed with hypofunction of the parathyroid gland is expected to have muscle cramps and irritability; therefore, the nurse should not assess this client first. Bleeding and loss of airway are the priority over an expected symptom of the disease process, which is not as immediately life threatening.

4. Addison's disease, hypofunction of the adrenal gland, causes the client weakness, fatigue, and anorexia. These signs or symptoms are expected; therefore, the nurse should not assess this client first.

CLINICAL JUDGMENT GUIDE: The test taker must determine which sign or symptom is not expected for the disease process. If the sign or symptom is not expected, then the nurse should assess the client first. This type of question is determining if the nurse is knowledgeable of signs and symptoms of a variety of disease processes.

18. 1. The nurse should obtain the client's baseline weight but it is not the priority intervention over restoring the client's circulatory status.

2. Desmopressin acetate (DDAVP), an analog of the antidiuretic hormone, is the hormone replacement of choice for central DI. It is not the first intervention because restoring circulatory volume is the priority.

3. **In acute DI, hypotonic saline is administered intravenously and is titrated to replace urinary output. Restoring circulatory volume is the priority intervention. Remember Maslow's Hierarchy of Needs; physiological needs are the priority.**

4. Monitoring the client's intake and output is an appropriate nursing intervention but not a priority over restoring circulatory volume.

CLINICAL JUDGMENT GUIDE: All options are plausible in questions that ask the test taker to identify a priority intervention. The test taker must identify the most important intervention.

19. 1. The beta-adrenergic blocker propranolol (Inderal) is used to treat thyrotoxicosis, a thyroid storm, but it is not the nurse's first intervention.

2. The nurse should notify the health-care provider of this rare condition, thyrotoxic crisis, but the nurse should first assess the client before calling the HCP.

3. Because the UAP gave the RN this information, the nurse must assess the client before taking any further action.

4. The nurse should administer acetaminophen (Tylenol) PO STAT to help decrease the fever, but the RN should first assess the client because the UAP gave the nurse the information.

CLINICAL JUDGMENT GUIDE: Any time a nurse receives information from another staff member about a client who may be experiencing a complication, the RN must assess the client. A nurse should not make decisions about the client's needs based on another staff member's information.

20. 1. The UAP cannot sit for an extended period of time with a grieving client.

2. A chaplain is a spiritual adviser who can stay with the client until a family member or the client's personal spiritual adviser can come to the hospital to be with the client.

3. The client should not be sedated. Grieving is a natural process that must be worked through. Sedating the client will delay the grieving process. The nurse should allow the client to vent her feelings to foster the grieving process, not numb the client.

4. The client may request to be left alone, but the nurse should refer the client for spiritual support first and not assume the client wants to be left alone. Most clients feel the need for someone's presence.

CLINICAL JUDGMENT GUIDE: The test taker must be knowledgeable of the role of all members of the multidisciplinary health-care team as well as HIPAA rules and regulations. These will be tested on the NCLEX-RN® examination.

21. **1. The client is exhibiting signs of hypoglycemia; therefore, the nurse should treat the client's symptoms with a simple carbohydrate, such as glucose tablets. This is the first intervention.**

2. The nurse should provide the client with complex carbohydrates so another episode of hypoglycemia will not occur.

3. The nurse could obtain a glucometer reading at the bedside, but having the laboratory draw a serum blood glucose level should not be the nurse's first intervention.

4. The nurse should determine the last time the client received insulin, but it is not the first intervention. Remember: The nurse should not assess if the client is in distress.

CLINICAL JUDGMENT GUIDE: When the question asks which intervention should be implemented first, it means all the options are something a nurse could implement, but only one should be implemented first. The test taker should use the nursing process to determine the appropriate response: If the client is in distress, do not assess; if the client is not in distress, then the nurse should assess.

22. 1. The client has not reported claustrophobia. The client has some type of neurological abnormality.

2. A vest restraint will not keep the client's head still during the MRI.

3. The nurse should make sure that the client does not have any medical device implanted that could react with the magnetic field created by the MRI scanner. An implanted ECG device could prevent the client from having an MRI, depending on the age of the pacemaker and the material with which it was made.

4. Family members are requested to stay outside of the area where the MRI is performed.

CLINICAL JUDGMENT GUIDE: The nurse must be knowledgeable of normal diagnostic tests pre- and post-procedure. These interventions must be memorized and the nurse must be able to determine if the client is able to have the diagnostic procedure and post-procedure care to ensure the client is safe.

23. 1. The nurse needs as much information as possible in order to provide care for the client. The client may or may not have a significant other to be contacted. This is not the best way to try to get information about the client.

2. The ambulance workers will only be able to give a cursory report based on the limited information that was provided to them. This is not the best place to try to get information about the client.

3. The nursing home should send a transfer form with the client that details current medications and diagnoses as well as hygiene needs. Previous hospital records will include a history and physical examination and a discharge summary. This is

the best place to start to glean information regarding the client.

4. The HCP orders may contain a current diagnosis but will not contain any information
about the client's medical history. This is not
the best place to try to get information about
the client.

CLINICAL JUDGMENT GUIDE: Assessment is the
first step of the nursing process, and the test
taker should use the nursing process or some
other systematic process to assist in determining
priorities. The nurse should access documentation that has objective data about the client's
condition.

24. 1. The nurse asked the client her name, and
the client replied that she was a different
person.
   2. **The step the nurse did not take was to
verify the client's armband against the
MAR. Checking the identification band
against the MAR would have prevented
the error.**
   3. This is not the step that was overlooked.
   4. This is not the step that was missed.

CLINICAL JUDGMENT GUIDE: The NCLEX-RN®
test plan includes the category Medication
Administration under Physiological Integrity:
Pharmacological and Parenteral Therapies. This
is a knowledge-based question.

25. Correct answers are 1, 2, 3, and 4.
   1. **Health promotion activities that help
prevent UTIs include emptying the
bladder; bacteria can grow in stagnated
urine in the bladder, and emptying the
bladder will help prevent this.**
   2. **Enzymes found in cranberries inhibit
attachment of urinary pathogens
(especially *E. coli*) to the bladder
epithelium. Daily cranberry juice helps
prevent UTIs.**
   3. **Women diagnosed with diabetes are two
to three times more likely to have bacteria in their bladders than women without
diabetes. Taking hypoglycemic medication is important to maintain appropriate
blood sugar levels.**
   4. **Antibiotic therapy is a priority intervention for the client with a diagnosed UTI.**
   5. Measuring urine output will not prevent the
development of urinary tract infections.

CLINICAL JUDGMENT GUIDE: This is an alternate
type of question included in the NCLEX-RN®

examination. The nurse must be able to select all
the options that answer the question correctly.

26. 1. Steroids do not affect the client's potassium
level.
   2. Glucocorticoids do not affect the client's
sodium level.
   3. Steroids do not affect the client's liver
enzymes.
   4. **Methylprednisolone (Solu-Medrol), a
glucocorticoid steroid, is excreted as glucocorticoids from the adrenal gland and
are responsible for insulin resistance by
the cells, which may cause hyperglycemia;
therefore, the nurse should monitor the
glucose level.**

CLINICAL JUDGMENT GUIDE: The nurse must be
knowledgeable of laboratory values affected by
medication. These values must be memorized
and the nurse must be able to determine if the
laboratory value is normal for the client's disease
process or medications the client is taking.

27. 1. A 6-pound weight gain between dialysis
treatments is expected; therefore, the nurse
would not need to notify the client's HCP.
   2. In the early stage of renal insufficiency, polyuria results from the inability of the kidneys
to concentrate urine, which most often happens at night (nocturia). The nurse would
not notify the client's HCP.
   3. The nurse should call this client, but psychosocial problems do not take priority over
physiological, potentially life-threatening
problems.
   4. **These are signs of an acute transplant
rejection, which is potentially a life-
threatening problem; therefore, the nurse
should notify the health-care provider
about this client.**

CLINICAL JUDGMENT GUIDE: The nurse should
ask, "Are the assessment data normal?" for the
disease process. If they are normal for the disease process, then the nurse would not need to
intervene; if they are not normal for the disease
process, then this warrants intervention by the
nurse.

28. 1. **This client should be seen first because
clear nasal drainage could be cerebrospinal fluid (CSF), which is a potentially
life-threatening complication from surgery. The nurse needs to determine if the
drainage has glucose. If it does, it is CSF
and the surgeon needs to be notified.**

2. The client diagnosed with Graves' disease has exophthalmos (protruding eyes) and bruits (swishing sound) over the thyroid gland so the nurse would not assess this client first.
3. The client diagnosed with hyperparathyroidism is expected to have weakness, loss of appetite, and constipation; therefore, the nurse would not assess this client first.
4. The client diagnosed with Addison's disease is expected to have orthostatic hypotension, nausea, and vomiting; therefore, the nurse would not assess this client first.

CLINICAL JUDGMENT GUIDE: The test taker must determine which sign or symptom is not expected for the disease process. If the sign or symptom is not expected, then the nurse should assess the client first. This type of question is determining if the nurse is knowledgeable of signs and symptoms of a variety of disease processes.

29. 1. A case manager is assigned to a client diagnosed with a chronic illness; therefore, a client diagnosed with a renal calculi who had lithotripsy would not be appropriate for a case manager.
2. **It would be appropriate to assign this client to a case manager because this client has two chronic illnesses, often having multiple hospitalizations and chronic complications, and requires long-term health care.**
3. Hypothyroidism is not a disease process resulting in multiple hospitalizations or chronic complications.
4. A client diagnosed with Addison's disease on corticosteroid therapy would not be a client referred to a case manager.

CLINICAL JUDGMENT GUIDE: Diabetes and CAD are well-known chronic disease processes and should make the test taker look at this option as the correct answer. Postoperative clients, for the most part, return to their normal life, which would not require a case manager.

30. 1. This client would benefit from a home health nurse but not a parish nurse.
2. **A parish nurse is a registered nurse with a minimum of 2 years of experience who works in a faith community, addressing health issues of its members as well as those in the broader community or neighborhood. Parish nursing was recognized as a specialty in 1998 by the American Nurses Association. The client**

is a Catholic, so that is the reason the parish nurse should care for this client.
3. This option has no faith base; therefore, the parish nurse should not be assigned this client.
4. The client diagnosed with chronic renal disease and the caregiver need assistance in the home, but the parish nurse does not need to offer it.

CLINICAL JUDGMENT GUIDE: The nurse must be knowledgeable of the roles and responsibilities of different nurses working in different areas of the hospital and the community.

31. 1. The UAP should not remove anything from the room. The nuclear medicine personnel will check the waste from the room for radioactivity before the removal and, if radioactive, will arrange for disposal in a way that protects the environment.
2. The UAP is hired to care for clients in the ambulatory care unit, not to take a client out to smoke. Clients in ambulatory care should not be smoking before or after surgery or procedures.
3. The UAP cannot assess the client's surgical dressing.
4. **The UAP can obtain a glucometer reading on a client who is stable, and clients in the ambulatory care unit are stable.**

CLINICAL JUDGMENT GUIDE: The RN cannot delegate assessment, teaching, evaluation, medications, or an unstable client to the UAP.

32. **Answer: 125 gtt/min.**
   A microdrip delivers 60 gtt/mL. The formula for this dosage problem is as follows:
   1,000 mL divided by 8 = 125 mL per hour
   125 times 60 = 7,500 gtt per hour
   7,500 divided by 60 minutes = 125 gtts per minute

CLINICAL JUDGMENT GUIDE: This is an alternate type of question included in the NCLEX-RN®. The nurse must know how to perform math calculations.

33. **Correct answers are 1, 2, 4, and 5.**
1. Some herbal remedies commonly recommended for hypothyroid conditions include: *Equisetum arvense, Avena sativa, Centella asiatica, Coleus forskohlii,* and *Fucus vesiculosus.* This is an example of an herbal CAM, a healing practice that does not fall within the realm of conventional medicine.

2. **Cinnamon is a popular spice and flavoring that has shown considerable evidence of lowering blood sugar. This is an example of a CAM, a healing practice that does not fall within the realm of conventional medicine.**

3. Daily baby aspirin is a medically accepted practice and prescribed by medical doctors. This is not an example of a CAM.

4. **This is an example of a CAM, a healing practice that does not fall within the realm of conventional medicine. Acupuncture is a type of traditional Chinese medicine.**

5. **Hypnosis is used in clients for concentration and memory improvement. This is an example of a CAM.**

CLINICAL JUDGMENT GUIDE: The NCLEX-RN® tests candidates on complementary alternative medicine, so the test taker should be knowledgeable of types of CAMs. Many clients use these along with conventional medical interventions.

34. 1. This is an example of community-based nursing wherein nurses care for an individual client living in the community.

2. **Community-oriented, population-focused nursing practice involves the engagement of nursing in promoting and protecting the health of populations, not individuals in the community. Therefore, this is an example of community-oriented, population-focused nursing.**

3. This is an example of community-based nursing wherein nurses care for an individual client living in the community.

4. This is an example of community-based nursing wherein nurses care for an individual client living in the community.

CLINICAL JUDGMENT GUIDE: The test taker should note options 1, 3, and 4 all address an individual client, but option 2 is the "odd man out" and addresses a group of clients; this should cause the test taker to select this option as the correct answer.

35. 1. The client should keep a written record of the results but it is not a priority.

2. The glucometer readings should be done in the morning when the client has not had anything to eat, but it can be done several times a day. This is not a priority.

3. **Have the client demonstrate the skill to ensure the client can correctly perform**

the glucometer reading. This is the priority when teaching about glucometer tests.

4. Proper disposal of lancets and strips with blood on them is important, but not a priority over the client demonstrating the skill.

CLINICAL JUDGMENT GUIDE: In questions that ask the nurse to identify a priority intervention, all the options are plausible. The priority intervention when teaching the client any skill is having the client perform the skill in front of the nurse.

36. 1. **Acupressure applies pressure along the body's energy meridian. Applying pressure on the medial forearm helps decrease the client's feeling of nausea.**

2. This client must have medical interventions and would not benefit from acupressure.

3. Sheehan syndrome is a postpartum condition of pituitary necrosis and hypopituitarism that occurs after circulatory collapse from uterine hemorrhaging. This client would not be treated with acupressure.

4. The client diagnosed with hypertension needs medications and would not benefit from acupressure.

CLINICAL JUDGMENT GUIDE: The NCLEX-RN® tests complementary alternative medicine (CAM), so the nurse must be familiar with the different types of activities and therapies used for clients.

37. 1. Moving the staff members to another room will just allow the argument to continue. This is not the director's first intervention.

2. **The nursing supervisor should intervene and listen to both staff members' concerns and attempt to help resolve the disagreement. This is the director's first intervention.**

3. The director should not ask another staff member to intervene in the argument. The director should address the professional staff about unprofessional behavior.

4. The director should not act unprofessionally and correct the staff in front of everyone in the office. This should be done in private.

CLINICAL JUDGMENT GUIDE: In any business, including a health-care facility, arguments or discussions of confidential information should not occur among staff of any level where the customers or other staff can hear or see it.

38. 1. **These are signs of myxedema coma, which is characterized by subnormal**

temperature, hypotension, and hypoventilation. This client should be seen first by the nurse.
2. The client diagnosed with hypoparathyroidism is expected to have a positive Chvostek's sign (twitching of the facial muscles when the facial nerve is tapped); therefore, the nurse should not assess this client first.
3. Hoarseness is expected for 3 to 4 days after surgery because of edema; therefore, the nurse should not assess this client first.
4. The client diagnosed with diabetes insipidus has polyuria and compensates for the fluid loss by drinking great amounts of water; therefore, the nurse should not assess this client first.

CLINICAL JUDGMENT GUIDE: The test taker must determine which sign or symptom is not expected for the disease process. If the sign or symptom is not expected, then the nurse should assess the client first. This type of question is determining if the nurse is knowledgeable of signs and symptoms of a variety of disease processes.

39. Correct answers are 1, 3, 4, and 5.
    1. **This is an example of an activity the home health nurse would implement in the home.**
    2. Preoperative teaching is not an activity the home health nurse performs in the home. This is usually completed by the preoperative nurse.
    3. **This is an example of an activity the home health nurse would implement in the home.**
    4. **This is an example of an activity the home health nurse would implement in the home.**
    5. **This is an example of an activity the home health nurse would implement in the home.**

CLINICAL JUDGMENT GUIDE: This is an alternate type of question included in the NCLEX-RN®. The nurse must be able to select all the options that answer the question correctly. There are no partially correct answers.

40. 1. The client is exhibiting Trousseau's sign indicating hypoparathyroidism and is treated with IV calcium gluconate, but it is not the nurse's first intervention. The nurse must first assess the client before taking any action.
    2. **When the UAP gives information to the RN about a client, the nurse must first assess the client before taking any action.**

3. The client is exhibiting signs and symptoms of hypoparathyroidism, which makes this client unstable, and the RN should not delegate any task to the UAP for the client who is unstable.
4. The nurse will need to notify the HCP, but not before assessing the client first.

CLINICAL JUDGMENT GUIDE: Any time the RN receives information from another staff member about a client who may be experiencing a complication, the nurse must assess the client. A nurse should not make decisions about the client's needs based on another staff member's information.

41. 1. The client must need intermittent professional skilled care (such as nursing), not constant care.
    2. The client does not have to have a family member living in the home to be eligible for home health care.
    3. **The client must be confined to the home or require a considerable and taxing amount of effort to leave the home for brief periods to be eligible for home health care.**
    4. The client can be referred directly from a health-care provider's office or a long-term care facility, and clients may also request home health care for themselves.

CLINICAL JUDGMENT GUIDE: The nurse must be knowledgeable of the areas of nursing, and how and why the client would qualify for the care. The nurse must be a resource and advocate for the client.

42. 1. **This is an example of meditation.**
    2. Imagery uses the client's mind to generate images to help have a calming effect on the body.
    3. Aromatherapy, a biologically based therapy, involves the use of plants' essential oils for their beneficial effect.
    4. Acupressure is a manipulative and body-based method applying finger and hand pressure to specific areas of the body.

CLINICAL JUDGMENT GUIDE: The NCLEX-RN® tests complementary alternative medicine (CAM), so the nurse must be familiar with the different types of activities and therapies used for clients.

43. 1. **The priority intervention is to restrict fluids to help prevent weight gain, edema, or a serum sodium decline.**

2. This position enhances venous return to the heart and increases left atrial filling pressure, reducing ADH release, but it is not a priority over fluid restriction.
3. The edematous skin is fragile and at risk for skin breakdown, and turning every 2 hours is a pertinent intervention, but it is not a priority over fluid retention.
4. The client needs oral hygiene, but it is not a priority over fluid restriction.

CLINICAL JUDGMENT GUIDE: Physiological problems have the highest priority when deciding on a course of action. The nurse should use Maslow's Hierarchy of Needs; fluid and electrolyte balance is the priority.

44. 1. Dyspnea and confusion are not expected in a client diagnosed with Cushing's syndrome; therefore, this client would warrant a more experienced nurse to assess the reason for the complications.
2. The client with financial problems should be assigned to a social worker, not to a nurse.
3. A full-thickness (third-degree) burn is the most serious burn and requires excellent assessment skills to determine whether complications are occurring. This client should be assigned to a more experienced nurse.
4. **The client diagnosed with diabetic neuropathy would be expected to have pain; therefore, this client could be assigned to a nurse new to home health nursing. The client is not exhibiting a complication or an unexpected sign or symptom.**

CLINICAL JUDGMENT GUIDE: When the test taker is deciding which client should be assigned to a new graduate, the most stable client should be assigned to the least experienced nurse.

45. 1. The client who is 1-day postoperative transsphenoidal hypophysectomy is able to feed him- or herself; therefore, this task should not be delegated.
2. **The UAP is able to obtain a urine specimen from the client. This task is not assessment, teaching, evaluation, medications, or the care of an unstable client.**
3. The client diagnosed with myxedema coma is unstable; therefore, this task cannot be delegated.
4. The UAP cannot assess, and the client diagnosed with an Addisonian crisis is not stable; therefore, this task cannot be delegated.

CLINICAL JUDGMENT GUIDE: This is an "except" question. The test taker could ask which task is appropriate to delegate to the UAP; three options would be appropriate to delegate and one would not. Remember: The RN cannot delegate assessment, teaching, evaluation, medications, or an unstable client to the UAP.

46. 1. This statement does not allow the nurses to have any input into the assignments; therefore, this is the statement of an autocratic manager. These managers use an authoritarian approach to direct the activities of others.
2. Laissez-faire managers maintain a permissive climate with little direction or control. Allowing the assistants to have total control is laissez-faire management. Supporting the assistants in front of the charge nurse is an appropriate action, but it does not address the needs of the field nurses.
3. This statement does not support a democratic leadership style. It is more autocratic: The director is going to take care of the problem.
4. **Democratic managers are people oriented and emphasize efficient group functioning. The environment is open, and communication flows both ways. Meetings to discuss concerns illustrate a democratic leadership style.**

CLINICAL JUDGMENT GUIDE: There will be management questions on the NCLEX-RN®. Concepts of Management is included under the category Safe and Effective Care Environment and the subcategory Management of Care.

47. 1. The client may be diagnosed with diabetes, but at the end of life this is not the priority nursing diagnosis. In fact, as a comfort measure, many clients are allowed to eat whatever they wish occasionally without regard to carbohydrates.
2. This is a psychosocial diagnosis and not a priority over the physiological problems.
3. **The client has peripheral neuropathy, which produces shooting pain in the extremities. The priority at the end of life is to keep the client comfortable.**
4. This is a psychosocial diagnosis and not a priority over the physiological problems.

CLINICAL JUDGMENT GUIDE: The test taker must be aware of the setting, which dictates the appropriate intervention. The "hospice nurse" tells the test taker that this client has a prognosis of

less than 6 months to live. Comfort measures are very important at the end of life.

48. 1. This type of breathing is called Cheyne-Stokes respirations, a pattern of breathing characterized by alternating periods of apnea and deep-rapid breathing. This is not the nurse's first intervention.
2. The nurse should notify the chaplain but it is not the nurse's first intervention.
3. **The RN must first assess the client because the UAP gave the nurse the information.**
4. The family should be contacted but not before assessing the client.

CLINICAL JUDGMENT GUIDE: Whenever any other person gives the RN information about a client, the nurse must first assess the client before taking any other action.

49. Correct answers are 1, 2, and 5.
1. **This is an intervention the nurse should establish with every client.**
2. **Exercises with large muscles allow the release of nervous tension and restlessness. Tremors can interfere with small-muscle coordination.**
3. The UAP should use light coverings, not heavy coverings, because the client diagnosed with hyperthyroidism feels hot.
4. The client diagnosed with hyperthyroidism is not terminal and there is no reason the caregiver cannot leave the client's bedside.
5. **A calm, quiet, cool room should be provided because increased metabolism causes sleep disturbances and the feeling of being hot.**

CLINICAL JUDGMENT GUIDE: The test taker will have alternate types of questions on the NCLEX-RN®. The test taker must select all the correct options to get the question correct.

50. 1. This statement indicates the client understands the teaching and the client does not need more teaching. The exophthalmos that occurs with the disease allows the eyes to dry out, making them uncomfortable, and exposes the client to a risk of sclera damage.
2. The client should wear dark glasses; therefore, the client understands the teaching.
3. **To maintain flexibility, the client should exercise the intraocular muscles several times a day by turning the eyes in the complete range of motion. This**

statement indicates the client needs more teaching.
4. The client should tape the eyes shut; therefore, this client understands the client teaching.

CLINICAL JUDGMENT GUIDE: This is an "except" question. Three of the comments indicate the client understands the teaching and one indicates the client does not understand the teaching. These are occasionally found on the NCLEX-RN® and are worded in this manner. The test taker must realize that the reverse of the usual is in place. A hint: If the test taker is sure more than one option is correct, then the test taker should re-read to make sure that a word or words such as "inappropriate" or "needs more teaching" have not been overlooked.

51. 1. Conserving the energy of the client who is dying is an appropriate intervention and does not warrant intervention by the hospice nurse.
2. Applying lubricant to the client's dry lips and mouth is an appropriate intervention and does not warrant intervention by the hospice nurse.
3. **This is a form of restraint, and the UAP cannot restrain the client in the home or in the acute care setting. This behavior warrants intervention by the RN.**
4. This is an appropriate action to help with shortness of breath or dyspnea. This action would not warrant intervention by the nurse.

CLINICAL JUDGMENT GUIDE: The RN must ensure the UAP can perform any tasks delegated. It is the nurse's responsibility to demonstrate to or teach the UAP how to perform the task, and then evaluate the task.

52. 1. The LPN cannot perform assessments on new admissions.
2. The RN cannot assign evaluation of the client's medical regimen to the LPN.
3. The wound care RN should perform care for a stage 4 pressure ulcer, not the LPN.
4. **The LPN can contact medical supply companies and request durable medical equipment (DME); therefore, this is the most appropriate task to assign the LPN.**

CLINICAL JUDGMENT GUIDE: The RN cannot assign assessment, teaching, evaluation, or an unstable client to the LPN in the home or in the acute care setting.

53. 1. The client diagnosed with hypoparathyroidism is expected to have a decreased serum calcium level; therefore, the nurse would not contact the client's HCP.
2. The client diagnosed with Cushing's syndrome is expected to have a urine cortisol level of 50 to 100 mcg/day; therefore, the nurse would not notify the client's HCP.
3. The client diagnosed with diabetes insipidus is expected to have a low urine specific gravity (lower than 1.005); therefore, the nurse would not notify the client's HCP.
4. **The client diagnosed with hyperthyroidism should have a decreased TSH level; therefore, the nurse should notify the client's HCP.**

CLINICAL JUDGMENT GUIDE: The nurse must be knowledgeable of normal laboratory values. These values must be memorized and the nurse must be able to determine if the laboratory value is normal for the client's disease process or medications the client is taking.

54. 1. The nurse would expect to administer the hormone levothyroxine (Synthroid) to the client diagnosed with hypothyroidism.
2. **Metformin (Glucophage) must be held 24 hours after a client has received any type of contrast dye, because it can cause renal failure. This medication should be questioned by the nurse.**
3. The client diagnosed with DM should receive his or her prescribed (human recombinant) insulin (Humulin N) as soon as he or she is no longer NPO.
4. The client diagnosed with Addison's disease would be receiving the steroid prednisone; therefore, the nurse would not question administering this medication.

CLINICAL JUDGMENT GUIDE: The nurse must be aware of interventions that must be implemented before administering medications. The nurse must know what to monitor before administering medications because untoward reactions and possibly death can occur.

55. Correct answers are 1, 2, 3, and 5.
1. **The client with a unilateral adrenalectomy should be ambulated to prevent postoperative complications. This task could be delegated to the UAP.**
2. **The UAP can change linens for a client. Acute thyrotoxicosis is not a life-threatening condition.**

3. **The client diagnosed with DI is very thirsty and craves ice water; therefore, this task can be delegated to the UAP.**
4. The client just returning from surgery and the PACU should be assessed immediately by the RN. The UAP is not qualified to identify an unstable situation.
5. **The UAP can deliver meal trays to clients receiving regular insulin on a sliding scale.**

CLINICAL JUDGMENT GUIDE: The RN must ensure the UAP can perform any tasks that are delegated. It is the nurse's responsibility to demonstrate to or teach the UAP how to perform the task, and evaluate the task.

56. 1. **The manager should assess the abilities of each staff member for the needs of the unit before deciding which staff member to transfer.**
2. This may be the method used by many managers, but the best action is to evaluate the needs of the unit and the abilities of the staff.
3. In many instances, the unit manager must make hard decisions without consulting the staff members. Asking for the staff members' input could cause tension among the staff; therefore, this is not an appropriate intervention.
4. This will be completed after the decision has been made and the staff member is notified.

CLINICAL JUDGMENT GUIDE: There will be management questions on the NCLEX-RN®. Concepts of Management is included under the category Safe and Effective Care Environment and subcategory Management of Care.

57. 1. **Children are being diagnosed with type 2 diabetes mellitus because of excessive intake of calories and lack of exercise. This is the priority problem. Many states are performing screening activities to identify children at risk for developing type 2 DM so that interventions can be made to delay or prevent the child being diagnosed with type 2 DM. Acanthosis nigricans (hyperinsulinemia) can be identified with simple, non-invasive screening.**
2. The client has a risk of low self-esteem because of the excess weight, but if the client and parents adhere to the recommended treatment regimen for weight control, diet, and exercise, the client's self-esteem should improve.

3. The client's problem is hyperglycemia, not hypoglycemia.
4. Amputation is a chronic problem associated with diabetes and occurs after years of uncontrolled blood glucose levels. This is not the priority problem at this time.

CLINICAL JUDGMENT GUIDE: The NCLEX-RN® integrates the nursing process throughout the Client Needs categories and subcategories. The nursing process is a scientific, clinical reasoning approach to client care that includes assessment, analysis, planning, implementation, and evaluation. The nurse will be responsible for identifying nursing diagnoses for clients.

58. 1. On a floor not directly affected by the fire, the oxygen is turned off only at the instruction of the administrative supervisor or plant operations director.
2. The clients are safer on the floor where they are, not in an area closer to the fire.
3. **The first action in a Code Red (actual fire) is to Rescue (R) the clients in immediate danger, followed by confine (C), closing the doors. Doors in a hospital must be fire rated to confine a blaze for an hour and a half.**
4. This could be done, but it is a charge nurse's responsibility that is not called for at this time.

CLINICAL JUDGMENT GUIDE: The nurse must be knowledgeable of emergency preparedness. Employees receive this information in employee orientation and are responsible for implementing procedures correctly. The NCSBN NCLEX-RN® test plan includes questions on promoting a Safe and Effective Care Environment.

59. 1. The nurse should check the laboratory tests to determine the thyroid levels, but this is not the first intervention.
2. Assessing the client for diarrhea could be done, but it is more important not to worsen the problem, and, therefore, the nurse should hold the thyroid medication first.
3. Documentation of the client's symptoms is always important, but it is not the first intervention.
4. **The client is describing symptoms of hyperthyroidism. Because the client is diagnosed with hypothyroidism, has been prescribed thyroid hormone replacement, and now has symptoms of hyperthyroidism, it can be assumed that the client now has an excess of thyroid**

hormone. Therefore, the nurse should hold the thyroid medication and check the client's thyroid profile.

CLINICAL JUDGMENT GUIDE: The nurse must be aware of expected actions of medications. The nurse must be aware of assessment data indicating whether the medication is effective or whether the medication is causing a side effect or an adverse effect.

60. 1. Propylthiouracil (PTU) blocks peripheral conversion of T_4 to T_3 and is prescribed for the client diagnosed with hyperthyroidism. The nurse would not question administering this medication.
2. Desmopressin acetate (DDAVP) is the treatment of choice for the client diagnosed with central diabetes insipidus.
3. Somatropin (Genotropin), a growth hormone, is the treatment of choice for clients diagnosed with hypofunction of the pituitary gland.
4. **The client diagnosed with hypothyroidism has a decreased pulse rate; therefore, the nurse should not administer a beta blocker, which could further decrease pulse rate. The client diagnosed with thyrotoxicosis (hyperthyroidism) would receive propranolol (Inderal). The nurse should question administering this medication.**

CLINICAL JUDGMENT GUIDE: The nurse must be aware of medications prescribed for specific conditions and disease processes. The nurse is the last person who ensures the client receives the correct medications.

61. 1. **A terminally ill client should be allowed comfort measures even when the activity would normally not be encouraged or allowed. The client can receive sliding-scale insulin, if needed, to cover the ice cream.**
2. The nurse could do this after the ice cream has been metabolized to determine whether an insulin injection is needed.
3. The nurse should tell the client that food such as ice cream may be consumed in moderation and with the appropriate coverage.
4. Low-fat sweets may be a good substitute for some of the foods the client may want to eat.

CLINICAL JUDGMENT GUIDE: The NCLEX-RN® addresses questions concerned with end-of-life care. This is included in the Psychosocial Integrity section of the test plan. Supporting the client's choice is an appropriate option when working with clients who are dying.

62. 1. The HOB should be elevated 30 degrees because the elevation avoids pressure on the sella turcica and decreases headaches, a frequent postoperative problem.
2. A hypophysectomy is surgery that removes the pituitary gland by making an incision in the inner aspect of the upper lip and gingiva. The client should avoid vigorous coughing, sneezing, and straining at stool.
3. **A hypophysectomy is surgery that removes the pituitary gland by making an incision in the inner aspect of the upper lip and gingiva. The sella turicica is entered through the floor of the nose and sphenoid sinuses. There are no visual incisions and the nose cannot be splinted.**
4. The UAP can take the client's vital signs. This would not warrant intervention by the RN.

CLINICAL JUDGMENT GUIDE: The RN must ensure the UAP can perform any tasks that are delegated. It is the nurse's responsibility to demonstrate to or teach the UAP how to perform the task, and evaluate the task performed.

63. 1. The client needs preoperative teaching and the charge nurse should not request a discharge for a client having surgery in the morning.
2. **This client is stable and could be prescribed oral pain medication. She could be discharged home and followed by home health nursing if needed. This client is the most appropriate client for the charge nurse to request to be discharged.**
3. This client is experiencing a complication of surgery and is hemorrhaging; the Hgb/Hct is very low. Therefore, this client cannot be discharged home.
4. This client may be showing signs of acute rejection; therefore, this client cannot be discharged home.

CLINICAL JUDGMENT GUIDE: When the nurse is deciding which client should be discharged home, the most stable client should be discharged.

64. 1. This is a normal potassium level, and the HCP does not need to be notified.

2. This level is within therapeutic range, and the HCP does not need to be notified.
3. A BUN of 84 mg/dL is an abnormal laboratory value, but it would be expected in a client diagnosed with ESRD. The HCP does not need to be notified.
4. **This is a very high blood glucose level, and the client diagnosed with type 1 diabetes will be catabolizing fats at this level and is at risk for diabetic ketoacidosis (DKA) coma.**

CLINICAL JUDGMENT GUIDE: The nurse must be knowledgeable of normal laboratory values. These values must be memorized and the nurse must be able to determine if the laboratory value is normal for the client's disease process or medications the client is taking.

65. 1. The client diagnosed with DKA would have fruity breath; therefore, this nursing intervention does not have priority.
2. Glucose levels are monitored at least every hour.
3. The pulse oximeter reading is not a priority for a client in DKA.
4. **The client will be on a regular insulin drip, which must be maintained at the prescribed rate on an intravenous pump device. Decreasing the client's blood glucose level is the priority nursing intervention.**

CLINICAL JUDGMENT GUIDE: The nurse should remember if a client is in distress and the nurse can do something to relieve the distress, it should be done first, before assessment. The test taker should select an option that directly helps the client's condition.

66. 1. The client's hemoglobin A1C is a test that reveals the average blood glucose for the previous 2 to 3 months. The current blood glucose level may or may not be in the desired range, but the client's diabetes with this level of hemoglobin A1C is not controlled.
2. The nurse should assess for complications of diabetes, but this is not the first intervention. Getting the client to realize the meaning of a high hemoglobin A1C is the priority at this time.
3. **The client must be taught the long-term effects of hyperglycemia. A hemoglobin A1C of 11 indicates an average blood glucose of 269 mg/dL. Over time, a level higher than 120 to 140 mg/dL can lead to damage to many body systems.**

4. Monitoring blood work is not a priority over teaching the client about complications of diabetes when having such a high A1C.

CLINICAL JUDGMENT GUIDE: The nurse must be knowledgeable of normal laboratory values. These values must be memorized and the nurse must be able to determine if the laboratory value is normal for the client's disease process or medications the client is taking.

67. 1. **This client has an elevated WBC count, which could indicate an infection. The HCP should be made aware of this client first.**
    2. These are normal laboratory values.
    3. These are normal laboratory values.
    4. These are normal laboratory values.

CLINICAL JUDGMENT GUIDE: This is an alternate type of question included in the NCLEX-RN® test plan. The test taker must be able to read an electronic health record (EHR), be knowledgeable of laboratory data, and make decisions concerning the nurse's most appropriate action.

68. **The nurse should administer 8 units of regular insulin, a pancreatic hormone, because 249 is between 201 and 250.**

CLINICAL JUDGMENT GUIDE: A fill-in-the-blank question is an alternate type of question included in the NCLEX-RN®. The test taker must use the number keyboard to answer fill-in-the-blank questions.

69. Correct answers are 1, 2, and 3.
    1. The UAP can escort the client to the examination room and take the initial vital signs.
    2. The UAP can weigh the client and document the weight.
    3. The UAP can prepare the examination room for the next client.
    4. Discussing prescriptions is teaching and the RN cannot delegate teaching.
    5. Calling the pharmacy requires knowledge of medications and medication administration. This task cannot be delegated to a UAP.

CLINICAL JUDGMENT GUIDE: This is an alternate type of question included in the NCLEX-RN®. The nurse must be able to select all the options that answer the question correctly. There are no partially correct answers. The registered nurse cannot delegate assessment, teaching, evaluation, medications, or an unstable client to the UAP.

70. Correct order is 1, 3, 4, 2, 5.
    1. This client may have overdosed accidentally or on purpose. This is a physiological problem and the nurse must determine which intervention is required next. This is a potentially life-threatening situation, so the nurse should return this phone call first.
    3. The client diagnosed with hypothyroidism is reporting signs of hyperthyroidism, indicating the client is overdosing on the thyroid hormone replacement and needs to be seen in the clinic. This is a physiological problem; therefore, the nurse should call this client second.
    4. The pharmacist needs to know if the substitution can be made in order to fill this prescription. This call should be returned third.
    2. The nurse needs to discuss the prescribed medication with the HCP to see if a different, less expensive medication would work as well for the client, or if there is an alternative medication program that could be discussed with the client. This phone call should be returned fourth.
    5. The nurse must first determine where the breakdown in the communication of the results of the MRI occurred, then obtain the results and provide them to the HCP before returning the call. This phone call can be returned last.

CLINICAL JUDGMENT GUIDE: This is an alternate type of question that requires the nurse to assess clients in order of priority. This requires the nurse to evaluate each client's situation and determine which situations are life threatening, which situations are expected for the client's situation, and which client has a psychosocial problem.

The correct answer number and rationale for why it is the correct answer are given in **boldface type.** Rationales for why the other possible answer options are incorrect also are given, but they are not in boldface type.

1. **Correct answers are 1, 2, 3, and 5.**
   1. **This is an assessment question and is needed to determine the extent of the current situation.**
   2. **Knowing the blood glucose level is important for the nurse to determine if the client is at risk for diabetic ketoacidosis (DKA).**
   3. **This will determine what has been tried and what the next step will be.**
   4. The client should drink liquids that provide calories, such as sports drinks, and alternate with water to maintain hydration.
   5. **The client will still need to take insulin. Without insulin the client's body will begin to break down fats. A by-product of fat catabolism is acid. The buildup of acid in the body will result in diabetic ketoacidosis (DKA), which can lead to coma and death.**

2. **Correct answers are 1, 3, 4, and 5.**
   1. **The client should monitor for urine ketones. The body usually does not spill ketones in the urine until after the blood glucose levels reach 240 and above. Urine ketones indicate the client's body will begin to break down fats; ketones are the by-product of fat metabolism.**
   2. The client should try to practice "sick day rules" to manage diabetes mellitus during times of illness. It is not necessary for clients to immediately go to the emergency department with an illness.
   3. **Over-the-counter (OTC) medications to control cough and nasal congestion are safe but the client should be taught to avoid those OTC medications containing sugar.**
   4. **If the client is "spilling" ketones in the urine, then the health-care provider will need to adjust the insulin dosage.**
   5. **In order to prevent DKA, the client must continue to take insulin. To prevent hypoglycemia, the client should attempt to ingest calories to balance the insulin. The antidote for insulin is food.**

3. **Correct answers are 1, 2, 3, 4, and 5.**
   1. **The client should be assessed for fluid volume deficit and electrolyte imbalance. Intake and output should be strictly monitored.**
   2. **Bedside glucose assessments should be monitored at least hourly to evaluate the client's response to treatments.**
   3. **Intravenous fluids and regular insulin are initial treatments for DKA.**
   4. **The client was admitted for nausea and vomiting, so oral care is an important intervention for the nurse to perform.**
   5. **The client in DKA loses potassium from increased urinary output, acidosis, catabolic state, and vomiting. Monitoring and replacement is essential for preventing cardiac dysrhythmias secondary to hypokalemia.**

4. 1. The client should be cleaned with warm water and mild soap.
   2. The client's feet should be thoroughly dried by patting, not rubbing of the skin.
   3. **Lotion can be applied to the feet but should not be applied between the toes. The moisture of the lotion can cause skin breakdown. The nurse should intervene.**
   4. The client should wear cotton or wool socks, which are moisture resistant, and avoid going barefoot.

5. **Correct answers are 1, 2, 3, and 5.**
   1. **The client should be taught about "sick day rules" to ensure blood sugar remains stable during illness.**
   2. **Regular monitoring of blood glucose should be reinforced with the client.**
   3. **Diabetes affects all the tissues in the body and the feet are particularly at risk for the development of foot ulcers.**
   4. Type 1 diabetes occurs in young clients who have no production of insulin from the beta cells of the pancreas. These clients are usually underweight. This teaching is not indicated.
   5. **The client should have regular examinations with the diagnosis of type 1 diabetes.**

6. 1. There is no indication that the client recovering from DKA needs a physical therapist.

2. There is no indication that the client newly diagnosed with type 1 diabetes would need a referral to a hospice organization.

3. **A diabetes educator can educate and support this client with the new diagnosis. This is an appropriate referral.**

4. There is no indication that the client needs a fitness trainer.

7. 1. CGM gives glucose readings every 5 minutes; fingerstick tests are still required, but less often.

2. The CGM system is more expensive than performing fingerstick tests.

3. The CGM is a blood glucose monitoring system only, but it can be used in conjunction with an insulin pump for better maintenance of blood sugar.

4. **The continuous glucose monitoring (CGM) system is designed to show real-time blood glucose measurements and trends over a period of time, allowing for better understanding of the fluctuations in the client's glucose level. Many continuous glucose monitoring systems can send information and alerts directly to the client's smartphone.**

8. 1. The client can place the pump on the bed or attach it to his or her clothing or pillow. This statement indicates the client understands the teaching.

2. An insulin pump allows the client to administer a continuous dose of insulin and bolus doses to cover meals high in carbohydrates. This helps to avoid large fluctuations in blood glucose levels. This statement indicates the client understands the teaching.

3. The client must continue to monitor blood glucose levels to ensure the insulin pump is working correctly. If the insulin pump malfunctions, the client could experience diabetic ketoacidosis (DKA). This statement indicates the client understands the teaching.

4. **An insulin pump allows the client to match insulin to exercise and activities.**

When performing some types of exercise, such as swimming or contact sports, the insulin pump should be disconnected to avoid damage to the pump or injury to the client. This statement indicates the client needs more teaching.

9. 1. **Lipohypertrophy is an abnormal fat accumulation under the surface of the skin and is most often associated with repeated injections at the same location. The priority intervention is to rotate catheter insertion sites to avoid lipohypertrophy.**

2. The client should be taught to perform frequent hand washing to prevent an infection at the catheter insertion site; however, the priority intervention is to rotate insertion sites.

3. The client should be taught to avoid inserting the insulin pump catheter in the inner thigh. The inner thigh has many nerves and blood vessels, which can cause increased discomfort and reduce insulin absorption. This is not the priority intervention to avoid lipohypertrophy.

4. The client should be instructed to complete the prescribed course of antibiotics to treat the lipohypertrophy, but this will not prevent the reoccurrence. The priority intervention is to prevent lipohypertrophy by rotating catheter insertion sites.

10. **Correct order is 4, 3, 5, 1, 2.**

4. **The nurse should wash hands and don nonsterile gloves.**

3. **The nurse should wash the insertion area with an antibacterial soap and let dry thoroughly.**

5. **The nurse should then cleanse the area with an antibacterial solution and let dry thoroughly.**

1. **The next step is to apply an antiseptic and adhesive wipe to the area.**

2. **The final step is to insert the catheter in a slow, continuous motion.**

Integumentary Management

9

Believe you can and you're halfway there.

—Theodore Roosevelt

QUESTIONS

1. The nurse received the a.m. shift report on the following clients. Which client should the nurse assess **first?**
   1. The client with a right total knee replacement who wants to be removed from the continuous passive motion (CPM) machine
   2. The client diagnosed with chronic low back pain who is crying and upset about being discharged home
   3. The client who is 1 week postoperative for right total hip replacement (THR) who has a temperature of 100.4°F
   4. The client who has full-thickness burns who needs to be medicated before being taken to whirlpool

2. The nurse is working in an orthopedic unit. Which client should the nurse assess **first?**
   1. The client who is 2 weeks postoperative open reduction and external fixation (ORIF) of the right hip who is reporting pain when ambulating
   2. The client who is 10 days postoperative for left total knee replacement (TKR) who is refusing to use the continuous passive motion (CPM) machine
   3. The client who is 1 week postoperative for L3–L4 laminectomy who is reporting numbness and tingling of the feet
   4. The client who is being admitted to the rehabilitation unit from the orthopedic surgical unit after a motor vehicle accident (MVA)

3. The client is 1 week postoperative for right below-the-knee amputation secondary to arterial occlusive disease. The nurse is unable to assess a pedal pulse in the left foot. Which intervention should the nurse implement **first?**
   1. Assess for paresthesia and paralysis.
   2. Utilize the Doppler device to auscultate the pulse.
   3. Place the client's leg in the dependent position.
   4. Wrap the client's left leg in a warm blanket.

4. The client who has a history of cerebrovascular accident (CVA) is admitted to the orthopedic unit diagnosed with a fractured right hip. The client is reporting bleeding when brushing his teeth. The nurse reviews the client's medication administration record (MAR). Which intervention should the nurse implement **first?**

Client's Name: P.W. Height: 72 inches	Account Number: 1230456 Weight: 240 pounds	Allergies: NKDA Date:
Medication	0701–1900	1901–0700
Levothyroxine 1 tablet PO qd	0900 DN	
Atenolol 50 mg PO qd	0900 DN AP 72	
Warfarin 5 mg PO 1700	1700 DN	
Hydrocodone 5 mg/500 mg PO q 4–6 hours PRN for pain		
Signature/Initials	Day Nurse RN/DN	Night Nurse RN/DN

1. Prepare to administer vitamin K.
2. Determine whether the client is using a soft-bristle toothbrush.
3. Check the client's apical pulse and blood pressure.
4. Request the laboratory to draw a STAT INR.

5. The nurse is preparing to administer morning (a.m.) medications to the following clients. Which medication should the nurse administer **first?**
1. The NSAID to the client diagnosed with osteoarthritis
2. The IV antibiotic to the client diagnosed with cellulitis
3. The antiviral agent to the client diagnosed with herpes zoster (shingles)
4. The antihistamine to the client diagnosed with urticaria and pruritus

6. The client tells the nurse, "I have a mole on my back that is darker and getting larger." Which intervention should the nurse implement **first?**
1. Tell the client to use corticosteroid cream on the area.
2. Recommend the client use SPF 15 or higher when in the sun.
3. Instruct the client to notify his or her health-care provider immediately.
4. Encourage the client to wear dark, woven clothing when outside.

7. The nurse is at a local playground and her 10-year-old son falls and reports that his left ankle and foot are hurting. Which intervention should the nurse implement **first** at the scene of the accident?
1. Instruct her son not to move the left leg.
2. Elevate the left leg on two rolled towels.
3. Apply an ice pack to the left ankle.
4. Check her son's pedal pulse bilaterally.

8. The nurse is preparing to change a dressing on an 82-year-old client diagnosed with a stage III pressure ulcer. Which intervention should the nurse implement **first?**
1. Obtain the needed equipment to perform the procedure.
2. Remove the client's old dressing with nonsterile gloves.
3. Explain the procedure to the client in understandable terms.
4. Check to determine whether the client has received pain medication.

9. Which client should the charge nurse on the rehabilitation unit assess **first** after receiving the a.m. shift report?
    1. Mr. J.L., who is postoperative open reduction and internal fixation (ORIF) of the right hip

Client Name: J.L.	Account Number: 1133557		Allergies: PCN
Laboratory Report			
Laboratory Test	**Client Value**	**Normal Value**	
WBC	9.1	4.5 to 11.1 10³/microL	
Hgb	8	Male: 14 to 17.3 g/dL	
		Female: 11.7 to 15.5 g/dL	
Hct	24	Male: 42% to 52%	
		Female: 36% to 48%	
Glucose	89	Fasting: Less than 100 mg/dL	
		Random: Less than 200 mg/dL	
Rheumatoid factor	12	Less than 14 IU/mL (international units per mL)	

2. Ms. M.P., who is diagnosed with rheumatoid arthritis

Client Name: M.P.	Account Number: 2299483		Allergies: NKDA
Laboratory Report			
Laboratory Test	**Client Value**	**Normal Value**	
WBC	8.2	4.5 to 11.1 10³/microL	
Hgb	12	Male: 14 to 17.3 g/dL	
		Female: 11.7 to 15.5 g/dL	
Hct	36	Male: 42% to 52%	
		Female: 36% to 48%	
Glucose	95	Fasting: Less than 100 mg/dL	
		Random: Less than 200 mg/dL	
Rheumatoid factor	20	Less than 14 IU/mL (international units per mL)	

3. Mr. P.G., who is diagnosed with a stage IV pressure ulcer

Client Name: P.G.	Account Number: 8833774		Allergies: NKDA
Laboratory Report			
Laboratory Test	**Client Value**	**Normal Value**	
WBC	14	4.5 to 11.1 10³/microL	
Hgb	14	Male: 14 to 17.3 g/dL	
		Female: 11.7 to 15.5 g/dL	
Hct	42	Male: 42% to 52%	
		Female: 36% to 48%	
Glucose	99	Fasting: Less than 100 mg/dL	
		Random: Less than 200 mg/dL	
Rheumatoid factor	10	Less than 14 IU/mL (international units per mL)	

4. Ms. K.C., who is diagnosed with systemic allergies and taking a prednisone dose pack

Client Name: K.C.	Account Number: 2255449		Allergies: NKDA
Laboratory Report			
Laboratory Test	**Client Value**	**Normal Value**	
WBC	8.5	4.5 to 11.1 10^3/microL	
Hgb	12.3	Male: 14 to 17.3 g/dL	
		Female: 11.7 to 15.5 g/dL	
Hct	36	Male: 42% to 52%	
		Female: 36% to 48%	
Glucose	189	Fasting: Less than 100 mg/dL	
		Random: Less than 200 mg/dL	
Rheumatoid factor	8	Less than 14 IU/mL (international units per mL)	

10. The client ambulating down the orthopedic hallway unassisted fell to the floor. Which action should the nurse implement **first?**
   1. Complete an adverse occurrence report.
   2. Notify the clinical manager on the unit.
   3. Determine whether the client has any injuries.
   4. Ask why the client was in the hall alone.

11. The RN rehab nurse and the unlicensed assistive personnel (UAP) are caring for clients on a rehabilitation unit. Which nursing task is **most** appropriate for the RN to delegate to the UAP?
   1. Flush the triple-lumen lines on a central venous catheter.
   2. Demonstrate for the client how to ambulate with a walker.
   3. Assist with bowel training by escorting the client to the bathroom.
   4. Apply corticosteroid cream to the client diagnosed with allergic dermatitis.

12. The unlicensed assistive personnel (UAP) tells the RN primary nurse the client with a right above-the-knee amputation has a large amount of bright red blood on the right leg residual limb. Which action should the nurse implement?
   1. Assess the client's residual limb dressing.
   2. Tell the UAP to take the client's pulse and blood pressure.
   3. Remove the dressing to assess the incision.
   4. Request the UAP to reinforce the dressing.

13. Which action by the unlicensed assistive personnel (UAP) warrants **immediate** intervention by the RN staff nurse?
   1. The UAP tied the confused client to a chair with a sheet.
   2. The UAP escorted the client downstairs to smoke a cigarette.
   3. The UAP bought the client a carbonated beverage from the cafeteria.
   4. The UAP assisted the client to ambulate to the dayroom area.

14. The RN charge nurse, a licensed practical nurse (LPN), and two unlicensed assistive personnel (UAPs) are caring for clients. Which action is **most** appropriate for the charge nurse to assign or delegate?
   1. Ask the UAP to apply warm compresses to the client diagnosed with tinea corporis.
   2. Request the LPN to apply antifungal cream to the client diagnosed with tinea pedis.
   3. Tell the UAP to remove the toenail of the client diagnosed with onychomycosis.
   4. Instruct the LPN to administer isotretinoin to the client who is pregnant.

15. The RN staff nurse in the rehabilitation unit is caring for clients along with an unlicensed assistive personnel (UAP). Which action by the UAP warrants **immediate** intervention?
1. The UAP assists a client 1 week postoperatively to eat a regular diet.
2. The UAP calls for assistance when taking a client to the shower.
3. The UAP is assisting the client who weighs 181 kg to the bedside commode.
4. The UAP places the call light within reach of the client who is sitting in the chair.

16. The unlicensed assistive personnel (UAP) on the rehabilitation unit is placing the client with a left above-the-knee amputation in the prone position. Which action should the RN rehab nurse implement?
1. Tell the UAP to place the client on the back.
2. Praise the UAP for positioning the client prone.
3. Report this action verbally to the charge nurse.
4. Explain to the UAP that the client should not be placed on the stomach.

17. The unlicensed assistive personnel (UAP) is applying elastic compression stockings to the client. Which action by the UAP indicates to the RN primary nurse the UAP understands the correct procedure for applying the elastic compression stockings?
1. The UAP applies the stockings while the client is sitting in a chair.
2. The UAP is unable to insert two fingers under the proximal end of the stocking.
3. The UAP had the client elevate the legs before putting on the stockings.
4. The UAP places the toe opening of the elastic stocking on top of the client's foot.

18. The charge nurse on the acute care rehabilitation unit is making assignments for the shift. Which client should the charge nurse assign to the **most** experienced nurse?
1. The client diagnosed with a full-thickness burn who is refusing to go to therapy
2. The client diagnosed with osteomyelitis who has bone pain and a fever
3. The client diagnosed with a fractured tibia who has deep, unrelenting pain
4. The client diagnosed with low back pain radiating down the left leg

19. The RN charge nurse on the busy 36-bed rehabilitation unit must send one staff member to the emergency department (ED). Which staff member is the **most** appropriate person to send?
1. The LPN who has worked on the rehabilitation unit for 3 years
2. The RN who has been employed on the rehabilitation unit for 8 years
3. The UAP who is completing the 4-week orientation to the rehabilitation unit
4. The RN who transferred to the rehabilitation unit from the medical unit

20. Which task should the RN rehabilitation nurse delegate to the unlicensed assistive personnel (UAP)?
1. Tell the UAP to show the client how to perform self-catheterization.
2. Ask the UAP to place the newly confused client in the inclusion bed.
3. Request the UAP give the client 30 mL of magnesium hydroxide, aluminum hydroxide.
4. Encourage the UAP to attend the multidisciplinary team meeting.

21. The client is 8 hours postoperative spinal surgery. Which **priority** intervention should the nurse implement?
1. Evaluate how much pain medication the client is using via the patient-controlled analgesia (PCA) pump.
2. Logroll the client with three staff members when turning the client side to side.
3. Assist the client to ambulate to the bathroom using an elevated commode seat.
4. Place pillows under the thighs of each leg when the client is in supine position.

22. The elderly wife of a client with a total hip replacement who is being discharged home tells the nurse, "I am really worried about taking my husband home. I don't know how I will be able to take care of him." Which intervention is **most** appropriate for the nurse?
    1. Refer the client to the home health nurse.
    2. Discuss the possibility of placing her husband in a nursing home.
    3. Request the client's health-care provider to talk to the wife.
    4. Allow the client's wife to vent her feelings about the situation.

23. The male nurse who has been told by the female nurse on previous occasions not to talk to her about her body says, "You really look hot in those scrubs. You have a great-looking body." Which action should the female nurse take **next?**
    1. Document the comment in writing and file a formal grievance.
    2. Tell the male nurse this makes her feel very uncomfortable.
    3. Notify the clinical manager of the sexual harassment.
    4. Discuss the male nurse's behavior with the hospital lawyer.

24. The client who was admitted to the rehabilitation unit because of a debilitative state asks the nurse, "Why do I have to go to physical therapy every day?" Which statement is the nurse's **best** response?
    1. "The physical therapy will help you become **more** independent in caring for yourself."
    2. "You must have at least 3 hours of therapy a day to be able to stay in this rehab unit."
    3. "The multidisciplinary team determined that you should be in physical therapy daily."
    4. "The physical therapist will help you with exercises to improve your muscle strength."

25. The client diagnosed with a fractured right ankle needs to be instructed on crutch walking. Which member of the multidisciplinary team should address this problem?
    1. The physical therapist
    2. The social worker
    3. The occupational therapist
    4. The rehabilitation physician

26. The client with bilateral amputations tells the nurse, "I was told I can't go back to my job because they do not have handicap accessible bathrooms or ramps." Which action by the nurse is **most** helpful to the client?
    1. Discuss the situation with the multidisciplinary health-care team.
    2. Explain the Americans with Disabilities Act (ADA) to the client.
    3. Contact the client's employer via telephone and discuss the situation.
    4. Encourage the client to hire an attorney and sue the employer.

27. Which action by the RN primary nurse would warrant **immediate** intervention by the RN charge nurse on the rehabilitation unit?
    1. The primary nurse tells the unlicensed assistive personnel (UAP) to escort a client to the swimming pool.
    2. The primary nurse evaluates the client's plan of care with the family member.
    3. The primary nurse asks another nurse to administer an injection he prepared.
    4. The primary nurse requests another nurse to watch her clients for 30 minutes.

28. The client in a motor vehicle accident (MVA) is in critical condition diagnosed with a pelvic fracture, flail chest, bilateral arm fractures, and a left hip fracture. The client tells the nurse, "I just want to die. I can't feed myself or clean myself." Which statement is the nurse's **best** response?
    1. "I know this must be hard for you but you can have a life."
    2. "I can see you must feel helpless; I am here to listen."
    3. "Have you thought about killing yourself?"
    4. "You are in shock but in time things will get better."

29. The nurse on the surgical unit is being sent to the neonatal intensive care unit (NICU) to work because the unit is short staffed. The nurse has never worked in the NICU. Which response by the nurse supports the ethical principle of nonmaleficence?
    1. The nurse requests not to be floated to the NICU.
    2. The nurse accepts the assignment to the NICU.
    3. The nurse asks why another nurse can't go to the NICU.
    4. The nurse talks another nurse into going to the NICU.

30. The client's husband is frustrated and tells the nurse, "Everyone is telling me something different as to when my wife is going to be able to go home. I don't know whom to believe." Which statement is the rehabilitation nurse's **best** response?
    1. "I can see you are frustrated. Do you want to talk about how you feel?"
    2. "I will contact the case manager and have her talk to you as soon as possible."
    3. "Do not worry. Your wife won't go home until you and she are both ready."
    4. "Your wife's health-care provider should be able to give you that information."

31. The client with an upper extremity amputation tells the nurse, "I do everything with my right hand and now it is gone. I have no idea what I am going to do after I get discharged. How will I support my family? I will need to get a new job." Which statement is the nurse's **best** response?
    1. "With time you will be able to do everything with your left hand."
    2. "The state rehabilitation commission will help retrain you."
    3. "You should ask the social worker about applying for disability."
    4. "You are worried about how you will be able to support your family."

32. The client tells the nurse, "I do not like my doctor and I want another doctor." Which statement is the nurse's **best** response?
    1. "You should tell your doctor you are not happy with his care."
    2. "Can you tell me what you don't like about your doctor's care?"
    3. "I will notify my nursing supervisor and report your concern."
    4. "I am sorry, but you really must keep this doctor until you are discharged."

33. The RN staff nurse and the unlicensed assistive personnel (UAP) are caring for a 74-year-old client who is 3 days postoperative right total hip replacement (THR). Which nursing task should be delegated to the UAP?
    1. Place the abductor pillow between the client's legs.
    2. Ensure the client stays on complete bedrest.
    3. Feed the client the evening meal.
    4. Check the client's right hip surgical dressing.

34. The RN staff nurse tells the unlicensed assistive personnel (UAP) to assist the client who is 1 day postoperative spinal surgery with a.m. care. Which action by the UAP warrants **immediate** intervention?
    1. The UAP closes the door and cubicle curtain.
    2. The UAP requests the client to turn to the side.
    3. The UAP checks the temperature of the bathing water.
    4. The UAP puts the side rails up when bathing the client.

35. The client with a right below-the-knee amputation who also has impetigo is admitted to a rehabilitation unit. Which interventions should be included in the nursing care plan? **Select all that apply.**
    1. Elevate the client's right leg on two pillows.
    2. Refer the client to occupational therapy daily.
    3. Encourage the client to push the residual limb against a pillow.
    4. Use warm soap and water to remove the crusts secondary to impetigo.
    5. Ensure all staff members wear gloves when caring for a client.

36. The overhead page has issued a Code Black, indicating a tornado in the area. Which intervention should the charge nurse implement?
    1. Instruct the hospital staff to assist the clients and visitors to the cafeteria.
    2. Request the client and visitors go into the bathroom in the client's room.
    3. Have the clients and visitors remain in the hallway with the doors closed.
    4. Tell the client and any visitors to remain in the client's room with the door open.

37. The male client is placed in a double hip spica cast for 3 months. The client's wife tells the nurse, "My husband said we are supposed to talk to his case manager. What is a case manager?" Which statement is the nurse's **best** response?
    1. "A case manager discusses the cost and insurance issues concerning the rehabilitation."
    2. "The case manager is responsible for the medical treatment regimen for your husband."
    3. "The case manager is a member of the team who will assist your husband in finding another job."
    4. "The case manager is a nurse who will coordinate the rehabilitation team and keep you informed."

38. The 28-year-old male client who sustained traumatic bilateral amputations secondary to a motor vehicle accident (MVA) is being discharged home to live with his wife and 3-year-old son. Which **priority** psychosocial intervention should the rehabilitation nurse discuss with the client?
    1. Ask the client whether he has any sexual concerns he needs to discuss.
    2. Determine whether the home is safe for ambulating with prosthetic devices.
    3. Discuss the procedure for obtaining a specially equipped car.
    4. Explain the importance of getting psychological counseling.

39. The RN primary nurse overhears the unlicensed assistive personnel (UAP) telling a family member of a client, "One of the clients will be going to prison because that person was charged with vehicular manslaughter. Two people in the motor vehicle accident died." Which action should the primary nurse implement **first?**
    1. Apologize to the family member for the UAP's comments.
    2. Tell the UAP that the comment is a violation of HIPAA.
    3. Allow the UAP to complete the conversation and then discuss the situation.
    4. Interrupt the conversation and tell the UAP to go to the nurse's station.

40. The clinical nurse manager has verbally warned a staff nurse about being late to work on two previous occasions. The nurse was 35 minutes late for today's shift. Which action should the charge nurse take?
    1. Ask the staff nurse why he or she was late again today.
    2. Notify the human resources department in writing.
    3. Initiate the hospital policy for unacceptable behavior.
    4. Do not allow the staff nurse to work on the unit today.

41. The RN charge nurse on the rehabilitation unit is making assignments for the day shift. Which assignment would be **most** appropriate for the licensed practical nurse (LPN)?
    1. Have the LPN call the HCP to obtain an order for a diet change.
    2. Instruct the LPN to complete the admission assessment.
    3. Ask the LPN to teach the client about a high-fiber diet.
    4. Request the LPN to obtain the intake and output for the clients.

42. The charge nurse received laboratory data on the following clients. Which client warrants **immediate** intervention by the charge nurse?
    1. The client diagnosed with COPD who has ABGs of pH, 7.35; Pao_2, 77; $Paco_2$, 57; Hco_3, 24
    2. The client diagnosed with bilateral TKR who has a WBC count of 10,400
    3. The client on antibiotic therapy who has a serum potassium level of 3.3 mEq/L
    4. The client receiving TPN who has a glucose level of 145 mg/dL

43. The client tells the primary nurse, "I just finished completing my living will and I need you to witness my signature." Which action should the nurse implement?
   1. Witness the client's living will using an ink pen.
   2. Explain that the nurse cannot witness this document.
   3. Tell the client the document does not need a witness's signature.
   4. Offer to have the hospital attorney to come notarize the form.

44. The nurse is preparing to ambulate the client diagnosed with full-thickness burns on the lower extremities down the hall. Which **priority** intervention should the nurse implement?
   1. Place rubber-soled shoes on the client.
   2. Put a gait belt around the client's waist.
   3. Explain the procedure to the client.
   4. Provide a clear path for the client to walk.

45. The client in the rehabilitation unit tells the nurse, "I will not go to physical therapy again because it hurts so much when I do the exercises." Which statement **supports** the nurse's role as a client advocate?
   1. "You do not have to go to physical therapy if it causes you pain."
   2. "I will talk to the physical therapist (PT) about the exercises that cause you pain."
   3. "Let me check and see if you can receive pain medication before therapy."
   4. "I will discuss your concerns at the next multidisciplinary team meeting."

46. The rehabilitation nurse enters the client's room and the client is talking on the phone. The client asks the nurse to talk to his wife because she has some questions. Which action should the nurse take?
   1. Explain that HIPAA regulations prevent the nurse from talking to the wife.
   2. Tell the client it would be best for the nurse to talk to the wife in person.
   3. Request the client's wife to come to the weekly team meeting to ask questions.
   4. Honor the client's request and answer any questions the wife has on the phone.

47. The school nurse notes the child has impetigo. Which interventions should the nurse implement? **Select all that apply.**
   1. Administer an antibiotic ointment four times a day.
   2. Instruct the parents to keep the child at home until lesions crust over.
   3. Tell the parents to use separate towels for the child.
   4. Do not remove the crusts from the skin lesions.
   5. Tell the parents to have the child wear non-latex sterile gloves over both hands until no crusting is present.

48. Which action by the primary nurse requires **immediate** intervention by the charge nurse?
   1. The nurse is teaching the client how to use a glucometer.
   2. The nurse leaves the computer screen open to the EHR at the nurse's station.
   3. The nurse is discussing a client situation on the phone with the HCP.
   4. The nurse contacts the chaplain to come and talk to a client.

49. The nurse is triaging phone calls in a dermatological clinic. Which client **warrants** the nurse making an appointment **immediately?**
   1. The client reports having white spots on both of the hands.
   2. The client reports redness and itching on the hands.
   3. The client reports a cherry angioma on the right lower leg.
   4. The client reports red patches on one side of the body.

50. The client has an area on the skin the dermatologist thinks may be basal cell carcinoma. Which intervention will the nurse implement to confirm the diagnosis?
   1. Refer the client for the magnetic resonance imaging (MRI).
   2. Explain how to obtain a washing of the abnormal skin area.
   3. Prepare the client for a biopsy of the abnormal skin growth.
   4. Tell the client there is no way to definitively confirm the diagnosis.

QUESTIONS

51. The nurse is assisting the client to use a cane when ambulating. **Rank in order of performance.**
1. Request the client to move the cane forward.
2. Move the weaker leg one step forward.
3. Ensure the client places the cane in the strong hand.
4. Move the stronger leg one step forward.
5. Apply a gait belt around the client's waist.

52. Which **priority** intervention should the nurse implement to help prevent pressure ulcers in the client who is on strict bedrest?
1. Provide adequate skin care for the client.
2. Turn the client every 2 hours or more often.
3. Ensure sufficient nutritional intake.
4. Use pressure-relieving devices such as waterbeds.

53. Which intervention should the nurse implement **first** for the client diagnosed with a fractured femur who is suspected of having a fat embolism?
1. Assess the client's bilateral breath sounds.
2. Encourage the client to cough and deep breathe.
3. Administer oxygen via nasal cannula.
4. Prepare to administer IV heparin therapy.

54. The client diagnosed with an electrical burn is brought to the emergency department (ED). The entrance wound is on the right hand and the exit wound is on the left foot. Which intervention should the nurse implement **first?**
1. Place sterile gauze on the entrance and exit wounds.
2. Assess the client's vital signs.
3. Monitor the client's pulse oximetry.
4. Place the client on cardiac telemetry.

55. The nurse is using an electric client lift to transfer the client from the bed to a stretcher. Which **priority** intervention should the nurse implement?
1. Have two staff members assist when using the lift.
2. Ensure the client is correctly placed in the lift before moving.
3. Lift the client slowly off the bed when turning on the lift.
4. Ensure the stretcher is in the correct position and locked.

56. The RN staff nurse is assessing the functional ability of a client using the Katz Index of Activities of Daily Living (ADLs). Which assessment score would require the nurse to delegate feeding, bathing, and toileting to the unlicensed assistive personnel (UAP)?
1. Katz Index of ADLs score 6
2. Katz Index of ADLs score 4
3. Katz Index of ADLs score 3
4. Katz Index of ADLs score 2G

57. The client has cellulitis on the right lower leg. Which intervention should the nurse implement?
1. Place the client's right arm in the dependent position.
2. Apply warm moist heat to the affected area.
3. Wash the affected area with anti-staphylococcal soap.
4. Wrap the right arm with elastic bandages.

58. The unlicensed assistive personnel (UAP) is transferring the client from the bed to the chair. Which interventions should the RN primary nurse ensure the UAP implements during this procedure? **Rank in order of priority.**
1. Assist the client to sit when the client's legs touch the edge of the chair.
2. Place the wheelchair at an angle on the client's strong side.
3. Assist the client to stand and put the strong hand on the wheelchair armrest.
4. Keep the client's weight forward and pivot the client.
5. Lock the wheelchair brakes and secure the chair position.

59. The RN charge nurse on the rehabilitation unit is assigning and delegating tasks to the unlicensed assistive personnel (UAP) and licensed practical nurse (LPN). Which task is **most** appropriate for the RN to delegate or assign?
    1. Tell the UAP to elevate the client's residual limb above the heart.
    2. Instruct the LPN to give the diabetic clients their HS snacks.
    3. Request the UAP to insert an indwelling urinary catheter.
    4. Ask the LPN to assess the client who may have herpes zoster.

60. The RN burn unit nurse is caring for a client diagnosed with a full-thickness burn over the right lower extremity. Which task should the nurse delegate to the UAP?
    1. Instruct the UAP to check the client's right dorsalis pedal pulse.
    2. Ask the UAP to cleanse the client's dentures and place in the container.
    3. Request the UAP to perform passive range-of-motion (ROM) exercises.
    4. Tell the UAP to keep the client's right leg in the dependent position.

61. The client is admitted to the emergency department (ED) diagnosed with a third-degree burn over the front of both legs. Which **priority** intervention should the nurse implement?
    1. Maintain a sterile environment when caring for the client.
    2. Insert two large-bore intravenous access routes.
    3. Administer intravenous antibiotic therapy.
    4. Assess the client's pain level on a 1 to 10 pain scale.

62. The day nurse is preparing to administer medications to the client who is reporting light-headedness when getting out of bed. Which medication should the day nurse **question** administering?

Client's Name: J.S. Weight: 75 kg	Account Number: 1032456 Date:	Height: 72 inches
Medication	**0701–1900**	**1901–0700**
Atenolol 50 mg PO qd	0900	
Ceftriaxone 150 mg IVBP q 12 hours	0900	
Bisacodyl 2 PO PRN constipation		
Hydrocodone 5 mg/500 mg PO q 4–6 hours PRN for pain		
Signature/Initials	Day Nurse RN/DN	Night Nurse RN/DN

    1. Atenolol 50 mg PO
    2. Ceftriaxone 150 mg IVPB
    3. Bisacodyl 2 PO
    4. Administer all medications as ordered

63. The nurse is discussing complementary and alternative medicine (CAM) with a client on the rehabilitation unit. Which therapies should the nurse discuss with the client? **Select all that apply.**
    1. Acupuncture
    2. Guided imagery
    3. Compression sequential devices
    4. Music therapy
    5. Muscle-strengthening exercises

64. The nurse tells the client, "I am going to refer you to the vocational counselor." The client asks the nurse, "Why are you making this referral?" Which statement is the nurse's **best** response?
    1. "The counselor will assist you with job placement, training, or further education."
    2. "The counselor specializes in rehabilitative medicine and will help you get better."
    3. "The counselor will help develop your fine motor skills to help perform ADLs."
    4. "The counselor will help you continue or develop hobbies or interests."

QUESTIONS

65. The nurse is assessing the client's daily schedule and habits. Which question is **most** appropriate for the nurse to ask the client?
    1. "Do you have a family member who can assist you when you go home?"
    2. "What time do you prefer bathing and do you take a tub bath or a shower?"
    3. "Do you have insurance to help with the cost of rehabilitation?"
    4. "Do you have concerns about the care you are receiving here?"

66. The nurse is administering medication to the client diagnosed with a third-degree burn on the chest area. Which medication requires a laboratory test?

Client Name: A.M. Height: 68 inches Date of Birth: 05/09/1941	Account Number: 1432223 Weight in pounds: 140 Date:		Allergies: NKDA Weight in kg: 63.63
Medication		1901–0700	0701–1900
Vancomycin IVPB 500 mg qd			
Pantoprazole 40 mg IVPB qd			
Silver sulfadiazine topical ointment to burn tid			
Morphine 2 to 5 mg IVP PRN pain			
Signature/Initials		Night Nurse RN/NN	Day Nurse RN/DN

   1. The vancomycin medication
   2. The pantoprazole medication
   3. The silver sulfadiazine topical ointment
   4. The morphine medication

67. The home health (HH) nurse is arranging for the spouse of an elderly client diagnosed with heart failure to administer furosemide. The medication is to be administered 20 mg on Monday/Wednesday/Friday and 40 mg on Sunday/Tuesday/Thursday/Saturday. The prescription is for 40 mg scored tablets. How many tablets should the nurse teach the spouse to administer on Sundays?

   [   ]

68. The RN home health (HH) nurse has arranged for a home health aide (HHA) to assist a 79-year-old client diagnosed with Alzheimer's disease. Which interventions should the nurse delegate to the HHA? **Select all that apply.**
    1. Weigh the client once a week and document the weight on the client record.
    2. Stay with the client twice a week while the spouse goes out to run errands.
    3. Take and record the client's vital signs.
    4. Take the client to the bank and store to perform personal business.
    5. Listen to the client's heart sounds and notify the HCP if abnormal sounds are heard.

69. The nurse is at the local mall and a young woman starts having shortness of breath, has hives on her face and arms, and is reporting itching. Which intervention should the nurse implement **first?**
    1. Tell a bystander to call 911 immediately.
    2. Ask the woman if she has an epinephrine auto-injector.
    3. Check the client for a medical alert bracelet.
    4. Place a soft cushion under the client's head.

70. The home health (HH) nurse is planning to make rounds for the day. **Rank in order of priority.**
1. The 29-year-old client diagnosed with spinal cord injury (SCI) post–motor vehicle accident (MVA) who needs a dressing changed on a stage IV pressure area
2. The 56-year-old client diagnosed with breast cancer who needs an injection of filgrastim subcutaneously
3. The 67-year-old client diagnosed with emphysema who called to report that the sputum is a rusty color this morning
4. The 80-year-old client diagnosed with Alzheimer's disease who is confused and wandering around the house
5. The 72-year-old client diagnosed with atrial fibrillation who needs a prothrombin time performed and called to the HCP

INTEGUMENTARY CLINICAL SCENARIO

The RN charge nurse is on the 7 p.m. to 7 a.m. shift for the 10-bed burn unit in a level I trauma adult and pediatric teaching hospital with culturally diverse clients of all ages. There are three additional RNs with four UAPs and a unit secretary. There are no LVNs in the burn unit but there are burn techs—specially trained paraprofessionals who maintain the whirlpool baths and perform other appropriately delegated client care tasks.

1. The male client is admitted to the burn unit after a boiling pot of hot water accidentally spilled on his lower legs. The assessment reveals blistered, mottled red skin, and both feet are edematous. Which depth of burn should the nurse document?
   1. Superficial partial thickness
   2. Deep partial thickness
   3. Full thickness
   4. First degree

2. The nurse is caring for a client who experienced a full-thickness burn to 65% of the body 12 hours ago. After establishing a patent airway, which nursing intervention is the **priority** for the client?
   1. Replace the client's fluids and electrolytes.
   2. Prevent the client from developing Curling's ulcers.
   3. Implement interventions to prevent infection.
   4. Prepare to assist with an escharotomy.

3. The charge nurse is developing a nursing care plan for a client who experienced a full-thickness burn and deep partial-thickness burns over half the body 4 days ago. Which client problem should the charge nurse make a **priority?**
   1. High risk for infection
   2. Pain
   3. Impaired physical mobility
   4. Fluid and electrolyte imbalance

4. Which nursing interventions should be included for the client who has full-thickness and deep partial-thickness burns to 50% of the body? **Select all that apply.**
   1. Perform meticulous hand hygiene.
   2. Screen visitors for infections.
   3. Provide a low-cholesterol, low-protein diet.
   4. Change invasive lines once a week.
   5. Administer prophylactic antibiotics as prescribed.

5. Which nursing task should the RN delegate to a UAP for the client diagnosed with full-thickness burns over the right leg?
   1. Instruct the UAP to take the client's pulse oximeter reading.
   2. Tell the UAP to change the dressing on the right leg.
   3. Ask the UAP to apply mafenide acetate to the right leg.
   4. Request the UAP to complete the admission assessment.

6. The nurse is caring for a client diagnosed with deep partial-thickness and full-thickness burns to the chest area. Which assessment data **warrants** notifying the health-care provider?
   1. The client is reporting pain rated 9 on a 1 to 10 pain scale.
   2. The client's pulse oximeter reading is 90%.
   3. The client has a T 100.4°F, P 100, R 24, and BP 102/60.
   4. The client's urinary output is 150 mL in 4 hours.

7. The charge nurse is teaching a group of community members about fire safety. A participant asks, "What should I do if I get hot grease burns on my hand?" Which statement is the nurse's **best** response?
   1. "Apply an ice pack directly to the hand."
   2. "Place the hand under cool tap water."
   3. "Put burn ointment on the hand."
   4. "Go immediately to the doctor's office."

8. The RN charge nurse is teaching a group of new UAPs about burn care. Which information regarding skin care should be emphasized?
   1. Keep the skin moist by leaving the skin damp after the bath.
   2. Ensure the client is premedicated before the whirlpool.
   3. Tell the UAPs to turn the client from side to side at least every 2 hours.
   4. Instruct the UAPs to not implement any interventions regarding skin care.

9. Which action by the UAP **warrants** intervention by the RN charge nurse?
   1. The UAP decreases the IV rate of the client whose total parenteral nutrition is almost empty.
   2. The UAP elevates the head of the bed for a client who is receiving a continuous tube feeding.
   3. The UAP assists the client diagnosed with full-thickness burns to the upper extremities to eat a high-protein meal.
   4. The UAP mixes a thickener into a glass of water for a client who has difficulty swallowing.

10. The charge nurse is caring for clients on the burn unit. After the shift report, which client should the charge nurse assess **first**?
    1. The client diagnosed with full and deep partial-thickness burns who has pain rated 8 on a 1 to 10 pain scale
    2. The client diagnosed with full-thickness burns who has a urinary output of 120 mL in the past 8 hours
    3. The client diagnosed with full-thickness burns on the chest who is having difficulty breathing
    4. The client who has full-thickness burns to the right leg with no palpable pedal pulse

The correct answer number and rationale for why it is the correct answer are given in **boldface type**. Rationales for why the other possible answer options are incorrect also are given, but they are not in boldface type.

1. 1. This client needs assistance being removed from the CPM machine but it is not a priority over a client who needs pain medication before a very painful procedure. Equipment is not a priority over the client's body.
   2. This is a psychosocial need and should be addressed, but it is not a priority over a physiological need.
   3. This temperature is elevated and the client should be seen, but the nurse should medicate the client going to the whirlpool first, then assess this client. Pain is a priority over an elevated temperature.
   4. **The client must be medicated with a narcotic medication before being taken to the whirlpool, which is a physiological need; therefore, the nurse should see this client first.**

CLINICAL JUDGMENT GUIDE: When deciding which client to assess first, the nurse should utilize Maslow's Hierarchy of Needs, in which physiological needs are the priority over psychosocial needs. The alleviation of pain, actual or potential, is a priority need.

2. 1. The client having pain when ambulating after an open reduction and external fixation (ORIF) of the hip is expected; this client would not need to be assessed first.
   2. The client should be ambulating and moving the left leg while in bed and would not need to be in the CPM machine 10 days postoperatively.
   3. **Numbness and tingling of the legs are signs of possible neurovascular compromise. This client should be assessed first.**
   4. The client being transferred should be assessed but would be considered stable; therefore, this client would not be assessed before a client experiencing possible neurovascular compromise.

CLINICAL JUDGMENT GUIDE: The nurse must determine which sign or symptom is not expected for the disease process or surgical procedure. If the sign or symptom is not expected, then the nurse should assess the client first. This type of question is determining if the nurse is knowledgeable of the signs and symptoms of a variety of disease processes.

3. 1. **An absent pulse is not uncommon in a client diagnosed with arterial occlusive disease. If the client can move the toes and denies tingling or numbness, then no further action should be taken.**
   2. To identify the location of the pulse, the nurse should use a Doppler device to amplify the sound, but this is not the first intervention if the client is able to move the toes and denies numbness and tingling.
   3. Placing the client's leg in a dependent position will increase blood flow and may help the nurse palpate the pulse, but it is not the nurse's first intervention.
   4. Warming will dilate the arteries and may help the nurse to find the pedal pulse, but this is not the first intervention. (Cooling, in contrast, causes vasoconstriction and decreases the ability to palpate the pulse.)

CLINICAL JUDGMENT GUIDE: When the question asks which intervention should be implemented first, it means all the options are something a nurse could implement, but only one should be implemented first. The nurse should use the nursing process to determine the appropriate intervention: If the client is in distress, do not assess; if the client is not in distress, then the nurse should assess.

4. 1. If the client's International Normalized Ratio (INR) is elevated, the antidote for the oral anticoagulant warfarin (Coumadin) is vitamin K (AquaMephyton), but this is not the nurse's first intervention.
   2. The client should be using a soft-bristle toothbrush, but this is not the nurse's first intervention.
   3. The nurse can always check the client's vital signs, but it is not the first intervention when addressing the client's report of gums bleeding.
   4. **The nurse should first check the client's INR to determine whether the bleeding is secondary to an elevated INR level. An INR level above 3 or 3.5, in the case of a mechanical valve, can cause bleeding.**

CLINICAL JUDGMENT GUIDE: This is an alternate type of question included in the NCLEX-RN® test plan. The test taker must be able to read a medication administration record (MAR), be knowledgeable of medications, and be able to make an appropriate decision as to the nurse's most appropriate intervention.

5. 1. The nonsteroidal anti-inflammatory drug (NSAID) is a routine medication and is not a priority medication.
2. The client needs to receive the IV antibiotic but this is not a priority over the client who is reporting an acute problem of itching and hives.
3. The client should receive the antiviral agent but not before a client who is exhibiting hives and itching, which is an acute problem.
4. **The client diagnosed with urticaria (hives) and pruritus (itching) is having some type of allergic reaction and should receive the antihistamine first.**

CLINICAL JUDGMENT GUIDE: The client who is exhibiting an acute reaction or problem should receive medical treatment first. Routine scheduled medications are not a priority over medications addressing acute client needs.

6. 1. Corticosteroid cream will not treat potential melanoma, which is what the client is explaining to the nurse.
2. SPF 15 is recommended to help prevent skin cancer but it will not help treat a melanoma.
3. **The client should consult his or her HCP immediately if a mole or lesion shows any signs of melanoma—asymmetry, border irregularity, color change or variation, and diameter of 6 mm or more (ABCD).**
4. Dark, woven clothing helps prevent skin cancer but it will not do anything for a change in a mole.

CLINICAL JUDGMENT GUIDE: The test taker needs to read all the options carefully before choosing the option that says, "Notify the HCP." If any of the options will provide information the HCP needs to know in order to make a decision, the test taker should choose that option. If, however, the HCP does not need any additional information to make a decision and the nurse suspects the condition is serious or life threatening, the priority intervention is to notify the HCP.

7. 1. **The nurse should implement the first intervention, ensuring the client does not move the leg, because doing so may cause further injury. The client should not attempt to move or stand on the injured extremity.**
2. The client should elevate the leg to decrease edema but it is not the first intervention—remember to do no harm.

3. The application of ice will help decrease edema and pain but the first intervention is to do no harm.
4. Assessment is usually the first intervention, but when at the scene of an accident, the nurse should ensure the accident victim does not cause further injury before assessing.

CLINICAL JUDGMENT GUIDE: The nurse should use the nursing process when answering questions that ask which intervention to implement first. Assessment is the first step in the nursing process, but in an emergency situation, remember the nurse should ensure the client does not further injure him- or herself.

8. 1. The nurse should obtain the needed equipment, but that is not the first intervention.
2. The nurse should remove the old dressing with nonsterile gloves, but not before determining whether the client has been premedicated.
3. The nurse should explain the procedure before performing the dressing change, but that is not the first intervention.
4. **Dressing changes for a stage III pressure ulcer will be painful for the client. The nurse should make sure the client has received pain medication at least 30 minutes before the procedure. This is showing client advocacy.**

CLINICAL JUDGMENT GUIDE: There will be management questions on the NCLEX-RN® addressing client advocacy. A client advocate acts as a liaison between clients and health-care providers to help improve or maintain a high quality of health care.

9. 1. **The H&H is low, which requires the nurse to assess this client first. The nurse must take the client's vital signs, check the surgical dressing, and determine whether the client is symptomatic for hypovolemia.**
2. The client diagnosed with rheumatoid arthritis should have a positive rheumatoid factor (RF). The positive RF factor confirms the diagnosis of this disease process.
3. A client diagnosed with a stage IV pressure ulcer would frequently have an infection; therefore, the nurse would expect an elevated white blood cell (WBC) count.
4. Corticosteroids elevate the client's glucose level; therefore, the nurse would not assess this client first.

CLINICAL JUDGMENT GUIDE: The nurse must be knowledgeable of normal laboratory values. These values must be memorized and the nurse must be able to determine if the laboratory value is normal for the client's disease process or medications the client is taking.

10. 1. The nurse should complete a report documenting the client's fall, but this is not the first intervention.
    2. The nurse should notify the clinical manager, but this is not the nurse's first intervention.
    3. **The nurse must first determine whether the client has any injuries before taking any other action. This is the first intervention the nurse must implement before moving the client.**
    4. The nurse should determine why the client was ambulating alone, but it is not the priority nursing intervention. Determining whether the client has any injuries is the most important intervention.

CLINICAL JUDGMENT GUIDE: Assessment is the first step of the nursing process, and the test taker should use the nursing process or some other systematic process to assist in determining priorities.

11. 1. The triple-lumen lines should be flushed with 100 units/mL of heparin solution, and this task should not be delegated to a UAP.
    2. This is teaching, and the nurse should not delegate teaching the client.
    3. **The UAP can assist the client to the bathroom as part of the bowel training; the RN is responsible for the training, but the nurse can delegate this task.**
    4. Corticosteroid cream is a medication and the RN cannot delegate medicating to a UAP.

CLINICAL JUDGMENT GUIDE: The RN cannot delegate assessment, evaluation, teaching, administering medications, or an unstable client to a UAP.

12. 1. **Because the UAP is informing the RN of pertinent information, the nurse should assess the client to determine which action to take.**
    2. The client may be hemorrhaging; therefore, the nurse cannot delegate assessing vital signs on an unstable client.
    3. The nurse should not remove the dressing. The nurse should reinforce the dressing and notify the HCP if bleeding does not stop or if the client is showing signs of hypovolemia.

Reinforcing the dressing would help decrease bleeding, but the nurse must assess first.
    4. The client is potentially unstable; therefore, the RN should not delegate any care to the UAP.

CLINICAL JUDGMENT GUIDE: Any time the nurse receives information from another staff member about a client who may be experiencing a complication, the nurse must assess the client. The nurse should not make decisions about a client's needs based on another staff member's information.

13. 1. **Tying a client to a chair is a form of restraint, and the client cannot be restrained without an HCP order; therefore, the nurse should immediately free the client. This is a legal issue.**
    2. The UAP is not hired to smoke with the client and the RN should talk to the UAP, but this does not warrant an immediate response. The client being illegally restrained warrants immediate intervention.
    3. Bringing a beverage to the client would not warrant immediate intervention.
    4. The UAP can assist the client to ambulate.

CLINICAL JUDGMENT GUIDE: Delegation means the RN is responsible for the UAP's actions and performance. The nurse must correct the UAP's performance to ensure the client is cared for safely and legally in the hospital or the home.

14. 1. Tinea corporis is commonly known as "ringworm" and should have cool compresses applied, not warm compresses.
    2. **The LPN can apply medication to the client's athlete's foot; therefore, this is an appropriate assignment for the LPN.**
    3. Onychomycosis is a fungal infection of the toenails (crumbly, discolored, and thickened nails); the HCP, not the UAP, should remove the toenail.
    4. Isotretinoin (Accutane) used to treat acne is contraindicated in women who are pregnant or who are intending to become pregnant while on the drug.

CLINICAL JUDGMENT GUIDE: When the test taker is deciding which option is the most appropriate task to delegate or assign, the test taker should choose the task that allows each member of the staff to function within his or her full scope of practice. Do not assign a task to a staff member that requires a higher level of expertise than the staff member has.

ANSWERS

15. 1. The UAP can assist a client to eat a regular meal; this would not warrant immediate action.
2. The UAP's request for assistance is appropriate because it is ensuring client safety. This action would not warrant immediate intervention.
3. **The UAP is attempting to move a client who weighs 400 pounds to the bedside commode. The UAP should request assistance to ensure client safety as well as to protect the UAP's back. This is a dangerous situation and requires intervention by the RN.**
4. This action ensures client safety and does not require immediate intervention by the nurse.

CLINICAL JUDGMENT GUIDE: Delegation means the RN is responsible for the UAP's actions and performance. The nurse must correct the UAP's performance to ensure the client is cared for safely and legally in the hospital or the home.

16. 1. The client with a lower extremity amputation should be placed in the prone position to prevent contractures.
2. **The RN should praise the UAP for taking the initiative and placing the client in the prone position. The prone position will help prevent contractures of the residual limb, which will make it easier to apply a prosthetic device.**
3. This action is appropriate and should not be reported to the charge nurse. The RN should first praise the UAP, and then report this behavior to the charge nurse to reward the UAP for appropriate behavior.
4. The client with a lower extremity amputation presents one of the few times a client should be placed on the stomach, the prone position.

CLINICAL JUDGMENT GUIDE: Delegation means the RN is responsible for the UAP's actions and performance. The nurse should praise the UAP's action when warranted or must correct the UAP's performance to ensure the client is cared for safely and legally in the hospital or the home.

17. 1. Stockings should be applied after the legs have been elevated for a period of time when the amount of blood in the leg vein is at its lowest. Applying the stockings when the client is sitting in a chair indicates that the UAP does not understand the correct procedure for applying the elastic compression stockings.
2. The top of the stocking should not be too tight. The UAP should be able to insert two to three fingers under the proximal end of the stocking. Not allowing this much space indicates the UAP does not understand the correct procedure for applying compression stockings.
3. **Stockings should be applied after the legs have been elevated for a period of time when the amount of blood in the leg vein is at its lowest. Having the client elevate the legs before placing the stockings on the legs indicates that the UAP understands the procedure for applying the elastic compression stockings.**
4. The toe opening should be positioned on the bottom of the foot; therefore, this indicates the client does not understand the correct procedure for applying the elastic compression stockings.

CLINICAL JUDGMENT GUIDE: Delegation means the RN is responsible for evaluating the UAP's actions and performance. The nurse should praise the UAP's action when warranted or must correct the UAP's performance to ensure the client is cared for safely and legally in the hospital or the home.

18. 1. The client needs to be told the importance of therapy, but this is not the most critical client; therefore, this client does not need to be assigned to the most experienced nurse.
2. Bone pain and fever are expected clinical manifestations of the client diagnosed with osteomyelitis, so this client is stable and does not need to be assigned to the most experienced nurse.
3. **Deep, unrelenting pain is a sign of compartment syndrome, an acute, potentially life-threatening complication, in a client diagnosed with a fracture; therefore, this client should be assigned to the most experienced nurse.**
4. The client diagnosed with low back pain and radiating pain should be assessed, but this is not a sign of an acute complication; therefore, this client does not need to be assigned to the most experienced nurse.

CLINICAL JUDGMENT GUIDE: The test taker must determine which client is the most unstable and would require the most experienced nurse, thus making this type of question an "except" question. Three clients are either stable or have non–life-threatening conditions.

19. 1. The LPN should not be sent to the emergency department because the LPN's expertise is needed to care for the clients on the busy rehabilitation unit.
2. The RN has 8 years of experience on the rehabilitation unit, and the charge nurse does not want to send a nurse who is a vital part of the rehabilitation team.
3. The UAP who is completing orientation should stay on the unit, and a UAP would not be able to do as much in the emergency department as a licensed nurse.
4. **The RN with medical unit experience would be the most appropriate nurse to send to the emergency department because this nurse has experience that would be helpful in the ED. The nurse is also an RN, who would be more helpful in the ED than a UAP or an LPN.**

CLINICAL JUDGMENT GUIDE: The charge nurse must be able to determine which staff member is most appropriate to float to another unit. The charge nurse does not want to leave his or her unit unsafe by sending the most experienced nurse, but wants to send the staff member who will be most helpful on the other unit.

20. 1. The UAP cannot teach the client; therefore, this task cannot be delegated.
2. The client is confused and should be assessed before being placed in an inclusion bed, which is used when a client wanders. The client should be assessed, and assessment cannot be delegated.
3. The UAP cannot administer medications; therefore, this task cannot be delegated.
4. **The UAP is a vital part of the health-care team and should be encouraged to attend the multidisciplinary team meeting and provide input into the client's care.**

CLINICAL JUDGMENT GUIDE: The test taker must be knowledgeable of the role of all members of the multidisciplinary health-care team as well as HIPAA rules and regulations. These will be tested on the NCLEX-RN® examination.

21. 1. The nurse should monitor the PCA pump but remember that equipment is not a priority over the client's body.
2. **Logrolling clients when turning is essential and a priority to maintain proper body alignment.**
3. The client with spinal surgery is on bedrest until the first postoperative day; therefore, this is not a priority intervention.

4. The nurse can place pillows under the client's thighs, but the priority postoperative intervention is to prevent postoperative complications; this means ensuring the client is logrolled when turning.

CLINICAL JUDGMENT GUIDE: When answering questions about a specific type of surgery or procedure, the nurse should identify an intervention that is specific to the surgery or procedure.

22. 1. **This client would benefit from a home health-care nurse's evaluation of the client's home and the wife's ability to care for the client.**
2. The nurse should help the client care for her husband in the home. Placing him in a nursing home may be a possibility if she is unable to care for him, but the most appropriate response would be trying to help the wife care for her husband in the home.
3. The HCP can talk to the wife but will not be able to address her concerns of taking care of her husband when he is discharged home.
4. The nurse could allow the wife to vent feelings, but the first intervention is to address her concerns and do something to alleviate her concern.

CLINICAL JUDGMENT GUIDE: The test taker must be knowledgeable of the role of all members of the multidisciplinary health-care team as well as HIPAA rules and regulations. These will be tested on the NCLEX-RN® examination.

23. 1. This is a formal step in filing a grievance, but the nurse's next action should be to follow the chain of command and place an informal complaint with the clinical manager.
2. The female nurse has already told the male nurse this makes her feel uncomfortable; therefore, this action is not appropriate.
3. **If a direct request to the perpetrator does not stop the comments, then an informal complaint may be effective, especially if both parties realize a problem exists. The female nurse should utilize the chain of command and notify the clinical manager.**
4. The female nurse should follow the chain of command and notify the clinical manager as the next action.

CLINICAL JUDGMENT GUIDE: The nurse is responsible for knowing and complying with local, state, and federal standards of care, especially sexual harassment.

ANSWERS

24. 1. Assisting the client to become independent in self-care is the role of the occupational therapist.
   2. The client must be in therapy at least 3 hours a day, but the 3-hour period includes all types of therapy, not just physical therapy. This is a true statement, but it does not answer the client's question.
   3. A multidisciplinary team decides which therapy the client should be receiving, but this does not answer the client's question.
   4. **The physical therapist will assist in improving the circulation, strengthening muscles, and ambulating and transferring the client from a bed to a chair. This is the nurse's best response to explain why the client goes to physical therapy daily.**

CLINICAL JUDGMENT GUIDE: The test taker must be knowledgeable of the role of all members of the multidisciplinary health-care team as well as HIPAA rules and regulations. These will be tested on the NCLEX-RN® examination.

25. 1. **The physical therapist addresses crutch walking, how to use a walker, gait training, or transferring techniques. This is the most appropriate team member to address the problem.**
   2. The social worker addresses the client's concerns that are usually outside the acute care arena, such as financial concerns or referrals.
   3. The occupational therapist addresses the upper extremity activities of daily living, not walking difficulties.
   4. The HCP can order the physical therapist to see the client to teach the client about crutch walking, but would not be the one doing the instruction.

CLINICAL JUDGMENT GUIDE: The test taker must be knowledgeable of the role of all members of the multidisciplinary health-care team as well as HIPAA rules and regulations. These will be tested on the NCLEX-RN® examination.

26. 1. The nurse can discuss this situation with the health-care team, but the most helpful intervention is to explain the rights of the disabled according to the ADA.
   2. **The ADA was passed in 1990 and ensures that a client diagnosed with a disability has a right to be employed. Employers must make "reasonable accommodations," such as equipment or access ramps to facilitate employment of a person diagnosed with a disability.**

3. The nurse should not interfere and contact the client's employer. The nurse should empower clients to care independently for themselves.
4. This client might be able to do this, but the most helpful intervention is to contact the ADA. The employer is violating the 1990 Americans with Disabilities Act.

CLINICAL JUDGMENT GUIDE: The nurse is responsible for knowing and complying with local, state, and federal standards of care.

27. 1. The UAP can escort clients to the different rehabilitation therapies. This action would not warrant immediate intervention.
   2. The family members are an integral part of the health-care team. This action would not warrant intervention by the charge nurse.
   3. **The primary nurse cannot ask another nurse to administer medication that he prepared. The nurse preparing the injection must administer the medication. This action requires the charge nurse to intervene.**
   4. Making sure someone watches the nurse's assigned clients is an appropriate action and would not require intervention by the charge nurse.

CLINICAL JUDGMENT GUIDE: There will be management questions on the NCLEX-RN®. Concepts of Management is included under the category Safe and Effective Care Environment and subcategory Management of Care.

28. 1. This response does not address the client's fears and concerns.
   2. **This statement will allow the client to vent feelings of helplessness and fear. It is the nurse's best response.**
   3. The client is not verbalizing that he will kill himself; therefore, this is not the nurse's best response.
   4. This is negating the client's feelings; the client has a C-6 SCI so the situation may not improve much. Therefore, this is not the nurse's best response.

CLINICAL JUDGMENT GUIDE: The NCLEX-RN® test plan includes Therapeutic Communication as a subcategory under Psychosocial Integrity. The nurse should allow clients and family to vent feelings.

29. 1. Nonmaleficence is the duty to prevent or avoid doing harm. The nurse asking not to be assigned to the NICU because of lack of experience in caring for critically ill infants is supporting the ethical principle of nonmaleficence.
   2. The NICU is a very specialized unit requiring the nurse to be knowledgeable of equipment and caring for critically ill infants. Accepting the assignment may cause harm to one of the neonates.
   3. This is challenging the charge nurse's assignment, and this does not support the ethical principle of nonmaleficence.
   4. This is blatantly violating the charge nurse's authority and does not support the ethical principle of nonmaleficence.

CLINICAL JUDGMENT GUIDE: The NCLEX-RN® test plan includes nursing care addressing ethical principles, including autonomy, beneficence, justice, and veracity, to name a few.

30. 1. This is a therapeutic response that encourages the husband to vent feelings, but the client's husband needs specific information.
   2. **According to the NCSBN, case management is content included in the management of care. The case manager is responsible for collaborating with and coordinating the services provided by all members of the health-care team, including the home health-care nurse who will be responsible for directing the client's care after discharge from the rehabilitation unit. This is the nurse's best response.**
   3. This is not addressing the husband's concern, and sometimes the client is discharged when the family and client are not ready in the client's opinion. This is a false reassurance and is not the nurse's best response.
   4. In rehabilitation, the HCP is part of the team and is not the only team member to determine the discharge date. This is not the nurse's best response.

CLINICAL JUDGMENT GUIDE: The test taker must be knowledgeable of the role of all members of the multidisciplinary health-care team as well as HIPAA rules and regulations. These will be tested on the NCLEX-RN® examination.

31. 1. The nurse's comment does not address the client's question and concern. This is not an appropriate response.

2. The rehabilitation commission of each state will help evaluate and determine whether the client can receive training or education for another occupation after injury.
   3. This client is not asking about disability. The client is concerned about employment. The nurse needs to refer the client to the appropriate agency.
   4. This does not address the client's concern about gainful employment. This is a therapeutic response that will allow the client to vent feelings, but the client is asking for information.

CLINICAL JUDGMENT GUIDE: There will be management questions on the NCLEX-RN®. In many instances, there is no test-taking strategy. The nurse must be knowledgeable of management issues and must comply with local, state, and federal requirements.

32. 1. The client is confiding in the nurse about a doctor, and the nurse should address the client's concern, not tell the client to talk to the doctor. Many clients do not feel comfortable talking to a doctor.
   2. **The nurse should determine what is concerning the client. It could be a misunderstanding or a real situation in which the client's care is unsafe or inadequate.**
   3. After the nurse determines whether the client's concern warrants a new doctor, the nurse should talk to the nursing supervisor and help the client get a second opinion. The nurse is the client's advocate.
   4. The choice of doctor is ultimately the client's, and the client has a right to another doctor.

CLINICAL JUDGMENT GUIDE: The nurse should always try and support the client's or the family's request if it does not violate any local, state, or federal rules and regulations. The client has a right to request a second opinion if the client does not like the health-care provider's care.

33. 1. **An abductor pillow is used for a client with a total hip replacement (THR) to help prevent hip dislocation; the UAP can place the pillow between the client's legs. This task is appropriate to delegate.**
   2. The client should be out of bed and ambulating by the third day post-op to help prevent complications secondary to immobility, such as deep vein thrombosis (DVT) or pneumonia.

3. Just because the client is elderly does not mean the client must be fed. There is nothing in the stem of the question that would indicate the client could not feed him- or herself. The RN should encourage independence as much as possible and delegate feeding the client to a UAP only when it is necessary.

4. The RN cannot delegate assessment to the UAP; therefore, checking the surgical dressing is not appropriate delegation.

CLINICAL JUDGMENT GUIDE: A registered nurse cannot delegate assessment, teaching, evaluation, medications, or an unstable client to a UAP. Tasks that cannot be delegated are nursing interventions requiring nursing judgment.

34. 1. Closing the door and cubicle curtain protects the client's privacy and would not warrant immediate intervention from the nurse.

2. **The client with spinal surgery should be logrolled with at least two if not three staff members assisting with the turning from side to side. Logrolling the client ensures proper body alignment. Asking the client to turn would warrant intervention by the nurse.**

3. Checking the temperature of the bathwater prevents scalding the client with water that is too hot or making the client uncomfortable with water that is too cold. This action would not warrant immediate intervention.

4. The UAP must perform the skill safely; putting the side rails in an upright position ensures the client will not fall out of the bed.

CLINICAL JUDGMENT GUIDE: The RN must ensure the UAP can perform any tasks that are delegated. It is the nurse's responsibility to demonstrate to or teach the UAP how to perform the task, and then evaluate the task performed.

35. Correct answers are 3, 4, and 5.

1. The right leg should not be elevated in the rehabilitation unit because it can cause a contracture of the right leg, which can lead to the prosthetic leg not fitting properly. The leg should be elevated the first 48 hours to decrease edema and then kept straight.

2. The occupational therapist addresses the client's activities of daily living and upper extremity problems, not lower extremity problems.

3. **Pushing the residual limb against a pillow will help toughen the end of the limb, which is needed when wearing a prosthetic limb.**

4. **The expected treatment for a client diagnosed with impetigo is warm saline followed by soap and water for removal of crusts, followed by topical antibiotic cream.**

5. **Impetigo is very contagious, so wearing gloves and meticulous hygiene is essential when caring for this client.**

CLINICAL JUDGMENT GUIDE: This is an alternate type of question included in the NCLEX-RN®. The nurse must be able to select all the options that answer the question correctly. There are no partially correct answers.

36. 1. The procedure for tornadoes is to have all clients, staff, and visitors stay in the hallway and close the doors to all the rooms. This will help prevent any flying debris or glass from hurting anyone.

2. This may be recommended for individuals in the home, but it is not the hospital protocol for tornadoes.

3. **The procedure for tornadoes is to have all clients, staff, and visitors stay in the hallway and close the doors to all the rooms. This will help prevent any flying debris or glass from hurting anyone.**

4. The client and visitors should be in the client's room with the door closed for a fire, but this is not the correct procedure for a tornado.

CLINICAL JUDGMENT GUIDE: The nurse must be knowledgeable of emergency preparedness. Employees receive this information during employee orientation and are responsible for implementing procedures correctly. The NCSBN NCLEX-RN® test plan includes questions on a Safe and Effective Care Environment.

37. 1. The finance office is responsible for discussing the cost and insurance issues with the client.

2. The physiatrist is a medical health-care provider who cares for clients in the rehabilitation area.

3. The vocational counselor would assist the client with employment training if needed.

4. **The case manager is responsible for coordinating the total rehabilitative plan and collaborating with and coordinating the services provided by all members of the health-care team, including the home health-care nurse who will be responsible for directing the client's care after discharge from the rehabilitation unit.**

CLINICAL JUDGMENT GUIDE: The test taker must be knowledgeable of the role of all members of the multidisciplinary health-care team as well as HIPAA rules and regulations. These will be tested on the NCLEX-RN® examination.

38. 1. **The rehabilitation nurse must recognize and address sexual issues in order to promote feelings of self-worth that are essential to total rehabilitation. The age of the client should not matter, but this client is young; therefore, this is a priority.**
    2. This is not a psychosocial intervention, and the social worker or occupational therapist usually addresses the home situation.
    3. This is not necessarily a psychosocial intervention, but it should be addressed so the client can be independent. The social worker usually addresses transportation.
    4. The client may or may not need psychological counseling, but the priority psychosocial intervention of the rehabilitation nurse is to discuss the client's sexuality needs.

CLINICAL JUDGMENT GUIDE: The NCLEX-RN® test plan includes Therapeutic Communication as a subcategory of Psychosocial Integrity. The nurse should allow clients and family to vent feelings and address psychosocial concerns.

39. 1. The RN could apologize for the UAP's comments, but this is not the first intervention.
    2. This is a violation of HIPAA and the RN should tell this to the UAP, but it is not the first intervention.
    3. The RN should not allow the conversation to continue. The UAP is violating confidentiality and is gossiping about another client.
    4. **The RN should stop the conversation immediately and ask the UAP to go to the nurse's station so as not to embarrass the UAP. Gossiping about clients is a violation of their privacy, and a breach of protected health information under HIPAA.**

CLINICAL JUDGMENT GUIDE: There will be management questions on the NCLEX-RN®. In many instances, there is no test-taking strategy. The nurse must be knowledgeable of management issues. The Health Insurance Portability and Accountability Act (HIPAA) was passed into law in 1996 to standardize the exchange of information between health-care providers, and to ensure client record confidentiality.

40. 1. After two verbal warnings, the clinical manager should document the behavior and start formal proceedings to correct the staff nurse's behavior.
    2. The human resources department would not need to be notified until the clinical manager has decided to terminate the staff nurse's employment.
    3. **Every hospital has a procedure for termination if the employee is not performing as expected. After two verbal warnings, the clinical manager should document the employee's actions in writing and implement the hospital policy for possible termination.**
    4. The clinical manager cannot allow the nurse to go home because this will affect the care of the clients during the shift and cause a hardship on the other staff members.

CLINICAL JUDGMENT GUIDE: There will be management questions on the NCLEX-RN®. In many instances, there is no test-taking strategy. The nurse must be knowledgeable of management issues.

41. 1. **The LPN's scope of practice allows the LPN to take telephone orders.**
    2. The LPN's scope of practice does not include an admission assessment.
    3. The registered dietitian would be the most appropriate team member to teach about diets.
    4. The unlicensed assistive personnel (UAP) could obtain the intake and output; therefore, this is not an appropriate assignment for an LPN.

CLINICAL JUDGMENT GUIDE: The RN cannot assign assessment, teaching, evaluation, or an unstable client to an LPN. The LPN can transcribe HCP orders and can call HCPs on the phone to obtain orders for a client.

42. 1. The client diagnosed with COPD would be expected to have low oxygen and high CO_2 levels in the arterial blood; therefore, this laboratory result would not warrant intervention from the charge nurse.
    2. This WBC level is within normal limits; therefore, this client does not warrant immediate intervention from the charge nurse.
    3. **Antibiotic therapy can result in a superinfection that destroys the normal bacterial flora of the intestines and produces diarrhea. Diarrhea, in turn, causes**

an increased excretion of potassium, resulting in hypokalemia. This K_+ level is below normal, and the charge nurse should notify the health-care provider.

4. This glucose level is slightly elevated, and TPN is high in glucose; therefore, this laboratory result does not require immediate intervention.

CLINICAL JUDGMENT GUIDE: The nurse must be knowledgeable of normal laboratory values. These values must be memorized and the nurse must be able to determine if the laboratory value is normal for the client's disease process or medications the client is taking.

43. 1. The nurse is an employee of the hospital and cannot witness documents for clients.
   2. **This is the correct action to take; the nurse is an employee of the hospital directly involved in providing care and cannot witness documents for clients.**
   3. This is incorrect information; the document should be witnessed by individuals who are not family members or employees of the hospital providing direct care.
   4. The living will must be witnessed by two individuals when the client is signing it, but it does not have to be notarized.

CLINICAL JUDGMENT GUIDE: The NCLEX-RN® test plan includes nursing care that is ruled by legal requirements. The nurse must be knowledgeable of these issues.

44. 1. The nurse should ensure the client has appropriate shoes when ambulating, but the priority is safety of the client, which means using a gait belt.
   2. **The nurse's priority is to ensure the safety of the client, and placing a safety gait belt around the client's waist before ambulating the client helps to ensure safety. The gait belt provides a handle to hold onto the client securely during ambulation.**
   3. The nurse should explain the procedure to the client, but it is not a priority over ensuring safety for the client while walking in the hall.
   4. The nurse should make sure there is a clear path to walk, but the priority intervention is to protect the client if he or she falls, and that can be prevented by placing a gait belt around the client's waist.

CLINICAL JUDGMENT GUIDE: The NCLEX-RN® test plan includes adhering to safety standards when caring for clients.

45. 1. Being a client advocate means the nurse will support the client's wishes, but in some situations the nurse must adhere to the medical regimen. Saying the client does not have to attend therapy is detrimental to the client's recovery and is not being a client advocate.
   2. Being a client advocate means the nurse will support the client's wishes, but in some situations the nurse must adhere to the medical regimen. Talking to the physical therapist will not help the client's recovery.
   3. **Finding ways for the client to perform the exercises with the physical therapist is supporting the medical regimen. This action supports client advocacy. PTs cannot prescribe.**
   4. Discussing the client concerns does not help the client's recovery; therefore, this statement does not support client advocacy.

CLINICAL JUDGMENT GUIDE: There will be management questions on the NCLEX-RN® addressing client advocacy. A client advocate acts as a liaison between clients and health-care providers to help improve or maintain a high quality of health care.

46. 1. As long as the client gives permission, the nurse can discuss the client's condition with anyone.
   2. The nurse can answer questions over the phone with the client's permission. It may be difficult for the client's wife to come to the rehabilitation unit.
   3. The client and wife are allowed and encouraged to come to the multidisciplinary team meeting, but the nurse should talk to the wife on the phone.
   4. **The nurse can talk to anyone the client requests. This is not a violation of HIPAA as long as the client gives permission for the nurse to share information.**

CLINICAL JUDGMENT GUIDE: There will be management questions on the NCLEX-RN®. In many instances, there is no test-taking strategy. The nurse must be knowledgeable of management issues.

47. Correct answers are 1, 2, and 3.
   1. **An antibiotic ointment, such as Polysporin, should be applied thinly four times daily. Polysporin can be purchased without a prescription.**

2. **Children should be kept home from school until the lesions crust over.**
3. **Use separate towels for the client. The client's towels, pillowcases, and sheets should be changed after the first day of treatment. The clothing should be changed and laundered daily for the first 2 days.**
4. Crusts should be removed before the ointment is applied. Soak a soft, clean cloth in a mixture of one-half cup of white vinegar and a quart of lukewarm water. Press a cloth on the crusts for 10 to 15 minutes three or four times daily. Then gently wipe off the crusts and apply a little antibiotic ointment.
5. The child does not have to wear sterile gloves.

CLINICAL JUDGMENT GUIDE: This is an alternate type of question included in the NCLEX-RN®. The nurse must be able to select all the options that answer the question correctly. There are no partially correct answers.

48. 1. The nurse's scope of practice includes teaching the client how to use equipment.
    2. **This is a violation of HIPAA. The client's right to confidentiality is being compromised because anyone could read the client's record on the computer. The charge nurse should intervene.**
    3. The nurse can discuss a client situation with the HCP; therefore, this action does not require intervention.
    4. The nurse should refer a client with a spiritual need to the chaplain. It is not necessary to know what the need is, only that the chaplain needs to see the client.

CLINICAL JUDGMENT GUIDE: There will be management questions on the NCLEX-RN®. In many instances, there is no test-taking strategy; the nurse must be knowledgeable of management issues. The Health Insurance Portability and Accountability Act (HIPAA) was passed into law in 1996 to standardize the exchange of information between health-care providers, and to ensure client record confidentiality.

49. 1. Vitiligo is a common skin disorder in which white spots appear on the skin, usually occurring on both sides of the body in the same location. The client would not need an immediate appointment.
    2. **Allergic contact dermatitis occurs when skin comes in contact with an allergen the client is sensitive or allergic to. Symptoms**

include redness, swelling, blistering, itching, and weeping. This client has an acute dermatological condition and should be seen immediately.
3. Angiomas are not dangerous or contagious. Angiomas do not need to be treated unless they bleed or bother the client. This client does not need an immediate appointment.
4. The client may have shingles but it cannot be determined at this time. The rash of shingles begins as red patches that soon develop blisters, often on one side of the body. It is treated with acyclovir (Zovirax) but at this time the nurse would not need to make an appointment immediately.

CLINICAL JUDGMENT GUIDE: The test taker must determine which sign or symptom is not expected for the disease process. If the sign or symptom is not expected, then the nurse should assess the client first. This type of question is determining if the nurse is knowledgeable of signs and symptoms of a variety of disease processes.

50. 1. An MRI is not the diagnostic test used to confirm the diagnosis of basal cell carcinoma.
    2. A washing is not used to confirm the diagnosis of basal cell carcinoma.
    3. **The only way to tell for sure if a skin growth is cancerous is to biopsy it.**
    4. A biopsy will definitively diagnose the skin cancer.

CLINICAL JUDGMENT GUIDE: The nurse must be knowledgeable of normal diagnostic tests pre- and post-procedure. These interventions must be memorized, and to ensure the client is safe, the nurse must be able to determine if the client is able to have the diagnostic procedure and post-procedure care.

51. **Correct order is 5, 3, 1, 2, 4.**
    These are the best practices for helping a client use a cane when ambulating.
    5. **The gait belt is applied to ensure safety of the client and the person assisting the client to ambulate.**
    3. **The client should use the strong hand to control the assistive device.**
    1. **The client should move the cane forward to provide a stable support for the weaker leg when it is moved.**
    2. **The client should move the weaker leg even with the supportive cane while maintaining the stronger leg in place.**
    4. **Finally, the stronger leg can move to a position even with the weak leg and cane.**

CLINICAL JUDGMENT GUIDE: The NCLEX-RN® has alternate types of questions including putting interventions in rank order. The test taker must put the interventions in the correct order to get the answer correct.

52. 1. Adequate skin care is an appropriate intervention to help prevent pressure ulcers, but it is not the priority intervention.
    2. **The priority intervention to prevent skin impairment is frequent position changes along with skin care and nutritional support.**
    3. Sufficient nutritional intake will help prevent pressure ulcers but it is not the priority intervention.
    4. The use of any mechanical device does not eliminate the need for turning and repositioning the client to help prevent pressure ulcers.

CLINICAL JUDGMENT GUIDE: Test questions asking the test taker to select the priority intervention mean all the options may be plausible. The test taker has to determine the most important.

53. 1. Assessing the client's breath sounds is an appropriate intervention, but if the client is in distress the nurse should intervene to help the client's body.
    2. The client should be encouraged to cough and deep breathe, but it will not help oxygenate the client, which is the priority for the client diagnosed with a fat embolism.
    3. **Oxygen must be administered to treat hypoxia, which occurs after a fat embolism; therefore, this is the nurse's first intervention.**
    4. The HCP may or may not administer heparin therapy, but it would not be the first intervention the nurse would implement.

CLINICAL JUDGMENT GUIDE: The nurse should use the nursing process when answering questions asking which intervention the nurse should implement first. If the client is in distress, do not assess; the nurse needs to address the client's physiological needs. The nurse should use Maslow's Hierarchy of Needs, which states that oxygenation needs are the priority.

54. 1. The wounds need to be kept sterile to decrease the chance of infection, but the priority for electrical burn wounds is to monitor for cardiac problems.
    2. All clients need to have vital signs assessed, but the priority for electrical burn wounds is to monitor for cardiac problems.
    3. The client's oxygenation level should be monitored, but the priority for electrical burns is cardiac problems.
    4. **The electrical current in the body bounces off bone and goes through muscle. The heart is a muscle; therefore, the priority intervention is for the nurse to apply cardiac monitors to assess for lethal dysrhythmias that may occur.**

CLINICAL JUDGMENT GUIDE: The test taker should try to determine what is different about the client's disease process or disorder. All clients need to have vital signs assessed and oxygenation levels monitored—what is different for the client diagnosed with an electrical burn?

55. 1. The nurse should have another staff member to assist with the lift, but it is not a priority over the safety of the client in the equipment.
    2. **This is a priority because the safety of the client must be ensured. If the client is not placed correctly in the lift sleeve, the client could fall. Electric client "Hoyer" lifts are powered either through a standard electrical outlet or by a rechargeable battery. The lifting is completely controlled through a hand control, eliminating any physical exertion by the caregiver.**
    3. The nurse should lift the client slowly but it is not a priority.
    4. The stretcher should be locked and ready for the transfer, but the client is the priority.

CLINICAL JUDGMENT GUIDE: If the test taker is trying to determine the correct answer between option 2 and 4, the test taker should select the client's body over any type of equipment. All these options are plausible for a nurse to implement, but safety of the client is the priority.

56. 1. Grade 6 indicates the client is independent in feeding, bathing, and toileting.
    2. Grade 4 indicates the client has some functioning areas of ADLs.
    3. Grade 3 indicates the client will need more assistance with ADLs.
    4. **Grade 0 indicates the client is dependent in all six functions: bathing, feeding, toileting, continence, dressing, and transferring. This client would require the RN to delegate activities of daily living to the UAP.**

CLINICAL JUDGMENT GUIDE: This is a knowledge-based question but pertinent to rehabilitation nursing. The test taker must realize either a score of 6 or 0 would be the answer because in most scales, but not all, the higher the number, the more severe the condition.

57. 1. The arm should be elevated to decrease edema, not placed in the dependent position, which is lower than the heart.
    2. **Moist heat, immobilization, elevation, and systemic antibiotics are the treatments for cellulitis, which is an inflammation of subcutaneous tissue.**
    3. Anti-staphylococcal soap (Hibiclen, Lever 2000, Dial) is prescribed for staph infection.
    4. The affected area should be left open to air, not wrapped by elastic (ACE) bandages.

CLINICAL JUDGMENT GUIDE: The nurse must know the expected medical treatment for the client. This is a knowledge-based question.

58. **Correct order is 2, 5, 3, 4, 1.**
    This is the procedure in correct order when transferring a client from the bed to a wheelchair.
    2. **The wheelchair should be ready for the client to transfer to and is the first step.**
    5. **The brakes should be locked so the chair will not move during the transfer.**
    3. **The client should use the stronger side of the body for support when moving.**
    4. **The client next shifts the weight forward to pivot into the chair.**
    1. **The client should not attempt until the chair is felt on the back of the legs so the client knows where the chair is.**

CLINICAL JUDGMENT GUIDE: The NCLEX-RN® has alternate types of questions including ranking interventions in priority order. The test taker must put the interventions in the correct order to get the answer correct.

59. 1. **The residual limb of an AKA should be elevated after 48 hours to help prevent contractures. Because the client is in the rehabilitation unit, it is past 48 hours.**
    2. The LPN could give the HS snacks to the clients but the UAP could also do this; therefore, it is not appropriate for the LPN to do this task.
    3. The UAP cannot perform sterile procedures, so this cannot be delegated to a UAP.
    4. The RN cannot assign assessment to the LPN.

CLINICAL JUDGMENT GUIDE: The RN cannot delegate assessment, teaching, evaluation, medications, or an unstable client to the UAP. The RN cannot assign assessment, teaching, evaluation, or an unstable client to the LPN.

60. 1. The RN cannot delegate assessment to the UAP.
    2. **The UAP can clean the client's dentures, so this task should be delegated.**
    3. The UAP should not perform passive range-of-motion exercises because it could lead to harm if not done correctly. The RN should perform passive ROM.
    4. The client's right leg should be elevated to decrease edema, not in a dependent position, which is hanging off the bed.

CLINICAL JUDGMENT GUIDE: The RN cannot delegate assessment, teaching, evaluation, medication, or an unstable client to a UAP. The nurse must be knowledgeable about interventions that cannot be delegated, and in some cases, the intervention should not be implemented at all—such as option 1.

61. 1. A sterile environment should be maintained, but the priority is fluid volume because the client is at risk for hypovolemia.
    2. **The priority intervention in the first 24 hours for the client diagnosed with a third-degree burn is maintaining intravascular volume so the client will not die from hypovolemic shock.**
    3. Preventing infection is important but initially maintaining fluid volume is the priority.
    4. The nurse should assess the client's pain, but for a client diagnosed with third-degree burns over both the legs the priority is maintaining fluid volume.

CLINICAL JUDGMENT GUIDE: The nurse must know the expected medical treatment for the client. This is a knowledge-based question.

62. 1. **Orthostatic hypotension is a side effect of administering the beta blocker medication atenolol (Tenormin); therefore, this medication should be questioned.**
    2. Ceftriaxone (Rocephin) is an antibiotic and these signs and symptoms would not warrant questioning this medication.
    3. Bisacodyl (Dulcolax) is a laxative and light-headedness would not warrant questioning this medication.
    4. Light-headedness is a side effect of beta blockers and should not be administered until further assessment and notification of the health-care provider.

ANSWERS

CLINICAL JUDGMENT GUIDE: The NCLEX-RN® has alternate types of questions such as this one. It is an application-style question and the test taker needs to be able to read a medication administration record (MAR) as well as know the side effects of medications.

63. Correct answers are 1, 2, and 4.
    1. **Acupuncture is traditional Chinese medicine, which involves the use of sharp, thin needles that are inserted in the body at very specific points and is believed to adjust and alter the body's energy flow into healthier patterns.**
    2. **Guided imagery is the use of relaxation and mental visualization to improve mood or physical well-being.**
    3. A compression sequential device is a pneumatic device used to prevent DVT from the legs and arms. This is medically approved and is not a CAM.
    4. **Music therapy is a technique of complementary alternative medicine that uses music prescribed in a skilled manner by trained therapists. Programs are designed to help clients overcome physical, emotional, intellectual, and social challenges.**
    5. Muscle-strengthening exercises are not a CAM. It is performed as physical therapy and is a medical treatment.

CLINICAL JUDGMENT GUIDE: This is an alternate type of question in which the test taker must select all options to get the question correct. The NCLEX-RN® tests complementary alternate medicine (CAM) according to the test plan.

64. 1. **This is the reason for referring a client to a vocational counselor.**
    2. This describes the physiatrist who is a physician specializing in rehabilitative care.
    3. This is the reason for referring a client to an occupational therapist.
    4. This is the reason for referring a client to the recreational therapist.

CLINICAL JUDGMENT GUIDE: The nurse must know the role of the client's multidisciplinary team in rehabilitation. The nurse must be able to refer to the appropriate team member to help with rehabilitation for the client.

65. 1. This question may be asked but it is not assessing daily schedules and habits.
    2. **Assessment of daily schedules and habits includes questions concerning hygiene practices, eating, elimination, sexual activity, sleep, work, exercise, and recreational activities.**
    3. Asking about insurance does not help the nurse assess the client's daily schedules and habits.
    4. This question can be asked but it does not address daily schedules and habits.

CLINICAL JUDGMENT GUIDE: The nurse must be able to ask appropriate questions when completing assessments, especially in rehabilitation nursing.

66. 1. **The vancomycin needs to have a peak and trough drawn every third or fourth dose depending on the HCP's order.**
    2. Pantoprazole (Protonix) does not have a required laboratory test on a routine basis.
    3. Silver sulfadiazine (Silvadene) does not have a required laboratory test on a routine basis.
    4. Morphine does not have a required laboratory test on a routine basis.

CLINICAL JUDGMENT GUIDE: This is an alternate type of question included in the NCLEX-RN® test plan. The test taker must be able to read a medication administration record (MAR), be knowledgeable of medications, and be able to make an appropriate decision as to the nurse's most appropriate intervention.

67. Answer: 1 tablet.
    The routine diuretic medication furosemide (Lasix) comes in 40 mg tablets. On M/W/F the client should receive 1/2 tablet, on Su/T/Th/Sa the client should receive 1 whole tablet.

CLINICAL JUDGMENT GUIDE: The NCLEX-RN® test plan includes dosage calculations under Pharmacological and Parenteral Therapies. This category is included under Physiological Integrity, which promotes physical health and wellness by providing care and comfort, reducing client risk potential, and managing health alterations.

68. Correct answers are 1, 2, and 3.
    1. **The HHA is capable of weighing a client and documenting the finding.**
    2. **An HHA can offer the SO time away from the home to do personal business.**
    3. **This is within the HHA's capabilities.**
    4. Taking the client to perform personal business in the HHA's vehicle is crossing boundaries, particularly when the business involves finances.
    5. The HHA is not capable of performing assessments and making nursing judgments based on the findings.

CLINICAL JUDGMENT GUIDE: This is an alternate type of question included in the NCLEX-RN®. The nurse must be able to select all the options that answer the question correctly. There are no partially correct answers.

69. 1. The emergency services need to come to the mall immediately. This woman is having an allergic reaction to something and this is a potentially life-threatening emergency.
    2. The nurse should determine if the woman has an epinephrine auto-injector (EpiPen) available that will save her life. If she doesn't, the nurse will have to wait for the ambulance.
    3. The client diagnosed with allergies should wear a medical alert bracelet to let anyone know what she is allergic to, but the first intervention is to try and save the woman's life by giving epinephrine to the client.
    4. The nurse should protect the client's head but it is not the priority intervention.

CLINICAL JUDGMENT GUIDE: When the question asks which intervention should be implemented first, it means all the options are something a nurse could implement but only one should be implemented first. The nurse should use the nursing process to determine the appropriate intervention: If the client is in distress, do not assess; if the client is not in distress, then the nurse should assess.

70. Correct order is 3, 1, 5, 2, 4.
    3. This client has a change in normal sputum production. Frequently, clients diagnosed with obstructive pulmonary diseases are placed on steroid therapy. Steroid therapy can mask an infection. The only symptom of an infection may be a change in the color of the sputum.
    1. This client has a deep wound that needs to be assessed.
    5. This test can be performed by the nurse with a portable machine. The HCP may need to adjust the client's medication based on the results.
    2. Filgrastim (Neupogen) is a medication to increase the client's WBC production.
    4. This is expected behavior for a client diagnosed with Alzheimer's disease.

CLINICAL JUDGMENT GUIDE: This is an alternate type of question that requires the nurse to assess clients in order of priority. This requires the nurse to evaluate each client's situation and determine which situations are life threatening, which situations are expected for the client's situation, or which client has a psychosocial problem.

CLINICAL SCENARIO ANSWERS AND RATIONALES

The correct answer number and rationale for why it is the correct answer are given in **boldface type.** Rationales for why the other possible answer options are incorrect also are given, but they are not in boldface type.

1. 1. Sunburn is an example of this depth of burn; a superficial partial-thickness burn affects the epidermis and the skin is reddened and blanches with pressure.
   2. Deep partial-thickness burns are scalds and flash burns that injure the epidermis, upper dermis, and portions of the deeper dermis. This causes pain, blistered and mottled red skin, and edema.
   3. Full-thickness burns are caused by flame, electric current, or chemicals, and include the epidermis, entire dermis, and sometimes subcutaneous tissue, and may also involve connective tissue, muscle, and bone.
   4. First-degree burn is another name for a superficial partial-thickness burn.

2. 1. **After airway, the most urgent need is preventing irreversible shock by replacing fluids and electrolytes.**
   2. This is important, but it is not a priority over fluid volume balance. Curling's ulcer is an acute peptic ulcer of the duodenum resulting as a complication from severe burns when reduced plasma volume leads to sloughing of the gastric mucosa.
   3. Prevention of infection is a priority but not before maintaining fluid and electrolyte balance for the first 48 to 72 hours. The client will die if fluid and electrolyte balance is not maintained.
   4. An escharotomy, an incision that releases the scar tissue, prevents the body from being able to expand and enables chest excursion

in circumferential chest burns. The client has not had time to develop eschar.

3. 1. This is a pertinent problem because the body's protective barrier, the skin, has been compromised and there is an impaired immune response, but it is not a priority over pain.

2. **Pain is the client's priority problem. The client has a full-thickness burn, which has no pain, but the deep partial-thickness burns are very painful.**

3. Burn wound edema, pain, and potential joint contractures can cause mobility deficits, but the first priority is preventing infection so wound healing can occur.

4. After the initial 48 to 72 hours, fluid and electrolyte imbalance is no longer a priority. This client is 4 days post–initial burn.

4. Correct answers are 1, 2, and 5.

1. **Hand washing is the number one intervention used to prevent infection, which is a priority for the client diagnosed with a burn.**

2. **The client is at risk for infection and visitors diagnosed with infections should not be allowed to visit the client.**

3. The client must have a high-protein diet to help with tissue growth.

4. Invasive lines and tubing should be changed daily.

5. **Prophylactic antibiotics are administered to help prevent infection.**

5. 1. **The UAP can put the pulse oximeter on the client's finger and record the number. The RN must evaluate the reading to determine if it is within normal limits.**

2. The dressing change is a sterile procedure; therefore, this cannot be delegated to the UAP.

3. Mafenide acetate (Sulfamylon) is a medication and the RN cannot delegate medication administration to a UAP.

4. The RN cannot delegate assessment to the UAP.

6. 1. Severe pain would be expected in a client diagnosed with these types of burns; therefore, it would not warrant notifying the health-care provider.

2. **A pulse oximeter reading greater than 93% is WNL. Therefore, a 90% reading indicates the client is in respiratory distress and requires the nurse to notify the health-care provider.**

3. The client's vital signs show an elevated temperature, pulse, and respiration, along with a low blood pressure, but these vital signs would not be unusual for a client diagnosed with severe burns.

4. Fluid and electrolyte balance must be evaluated to ensure the output is at least 30 mL an hour. This output is within normal limits; therefore, the data do not warrant notifying a HCP.

7. 1. Ice should never be applied to a burn because this will worsen the tissue damage by causing vasoconstriction.

2. **Cool water gives immediate and striking relief from pain and limits local tissue edema and damage.**

3. Burn ointment should not be applied until the burning has stopped. The client should first put the hand in cool water.

4. The client should be told to go to the emergency department, not the doctor's office, for burn care.

8. 1. The skin should be kept dry. The skin should be patted completely dry after each bath.

2. The client should be premedicated, but it is not the responsibility of the UAPs to ensure this intervention is implemented.

3. **Clients should be turned at least every 1 to 2 hours to prevent pressure areas on the skin. Prevention of pressure areas is a priority to a client diagnosed with a burn.**

4. All employees in any health-care facility are responsible for providing care within their scope of services. UAPs can turn clients to help prevent pressure ulcers.

9. 1. **The UAP cannot touch TPN; it is administered via a subclavian line and should be considered a medication. The RN cannot delegate assessment, teaching, evaluation, medications, or an unstable client.**

2. The UAP can care for a client receiving a continuous tube feeding and should elevate the HOB to prevent aspiration pneumonia.

3. The UAP can assist a client with a meal.

4. The UAP can add beverage thickener (Thick-It) to water before giving it to a client; it will help prevent the client from choking.

10. 1. The client diagnosed with full- and partial-thickness burns is expected to have pain and it should be assessed but not before a client having difficulty breathing.

2. The client does not have 30 mL urine output an hour (this should be 240 mL/8 hours) and the client should be assessed but not before a client diagnosed with airway problems.

3. When determining which client to see first, the charge nurse should use Maslow's Hierarchy of Needs and assess the client diagnosed with airway problems first.

4. No palpable pulse indicates neurovascular compromise but it is not a priority over airway problems.

Hematological and Immunological Management 10

You have brains in your head. You have feet in your shoes.
You can steer yourself any direction you choose.

—Dr. Seuss

QUESTIONS

1. The client diagnosed with breast cancer who is positive for the *BRCA* gene is requesting advice from the nurse about treatment options. Which statement is the nurse's **best** response?
   1. "If it were me in this situation, I would consider having a bilateral mastectomy."
   2. "What treatment options has your health-care provider (HCP) discussed with you?"
   3. "You should discuss your treatment options with your HCP."
   4. "Have you talked with your significant other (SO) about the treatment options available to you?"

2. The staff nurse answers the telephone on a medical unit and the caller tells the nurse that he has planted a bomb in the facility. Which actions should the nurse implement? **Select all that apply.**
   1. Do not touch any suspicious object.
   2. Call 911, the emergency response system.
   3. Try to get the caller to provide additional information.
   4. Immediately pull the red emergency wall lever.
   5. Write down exactly what the caller says.

3. The new graduate nurse working on a medical unit night shift is concerned that the charge nurse is drinking alcohol on duty. On more than one occasion, the new graduate has smelled alcohol when the charge nurse returns from a break. Which action should the new graduate nurse implement **first?**
   1. Confront the charge nurse with the suspicions.
   2. Talk with the night supervisor about the concerns.
   3. Ignore the situation unless the nurse cannot do her job.
   4. Ask to speak to the nurse educator about the problem.

4. The nurse is completing a head-to-toe assessment on a client diagnosed with breast cancer and notes a systolic murmur that the nurse was not informed of during report. Which action should the nurse implement **first?**
   1. Notify the HCP about the new cardiac complication.
   2. Document the finding in the client's EHR and tell the charge nurse.
   3. Check the EHR to determine whether this is the first time a murmur has been identified.
   4. Ask the client whether she has ever been told she has an abnormal heartbeat.

5. The nurse is reviewing the laboratory report for the female client diagnosed with lung cancer. Which action should the nurse implement?

Laboratory Report

Laboratory Test	Client Value	Normal Value
WBC	7.8	4.5 to 11.1 10^3/microL
Neutrophil	62%	40% to 75%
Hgb	13.4	Male: 14 to 17.3 g/dL
		Female: 11.7 to 15.5 g/dL
Hct	40.1%	Male: 42% to 52%
		Female: 36% to 48%

1. Place the client in reverse isolation.
2. Notify the HCP.
3. Make sure no flowers are taken into the room.
4. Continue to monitor the client.

6. The RN charge nurse observes two unlicensed assistive personnel (UAPs) arguing in the hallway. Which action should the nurse implement **first** in this situation?
1. Tell the manager to check on the UAPs.
2. Instruct the UAPs to stop arguing in the hallway.
3. Have the UAPs go to a private room to talk.
4. Mediate the dispute between the UAPs.

7. The graduate nurse (GN) is working with an unlicensed assistive personnel (UAP) who has been an employee of the hospital for 12 years. However, tasks delegated to the UAP by the GN are frequently not completed. Which action should the graduate nurse take **first**?
1. Tell the RN charge nurse the UAP will not do tasks as delegated by the nurse.
2. Write up a counseling record with objective data and give it to the manager.
3. Complete the delegated tasks and do nothing about the insubordination.
4. Address the UAP to discuss why the tasks are not being done as requested.

8. The client is diagnosed with laryngeal cancer and is scheduled for a laryngectomy next week. Which intervention would be a **priority** for the clinic nurse?
1. Assess the client's ability to swallow.
2. Refer the client to a speech therapist.
3. Order the client's preoperative laboratory work.
4. Discuss the client's operative permit.

9. The RN charge nurse is making assignments for the surgical unit. Which client should be assigned to the new graduate nurse (GN)?
1. The 84-year-old client who has a chest tube that is draining bright red blood
2. The 38-year-old client who is 1-day postoperative with a temperature of 101.2°F
3. The 42-year-old client who has just returned to the unit after a breast biopsy
4. The 55-year-old client who is reporting unrelenting abdominal pain

10. Which task is **most** appropriate for the RN surgical nurse to assign to the licensed practical nurse (LPN)?
1. Tell the LPN to administer the aminoglycoside antibiotic to the client.
2. Request the LPN to empty the client's indwelling urinary catheter.
3. Instruct the LPN to assess the client who was just transferred from the PACU.
4. Ask the LPN to determine if the client understands the discharge teaching.

11. The RN primary nurse informs the RN charge nurse that one of the unlicensed assistive personnel (UAPs) is falsifying vital signs. Which action should the shift manager implement **first?**
    1. Notify the unit manager of the potential situation of falsifying vital signs.
    2. Take the assigned client's vital signs and compare them with the UAP's results.
    3. Talk to the UAP about the primary nurse's allegation.
    4. Complete a counseling record and place it in the UAP's file.

12. The client tells the nurse, "I am not sure my surgeon is telling me the truth about my prognosis." The nurse knows the client has terminal cancer but the health-care provider is not telling the client per the family's request. Which statement is the nurse's **best** response?
    1. "I think you should know you have terminal cancer."
    2. "You do have a right to a second opinion."
    3. "You are concerned your surgeon is not telling you the truth."
    4. "I think you should talk to your surgeon about your concerns."

13. The nurse hung the wrong IV antibiotic for the postoperative client. Which intervention should the nurse implement **first?**
    1. Assess the client for any adverse reactions.
    2. Complete the incident or adverse occurrence report.
    3. Administer the correct intravenous antibiotic medication.
    4. Notify the client's health-care provider.

14. The 24-year-old male client diagnosed with testicular cancer is scheduled for a unilateral orchiectomy. Which **priority** intervention should the clinic nurse implement?
    1. Teach the client to turn, cough, and deep breathe.
    2. Discuss the importance of sperm banking.
    3. Explain about the testicular prosthesis.
    4. Refer the client to the American Cancer Society (ACS).

15. The female client in the preoperative holding area tells the nurse that she had a reaction to a latex diaphragm. Which intervention should the nurse perform **first?**
    1. Notify the operating room personnel.
    2. Label the client's EHR with the allergy.
    3. Place a red allergy band on the client.
    4. Inform the client to tell all HCPs of the allergy.

16. The RN critical care nurse, a licensed practical nurse (LPN), and the unlicensed assistive personnel (UAP) are caring for clients in a critical care unit. Which task would be **most** appropriate for the RN to assign or delegate?
    1. Instruct the UAP to obtain the client's serum glucose level.
    2. Request the LPN to change the central line dressing.
    3. Ask the LPN to bathe the client and change the bed linens.
    4. Tell the UAP to obtain urine output for the 12-hour shift.

17. Which task should the RN critical care nurse delegate to the unlicensed assistive personnel (UAP)?
    1. Check the pulse oximeter reading for the client on a ventilator.
    2. Take the client's sterile urine specimen to the laboratory.
    3. Obtain the vital signs for the client in an Addisonian crisis.
    4. Assist the HCP with performing a paracentesis at the bedside.

18. The critical care charge nurse is making client assignments. Which client should the charge nurse assign to the nurse who is pregnant?
    1. The client with intracavity radiation for cervical cancer who developed ARDS
    2. The client who is HIV positive and admitted for chest pain R/O myocardial infarction
    3. The client who is immunosuppressed and diagnosed with cytomegalovirus (CMV)
    4. The client receiving I131 iodine for hyperthyroidism who had a motor vehicle accident (MVA)

19. The intensive care nurse is caring for a client and notes blood oozing out from under the transparent dressing covering the peripheral intravenous site, bleeding gums, and blood in the indwelling urinary catheter bag. Which intervention should the nurse implement **first?**
    1. Check the client's hemoglobin/hematocrit (H&H) level.
    2. Monitor the client's pulse oximeter reading.
    3. Apply pressure to the intravenous site.
    4. Notify the client's health-care provider.

20. A client diagnosed with AIDS dementia is angry and yells at everyone entering the room. None of the critical care staff want to be assigned to this client. Which intervention would be **most** appropriate for the nurse manager to use in resolving this situation?
    1. Explain that this attitude is a violation of the client's rights.
    2. Request the HCP to transfer the client to the medical unit.
    3. Discuss some possible options with the nursing staff.
    4. Try to find a nurse who does not mind being assigned to the client.

21. Which situation would prompt the health-care team to utilize the client's advance directive when needing to make decisions for the client?
    1. The client diagnosed with a head injury who is exhibiting decerebrate posturing
    2. The client diagnosed with a C-6 SCI who is on a ventilator
    3. The client diagnosed with ESRD who is being placed on dialysis
    4. The client diagnosed with terminal cancer who is mentally retarded

22. Which staff nurse should the charge nurse in the intensive care unit (ICU) send to the medical unit?
    1. The nurse who has worked in the unit for 18 months
    2. The nurse who is orienting to the critical care unit
    3. The nurse who has been working at the hospital for 2 months
    4. The nurse who has 12 years' experience in this ICU unit

23. The confused client in the critical care unit (CCU) is attempting to pull out the IV line and the indwelling urinary catheter. Which action should the RN critical care nurse implement **first?**
    1. Ask a family member to stay with the client.
    2. Request the UAP to stay with the client.
    3. Place the client in a chest restraint.
    4. Notify the HCP to obtain a restraint order.

24. Which tasks should the RN long-term care nurse delegate to the unlicensed assistive personnel (UAP)? **Select all that apply.**
    1. Instruct the UAP to perform the a.m. care for the clients.
    2. Tell the UAP to wash the hair of the female clients.
    3. Ask the UAP to cut the toenails of the clients.
    4. Request the UAP to turn the clients every shift.
    5. Instruct the UAP to empty the clients' wastebaskets.

25. The RN long-term care nurse notes the unlicensed assistive personnel (UAP) tied a sheet around the client in the chair so the client will not fall out. Which action should the nurse implement **first?**
    1. Praise the UAP for being concerned about the safety of the client.
    2. Remove the sheet from the client immediately.
    3. Explain to the UAP the sheet is a form of restraint and cannot be tied around the client.
    4. Assess the client's need for restraints and notify the health-care provider for an order.

26. The RN charge nurse in the long-term care center is making assignments for licensed practical nurses (LPNs) and unlicensed assistive personnel (UAPs) on the day shift. Which task is **most** appropriate to assign to the LPN?
    1. Instruct the LPN to place anti-embolism hose on the client.
    2. Ask the LPN to escort the client outside to smoke a cigarette.
    3. Tell the LPN to administer the tube feeding to the client.
    4. Request the LPN to change the client's colostomy bag.

27. The RN staff nurse is caring for clients on a skilled nursing unit. Which task should the staff nurse delegate to the unlicensed nursing personnel (UAP)? **Select all that apply.**
    1. Instruct the UAP to apply sequential compression devices to the client on strict bedrest.
    2. Ask the UAP to assist the radiology tech to perform a STAT portable chest x-ray.
    3. Request the UAP to prepare the client for a wound debridement at the bedside.
    4. Tell the UAP to obtain the intakes and outputs for all the clients on the unit.
    5. Have the UAP help the client move from the bed to the chair for meals.

28. The older adult client receiving chemotherapy reports that food just does not taste the way it used to. Which intervention should the medical unit nurse implement **first?**
    1. Ask the dietitian to consult with the client on food preferences.
    2. Medicate the client before meals with an antiemetic medication.
    3. Ask the HCP to suggest an over-the-counter nutritional supplement.
    4. Check the client's current weight with the client's usual weight.

29. The nurse is assigned to a quality improvement committee to decide on a quality improvement project for the unit. Which issue should the nurse discuss at the committee meetings?
    1. Systems that make it difficult for the nurses to do their job
    2. How unhappy the nurses are with their current pay scale
    3. Collective bargaining activity at a nearby hospital
    4. The number of medication errors committed by another nurse

30. The nurse is discussing an upcoming surgical procedure with a 76-year-old client diagnosed with cancer. Which action is an example of the ethical principle of fidelity?
    1. The nurse makes sure the client understands the procedure before signing the permit.
    2. The nurse refuses to disclose the client's personal information to the CNO.
    3. The nurse tells the client his diagnosis when the family did not want him to know.
    4. The nurse tells the client that she does not know the client's diagnosis.

31. Which client laboratory data should the nurse report to the HCP **immediately?**
    1. The elevated amylase report on a client diagnosed with acute pancreatitis
    2. The elevated WBC count on a client diagnosed with a septic leg wound
    3. The urinalysis report showing many bacteria in a client receiving chemotherapy
    4. The serum glucose level of 235 mg/dL on a client diagnosed with type 1 diabetes

32. The RN charge nurse in a long-term care facility is reviewing the male resident's laboratory data. Which instructions should the nurse give to the unlicensed assistive personnel (UAP) caring for the client?

Laboratory Report

Laboratory Test	Client Value	Normal Value
WBC	5.25	4.5 to 11.1 10^3/microL
RBC	4.3	Male: 4.21 to 5.81 10^6 cells/microL
		Female: 3.61 to 5.11 10^6 cells/microL
Hgb	13	Male: 14 to 17.3 g/dL
		Female: 11.7 to 15.5 g/dL
Hct	39	Male: 42% to 52%
		Female: 36% to 48%
Platelets	39	150 to 450 (10^3 mm)

1. Place the client in reverse isolation immediately.
2. Administer oxygen during strenuous activities.
3. Do not shave the resident with a safety razor.
4. Check the resident's temperature every 4 hours.

33. The clinic RN manager is discussing osteoporosis with the clinic staff. Which activity is an example of a secondary nursing intervention when discussing osteoporosis?
    1. Obtain a bone density evaluation test on a female client older than 50.
    2. Perform a spinal screening examination on all female clients.
    3. Encourage the client to walk 30 minutes daily on a hard surface.
    4. Discuss risk factors for developing osteoporosis.

34. A client had an allergic reaction to penicillin and was admitted to the hospital 2 weeks ago. The client is being seen at the clinic for a follow-up visit. Which **priority** intervention should the nurse implement?
    1. Recommend the client wear a medical alert bracelet.
    2. Encourage the client to tell the pharmacy about the allergy.
    3. Tell the client not to be around any person taking penicillin.
    4. Allow the client to vent feelings about the hospitalization.

35. Which action would be **most** appropriate for the clinic nurse who suspects another staff nurse of stealing narcotics from the clinic?
    1. Confront the staff nurse with the suspicion.
    2. Call the state board of nurse examiners.
    3. Notify the director of nurses immediately.
    4. Report the suspicion to the clinic's HCP.

36. The clinic nurse administered 200,000 units of intramuscular penicillin to a client. Which **priority** intervention should the nurse implement?
    1. Place a bandage over the intramuscular injection site.
    2. Tell the client to put a warm compress over the injection site.
    3. Document the medication injection in the client's EHR.
    4. Inform the client to stay in the waiting room for 30 minutes.

37. The home health (HH) aide calls the office and reports pain after feeling a pulling sensation in her back when she was transferring the client from the bed to the wheelchair. Which **priority** action should the RN HH nurse tell the HH aide?
    1. Explain how to perform isometric exercises.
    2. Instruct the HH aide to go to the local emergency department.
    3. Tell the HH aide to complete an occurrence report.
    4. Recommend the HH aide apply an ice pack to the back.

38. The client diagnosed with osteoarthritis is 6 weeks postoperative for open reduction and internal fixation of the right hip. The home health (HH) aide tells the RN HH nurse the client will not get in the shower in the morning because she "hurts all over." Which action would be **most** appropriate by the HH nurse?
    1. Tell the HH aide to allow the client to stay in bed until the pain goes away.
    2. Instruct the HH aide to get the client up to a chair and give her a bath.
    3. Explain to the HH aide that the client should get up and take a warm shower.
    4. Arrange an appointment for the client to visit her health-care provider.

39. The RN home health (HH) nurse is discussing the care of a client with an HH aide. Which task can the HH nurse delegate to the HH aide?
    1. Instruct the HH aide to assist the client with a shower.
    2. Ask the HH aide to prepare the breakfast meal for the client.
    3. Request that the HH aide take the client to an HCP's appointment.
    4. Tell the HH aide to show the client how to use a glucometer.

40. The RN home health (HH) care agency director is teaching a class to the HH aides concerning safety in HH nursing. Which statement by the HH aide indicates the director needs to **re-teach** safety information?
    1. "It is all right to call the agency if I am afraid of going into the home."
    2. "I should wear my uniform and name tag when I go into the home."
    3. "I must take my cellular phone when visiting the client's home."
    4. "It is all right if I don't wear gloves when touching bodily fluids."

41. The home health (HH) agency RN director is making assignments. Which client should be assigned to the **most** experienced HH nurse?
    1. The client who is recovering from Guillain-Barré syndrome who reports being tired all the time
    2. The client who has multiple stage 3 and 4 pressure ulcers on the sacral area
    3. The client who is 2 weeks postoperative for laryngectomy secondary to laryngeal cancer
    4. The client who is being discharged from service within the next week

42. The home health (HH) nurse is visiting a female client diagnosed with colon cancer who has had a sigmoid colostomy. The client is crying and tells the nurse that she was told the cancer has spread and she will die very soon. Which intervention should the nurse implement?
    1. Discuss the possibility of being placed on hospice services.
    2. Contact the client's oncologist to discuss the client's prognosis.
    3. Ask the client whether she has planned her funeral services.
    4. Recommend the client get a second opinion concerning her prognosis.

43. The client tells the home health (HH) nurse, "My oncologist told me they can't do anything else for my cancer. I do not want my children to know, but I had to tell someone. You won't tell them, will you?" Which statement is the nurse's **best** response?
    1. "Because you told me about the prognosis, I must talk to your children."
    2. "I don't think it is a good idea not to tell your children; they should know."
    3. "I will not say anything to your children, but I will contact the HH doctor."
    4. "You are concerned I might talk to your children about your prognosis."

44. The home health (HH) hospice nurse is making rounds. Which client should the nurse assess **first?**
    1. The client diagnosed with end-stage heart failure who has increasing difficulty breathing
    2. The client whose family has planned to surprise her with an early birthday party
    3. The client who is reporting being tired and irritable all the time
    4. The client diagnosed with chronic lung disease who has not eaten for 3 days

45. A client diagnosed with cancer and receiving chemotherapy is brought to the emergency department (ED) after vomiting bright red blood. Which intervention should the nurse implement **first?**
   1. Check to see which antineoplastic medications the client has received.
   2. Start an IV of normal saline with an 18-gauge intravenous catheter.
   3. Investigate to see whether the client has a do not resuscitate (DNR) order written.
   4. Call the oncologist to determine what laboratory work to order.

46. The nurse is called to the room of a male client diagnosed with lung cancer by the client's wife because the client is not breathing. The client has discussed having a DNR order written but has not made a decision. Which interventions should the nurse implement **first?**
   1. Ask the spouse whether she wants the client to be resuscitated.
   2. Tell the spouse to leave the room and then perform a slow code.
   3. Assess the client's breathing and call a code from the room.
   4. Notify the oncologist the client has arrested.

47. The female client who is dying asks to see her son, but the son refuses to come to the hospital. Which action should the nurse implement **first?**
   1. Call the son and tell him he must come to see his mother before it is too late.
   2. Ask the social worker to call the son and see whether the son will come to the hospital.
   3. Check with the family to see whether they can discuss the issue with the son.
   4. Do nothing because to intervene in a private matter would be boundary crossing.

48. The nurse is caring for clients on an oncology unit. Which client should the nurse assess **first?**
   1. The client diagnosed with leukemia who is afebrile and has a white blood cell (WBC) count of 100,000 mm³
   2. The client who has undergone four rounds of chemotherapy and is nauseated
   3. The client diagnosed with lung cancer who has absent breath sounds in the lower lobes
   4. The client diagnosed with rule out (R/O) breast cancer who had a negative biopsy this a.m.

49. The nurse caring for clients on an oncology unit is administering medications. Which medication should the nurse administer **first?**
   1. The antinausea medication to the client who thinks he may get sick
   2. The pain medication to the client who has pain rated at a 2 on a 1 to 10 scale
   3. The loop diuretic to the client who had an output greater than the intake
   4. The nitroglycerin paste to the client who is diagnosed with angina pectoris

50. The staff nurse is caring for a client who was diagnosed with pancreatic cancer during an exploratory laparotomy. Which client problem is a **priority** for postoperative day 1?
   1. Ineffective coping
   2. Fluid and electrolyte imbalance
   3. Risk for infection
   4. Potential for suicidal thoughts

51. The male client who was just told he has 6 months to live tells the nurse, "This can't be happening. I am too young to die." Which statement is the nurse's **best** response?
   1. "I can contact the chaplain to come talk to you."
   2. "I will leave you alone and come back in a little while."
   3. "Is there anyone I can call to come be with you?"
   4. "If it is all right with you I am going to sit here with you."

52. The nurse administered pain medication 30 minutes ago to a client diagnosed with terminal cancer. Thirty minutes after the medication, the client tells the nurse, "I don't think you gave me anything. My pain is even worse than before." Which interventions should the nurse implement? **Select all that apply.**
1. Attempt to determine whether the client is experiencing spiritual distress.
2. Ask the client to rate the current pain on the numeric pain scale.
3. Reposition the client to relieve pressure on the pain site.
4. Call the HCP to request an increase in pain medication.
5. Explain to the client he or she should relax and let the medication take effect.

53. Which member of the health-care team should be assigned to a dying client who is having frequent symptoms of distress?
1. The unlicensed assistive personnel (UAP) who can be spared to sit with the client
2. The licensed practical nurse (LPN) who has grown attached to the family
3. The registered nurse (RN) who has experience as a hospice nurse
4. The registered nurse (RN) who graduated 2 months ago

54. During the morning assessment, the client diagnosed with cancer reports nausea most of the time. Based on the client's medication administration record (MAR), which intervention should the day nurse implement **first?**

Client's Name: Mr. B Height: 67 inches Diagnosis: Cancer of the pancreas	Admit Number: 543216 Date:	Allergies: NKDA Weight: 74.2 kg/163 pounds	
Medication		0701–1900	1901–0700
Morphine sulfate 2 mg q2 hours PRN IVP			
Promethazine 12.5 mg IVP q4 hours PRN			
Prochlorperazine 5 mg PO tid PRN			
Hydrocodone PO q4–6 hours PRN 5 mg			
Signature/Initials		Day Nurse DN/RN	Night Nurse NN/RN

1. Administer the prescribed promethazine PRN.
2. Administer the prescribed prochlorperazine ac.
3. Discuss changing the order for prochlorperazine to routine with the HCP.
4. Assess the client to see whether pain is the cause of the nausea.

55. The infection control nurse notices a rise in nosocomial infection rates on the surgical unit. Which action should the infection control nurse implement **first?**
1. Hold an in-service for the staff on the proper method of hand washing.
2. Tell the unit manager to decide on a corrective measure.
3. Arrange to observe the staff at work for several shifts.
4. Form a hospital-wide quality improvement project.

56. The unlicensed assistive personnel (UAP) is preparing to provide postmortem care to a client with a questionable diagnosis of anthrax. Which instruction is the **priority** for the RN staff nurse to provide to the UAP?
1. The UAP is not at risk for contracting an illness.
2. The UAP should wear a mask, gown, and gloves.
3. The UAP may skip performing postmortem care.
4. Ask whether the UAP is pregnant before she enters the client's room.

57. The client on a medical unit died of a communicable disease. Which information should the RN staff nurse provide to the mortuary workers?
1. No information can be released to the mortuary service.
2. The nurse should tell the funeral home the client's diagnosis.
3. Ask the family for permission to talk with the mortician.
4. Refer the funeral home to the HCP for information.

58. The RN med-surg nurse and unlicensed assistive personnel (UAP) are caring for a group of clients on a medical unit. Which action by the UAP warrants **immediate** intervention by the nurse?
    1. The UAP dons unsterile gloves before emptying a urinary catheter bag.
    2. The UAP places clean linen in all of the clients' rooms for the day.
    3. The UAP uses a different plastic bag for every client when getting ice.
    4. The UAP massages the client's trochanter when turning the client.

59. The charge nurse is making assignments on a surgical unit. Which client should be assigned to the **least** experienced nurse?
    1. The client who had a vaginal hysterectomy and still has an indwelling catheter
    2. The client who had an open cholecystectomy and has gray drainage in the tube
    3. The client who had a hip replacement and states something popped while walking
    4. The client who had a Whipple procedure and reports being thirsty all the time

60. The unit manager on an oncology unit receives a negative report about the care a client received from the assigned night shift nurse. Which action should the unit manager implement **first?**
    1. Ask the night charge nurse to make sure the nurse does the work.
    2. Request the nurse come in to discuss the care provided.
    3. Discuss the situation with the client making the report.
    4. Document this occurrence and place in the nurse's employee file.

61. The female client was admitted to the orthopedic unit for injuries received during an argument with her spouse. The client tells the nurse, "I am afraid my husband will kill me if I leave him. It was my fault anyway." Which statement is the nurse's **best** response?
    1. "What did you do to set him off that way?"
    2. "Do you have a plan for safety if you go back?"
    3. "Why do you think it was your fault?"
    4. "You should leave him before it is too late."

62. The husband of a client on the surgical unit comes to the desk and asks the nurse, "What is my wife's biopsy report?" Which intervention is the nurse's **best** action?
    1. Check the EHR to see whether the client has allowed the spouse to have information.
    2. Obtain the pathology report and tell the husband the results of the biopsy.
    3. Call the HCP and arrange a time for the husband to meet with the HCP.
    4. Inform the client and husband of the biopsy results at the same time.

63. The nurse is caring for a client diagnosed with acquired immunodeficiency syndrome (AIDS). Which client problem is **priority?**
    1. Body image disturbance
    2. Impaired coping
    3. Risk for infection
    4. Self-care deficit

64. The RN oncology nurse and licensed practical nurse (LPN) are caring for clients on an oncology unit. Which client should be assigned to the LPN?
    1. The client diagnosed with acute leukemia who is on a continuous infusion of antineoplastic medications
    2. The client newly diagnosed with cancer of the lung who is being admitted for placement of an implanted port
    3. The client diagnosed with an ovarian tumor weighing 22 pounds who is being prepared for surgery in the morning
    4. The client diagnosed with pancreatic cancer who reports frequent, unrelenting abdominal pain

65. The nurse has received the morning shift report on an oncology unit. Which client should the nurse assess **first?**
    1. The client diagnosed with leukemia who has a white blood cell (WBC) count of 1.2 (10^3)
    2. The client diagnosed with a brain tumor who has a headache rated as a 2 on a pain scale of 1 to 10
    3. The client diagnosed with breast cancer who is upset and crying
    4. The client diagnosed with lung cancer who is dyspneic on exertion

66. The RN staff nurse is caring for a female client diagnosed with systemic lupus erythematosus (SLE). Which client-reported data has **priority?**
    1. The client reports that she has trouble finding makeup to cover the rash across her nose.
    2. The client tells the unlicensed assistive personnel (UAP) to close the drapes because sunlight is bad for her.
    3. The client notices a bright red color in the bedside commode.
    4. The client reports joint stiffness and requests a pain medication.

67. The nurse caring for a client newly diagnosed with protein calorie malnutrition secondary to acquired immune deficiency syndrome (AIDS) writes a nursing problem of "altered nutrition: less than body requirements." Which nursing interventions should the nurse implement? **Select all that apply.**
    1. Place the client on daily weights.
    2. Have the client identify preferred foods.
    3. Refer to the dietitian.
    4. Monitor bedside glucose levels four times a day.
    5. Perform central line dressing changes every 72 hours.

68. The client diagnosed with congestive heart failure and iron deficiency anemia is prescribed a unit of packed red blood cells (PRBCs). **Rank in order of performance.**
    1. Administer furosemide between units.
    2. Check the client's hemoglobin and hematocrit.
    3. Assess the client's lung sounds and periphery.
    4. Have the client sign a permit to receive blood.
    5. Return the empty blood bags to the laboratory.

69. The nurse working in a rheumatology clinic is teaching a 34-year-old female client diagnosed with rheumatoid arthritis (RA) about methotrexate. Which information has the highest **priority?**
    1. Teach the client to take measures to ensure she does not become pregnant.
    2. Inform the client to keep the follow-up appointments with the clinic.
    3. Have the client see a dietitian if she loses her appetite.
    4. Tell the client to keep a diary of her symptoms to bring to appointments with her.

70. The 28-year-old female client in the outpatient clinic has been told that her test for the human immunodeficiency virus (HIV) is positive. Which interventions should the nurse implement? **Select all that apply.**
    1. Discuss having regular gynecological examinations.
    2. Assist the client to make her funeral arrangements.
    3. Refer the client to a social worker.
    4. Encourage the client to take the highly active antiretroviral therapy (HAART).
    5. Teach the client to follow a healthy lifestyle.

HEMATOLOGICAL AND IMMUNOLOGICAL CLINICAL SCENARIO

The RN charge nurse is on an inpatient oncology unit in a large university medical center located centrally to the metroplex. She is working with two RNs along with an LPN and two UAPs. They are working on Saturday from 0700 to 1900. There are 10 culturally diverse clients of all ages on the 15-bed intensive care oncology unit.

1. The RN oncology nurse and LPN are caring for clients. Which client should be assigned to the LPN?
   1. The 47-year-old client newly diagnosed with chronic lymphocytic leukemia
   2. The young adult client who is 4 hours post-procedure bone marrow biopsy
   3. The 30-year-old client who is receiving PRBCs with hemoglobin of 6
   4. The elderly client who is receiving antineoplastic medications

2. Which client should the charge nurse assign to the medical-surgical nurse who is being pulled to work on the oncology unit for this shift?
   1. The middle-age client diagnosed with non-Hodgkin's lymphoma who is having complications from daily radiation treatments
   2. The 36-year-old client diagnosed with Hodgkin's disease who is being prepared for a bone marrow transplant
   3. The malnourished client diagnosed with leukemia who has petechiae covering both anterior and posterior body surfaces
   4. The young adult female client diagnosed with ovarian cancer who is 1-day postoperative total abdominal hysterectomy

3. The RN oncology nurse and the UAP are caring for a group of clients. Which information provided by the UAP **warrants immediate** intervention by the nurse?
   1. The elderly male client diagnosed with bladder cancer has bright red blood in the urinal.
   2. The obese client receiving chemotherapy is reporting pain in the mouth.
   3. The 50-year-old client with a biological response modifier has a T 99.2°F, P 68, R 24, and BP of 198/102.
   4. The client receiving a steroid is reporting having a rounded swollen face.

4. The RN oncology nurse is caring for a middle-age male client who is 1-day postoperative sigmoid resection and notes bright red bleeding on the midline abdominal incision. Which intervention should the nurse implement **first?**
   1. Assess the client's vital signs.
   2. Reinforce the abdominal dressing.
   3. Notify the health-care provider.
   4. Place the client in the Trendelenburg position.

5. Which nursing task should the RN oncology nurse delegate to the UAP?
   1. Discontinue the elderly client's subclavian intravenous catheter.
   2. Empty the Jackson Pratt drainage tube and record the amount.
   3. Determine if the client's pain medication has been effective.
   4. Perform irrigation for the obese client who is 2 days post-op abdominoperineal resection.

6. The 79-year-old male client is 2 days post-ureterosigmoidostomy for cancer of the bladder. Which assessment data **warrants** the RN oncology nurse notifying the HCP?
   1. The client has excreted urine from the rectum.
   2. The client's abdominal incision is slightly reddened.
   3. The client has an apical rate of 98 and BP 114/80.
   4. The client has a low-grade fever and a hard, rigid abdomen.

7. The RN oncology nurse identifies a problem of "anticipatory grieving" for an elderly female client diagnosed with stage 4 ovarian cancer. Which nursing intervention is the **priority** for this client?
   1. Request the client is referred to hospice.
   2. Encourage the client to make plans for her funeral.
   3. Allow the client to verbalize feelings about having cancer.
   4. Discuss an advance directive and a power of attorney for health care.

8. The 57-year-old female client diagnosed with ovarian cancer has had five courses of chemotherapy. Which laboratory data **warrant immediate** intervention by the RN oncology nurse?
   1. Absolute neutrophil count (ANC) of 681 mm/dL
   2. Platelet count of 175,000
   3. Red blood cell count of 5.0×10^6
   4. Hemoglobin of 11.2 and hematocrit 37%

9. The RN oncology nurse is performing a head-to-toe assessment on an elderly client diagnosed with prostate cancer. The nurse notes an irregular-shaped lesion with some scabbed-over areas surrounding the lesion. Which intervention should the nurse implement **first?**
   1. Take no action because this is a common lesion found on the skin.
   2. Assess the lesion by completing the ABCDs of skin cancer.
   3. Document the findings in the client's EHR.
   4. Instruct the client to make sure the HCP checks the lesion.

10. The 39-year-old female client diagnosed with pancreatic cancer has an advance directive (AD) stipulating no cardiopulmonary resuscitation. Which intervention should the RN oncology nurse implement **first?**
    1. Notify the client's health-care provider about the AD.
    2. Determine if the client has discussed the AD with significant others.
    3. Scan a copy of the advance directive into the client's EHR.
    4. Give the original advance directive to the client.

The correct answer number and rationale for why it is the correct answer are given in **boldface type**. Rationales for why the other possible answer options are incorrect also are given, but they are not in boldface type.

1. 1. This is boundary crossing because the nurse does not have breast cancer. The nurse should assess what information the client is really seeking and then explain the treatment or refer the client, as appropriate.
2. **The nurse must assess what information the client actually needs. To do this, the nurse must know what treatment options have been suggested to the client. Assessment is the first step in the nursing process.**
3. This may be needed after the nurse further assesses the situation, but this is not the first intervention.
4. The client needs information about treatment options from a designated HCP; the significant other would not have such information or suggestions.

CLINICAL JUDGMENT GUIDE: The test taker should answer the question with factual information. Assessment is the first step of the nursing process and the nurse should assess the client's current understanding of treatment options.

2. Correct answers are 1, 3, and 5.
1. **The nurse should begin a systematic search of the unit after activating the bomb scare emergency plan, and if any suspicious objects are found the nurse should not touch them, and should notify the bomb squad.**
2. The nurse should notify the house supervisor and administration because they are responsible for notifying the police department.
3. **The nurse should stay calm and try to keep the caller on the telephone. The nurse should attempt to get as much information from the caller as possible. The nurse can jot a note to someone nearby to initiate the bomb scare procedure.**
4. The red emergency levers in hospitals are to notify the fire department of a fire, not a bomb scare.
5. **The nurse should try to transcribe exactly what the caller says; this may help identify who is calling and where a bomb might be placed.**

CLINICAL JUDGMENT GUIDE: The nurse must be knowledgeable of hospital emergency preparedness. Students as well as new employees receive this information in hospital orientations and are responsible for implementing procedures correctly. The NCLEX-RN® test plan includes questions on the Safe and Effective Care Environment.

3. 1. The new graduate nurse (GN) must work under this RN charge nurse; confronting the nurse would not resolve the issue because the nurse can choose to ignore the new graduate. Someone in authority over the charge nurse must address this situation with the nurse.
2. **The night supervisor or the unit manager has the authority to require the charge nurse to submit to drug screening. In this case, the supervisor on duty should handle the situation.**
3. The new graduate is bound by the nursing practice acts to report potentially unsafe behavior regardless of the position the nurse holds.
4. The nurse educator would not be in a position of authority over the charge nurse.

CLINICAL JUDGMENT GUIDE: When the nurse is deciding on a course of action involving other staff members, a rule of thumb is this: If the individual about which the nurse is concerned is superior in job title to the nurse, then the nurse should go through the chain of command to the next-level superior. If the individual is subordinate in job title to the nurse, then the nurse should confront the individual.

4. 1. This should be done if the murmur is a new finding; however, the nurse should investigate the finding further before notifying the HCP.
2. This should be done, but assessing the client's situation is the nurse's priority.
3. **Although the client was not admitted for a cardiac problem, she may have had a murmur for a while, and the previous nurse did not pick it up or did not mention it in the report because it was a long-standing physiological finding in this client. The nurse should research the EHR for a current history and physical to determine whether the HCP is aware of the condition.**
4. The nurse should not ask the client because this could scare or alarm the client needlessly.

CLINICAL JUDGMENT GUIDE: Assessment is the first step of the nursing process. The next step is for the nurse to investigate the assessment findings in the EHR without alarming the client.

5. 1. The client's laboratory work does not indicate an increased risk for infection. The client does not need to be placed in reverse isolation.
   2. The laboratory work is within normal limits. The nurse does not need to notify the HCP.
   3. The client is not at an increased risk for infection; therefore, the client may have flowers in the room.
   4. **This client's laboratory work is within normal limits. The nurse should continue to monitor the client.**

CLINICAL JUDGMENT GUIDE: This is an alternate type of question included in the NCLEX-RN® test plan. The test taker must be able to read an EHR, be knowledgeable of laboratory data, and make decisions concerning the nurse's most appropriate action.

6. 1. The nurse should stop the behavior from occurring in a public place. The RN charge nurse can discuss the issue with the UAPs and determine whether the manager should be notified.
   2. **The first action is to stop the argument from occurring in a public place. The RN charge nurse should not discuss the UAPs' behavior in public.**
   3. The second action is to have the UAPs go to a private area before resuming the conversation.
   4. The charge nurse may need to mediate the disagreement; this would be the third step.

CLINICAL JUDGMENT GUIDE: In any business, including a health-care facility, arguments or discussions of confidential information should not occur among staff of any level where clients, visitors, or other staff can see or hear it.

7. 1. The graduate nurse (GN) should handle the situation directly with the UAP first before notifying the RN charge nurse.
   2. This may need to be completed, but not before directly discussing the behavior with the UAP.
   3. The graduate nurse (GN) must address the insubordination with the UAP, not just complete the tasks that are the responsibility of the UAP.
   4. **The graduate nurse (GN) must discuss the insubordination directly with the UAP first. The nurse must give objective data as to when and where the UAP did not**

follow through with the completion of assigned tasks.

CLINICAL JUDGMENT GUIDE: When the nurse is deciding on a course of action involving other staff members, a rule of thumb is this: If the individual about which the nurse is concerned is superior in job title to the nurse, then the nurse should go through the chain of command to the next-level superior. If the individual is subordinate in job title to the nurse, then the nurse should confront the individual.

8. 1. The client's ability to swallow is not impaired before the surgical procedure.
   2. **The client will not be able to speak after the removal of the larynx; therefore, referral to a speech therapist who will be able to discuss an alternate means of communication is a priority.**
   3. The HCP, not the nurse, is responsible for ordering the preoperative laboratory work.
   4. The HCP, not the nurse, is responsible for discussing the operative permit.

CLINICAL JUDGMENT GUIDE: The test taker must be aware of the setting that ultimately dictates the appropriate intervention. The adjectives will clue the test taker to the setting. In this question, the words "clinic nurse" clue the test taker to the setting. The test taker must also remember the nurse's scope of practice and realize that options 3 and 4 are outside the nurse's scope of practice.

9. 1. This client is not stable and requires a more experienced nurse.
   2. An elevated temperature indicates a potential complication of surgery; therefore, this client requires a more experienced nurse.
   3. **Of the four clients, the one who is most stable is the client who has just undergone a breast biopsy; therefore, this client would be the most appropriate to assign to a new graduate nurse.**
   4. Unrelenting pain requires further assessment; therefore, the client should be assigned to a more experienced nurse.

CLINICAL JUDGMENT GUIDE: When the test taker is deciding which client should be assigned to a new graduate, the most stable client should be assigned to the least experienced nurse.

10. 1. The LPN can administer intravenous antibiotic medication according to the LPN scope of practice.

2. The UAP, not the LPN, should be instructed to empty the indwelling urinary catheter.

3. The LPN should not be assigned to assess a client.

4. The LPN should not be assigned to evaluate the client's understanding of the discharge teaching.

CLINICAL JUDGMENT GUIDE: The RN cannot assign assessment, teaching, evaluation, or an unstable client to an LPN.

11. 1. This should not be implemented until verification of the allegation is complete, and the RN charge nurse has discussed the situation with the UAP.

2. **The RN charge nurse should have objective data about the allegation of falsifying vital signs before confronting the UAP; therefore, the charge nurse should take the client's vital signs and compare them with the UAP's results before taking any other action.**

3. The RN charge nurse should not confront the UAP until objective data are obtained to support the allegation.

4. Written documentation should be the last action when resolving staff issues.

CLINICAL JUDGMENT GUIDE: There will be management and legal questions on the NCLEX-RN® examination. In many instances, there is no test-taking strategy; the nurse must be knowledgeable of management issues.

12. 1. If the nurse tells the client the truth at this time, the client may ask, "What happens now? How long do I have to live?" In this situation, the nurse should not tell the client the truth.

2. The client does have a right to a second opinion, but in this situation the nurse should encourage the client to talk to the surgeon.

3. This is a therapeutic response that encourages the client to vent his or her feelings, but the client needs answers. This is not the best response by the nurse.

4. **Because the nurse knows the client is terminal, it would be best for the nurse to encourage the client to talk to the surgeon. The client needs the truth and the surgeon is the person who should tell it to the client.**

CLINICAL JUDGMENT GUIDE: The nurse needs to be able to guide clients to the correct person

when they have questions about their health care.

13. 1. **The nurse should first assess the client before taking any other action to determine if the client is experiencing any untoward reaction.**

2. An incident report must be completed by the nurse, but not before taking care of the client.

3. The nurse should administer the correct medication, but not before assessing the client.

4. The client's HCP must be notified, but the nurse should be able to provide the HCP with pertinent client information, so this is not the first intervention.

CLINICAL JUDGMENT GUIDE: Whenever something happens to the client, the nurse should first assess the client before taking any other action.

14. 1. The client must be taught postoperative care, but this is not the priority intervention of the clinic nurse.

2. **Sperm banking will allow the client's sperm to be kept until the time the client wants to conceive a child. This is a priority because it must be done between the clinic visit and admission to the hospital for the procedure. The unilateral orchiectomy will not result in sterility, but the subsequent treatments may cause sterility.**

3. The nurse can discuss the testicular prosthesis, but this is not a priority over sperm banking because the prosthesis may or may not be inserted at the time of surgery.

4. A referral to the ACS is appropriate, but is not the most important information a 24-year-old male client needs at this time.

CLINICAL JUDGMENT GUIDE: All options are plausible in questions that ask the test taker to identify a priority intervention. The test taker must identify the most important intervention.

15. 1. **Because the client is in the preoperative holding area, the immediate safety need for the client is to inform the operating room personnel so that no latex gloves or equipment will come into contact with the client. Person-to-person communication for a safety issue ensures that the information is not overlooked.**

2. The nurse should document the allergy in the EHR, but because the client is in the

preoperative holding area, this is not the first intervention.

3. The nurse should place a red allergy band on the client, but because the client is in the preoperative holding area, this is not the first intervention.

4. The nurse should always teach the client, but at this time the first intervention is the client's safety, which is why the OR team should be notified.

CLINICAL JUDGMENT GUIDE: When the test question asks the test taker to determine which intervention should be implemented first, it means that all the options could be possible. In this situation, informing the operating room personnel ensures the client safety.

16. 1. The serum blood glucose level requires a venipuncture, which is not within the scope of the UAP's expertise. The laboratory technician would be responsible for obtaining a venipuncture.

2. This is a sterile dressing change and requires assessing the insertion site for infection; therefore, this would not be the most appropriate task to assign to the LPN.

3. The RN should ask the UAP to bathe the client and change bed linens because this is a task the UAP can perform. The LPN could be assigned higher-level tasks.

4. **The UAP can add up the urine output for the 12-hour shift; however, the RN is responsible for evaluating whether the urine output is what is expected for the client.**

CLINICAL JUDGMENT GUIDE: When the test taker is deciding which option is the most appropriate task to delegate or assign, the test taker should choose the task that allows each member of the staff to function at his or her full scope of practice. Do not assign a task to a staff member that requires a higher level of expertise than the staff member has, and do not assign a task to a staff member when another staff member with a lower level of expertise can do it.

17. 1. The client on the ventilator is unstable; therefore, the RN should not delegate any tasks to the UAP.

2. **The UAP can take specimens to the laboratory; it is not medications and not vital to the client.**

3. The client in an Addisonian crisis is unstable; therefore, the RN should not delegate any tasks to the UAP.

4. The UAP cannot assist the HCP with an invasive procedure at the bedside.

CLINICAL JUDGMENT GUIDE: The RN cannot delegate assessment, teaching, evaluation, medication, or an unstable client to a UAP.

18. 1. The client with intracavity radiation could cause problems with the pregnant nurse's fetus, so she should not be assigned to this client.

2. **The pregnant nurse can be assigned to a client who is HIV positive. The nurse must adhere to Standard Precautions.**

3. The cytomegalovirus could harm the nurse's fetus, so the pregnant nurse should not be assigned to this client.

4. The I131 is radioactive iodine and a pregnant nurse should not be near radiation.

CLINICAL JUDGMENT GUIDE: The NCLEX-RN® has questions asking the test taker to address making assignments on units. Nurses who are pregnant should not care for clients whose condition can harm the fetus.

19. 1. The nurse will need to check the client's H&H but not before notifying the HCP. The client is exhibiting signs of disseminated intravascular coagulation (DIC).

2. Monitoring the client's pulse oximeter reading would be an intervention the nurse could implement but it is not the first intervention for a client exhibiting signs of DIC.

3. Applying pressure to the IV site will not help stop the bleeding because the client's coagulation factors have been exhausted. The client must receive heparin therapy.

4. **The client is exhibiting signs of disseminated intravascular coagulation (DIC), which requires intravenous therapy. This is a life-threatening complication that requires immediate medical intervention, so the nurse must notify the HCP first.**

CLINICAL JUDGMENT GUIDE: When the stem of the question provides all the data needed to determine whether the client is in life-threatening distress, the nurse must contact the client's health-care provider.

20. 1. The feelings of the staff are not a violation of the client's rights. Refusing to care for the client is a violation of the client's rights.

2. Transferring the client to the medical unit solves the problem for the critical care unit, but the client's behavior should be addressed by the health-care team. This is not the most appropriate intervention for the nurse manager.

3. **This would be the most appropriate intervention because it allows the staff to have input into resolving the problem. When staff have input into resolving the situation, then there is ownership of the problem.**

4. One nurse cannot be on duty 24 hours a day. The nurse manager should try to allow the staff to identify options to address the client's behavior.

CLINICAL JUDGMENT GUIDE: There will be management questions on the NCLEX-RN® examination. In many instances, there is no test-taking strategy; the nurse must be knowledgeable of management issues.

21. 1. **The client must have lost decision-making capacity because of a condition that is not reversible, or must be in a condition that is specified under state law, such as a terminal, persistent vegetative state, irreversible coma, or as specified in the advance directive. A client who is exhibiting decerebrate posturing is unconscious and unable to make decisions.**

2. The client on a ventilator has not lost the ability to make health-care decisions. The nurse can communicate by asking the client to blink the eyes to yes or no questions.

3. The client receiving dialysis is alert and does not lose the ability to make decisions; therefore, the advance directive should not be consulted to make decisions for the client.

4. Mental retardation does not mean the client cannot make decisions unless the client has a legal guardian who has a durable power of attorney for health care. If the client has a legal guardian, then the client cannot complete an advance directive.

CLINICAL JUDGMENT GUIDE: There will be legal and management of care questions on the NCLEX-RN® examination. Advance directives are included under the category Safe and Effective Environment and subcategory of Management of Care.

22. 1. **This nurse should be sent to the medical unit because, with 18 months' experience,** the nurse is familiar with the hospital routine and would be helpful to the medical unit, but is not the most experienced ICU nurse on duty.

2. The nurse who is still orienting to the unit should not be sent to the medical unit. The nurse in orientation should be kept with the nurse preceptor.

3. The nurse who is new to the hospital should not be sent to a new unit that is unfamiliar.

4. The nurse with 12 years of experience should be kept on in the ICU because this level of expertise would be more helpful for client care than a nurse with 18 months of experience.

CLINICAL JUDGMENT GUIDE: The nurse needs to know management issues for the NCLEX-RN® examination. The nurse with experience in certain areas of nursing would be most appropriate to float to the areas with related types of clients, but the ICU must maintain appropriate staff levels and experience.

23. 1. The family may or may not be able to control the client's behavior, but the nurse should not ask a family member first. The CCU usually has mandated visiting hours.

2. **The nurse should first ensure the client's safety by having someone stay at the bedside with the client, and then call the HCP, and finally apply mitt restraints.**

3. This is a form of restraint and is against the law unless the nurse has a health-care provider's order. This is the least restrictive form of restraint but would not be helpful if the client is pulling at tubes.

4. The nurse must notify the health-care provider before putting the client in restraints; restraints must be used only in an emergency situation, for a limited time, and for the protection of the client.

CLINICAL JUDGMENT GUIDE: The nurse should address the client's safety needs first and be knowledgeable of legal compliance with local, state, and federal requirements, such as The Joint Commission Standards on Restraints and Seclusion.

24. Correct answers are 1 and 2.
1. **The UAP can perform a.m. care; therefore, this can be delegated to the UAP.**
2. **Washing the hair of female clients can be delegated to the UAP.**
3. The UAP should not cut the toenails of clients; this should be referred to a podiatrist.

4. The clients should be turned every 2 hours, not every shift.
5. The housekeeping department should empty the wastebaskets, not the UAP.

CLINICAL JUDGMENT GUIDE: The RN cannot delegate assessment, teaching, evaluation, medications, or an unstable client to the UAP.

25. 1. The RN can praise the UAP for safety concerns, but first the sheet must be removed because it is a form of restraint and is illegal.
    2. The nurse must remove the sheet because it is a restraint. There must be an HCP's order before restraining a client.
    3. The RN should discuss the restraint policy with the UAP but not before removing the restraint.
    4. The nurse should determine if the client needs restraints for safety and then call and obtain the order, but not before removing the sheet. A chest restraint could be used to secure the client to the chair if needed.

CLINICAL JUDGMENT GUIDE: The RN must ensure the UAP provides legal and ethical nursing care to the clients in the long-term care facility.

26. 1. The UAP could place anti-embolism hose on the client.
    2. The UAP should not escort the client outside to smoke a cigarette; the UAP will be off the unit, and this encourages poor health habits.
    3. The LPN, not the UAP, should administer a tube feeding.
    4. The UAP can change a colostomy bag on a client who has had it for an extended period of time, which is implied because the client is in a long-term care center.

CLINICAL JUDGMENT GUIDE: The RN charge nurse should not assign a task to the LPN that a UAP could implement.

27. Correct answers are 1, 2, 3, and 5.
    1. The UAP can apply sequential compression devices to the client on strict bedrest.
    2. The UAP can assist with a portable STAT chest x-ray as long as it is not a female UAP who is pregnant.
    3. The client will need to be premedicated for a wound debridement; therefore, this task cannot be delegated to the UAP.
    4. The UAP can obtain intake and output for clients.
    5. The UAP can assist the client to transfer from the bed to the chair.

CLINICAL JUDGMENT GUIDE: The RN cannot delegate assessment, teaching, evaluation, medications, and an unstable client to the UAP. The nurse cannot delegate premedicating the client.

28. 1. Asking the dietitian to consult with the client is a good intervention, but the nurse should assess the impact of the change in taste on the client.
    2. The client did not report nausea. Antiemetic medication is used to prevent nausea associated with food odors and attempting to eat.
    3. The nurse can recommend an over-the-counter supplement to increase nutrition, but the nurse should first assess the impact of the problem. Over-the-counter supplements are expensive, and the nurse should suggest the client try malts, milkshakes, and fortified soups. Then, if the client does not like or gets tired of the taste, a family member can consume the food and it is not wasted.
    4. Checking the client's weight change over a period of time is the first step in assessing the client's nutritional status and the impact of the taste changes on the client.

CLINICAL JUDGMENT GUIDE: The test taker should employ a systematic approach to problem-solving. The nursing process is a systematic approach, and assessment is the first step of the nursing process.

29. **1. A quality improvement project looks at the way tasks are performed and attempts to see whether the system can be improved. A medication delivery system in which it takes a long time for the nurse to receive a STAT or "now" medication is an example of a system that needs improvement and should be addressed by a quality improvement committee.**
    2. Financial reimbursement of the staff is a management issue, not a quality improvement issue.
    3. Collective bargaining is an administrative issue, not a quality improvement issue.
    4. The number of medication errors committed by a nurse is a management-to-nurse issue and does not involve a systems issue, unless several nurses have committed the same error because the system is not functioning appropriately.

CLINICAL JUDGMENT GUIDE: The NCLEX-RN® examination test plan includes management of care principles such as performance or quality

improvement. The nurse should be knowledgeable of research and quality improvement
initiatives.

30. 1. This is an example of autonomy. The client
needs all pertinent information before
making an informed choice.
2. **This is an example of fidelity. Fidelity
is the duty to be faithful to commitments and involves keeping information
confidential and maintaining privacy and
trust.**
3. This is an example of veracity, the duty to tell
the truth.
4. This is an example of nonmaleficence, the
duty to do no harm. This avoids telling a
client facing surgery that he has cancer.

CLINICAL JUDGMENT GUIDE: The NCLEX-RN®
test plan includes nursing care that addresses
ethical principles, including autonomy, fidelity,
veracity, and nonmaleficence, to name a few.

31. 1. An elevated amylase level would be expected
in a client diagnosed with acute pancreatitis.
The nurse would not need to call the HCP
immediately.
2. An elevated WBC would be expected in a
client diagnosed with a septic (infected) leg
wound. The nurse would not need to call the
HCP immediately.
3. **The urinalysis report showing many
bacteria is indicative of an infection.
Clients receiving chemotherapy are
at high risk of developing an infection. The nurse should notify the HCP
immediately.**
4. This blood glucose level is above normal
range but would not be particularly abnormal
for a client diagnosed with type 1 diabetes.
The nurse would not need to call the HCP
immediately.

CLINICAL JUDGMENT GUIDE: The nurse must
be knowledgeable of normal laboratory values.
These values must be memorized and the nurse
must be able to determine if the laboratory value
is normal for the client's disease process or medications the client is taking. The nurse must be
able to determine which laboratory values require immediate notification of the health-care
provider.

32. 1. The resident's WBC count is within normal
limits and indicates an ability to resist infection. The nurse should not place this resident
in reverse isolation.

2. The resident's H&H is slightly lower than
normal but not low enough to cause dyspnea
during activity. The resident does not need
oxygen.
3. **The resident's platelet count is very low
and could cause the resident to bleed.
The nurse should initiate bleeding
precautions that include not using sharp
blades to shave the resident and using
soft-bristle toothbrushes.**
4. The client is not at risk for developing an
infection. The client does not need his temperature checked every 4 hours.

CLINICAL JUDGMENT GUIDE: This is an alternate
type of question included in the NCLEX-RN®
test plan. The test taker must be able to read
the EHR, be knowledgeable of laboratory data,
and make decisions concerning the nurse's most
appropriate action.

33. 1. **A secondary nursing intervention includes
screening for early detection. The bone
density evaluation will determine the
density of the bone and is diagnostic for
osteoporosis.**
2. Spinal screening examinations are performed
on adolescents to detect scoliosis. This is a
secondary nursing intervention, but not to
detect osteoporosis.
3. Teaching the client is a primary nursing
intervention. This is an appropriate intervention to help prevent osteoporosis, but it is
not a secondary intervention.
4. Discussing risk factors is an appropriate intervention, but it is not a secondary nursing
intervention.

CLINICAL JUDGMENT GUIDE: The test taker
should be aware of primary, secondary, and
tertiary interventions. Primary nursing interventions are focused on prevention of a disease
or injury. Secondary nursing interventions are
aimed at early detection and treatment of a disease or injury. Tertiary nursing interventions are
centered on the management of chronic health
problems.

34. 1. **This is the nurse's priority intervention
because any emergency personnel who
may come into contact with the client
should be aware of the client's allergy.
Allergic reactions to penicillin, an
antibiotic, can kill the client.**
2. The client's pharmacy can be made aware of
the allergy, but this is helpful only when the
client is having prescriptions filled.

3. Unless the client has an allergy to penicillin dust, which is rare, coming into contact with another person taking penicillin will not cause the client to have an allergic reaction.

4. Therapeutic communication allows the client to vent feelings, which is an appropriate intervention, but it is not a priority over teaching the client how to prevent a potentially life-threatening reaction.

CLINICAL JUDGMENT GUIDE: All the options are plausible in questions that ask the test taker to identify a priority intervention. The test taker should identify the most important intervention.

35. 1. The clinic nurse should not confront the staff nurse without objective data that support the allegation.

2. The state board of nurse examiners cannot do anything to the nurse until the nurse has been convicted of the crime. Many states have programs to help addicted nurses, and some states may revoke the nurse's license to practice nursing.

3. **The clinic nurse should report the suspicions so that appropriate actions can be taken, such as a urine drug screen for the nurse, watching the nurse for the behavior, and possibly notifying the police department.**

4. The nurse should follow the chain of command, which does not include the HCP.

CLINICAL JUDGMENT GUIDE: There will be management and legal questions on the NCLEX-RN® examination. In many instances, there is no test-taking strategy; the nurse must be knowledgeable of management issues.

36. 1. The nurse can or cannot place a bandage over the injection site. This is not a priority intervention.

2. Warm compresses will help increase the absorption of the medication, but this is not the priority nursing intervention.

3. The medication injection must be documented in the client's EHR in a clinic, just as it must be in an acute care area, but documentation is not a priority over a possible life-threatening allergic reaction.

4. **The client is at risk for having an allergic reaction to the penicillin, which is a life-threatening complication. Therefore, the client must stay in the waiting room for at least 30 minutes so the nurse can**

determine whether an allergic reaction is occurring.

CLINICAL JUDGMENT GUIDE: The nurse must be knowledgeable of interventions when administering medications to clients and be able to make appropriate decisions to best evaluate the client's response to medications given.

37. 1. Isometric exercises such as weight lifting increase muscle mass. The RN HH nurse should not instruct the HH aide to do these types of exercises.

2. The HH aide may go to the emergency department, but the RN HH nurse should address the aide's back pain. Many times, the person with back pain does not need to be seen in the emergency department.

3. An occurrence report explaining the situation is important documentation and should be completed. It provides the staff member with the required documentation to begin a workers' compensation case for payment of medical bills. However, the RN HH nurse on the phone should help decrease the HH aide's pain, not worry about paperwork.

4. **The HH aide is in pain, and applying ice to the back will help decrease pain and inflammation. The RN HH nurse should be concerned about a coworker's pain. Remember: Ice for acute pain and heat for chronic pain.**

CLINICAL JUDGMENT GUIDE: The test taker should apply the nursing process in selecting the priority action. The HH aide is experiencing pain; therefore, the RN should offer an action to relieve the distress.

38. 1. Allowing the client to stay in bed is inappropriate because a client diagnosed with osteoarthritis should be encouraged to move, which will decrease the pain.

2. A bath at the bedside does not require as much movement from the client as getting up and walking to the shower. This is not an appropriate action for a client diagnosed with osteoarthritis.

3. **Movement and warm or hot water will help decrease the pain; the worst thing the client can do is not to move. The HH aide should encourage the client to get up and take a warm shower or bath.**

4. Osteoarthritis is a chronic condition, and the HCP could not do anything to keep the client from "hurting all over."

CLINICAL JUDGMENT GUIDE: This question requires the test taker to have a basic knowledge of disease processes and interventions to assist the client in recovery postoperatively.

39. **1. The HH aide's responsibility is to care for the client's personal needs, which include assisting with a.m. care.**
    2. The HH aide is not responsible for cooking the client's meals.
    3. The HH aide is not responsible for taking the client to appointments. This also presents an insurance problem, because the client is in the HH aide's car.
    4. Even in the home, the HH nurse should not delegate teaching.

CLINICAL JUDGMENT GUIDE: The RN cannot delegate assessment, evaluation, teaching, medications, or care of an unstable client to a UAP, including an HH aide.

40. 1. If the HH aide is fearful for any reason, the HH aide should not go into the home and should notify the agency. The employee's safety is important. This statement does not require re-teaching.
    2. For safety purposes, the HH aide should be clearly identified when entering the client's neighborhood and home. This statement does not require re-teaching.
    3. The HH aide should be able to contact the RN HH nurse or agency about any potential or actual concerns. This is for the safety of the client as well as the employee. This statement does not require re-teaching.
    4. Standard Precautions apply in the home as in the hospital. If the HH aide has the potential to touch the client's bodily fluids, then the aide should wear gloves and wash hands. The statement indicates the HH aide needs re-teaching.

CLINICAL JUDGMENT GUIDE: According to the NCLEX-RN® test plan, staff education and serving as a resource person to other staff is a component of the management of care.

41. 1. The client diagnosed with Guillain-Barré syndrome would have been on bedrest for days to weeks and would be in a debilitated state; therefore, reports of being tired all the time would be expected. This client would not require the most experienced nurse.
    2. The client diagnosed with pressure ulcers requires meticulous nursing care and a nurse who has experience with wounds.

The most experienced nurse should be assigned this client.
    3. The client with a laryngectomy has received teaching before and after the procedure and would not require extensive teaching or nursing care; therefore, this client would not require the most experienced nurse.
    4. Discharge teaching starts on admission into the home health-care agency; therefore, most of the teaching would have been completed, and this client would not need the most experienced nurse.

CLINICAL JUDGMENT GUIDE: The test taker must determine which client is the most unstable and would require the most experienced nurse.

42. **1. Hospice is a service for clients who have fewer than 6 months to live. If the client has been told she will die "very soon," then this is probably fewer than 6 months. If the client does not die within the 6 months, she will not automatically be discharged from hospice. Each client is assessed individually for the need to remain in hospice care. If the client does not want any heroic measures and wants to die at home, then hospice will provide these services. This intervention would be appropriate for the HH nurse.**
    2. The HH nurse is not responsible for discussing the client's prognosis. The oncologist would have to write a letter stating the client had fewer than 6 months to live to be placed on hospice services. The client should discuss this with the oncologist, not the HH nurse.
    3. Because the client is crying and upset, it would be more appropriate for the nurse to discuss a plan for living and hospice services than to discuss what is going to happen after she dies. At some point this should be done, but this is not an appropriate time.
    4. The client does have a right to a second opinion, but the nurse should not tell the client this unless the client is questioning the diagnosis.

CLINICAL JUDGMENT GUIDE: The test taker should be familiar with hospice and hospice services.

43. 1. The client is an adult and the nurse must respect the client's confidentiality. The nurse does not have to tell the children.
    2. This is giving advice and is not the nurse's role.

3. The nurse not telling the children respects the client's wishes and confidentiality, but the health-care providers should be told of new client circumstances, as the information applies to the client's care.

4. This is a therapeutic response, but the client did not indicate understanding that the nurse would talk about the client's status to the children. The client just wanted to tell someone.

CLINICAL JUDGMENT GUIDE: When the test taker is deciding on a therapeutic response, then the test taker must determine whether there is a response that directly addresses the problem or whether a therapeutic conversation is indicated.

44. 1. **This client may need oxygen or an intervention to keep the client comfortable. This client should be seen first.**

2. This client does not have priority over difficulty breathing.

3. This client does not have priority over difficulty breathing.

4. This client does not have priority over difficulty breathing.

CLINICAL JUDGMENT GUIDE: The test taker should apply some systematic approach when answering priority questions. Maslow's Hierarchy of Needs should be used when determining which client to assess first. The test taker should start at the bottom of the pyramid, where physiological needs are a priority.

45. 1. The medications are not important at this time. The client is bleeding.

2. **The client is at risk for shock. The nurse should take steps to prevent vascular collapse. Starting the IV is the priority.**

3. This is not important in the emergency department.

4. Prevention of circulatory collapse is the priority. The nurse could anticipate an order for a complete blood count (CBC) and a type and crossmatch.

CLINICAL JUDGMENT GUIDE: The test taker must be aware of the setting, which dictates the appropriate intervention. The adjectives will cue the test taker to the setting, in this case, the emergency department. The test taker must also remember the nurse's scope of practice. Starting an IV with normal saline is within a nurse's scope of practice.

46. 1. It is too late to ask this question. This decision must be made before an arrest situation.

2. The nurse should not hesitate to call a code, and a full code must be performed, not a slow code.

3. **These are the first steps of a code.**

4. This should be done by someone at the desk, not by the nurse responding to the emergency.

CLINICAL JUDGMENT GUIDE: The nurse must react immediately in an emergency situation and should not hesitate. The nurse should immediately begin cardiopulmonary resuscitation (CPR) and follow the hospital's protocol.

47. 1. The son has a right to refuse to come to the hospital regardless of what the nurse thinks the son should do. The nurse is unaware of the family dynamics that led to this dilemma.

2. This is only placing another health-care professional in the picture and would not be the best option.

3. **Other family members are more likely to understand the family dynamics and would be the best ones to intervene in the situation.**

4. The nurse should attempt to assist in reconciliation between the client and her son if possible.

CLINICAL JUDGMENT GUIDE: The nurse should always try and support the client if it does not violate any local, state, or federal rules and regulations. Presenting the client's request to the family does not violate any regulations.

48. 1. This is an expected laboratory value for a client diagnosed with leukemia. The client's bone marrow is overproducing immature white blood cells and clogging the bloodstream.

2. **This client is reporting nausea, which is an uncomfortable experience. The nurse should attempt to intervene and treat the nausea. This client should be seen first.**

3. Absent breath sounds are expected in a client diagnosed with lung cancer.

4. A negative biopsy is a good result. This client does not need to be seen first.

CLINICAL JUDGMENT GUIDE: When deciding which client to assess first, the test taker should determine whether the signs and symptoms the client is exhibiting are normal or expected for the client's situation. After eliminating the expected options, the test taker should determine which situation is unexpected or causing the client distress.

49. 1. **Anticipatory nausea is a very real problem for clients diagnosed with cancer**

and undergoing treatment. If this problem is not rectified quickly and progresses to vomiting, the client may not get relief. This medication should be administered first.

2. This is considered mild pain and can be treated after the anticipatory nausea.

3. This is expected and indicates the medication is working. This medication does not have priority.

4. This is a routine medication and can be administered after the nausea and pain medications. Sublingual nitroglycerin is administered for acute chest pain, or angina.

CLINICAL JUDGMENT GUIDE: The test taker should know which medications are a priority and should be administered first by the nurse.

50. 1. Ineffective coping is a psychological problem that would not have priority on the first day after major abdominal surgery.

2. **After major trauma, the body undergoes a fluid shift. The possibility of fluid and electrolyte imbalance is the top priority problem for 1 day after major abdominal surgery.**

3. This could be a priority, but a potential or risk is not a priority over an actual problem.

4. A potential psychological problem would not have priority on the first day after major abdominal surgery.

CLINICAL JUDGMENT GUIDE: When the test taker is deciding which client problem is a priority, physiological problems usually are a priority, and an actual problem is a priority over a potential problem.

51. 1. The nurse should address the client's spiritual faith, but at this time this is not the nurse's best response.

2. The nurse should not leave the client alone after receiving this type of news.

3. The nurse should ensure someone is with the client, but it is not the nurse's best response.

4. **The nurse's best response is to stay with the client and allow the client to vent feelings of denial, fear, and hopelessness.**

CLINICAL JUDGMENT GUIDE: The nurse needs to be able to address the client's psychosocial needs, and allowing the client to vent feelings is an appropriate intervention. A nurse who is a good listener is a very special nurse.

52. Correct answers are 1, 3, and 4.

1. **Spiritual distress can greatly affect the perception of pain. If the client is not**

receiving relief from pain medication, the nurse should explore other variables that could affect the perception of pain.

2. Clients experiencing chronic pain may or may not be able to rate their pain on a pain scale. The client has provided all the information about the pain that is currently needed. The pain is greater than it was before the medication.

3. **This is an alternative to medication that may provide some minimal relief while other interventions are being attempted.**

4. **The nurse should notify the HCP that the current pain regimen is not effective.**

5. This is a condescending statement and would tend to agitate the client more than help.

CLINICAL JUDGMENT GUIDE: This is an alternate type of question included in the NCLEX-RN®. The nurse must be able to select all the options that answer the question correctly. There are no partially correct answers.

53. 1. The RN charge nurse should not assign a UAP to care for a client in spiritual distress. This is outside of the UAP's functions.

2. The charge nurse should not delegate or assign care based on a personal relationship of the nurse with the family. The nurse most qualified to care for the client's needs should be assigned to the client.

3. **A hospice nurse has experience in managing symptoms associated with the dying process. This is the best nurse to care for this client.**

4. A new graduate would not have the experience or knowledge to manage the symptoms as effectively as an experienced hospice nurse.

CLINICAL JUDGMENT GUIDE: When the test taker is deciding which option is the most appropriate task to delegate or assign, the test taker should choose the task that allows each member of the staff to function within his or her full scope of abilities.

54. 1. The nurse could administer the antiemetic, promethazine (Phenergan), as a one-time medication administration or whenever the client asks for it, but this is not a proactive intervention.

2. **Administering the PRN antiemetic, prochlorperazine (Compazine), prophylactically before meals is a proactive stance and assists the client in**

maintaining nutrition goals. **This is the best action. If the client responds well to the regimen, the nurse should discuss changing the order to become a routine medication.**

3. If the client responds well to the PRN prochlorperazine (Compazine), the nurse should discuss changing the order to become a routine medication instead of just PRN.

4. The client did not report pain. Nausea can be caused by pain, but it can also be caused by any number of other reasons. The nurse should be concerned with controlling the symptom.

CLINICAL JUDGMENT GUIDE: This is an alternate type question included in the NCLEX-RN® test plan. The test taker must be able to read a medication administration record (MAR), be knowledgeable of medications, and be able to make decisions as to the nurse's most appropriate intervention.

55. 1. The infection control nurse should evaluate the problem fully before deciding on a course of action.

2. The infection control nurse should assess the staff member's delivery of care and use standard nursing practice before deciding on a course of action with the unit manager.

3. **This is an action that will allow the infection control nurse to observe compliance with standard nursing practices such as hand washing. Once the nurse has attempted to determine a cause, then a corrective action can be implemented.**

4. The entire hospital has not shown an increased infection rate; only one unit has shown an increase.

CLINICAL JUDGMENT GUIDE: The test taker should use a systematic process in determining priority interventions. Assessment is the first step in the nursing process. The infection control nurse should assess the surgical unit to determine possible causes of the increased nosocomial infection rates.

56. 1. The UAP may be at risk of contacting the illness.

2. **The UAP should wear appropriate personal protective equipment when providing any type of care.**

3. The UAP should not be told to skip performing assigned tasks.

4. The fetus is not affected by anthrax, so a pregnant nurse could care for the client,

taking the same precautions as a nurse who is not pregnant.

CLINICAL JUDGMENT GUIDE: The nurse must always put Standard Precautions as a priority when caring for all clients, especially when blood and body fluids are present.

57. 1. The mortuary service is considered part of the health-care team in this case. The personnel in the funeral home should be made aware of the client's diagnosis.

2. **The mortuary service is considered part of the health-care team. In this case, the personnel in the funeral home should be made aware of the client's diagnosis.**

3. The nurse does not need to ask the family for permission to protect the funeral home workers.

4. The nurse, not the HCP, releases the body to the funeral home.

CLINICAL JUDGMENT GUIDE: The test taker must be knowledgeable of the members and role of each member of the multidisciplinary health-care team as well as HIPAA rules and regulations. The client is being placed under the care of the mortuary service and should be aware of the client's diagnosis.

58. 1. This is the correct procedure when coming into contact with blood and body fluids. The nurse does not need to intervene.

2. This may be wasteful if the linens are not used because the client is discharged, but it does not warrant immediate intervention by the RN until the unit has a problem with linen overusage. This action saves the UAP time.

3. This is the correct procedure for getting ice. The nurse does not need to intervene.

4. **Massaging pressure points increases tissue damage and increases the risk of skin breakdown. The RN should intervene and stop this action by the UAP.**

CLINICAL JUDGMENT GUIDE: When the question asks, "Which warrants immediate intervention?" it is an "except" question. Three of the comments indicate the UAP is performing appropriate interventions, and one indicates the intervention is not correct and should be stopped. The RN must ensure the UAP is performing tasks correctly and intervene if the UAP is performing unsafely.

59. 1. **This client has had a common surgical procedure and is not experiencing a complication. The least experienced nurse could care for this client.**

2. Green bile in a T-tube is expected, but a gray tint to the drainage indicates an infection. An experienced nurse should be assigned to this client.

3. A popping feeling when ambulating indicates the hip joint may have dislocated. An experienced nurse should be assigned to this client.

4. A Whipple procedure involves removing most of the pancreas. The symptoms indicate the client is not metabolizing glucose (symptom of diabetes mellitus). An experienced nurse should be assigned to this client.

CLINICAL JUDGMENT GUIDE: The test taker must determine which client is the most stable to be assigned to the least experienced nurse.

60. 1. The unit manager should talk to the client first, not ask the night charge nurse to watch the nurse. This step may be needed if a doubt does surface about the nurse's performance.

2. This is the second step in this process if the manager determines the report is valid.

3. The first step is to discuss the report with the client. This step lets the client know that the client is being heard, and the manager is able to ask any questions to clarify the report.

4. The occurrence may need to be documented and placed in the employee's file, but this is not the unit manager's first intervention.

CLINICAL JUDGMENT GUIDE: The nurse needs to know management issues for the NCLEX-RN® examination. The first step is for the unit manager to seek further information from the client making the negative report.

61. 1. This is blaming the client. No one has the right to abuse the client.

2. The nurse must assess the client's risk from intimate partner violence (IPV) and provide the client a referral to a women's center. This is the nurse's best response.

3. The client does not owe the nurse an explanation of her feelings. This is not a good response to the client.

4. The nurse is advising. The decision whether to leave the abuser or not must be the client's decision.

CLINICAL JUDGMENT GUIDE: The nurse should assist the client to remain free from harm. The nurse should be knowledgeable about appropriate referrals and implement the referral to the most appropriate person or agency.

62. **1. Even though the spouse of the client is making the request, the nurse should still check to make sure that the client has listed the husband as being allowed to receive information. The Health Insurance Portability and Accountability Act (HIPAA) regulations do not allow for release of information to anyone not specifically designated by the client.**

2. The nurse cannot do this unless the client has designated that her husband is allowed to receive information.

3. The HCP as well as the nurse must abide by HIPAA.

4. The HCP is responsible for divulging biopsy results. If the spouse is present when the HCP enters the room and the client allows the spouse to stay, then consent for receiving information is implied.

CLINICAL JUDGMENT GUIDE: The nurse should be knowledgeable of the Health Insurance Portability and Accountability Act (HIPAA) and follow the guidelines related to the exchange of personal health-care information to ensure client medical record confidentiality.

63. 1. Clients diagnosed with acquired immunodeficiency syndrome (AIDS) may have body image disturbance issues related to weight loss and Kaposi's sarcoma lesions, but these are psychological problems, and physiological problems have priority.

2. Impaired coping is a psychological problem, and physiological problems are a priority.

3. The basic problem with a client diagnosed with AIDS is that the immune system is not functioning normally. This increases the risk for infection. This is the priority client problem.

4. Self-care deficit is a psychosocial problem, not a physiological problem.

CLINICAL JUDGMENT GUIDE: The NCLEX-RN® integrates the nursing process throughout the Client Needs categories and subcategories. The nursing process is a scientific, clinical reasoning approach to client care that includes assessment, analysis, planning, implementation and evaluation. The nurse will be responsible for identifying a nursing diagnosis for clients.

64. 1. The infusion of antineoplastic medications is limited to chemotherapy- and biotherapy-competent registered nurses. A qualified

registered nurse should be assigned to this client.

2. This client should be assigned to a registered nurse who can answer the client's questions about the cancer and cancer treatments.

3. **This client is pre-op, and the LPN can prepare a client for surgery. A 22-pound tumor indicates a benign ovarian cyst.**

4. An experienced registered nurse should be assigned to this client because the client is unstable, with unrelenting pain.

CLINICAL JUDGMENT GUIDE: The test taker must determine which client is the most stable to assign to the LPN. The expected care of the client should be included in the LPN's scope of practice.

65. 1. A low WBC count is expected in a client diagnosed with leukemia. This client does not need to be assessed first.

2. A client diagnosed with a brain tumor would be expected to have a mild headache. This client does not need to be assessed first.

3. **The client is upset and crying. When all the information in the options is expected and not life threatening, then psychological issues have priority. This client should be seen first.**

4. Dyspnea on exertion is expected in a client diagnosed with lung cancer. This client does not need to be assessed first.

CLINICAL JUDGMENT GUIDE: The nurse should use some tool as a reference to guide the decision-making process. In this situation, apply Maslow's Hierarchy of Needs. Physiological needs have a priority over psychosocial needs, but the other clients in the stem are not experiencing symptoms unrelated to their diagnosis, so the nurse can address the client with a psychosocial need first.

66. 1. A butterfly rash is one of the clinical manifestations of SLE; this statement does not alert the nurse to a new finding.

2. Photosensitivity is a clinical manifestation of SLE and does not alert the nurse to a new problem.

3. **Bright red in the bedside commode indicates blood, alerting the nurse to possible renal involvement. The health-care provider must be notified so that diagnostic tests can be ordered and steps taken to limit the damage to the kidneys.**

4. Joint stiffness is related to the SLE and is a clinical manifestation. The nurse will medicate the client for pain but the priority is to limit damage to the kidneys.

CLINICAL JUDGMENT GUIDE: When deciding on the priority, the test taker must decide between clinical signs and symptoms that are normally found in clients who have the diagnosis and are not life threatening and those that can be life threatening or life altering.

67. Correct answers are 1, 2, and 3.

1. **The client's daily weights will provide information as to fluid balance and nutrition deficits.**

2. **The client's preferred foods can be used to help increase the client's appetite and should be provided whenever possible on the meal trays.**

3. **The dietitian can be the nurse's best ally when caring for a client diagnosed with nutritional problems.**

4. Glucose levels are monitored when a client is on total parenteral nutrition (TPN), not for a client newly diagnosed with a nutritional problem.

5. This would be appropriate for a client on TPN.

CLINICAL JUDGMENT GUIDE: The test taker must note words that give a hint as to the extent of a problem, such as "newly," in the stem of the question. This eliminates options 4 and 5. Words matter. "Left" or "right," "only," "all"—words such as these can eliminate or define the option.

68. Correct order is 2, 4, 3, 1, 5.

2. **Of the steps listed, the nurse should check the client's hemoglobin and hematocrit. Most health-care facilities have a procedure to administer PRBCs only when the H/H are lower than 8 and 24, respectively. Blood is a scarce commodity, and unless the client is scheduled for surgery there are other means of providing care of the client without the administration of blood products.**

4. **The client must consent to receiving blood and blood products. If the client will not allow the blood to be administered, then the procedure stops there.**

3. **The nurse must determine the client's physical status before picking up the blood in case the nurse assesses a client situation that requires the nurse to get in touch with the health-care provider.**

1. If furosemide (Lasix), a loop diuretic, is ordered, it usually will be administered between the units of blood to prevent fluid volume overload.
5. The blood bags can be returned to the laboratory after the blood has infused.

CLINICAL JUDGMENT GUIDE: Rank order questions can be answered by test takers while "placing" themselves at the client's bedside and asking, "What would I really do first?"

69. **1. The disease-modifying antirheumatic drug methotrexate can cause fetal abnormalities or loss of the fetus. The client should be placed on birth control for the duration of administration of this medication and for 2 years post.**
2. This is a standard instruction for many disease processes, but it is not a priority over the prevention of pregnancy.
3. This medication can produce nausea and nutritional intake is important, but not over preventing a pregnancy and possible complications.
4. Keeping a diary of symptoms and questions is a good idea, but the priority is to prevent an unplanned pregnancy.

CLINICAL JUDGMENT GUIDE: If the stem of the question gives an age, then it is usually an important indication of what the question is actually asking. In this question an age and a gender, female, are both given. Any time the client is a female of childbearing age, the test taker must consider there may be another potential client, the fetus.

70. Correct answers are 1, 4, and 5.
    1. **Females who are HIV positive are at risk for multiple gynecological problems.**
    2. This is not in the scope of practice of a nurse, and clients newly diagnosed are living 20 years or longer with the virus.
    3. Nothing in the stem indicated a need for this referral.
    4. **HAART regimens are responsible for the improved prognosis of HIV-positive clients.**
    5. **A healthy lifestyle will improve the client's ability to maintain her health.**

CLINICAL JUDGMENT GUIDE: When answering "select all" questions, each option is answered as a true or false question. One option cannot rule out another.

CLINICAL SCENARIO ANSWERS AND RATIONALES

The correct answer number and rationale for why it is the correct answer are given in **boldface type.** Rationales for why the other possible answer options are incorrect also are given, but they are not in boldface type.

1. 1. The newly diagnosed client will need to be taught about the disease and about treatment options. The registered nurse cannot delegate teaching to an LPN.
   2. **This is post-procedure care for a stable client; therefore, the RN could assign the LPN to care for this client. The RN cannot assign assessment, teaching, evaluation, or an unstable client to the LPN.**
   3. This client has a hemoglobin of 6, which is extremely low; this client is not stable, and should not be assigned to the LPN.
   4. The LPN cannot administer antineoplastic (chemotherapy) medications to the client.

The chemotherapy nurse must be an RN with additional education in chemotherapy medication.

2. 1. This client is receiving treatments that can have life-threatening side effects; the nurse is not experienced with this type of client.
   2. Bone marrow transplants are very specific to oncology clients; therefore, this client would not be appropriate to assign to a float nurse.
   3. This is expected in a client diagnosed with leukemia, but it indicates a severely low platelet count; a nurse with more experience should care for this client.
   4. **A medical-surgical nurse should be able to care for a client who is 1-day post-operative abdominal surgery; therefore, this client can be assigned to a floating nurse.**

3. 1. This is expected from this client and does not warrant immediate attention.
   2. This is stomatitis and is expected with a client receiving chemotherapy.
   3. **Biological response modifiers that stimulate the bone marrow can increase the client's blood pressure to dangerous levels. This BP is very high and warrants immediate attention.**
   4. This client is experiencing steroid toxicity, which is called "moon" face and is expected; therefore, this client does not warrant immediate intervention.

4. 1. **The RN should assess the client's vital signs to determine if the client is hemorrhaging. Hypotension and tachycardia indicate hemorrhaging, potentially a life-threatening emergency.**
   2. The nurse may need to reinforce the dressing if the dressing becomes too saturated, but this would be after a thorough assessment is completed.
   3. The nurse should assess the situation before notifying the HCP.
   4. The client may be put in the Trendelenburg position.

5. 1. The UAP cannot discontinue a subclavian line; this is a higher level nursing intervention.
   2. **The UAP can empty the JP and reapply negative pressure. The RN cannot delegate assessment, teaching, evaluation, medications, or an unstable client.**
   3. Evaluation of the effectiveness of a PRN medication must be done by the nurse.
   4. The UAP should not do the initial colostomy irrigation, but the client would not have fecal output 2 days postoperative surgery.

6. 1. A ureterosigmoidostomy is a surgical procedure wherein the ureters, which carry urine from the kidneys, are diverted into the sigmoid colon. It is done as a treatment for bladder cancer, where the urinary bladder had to be removed. This is expected; therefore, it does not warrant notifying the HCP.
   2. This may indicate the client has an incisional infection, but the HCP can be notified of this on rounds because this is not life threatening.
   3. The AP and BP are within normal range; therefore, this does not warrant notifying the health-care provider.

4. **This client is exhibiting signs and symptoms of peritonitis, which is a life-threatening complication secondary to abdominal surgery; therefore, the nurse should notify the health-care provider.**

7. 1. Referral to hospice is an appropriate intervention for this client, but it does not apply to the identified problem of anticipatory grieving.
   2. At this time the client should consider funeral arrangements, but the priority intervention is to assist the client to deal with the loss of her life. That is accomplished by therapeutic communication.
   3. **Therapeutic communication is the priority intervention for a client diagnosed with stage 4 cancer and an identified problem of anticipatory grieving. Allowing the client to work through the steps of grieving is accomplished by encouraging the client to express feelings.**
   4. An advance directive and a durable power of attorney for health care are appropriate interventions for a client diagnosed with stage 4 cancer, but this does not address the problem of anticipatory grieving.

8. 1. **An absolute neutrophil count of 681 indicates the client does not have sufficient mature white blood cells or granulocytes to act as a defense against infections. This client needs to be placed in reverse isolation and receive pegfilgrastim (Neulasta), a biological response modifier.**
   2. A platelet count of 175,000 is within normal range. Thrombocytopenia is lower than 100,000; therefore, the RN does not need to intervene.
   3. A red blood cell count of 5,000,000 is within normal limits (3.61 to 5.11 [10^6 cells/microL]).
   4. This H&H is a little low, but it is not life threatening; therefore, this does not warrant intervention.

9. 1. The nurse should complete an assessment of the lesion. This is not a common lesion found on clients.
   2. **This is part of assessing the lesion and should be completed. The ABCDs of skin cancer detection include the following: (1) Asymmetry—Is the lesion balanced on both sides with an even surface? (2) Borders—Are the borders rounded and smooth or notched and indistinct? (3) Color—Is the color a uniform light**

brown or is it variegated and darker or reddish purple? (4) Diameter—A diameter exceeding 4–6 mm is considered suspicious.

3. The nurse should document the findings in the EHR, but it is not the RN's first nursing intervention.

4. Instructing the client to also notify the HCP to assess the lesion should be done, but does not have priority.

10. 1. **The HCP should be made aware of the AD so a do not resuscitate (DNR) order can be written. Only the HCP can write this order. The RN should notify the** HCP to get the DNR written immediately. The order must be written before an arrest occurs or CPR will be initiated.

2. The AD should be discussed between the client and the significant others, but the AD is still valid even if the significant others do not agree and the HCP can write the DNR order based on the client's wishes.

3. A copy is placed in the client's EHR to notify all health-care team members of the client's decisions, but this is not the priority intervention.

4. Giving the client a copy of the AD is good, but it is not the priority intervention.

Women's Health Management

The journey of a thousand miles begins with one step.

—Lao Tzu

QUESTIONS

1. Which client should the postpartum nurse assess **first** after receiving the a.m. shift report?
   1. The client who is reporting perineal pain when urinating
   2. The client who saturated multiple peri-pads during the night
   3. The client who is refusing to have the newborn in the room
   4. The client who is crying because the baby will not nurse

2. Which newborn infant would **warrant immediate** intervention by the nursery nurse?
   1. The 1-hour-old newborn who has abundant lanugo
   2. The 6-hour-old newborn whose respirations are 52
   3. The 12-hour-old newborn who is turning red and crying
   4. The 24-hour-old newborn who has not passed meconium

3. The client in labor is showing late decelerations on the fetal monitor. Which intervention should the nurse implement **first?**
   1. Notify the health-care provider (HCP) immediately.
   2. Instruct the client to take slow, deep breaths.
   3. Place the client in the left lateral position.
   4. Prepare for an immediate delivery of the fetus.

4. The nurse walks into the client's room to check on the mother and her newborn. The client states another nurse just took her baby back to the nursery. Which intervention should the nurse implement **first?**
   1. Initiate an emergency Code Pink, indicating an infant abduction.
   2. Ask the mother to describe the nurse who took the baby.
   3. Determine whether the infant was returned to the nursery.
   4. Ask the mother whether the nurse asked for the code word.

5. The nurse in the labor and delivery department is caring for a client whose abdomen remains hard and rigid between contractions and the fetal heart rate is 100. Which client problem is the **priority?**
   1. Alteration in comfort
   2. Ineffective breathing pattern
   3. Risk for fetal demise
   4. Fluid and electrolyte imbalance

6. The nurse working in a women's health clinic is returning telephone calls. Which client should the nurse contact **first?**
   1. The 16-year-old client who is reporting severe lower abdominal cramping
   2. The 27-year-old primigravida client who is reporting blurred vision
   3. The 48-year-old perimenopausal client who is expelling dark-red blood clots
   4. The 68-year-old client who thinks her uterus is falling out of her vagina

7. The charge nurse has received laboratory results for clients on the postpartum unit. Which client would **warrant** intervention by the nurse?
   1. The client whose white blood cell count is 18,000 mm³
   2. The client whose serum creatinine level is 0.8 mg/dL
   3. The client whose platelet count is 410,000 mm³
   4. The client whose serum glucose level is 280 mg/dL

8. The nurse on the postpartum unit is administering a.m. medications. Which medication should the nurse administer **first?**
   1. The sliding scale insulin to the client diagnosed with type 1 diabetes
   2. The stool softener to the client reporting severe constipation
   3. The non-narcotic analgesic to the client reporting a headache, rated as a 3 on a pain scale of 1 to 10
   4. The rectal suppository for the client reporting hemorrhoidal pain

9. The labor and delivery nurse is performing a vaginal examination and assesses a prolapsed cord. Which intervention should the nurse implement **first?**
   1. Place the client in the Trendelenburg position.
   2. Ask the father to leave the delivery room.
   3. Request the client not to push during contractions.
   4. Prepare the client for an emergency C-section.

10. Which newborn infant would the nursery nurse assess **first?**
    1. The 3-hour-old newborn who weighs 6 pounds and 2 ounces
    2. The 4-hour-old newborn delivered at 42 weeks' gestation
    3. The 6-hour-old newborn who is 22 inches long
    4. The 8-hour-old newborn who was born at 40 weeks' gestation

11. Which antepartum client should the charge nurse assign to the **most** experienced nurse?
    1. The 34-week gestation client who is receiving terbutaline and is on strict bedrest
    2. The 36-week gestation client in active labor whose fetus has a Biophysical Profile of 10
    3. The 38-week gestation client who is 10 cm dilated and 100% effaced
    4. The 42-week gestation client who has been pushing for 4 hours and has yellow amniotic fluid

12. A nurse has been floated from the medical unit to the postpartum unit. Which client should be assigned to this nurse?
    1. The 4-hour postpartum client whose fundus is not midline
    2. The 8-hour postpartum client who has saturated three peri-pads in 1 hour
    3. The 14-hour postpartum client who experienced eclampsia during delivery
    4. The 23-hour postpartum client who is being discharged home this morning

13. Which **priority** intervention should the nurse implement for the 38-week gestation client who is receiving epidural anesthesia?
    1. Place the client in the fetal position.
    2. Assess the client's respiratory rate.
    3. Pre-hydrate the client with intravenous fluid.
    4. Ensure the client has been NPO for 4 hours.

14. The 28-year-old female client is being scheduled for an emergency appendectomy. Which **priority** question should the emergency department nurse ask the client?
    1. "Are you currently breastfeeding?"
    2. "Have you ever had general anesthesia?"
    3. "Do you have any medication allergies?"
    4. "Is there any chance you are pregnant?"

15. Which client should the labor and delivery charge nurse assign to the **most** experienced nurse?
    1. The client who has a fetal heart rate of 130 bpm
    2. The client who has nonreassuring fetal heart rate patterns
    3. The client who is scheduled for a cesarean section
    4. The client having a vaginal birth who has been pushing for 1 hour

16. The female unlicensed assistive personnel (UAP) informs the RN postpartum nurse she has helped the 1-day postpartum client change her peri-pad three times in the last 4 hours. Which action should the nurse implement?
    1. Ask the UAP why the nurse was not notified earlier.
    2. Go to the room and check the client immediately.
    3. Instruct the UAP to massage the client's uterus.
    4. Document the finding in the client's EHR.

17. The unlicensed assistive personnel (UAP) is assisting the RN nursery nurse in the newborn nursery. Which action by the UAP would **warrant** intervention?
    1. The UAP swaddles the infant securely in a blanket.
    2. The UAP uses gloves when changing the infant.
    3. The UAP is bathing the newborn with a bar of soap.
    4. The UAP wipes down the crib with a disinfectant.

18. The charge nurse is making assignments in the labor and delivery department. Which client should be assigned to the **most** experienced nurse?
    1. The 26-week gestational client who is having Braxton Hicks contractions
    2. The 32-week gestational client who is having triplets and is on bedrest
    3. The 38-week gestational client whose contractions are 3 minutes apart
    4. The 39-week gestational client who has late decelerations on the fetal monitor

19. Which tasks should the RN postpartum nurse delegate to the unlicensed assistive personnel (UAP)? **Select all that apply.**
    1. Instruct the UAP to prepare a sitz bath for the client.
    2. Ask the UAP to call the laboratory for a STAT CBC.
    3. Tell the UAP to show the mother how to breastfeed.
    4. Direct the UAP to check the client's fundus.
    5. Have the UAP take the breakfast tray to the client.

20. A nurse from the medical-surgical unit is assigned to the postpartum unit. Which client should the charge nurse assign to the medical-surgical nurse?
    1. The client who has developed mastitis and is trying to breastfeed
    2. The client who had a vaginal hysterectomy and oophorectomy
    3. The client who is having difficulty bonding with her infant
    4. The unmarried client who is giving her child up for adoption

21. The unlicensed assistive personnel (UAP) responds to a code in the newborn nursery. Which task should the RN house supervisor delegate to the UAP?
    1. Tell the UAP to sit with the family in the waiting room.
    2. Give medication to the nurse from the crash cart.
    3. Assist the nurse anesthetist with intubation.
    4. Instruct the UAP to obtain supplies needed during the code.

22. Which action by the RN nursery nurse would **warrant immediate** intervention by the charge nurse?
    1. The nurse allows an experienced volunteer to rock an infant.
    2. The nurse puts a gloved finger into the newborn's mouth.
    3. The nurse performs the Ortolani maneuver on the newborn.
    4. The nurse requests the LPN to bathe the newborn infant.

23. The RN and unlicensed assistive personnel (UAP) are caring for clients on a postpartum unit. Which task would be **most** appropriate for the RN to assign to the UAP?
    1. Perform an in-and-out catheterization.
    2. Complete the client's discharge instructions.
    3. Escort the client to the car and check for a car seat.
    4. Spray anesthetic foam on the client's episiotomy.

24. The RN charge nurse is making assignments on the postpartum unit. Which client should be assigned to the licensed practical nurse (LPN)?
    1. The client who has delivered her sixth baby and has just returned to her room
    2. The client who had a C-section yesterday and is running a low-grade fever
    3. The client who had a vaginal delivery this morning and has foul-smelling lochia
    4. The client who is 1-day post–vaginal delivery who is ambulating in the hall

25. The RN nursery nurse and unlicensed assistive personnel (UAP) are caring for babies in the newborn nursery. Which action by the UAP would **warrant immediate** intervention?
    1. The UAP does not check the mother's identification (ID) band with the infant's ID band.
    2. The UAP brings the mother a full package of newborn diapers.
    3. The UAP applies baby lotion to the newborn while the mother is watching.
    4. The UAP tells the father to support the newborn's head.

26. Which tasks should the RN postpartum nurse delegate to the unlicensed assistive personnel (UAP)? **Select all that apply.**
    1. Tell the UAP to assess the vital signs of the client 4 hours post–vaginal delivery.
    2. Request the UAP to pass out the breakfast trays to the clients.
    3. Instruct the UAP to administer Rho(D) immune globulin to the client who is Rh-negative.
    4. Ask the UAP to remove the client's indwelling urinary catheter.
    5. Direct the UAP to assist the client to breastfeed her infant.

27. Which behavior by the unlicensed assistive personnel (UAP) **warrants immediate** intervention by the RN postpartum nurse?
    1. The UAP helped the client with an episiotomy apply an ice pack to the perineal area.
    2. The UAP pushes the PCA button for the 8-hour post-op C-section client.
    3. The UAP uses nonsterile gloves to remove the client's peri-pad.
    4. The UAP encourages the client to eat all the food on the breakfast tray.

28. The RN charge nurse is making assignments on a postpartum unit that has two registered nurses (RNs), two licensed practical nurses (LPNs), and two unlicensed assistive personnel (UAPs). Which task or assignment is **most** appropriate?
    1. Instruct the UAP to evaluate how the mother and infant are bonding.
    2. Tell the RN to change the sharps container in the medication room.
    3. Ask the LPN to administer ibuprofen to the client experiencing afterbirth pains.
    4. Request the LPN to care for the client who is 6 hours postpartum who had eclampsia.

29. The RN postpartum nurse instructed the unlicensed assistive personnel (UAP) to provide a sitz bath to the postpartum client diagnosed with hemorrhoids. Which **priority** intervention should the nurse implement?
    1. Document the sitz bath in the client's nurse's notes.
    2. Follow-up to ensure the UAP gave the sitz bath.
    3. Assess the client's hemorrhoids every 4 hours.
    4. Discuss the importance of not getting constipated.

30. Which newborn should the RN charge nurse in the nursery assign to the licensed practical nurse (LPN)?
    1. The 4-hour newborn who was born at 42 weeks
    2. The 8-hour newborn who is jittery and irritable
    3. The 18-hour newborn whose mother was addicted to heroin
    4. The 22-hour newborn who was born vaginally after 2 hours of pushing

31. The client being seen in the obstetric (OB) clinic tells the nurse, "I don't think it is right that the judge is making me get a contraceptive implant just because they don't think I am a good mother." Which ethical principle does the requirement violate?
    1. Autonomy
    2. Justice
    3. Fidelity
    4. Beneficence

32. The client in labor is diagnosed with gestational hypertension and has preeclampsia. Which interventions should the nurse implement? **Select all that apply.**
    1. Monitor the IV magnesium sulfate.
    2. Check the client's telemetry monitor.
    3. Assess the client's deep tendon reflexes.
    4. Administer furosemide intravenous push (IVP).
    5. Notify the nursery when delivery is imminent or has occurred.

33. The father of a newborn infant tells the nurse excitedly, "Someone just took our baby and they removed the infant security bracelet." Which action should the nurse implement **first?**
    1. Tell the father to remain calm and go back to his wife.
    2. Assign staff members to block all exits from the unit.
    3. Page a Code Pink, indicating an infant abduction.
    4. Question the father about what exactly happened in the room.

34. The client who delivered twins 3 days ago calls the women's health clinic and tells the nurse, "I am having hip pain that makes it difficult for me to walk." Which statement is the nurse's **best** response?
    1. "I am going to make you an appointment to see the HCP today."
    2. "This often occurs a few days after delivery and will go away with time."
    3. "Are you performing the Kegel exercises 10 to 20 times a day?"
    4. "The pain may decrease if you empty your bladder every 2 hours."

35. The 36-week gestational client has just delivered a stillborn infant. To whom should the nurse refer the client at this time?
    1. The sudden infant death syndrome (SIDS) support group
    2. The maternal child case manager
    3. The hospital chaplain
    4. Child Protective Services

QUESTIONS

36. The client who is 20 weeks' gestation comes to the women's health clinic, and the nurse notices bruises on her abdomen and back. Which response is **most** appropriate for the nurse?
    1. "Please tell me who is abusing you."
    2. "This could cause you to lose your baby."
    3. "How did you get these bruises?"
    4. "Do you feel safe in your home?"

37. The client's boyfriend comes to the postpartum unit and demands his girlfriend's room number. The nurse can smell alcohol on the man's breath, and he is acting erratically. Which action should the nurse implement?
    1. Explain to the client her boyfriend is causing problems.
    2. Give the boyfriend the client's room number.
    3. Contact hospital security to come to the unit.
    4. Tell the boyfriend that he can't be here if he is drunk.

38. The nurse is caring for a postpartum client who is a Jehovah's Witness and needs a Rho(D) immune globulin injection. Which question should the nurse ask the client?
    1. "Rho(D) immune globulin is a blood product. Do you want the injection?"
    2. "Do you know what type blood your husband has?"
    3. "Did you know that you have Rh-negative blood?"
    4. "Do you know whether your insurance will pay for the shot?"

39. The nurse is administering medications to clients on a postpartum floor. Which medication should the nurse **question** administering?
    1. The rubella vaccine to the postpartum client who has a negative titer
    2. The yearly flu vaccine to a client who reports an allergy to eggs
    3. The PPD to a client who suspects she was exposed to tuberculosis
    4. The hepatitis B vaccine to a client who is breastfeeding

40. Which client would the newborn nursery nurse assess **first** after receiving shift report?
    1. The newborn diagnosed with chignon
    2. The newborn diagnosed with caput succedaneum
    3. The newborn diagnosed with a cephalohematoma
    4. The newborn who has a port-wine stain

41. Which statement indicates to the postpartum nurse the discharge teaching to the first-time mother is **effective?**
    1. "I should contact my baby's doctor if she refuses two or more feedings."
    2. "My baby will have green liquid stools for at least 1 month after I take her home."
    3. "I must administer vitamin K elixir once a day with formula to my daughter."
    4. "If my daughter has thick, dark colored stool I will call her doctor."

42. Which primigravida client should the RN clinic nurse report to the certified nurse midwife?
    1. The 12-week gestation client reporting nausea and vomiting
    2. The 24-week gestation client reporting ankle edema
    3. The 32-week gestation client reporting facial edema
    4. The 38-week gestation client reporting urinary frequency

43. The nurse is caring for a postpartum client in the "taking in" phase. Which intervention is **most** appropriate for the nurse to implement?
    1. Ask the client to demonstrate how to change the infant's diaper.
    2. Determine if the client's blood is Rh-negative or Rh-positive.
    3. Allow the client to express feelings about the birth of her infant.
    4. Discuss the advantages of breastfeeding over bottle feeding.

44. Which data should the nurse assess on the 2-hour postpartum client who delivered vaginally? **Select all that apply.**
    1. Palpate the client's breasts.
    2. Check the client's vaginal discharge.
    3. Assess the client's pedal pulses.
    4. Inspect the client's surgical incision.
    5. Check the client's pupillary response.

45. Which interventions should the postpartum nurse teach the client who is breastfeeding her infant to avoid developing mastitis? **Select all that apply.**
    1. Clean nipples and breasts with soap before each breastfeeding.
    2. Ensure the infant latches on correctly to the breast when feeding.
    3. Apply a nipple shield between breastfeeding attempts.
    4. Perform hand washing before breastfeeding the infant.
    5. Wear a breast binder when not breastfeeding.

46. The nurse volunteering in a free clinic has been caring for a female client for several weeks. The client states, "My husband and I have been trying to have a baby for 6 years. What can we do?" Which statement is the nurse's **best** response?
    1. "You should discuss your concerns with the doctor when he comes in."
    2. "Infertility treatments are very expensive and you would have to pay for it."
    3. "You are concerned because you have not been able to get pregnant."
    4. "Have you tried the rhythm method to try and conceive a child?"

47. Which client should the labor and delivery nurse assess **first** after receiving report? **Rank in order of priority.**
    1. The client who is 10 cm dilated, 100% effaced, and "needing to push"
    2. The client who is exhibiting early decelerations on the fetal monitor
    3. The client who is vacillating about whether or not to have an epidural
    4. The client who is upset because her obstetrician is on vacation
    5. The client who is in the latent phase of labor and ambulating in the hallway

48. The nurse is caring for clients in a women's health clinic. Which client **warrants** intervention by the nurse?
    1. The pregnant client who has hematocrit and hemoglobin levels of 11/33
    2. The pregnant client who has a fasting blood glucose level of 100 mg/dL
    3. The pregnant client who has 3+ protein in her urine
    4. The pregnant client who has a white blood cell count of 11.5×10^3/microL

49. The client is 1-day postpartum, and the nurse notes the fundus is displaced laterally to the right. Which nursing intervention should be implemented **first?**
    1. Prepare to perform an in-and-out catheterization.
    2. Assess the bladder using the bladder scanner.
    3. Massage the client's fundus for 2 minutes.
    4. Assist the client to the bathroom to urinate.

50. While making rounds, the charge nurse notices an unattended workstation with the computer screen open to a client's electronic health record (EHR). Which actions should the charge nurse implement? **Select all that apply.**
    1. Ensure automatic locks are functioning for inactive workstations.
    2. Leave the EHR open and find the nurse using the workstation.
    3. Educate the unit staff that an unattended and exposed EHR could be a violation of HIPAA.
    4. Protect the workstation from unauthorized viewing of the EHR.
    5. Notify the Office of Civil Rights about a breach of client health information.

51. The 27-year-old female client is being scheduled for a chest x-ray. Which question should the nurse ask the client?
    1. "Have you ever had a chest x-ray before?"
    2. "Is there any chance you may be pregnant?"
    3. "When was the date of your last period?"
    4. "Do you have any allergies to shellfish?"

52. The clinical manager is reviewing hospital occurrence reports and notes that the nurse on the postpartum unit has documented three medication errors in the last 2 months. Which action should the clinical manager implement **first?**
    1. Initiate the formal counseling procedure for multiple medication errors.
    2. Continue to monitor the nurse for any further medication errors.
    3. Discuss the errors with the nurse to determine whether there is a medication system problem.
    4. Arrange for the nurse to attend a medication administration review course.

53. The nursery nurse is assessing newborns. Which newborn warrants **immediate** intervention by the nurse?
    1. The newborn who remains in the fetal position when lying supine
    2. The newborn whose toes flare out when the lateral heel is stroked
    3. The newborn whose head turns toward the cheek being stroked
    4. The newborn who extends the arms when hearing a loud noise

54. The client on the postpartum unit tells the nurse, "My husband thinks he is the father of my baby but he is not. What should I tell him?" Which response supports the ethical principle of nonmaleficence?
    1. "You should tell him the truth before he becomes attached to the infant."
    2. "How do you think your husband will feel if he knows he is not the father?"
    3. "I know my husband would want to know if my child was his or not."
    4. "Do you know what the real father is planning on doing about the baby?"

55. The chief nursing officer of the hospital instructed the RN clinical manager of the postpartum unit to research a change in the system of delivery of care. Which statement **best** describes modular nursing?
    1. Nurses are designated the primary responsible persons for client care.
    2. The RN and UAP are assigned a group of postpartum clients.
    3. Nursing staff members are divided into groups responsible for client care.
    4. Nurses are assigned specific tasks rather than specific clients.

56. Which action by the postpartum clinical manager would be **most effective** in producing a smooth transition to the new medication delivery system?
    1. Counsel any nurses who cannot adapt to the change.
    2. Ask the staff to vote on accepting the new system.
    3. Have an open-door policy to discuss the change.
    4. Send written documentation of the change by hospital e-mail.

57. During an interview, the pregnant client at the women's health clinic hesitantly tells the nurse, "I think I should let someone know that I can't stop eating dirt. I crave it all the time." Which action should the nurse implement **first?**
    1. Explain that the behavior is normal.
    2. Ask whether the client is taking the prenatal vitamins.
    3. Check the client's hemoglobin and hematocrit (H&H).
    4. Determine whether there is a history of pica in the family.

58. The client who is 16 weeks pregnant calls and tells the office nurse, "My husband's insurance has changed and they say I can't use you anymore." Which statement is the nurse's **best** response?
    1. "If we continue to see you it will cost you a lot more money."
    2. "Because you are already pregnant your insurance company must pay."
    3. "You are concerned you don't want to change doctors at this time."
    4. "Can your husband get a supplemental policy to cover this pregnancy?"

59. The 16-year-old mother of a 1-day-old infant wants her son circumcised. Which intervention should the nurse implement?
    1. Request the client's mother sign the permit.
    2. Determine whether the insurance will pay for the procedure.
    3. Refer the client to the social worker to apply for Medicaid.
    4. Have the 16-year-old client sign for informed consent.

60. The clinical manager is presenting a lecture on collective bargaining. One of the nurse participants asks, "What happens if nurses decide to go on strike?" Which statement is the RN clinical nurse manager's **best** response?
    1. "The UAPs and managers will have to take care of the clients."
    2. "If nurses go on strike it is considered abandonment of the clients."
    3. "The clients will get better care once the nurses' demands are met."
    4. "The nurses must give a 10-day notice before a strike takes place."

61. Which client should the newborn nurse refer to the hospital ethics committee?
    1. The newborn who is anencephalic whose parents want everything done
    2. The newborn whose 16-year-old mother wants to place the infant up for adoption
    3. The newborn whose mother is a known cocaine user and is HIV positive
    4. The newborn who needs a unit of blood and the parents are refusing consent

62. The client has delivered a 37-week gestation infant whose cord was wrapped around the neck. The infant died in utero. Which interventions should the nurse implement? **Select all that apply.**
    1. Allow the mother to hold and cuddle the infant.
    2. Have the mother transferred to the medical unit.
    3. Encourage the father to talk about his child to the nurse.
    4. Recommend to the parents that the child be cremated.
    5. Discourage the client from giving the infant a name.

63. Which action would be **most** important for the clinical manager to take regarding a primary nurse who has received numerous compliments from the clients and their families about the excellent care she provides?
    1. Ask the nurse what she does that makes her care so special.
    2. Document the comments on the nurse's performance evaluation.
    3. Acknowledge the comments with a celebration on the station.
    4. Take no action because excellent care is expected by all nurses.

64. The client asks the nurse in the women's health clinic, "I am so miserable during my premenstrual syndrome I can't even go to work. What can I do?" Which teaching interventions should the nurse implement? **Select all that apply.**
    1. Increase the amount of colas and coffee daily.
    2. Avoid simple sugars such as cakes and candy.
    3. Drink at least two glasses of red wine nightly.
    4. Decrease the intake of foods high in salt.
    5. Adhere to a regular schedule for sleep.

65. The nurse is completing the admission assessment on a 12-weeks-pregnant client who is visiting the women's health clinic. The client tells the nurse, "I am a vegan and will not drink any milk or eat any meat." Which intervention should the nurse implement?
    1. Recommend the client eat grains, legumes, and nuts daily.
    2. Suggest that the client eat at least two eggs every day.
    3. Discuss not adhering to the vegan diet during pregnancy.
    4. Explain that a vegan diet does not require iron supplements.

66. The charge nurse of the postpartum unit is making assignments. Which clients should be assigned to the medical-surgical nurse who has been assigned to the unit for the day? **Select all that apply.**
   1. The client who delivered 4 hours ago and is reporting pain
   2. The client who is being discharged and needs discharge teaching about breastfeeding
   3. The client who is being treated for HELLP syndrome
   4. The client who is 30 weeks' gestation on a fetal monitor
   5. The client who is gravida 8 and on a Pitocin drip

67. The labor and delivery nurse is preparing to assist the anesthetist to insert an epidural catheter in a client nearing delivery. Which picture indicates the correct position to assist the client to assume?
   1. Position 1

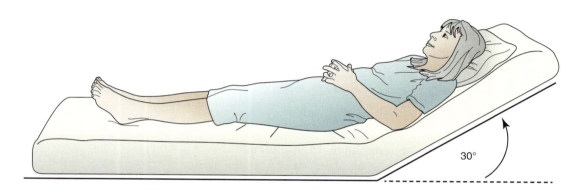

   2. Position 2

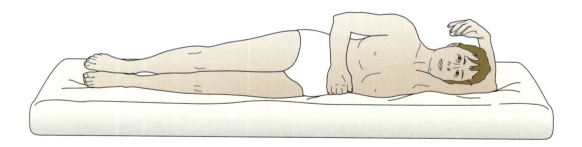

   3. Position 3

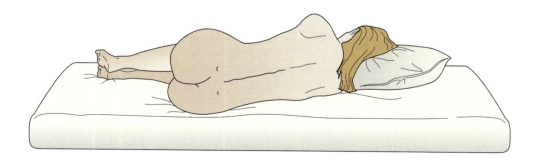

4. Position 4

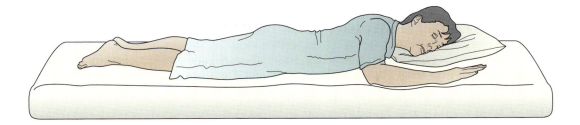

68. The 34-week pregnant client in the labor and delivery unit is on a magnesium sulfate intravenous drip for eclampsia. The labor and delivery nurse assesses the client's reflexes as absent with repeated stimulation. Which nursing intervention should the nurse implement **first?**

Deep Tendon Reflex Scale
0 = absent despite reinforcement
1 = present only with reinforcement
2 = normal
3 = increased but normal
4 = markedly hyperactive, with clonus

1. Notify the obstetrician.
2. Document the finding as absent.
3. Have another nurse assess the reflexes.
4. Turn off the magnesium drip.

69. The public health nurse is working at a sexually transmitted infection (STI) clinic. The female client has been diagnosed with gonorrhea. Which nursing interventions should the nurse implement? **Rank in order of performance**.
1. Notify the client's sexual partners of potential exposure to an STI.
2. Complete the report to the Centers for Disease Control and Prevention.
3. Teach the client safe sex procedures.
4. Administer the prescribed antibiotic to the client.
5. Ask the client to provide a list of sexual partners.

70. The emergency department nurse observed a motor vehicle accident (MVA) on the way home from work. The driver of one of the vehicles is obviously several months pregnant. Which nursing intervention should the nurse implement **first?**
1. Determine the length of gestation.
2. Assess the driver for signs of trauma.
3. Check to see if the client was wearing a seat belt.
4. Monitor for fetal heart tones.

MATERNAL-CHILD CLINICAL SCENARIO

The RN charge nurse is on the maternal child unit for the 7 a.m.–7 p.m. shift in a level II trauma, demographically diverse population, county hospital. She has three additional RNs and a new graduate nurse who has just completed a 3-month orientation along with one unlicensed assistive personnel (UAP) working on the unit. There are three labor and delivery clients, seven newborn nursery clients, and eight postpartum clients.

1. Which postpartum client should the charge nurse assign to the new graduate nurse?
   1. The client who has hemorrhoids and is reporting pain
   2. The client who saturated multiple peri-pads during the night
   3. The client who is refusing to have the newborn in the room
   4. The client who is crying because the baby will not nurse

2. Which newborn infant would **warrant immediate** intervention by the nursery nurse?
   1. The 1-hour-old newborn who has tiny, white, hard spots on the nose
   2. The 6-hour-old newborn who has a respiratory rate of 24
   3. The 12-hour-old newborn who is turning red and crying
   4. The 18-hour-old newborn who has a viscous, sticky tar, odorless stool

3. The laboring client is showing late decelerations on the fetal monitor. After placing the client in the left lateral position, which intervention should the labor and delivery nurse implement **first?**
   1. Notify the client's obstetrician immediately.
   2. Encourage the client to pant when the contraction occurs.
   3. Administer oxytocin intravenously.
   4. Prepare for an immediate delivery of the fetus.

4. The charge nurse is monitoring laboratory results for clients on the postpartum unit. Which client would **warrant** intervention by the postpartum nurse?
   1. The client who had a vaginal delivery and who has a white blood cell count of 15×10^3/microL
   2. The client who had a C-section who has a serum potassium level of 4.8 mEq/L
   3. The client diagnosed with preeclampsia who has a platelet count of 90×10^3/microL
   4. The client diagnosed with gestational diabetes who has a serum glucose level of 140 mg/dL

5. The charge nurse is making assignments in the labor and delivery department. Which client should be assigned to the **most** experienced nurse?
   1. The 26-week gestational client who is having Braxton Hicks contractions
   2. The 32-week gestational client who is having twins and is on bedrest
   3. The 38-week gestational client who is 100% effaced and 10 cm dilated
   4. The 39-week gestational client who has early decelerations on the fetal monitor

6. Which task should the RN postpartum nurse delegate to the unlicensed assistive personnel (UAP)?
   1. Instruct the UAP to take the client whose fundus is not midline to the bathroom.
   2. Ask the UAP to take the vital signs for the client diagnosed with HELLP syndrome.
   3. Tell the UAP to assist the mother with breastfeeding her newborn daughter.
   4. Request the UAP to administer Rho(D) immune globulin to the mother who is Rh-negative.

7. A float nurse from the medical-surgical unit is assigned to the postpartum unit. Which client should the charge nurse assign to the float nurse?
    1. The client who had a fetal demise at 34 weeks' gestation
    2. The client who has a boggy fundus that massaging has not helped
    3. The client who has had six saturated peri-pads in the last shift
    4. The unmarried client who is giving her child up for adoption

8. The postpartum nurse is administering medications to clients on a postpartum floor. Which medication should the nurse **question** administering?
    1. The yearly flu vaccine to a client who reports an allergy to tomatoes
    2. The hepatitis B vaccine to a client who is breastfeeding
    3. The Rho(D) immune globulin to the mother who is Rh-negative and whose infant is Rh-positive
    4. The rubella vaccine to the postpartum client who has a positive titer

9. Which client should the newborn nursery nurse assess **first** after receiving shift report?
    1. The Asian newborn who has purple-colored splotches on the lower back
    2. The Caucasian newborn with a purple-colored area on the right side of the face
    3. The Hispanic newborn who has a red rash, "flea bites," on the chest
    4. The African American newborn who has edema between suture lines

10. The nursery nurse is assessing newborns. Which newborn would require **further** assessment by the nurse?
    1. The newborn who remains in the fetal position when lying supine
    2. The newborn whose toes flare out when the lateral heel is stroked
    3. The newborn who acts as if he is walking when his feet are placed on a hard surface
    4. The newborn who grasps the finger when it is placed in his hand

The correct answer number and rationale for why it is the correct answer are given in **boldface type.** Rationales for why the other possible answer options are incorrect also are given, but they are not in boldface type.

1. 1. This pain may be related to an episiotomy or perineal tear, but this client is not a priority over a client who may be hemorrhaging.
   2. **Saturating multiple peri-pads indicates heavy bleeding, which may indicate hemorrhaging. The nurse should assess this client first.**
   3. The nurse needs to assess this client for possible maternal and infant bonding problems, but this is a psychosocial issue that should be addressed after a physiological issue, such as possible hemorrhaging.
   4. This client is going to require some time to be taught, but this is not a priority over a client who is hemorrhaging.

CLINICAL JUDGMENT GUIDE: The test taker should apply a systematic approach when answering a priority question. Maslow's Hierarchy of Needs should be used when determining which client to assess first. The test taker should start at the bottom of the pyramid, and physiological needs are the priority.

2. 1. The newborn diagnosed with lanugo is normal and would not warrant immediate intervention by the nurse.
   2. The normal respiratory rate for a newborn is 30 to 60; therefore, this would not warrant immediate intervention.
   3. The newborn who is turning red when crying is not in distress; therefore, this would not warrant immediate intervention.
   4. **The newborn who has not passed meconium 24 hours after birth must be evaluated for intestinal obstruction or a congenital abnormality. This could be caused by an imperforate anus, Hirschsprung's disease, cystic fibrosis, or several other possibilities. This newborn warrants immediate intervention.**

CLINICAL JUDGMENT GUIDE: When deciding which client to assess first, the test taker should determine whether the signs and symptoms the client is exhibiting are normal or expected for the client's situation. After eliminating the expected options, the test taker should determine which situation is more life threatening.

3. 1. The nurse should first intervene to increase blood supply to the fetus; therefore, notifying the HCP is not the nurse's first intervention.
   2. Slow, deep breaths may help decrease the mother's anxiety, but the nurse's first intervention is to increase blood supply to the fetus.
   3. **The left lateral position will improve placental blood flow and oxygen supply to the fetus. This should be the nurse's first intervention.**
   4. The nurse should prepare for an emergency C-section, but this is not the nurse's first intervention.

CLINICAL JUDGMENT GUIDE: When the test taker is deciding when to notify an HCP, the test taker should look at the other three options and determine whether one of the options should be implemented before notifying the HCP. Another option may, for example, provide information the HCP will need in order to make a decision.

4. 1. Once the nurse definitely determines the infant is not in the nursery, then a Code Pink should be initiated. This notifies all hospital personnel of a possible infant abduction.
   2. This will be done if the infant was not returned to the nursery, but this is not the first intervention.
   3. **The nurse should first determine whether another staff member returned the infant to the nursery. Most hospitals have infant security bracelets to prevent abduction from the hospital. The alarm has not sounded and the nurse should not call a false alarm.**
   4. There are many safety precautions to prevent infant abductions, and most facilities have a code word that is changed daily. The mother must ask anyone who wants to take the infant out of the mother's room for the code word. This is not the nurse's first intervention.

CLINICAL JUDGMENT GUIDE: The test taker should apply the nursing process when the question asks, "Which intervention should the nurse implement first?" All answers are plausible and the test taker must identify the most important intervention.

5. 1. Pain for the mother is a priority, but it is not a priority over potential death of the fetus.
   2. The client is not having trouble breathing; therefore, this would not be a priority problem. Altered gas exchange would be an appropriate problem for the fetus.

3. The client is exhibiting signs of abruptio placentae, and a decreased heart rate indicates a compromised fetus. This problem will lead quickly to the death of the fetus. Therefore, it is the priority problem.
4. All pregnant women experience an increase in fluid volume status and some resulting electrolyte imbalance; therefore, this is not a priority problem.

CLINICAL JUDGMENT GUIDE: The NCLEX-RN® integrates the nursing process throughout the examination. The nursing process is a scientific, clinical reasoning approach to client care that includes assessment, analysis, planning, implementation, and evaluation. The nurse will be responsible for identifying nursing diagnoses for clients.

6. 1. The client reporting severe lower abdominal cramping should be called to determine whether she is currently menstruating, but this is not a priority over a pregnant client with symptoms of preeclampsia.
2. **Blurred vision is a symptom of preeclampsia, and this is the client's first pregnancy. This client should be contacted first and told to come into the clinic for further evaluation.**
3. The expulsion of dark-red blood clots indicates the client is going through menopause. This is not a life-threatening situation because dark-red blood does not indicate frank bleeding.
4. This is uncomfortable for the client and indicates the need for a hysterectomy or instructions in the insertion and use of a pessary device to hold the uterus in place, but it is not life threatening.

CLINICAL JUDGMENT GUIDE: When deciding which client to assess first, the test taker should determine whether the signs and symptoms the client is exhibiting are normal or expected for the client's situation. After eliminating the expected options, the test taker should determine which situation is more life threatening.

7. 1. The white blood cell count rises normally during labor and postpartum—up to 25×10^3/microL; therefore, this does not warrant intervention.
2. The serum creatinine level is within normal limits; therefore, this client does not warrant immediate intervention.
3. Platelets show marked increase 3 to 5 days after birth, but the client who is 1 to 2 days postpartum would have a slightly increased

platelet count. Normal platelet count is 140 to 400×10^3/microL, so this client's count is within normal limits.
4. This glucose level is elevated, and the nurse should investigate further to determine why the glucose level is abnormal. The normal fasting glucose level is lower than 100 mg/dL and random lower than 200 mg/dL.

CLINICAL JUDGMENT GUIDE: The test taker must be knowledgeable of laboratory data and be able to make appropriate decisions based on the information.

8. 1. **The client diagnosed with type 1 diabetes must receive insulin before eating; therefore, this must be administered first.**
2. The stool softener will take several days to soften the stool; therefore, this medication does not need to be administered first.
3. The client reporting a headache is not a priority over a type 1 diabetic client who needs sliding scale coverage. This client should receive medication after the insulin-dependent diabetic receives insulin.
4. The rectal suppository is administered to shrink the hemorrhoids and has a local anesthetic effect, but it would not be a priority over the sliding scale insulin.

CLINICAL JUDGMENT GUIDE: The test taker should know which medications are a priority, such as life-sustaining medications, insulin, and mucolytics (Carafate). These medications should be administered first by the nurse.

9. 1. **A prolapsed cord is an emergency situation because the prolapsed cord could compromise the fetus's blood supply. Placing the client in the Trendelenburg position will cause the fetus to shift in the uterus and take the pressure off the umbilical cord. The safety of the fetus is the priority.**
2. In emergency situations, the nurse may need to request visitors to leave the delivery room, depending on how visitors are acting during the crisis, but this is not the first intervention.
3. This is an appropriate intervention, but the nurse's priority is getting pressure off the umbilical cord.
4. The fetus is in distress and the nurse must prepare for an emergency C-section, but it is not the nurse's first intervention.

CLINICAL JUDGMENT GUIDE: The test taker should apply the nursing process when the question asks the nurse, "Which intervention should be implemented first?" If the client is in distress, the nurse should do something. In this question, the fetus is in distress and the nurse should manipulate the position of the mother to increase blood flow through the umbilical cord.

10. 1. The newborn who weighs 6 pounds and 2 ounces is within normal weight for a newborn; therefore, the nurse would not need to assess this baby first.
    2. **The newborn delivered at 42 weeks is postmature and is at risk for hypoglycemia and hypothermia because the placenta begins to deteriorate after 40 weeks and subcutaneous fat is utilized to support the infant's life. The nurse should assess this baby first just because of the 42-week gestation.**
    3. The newborn who is 22 inches long is longer than most infants, but this infant would not need to be assessed first.
    4. The newborn delivered at 40 weeks' gestation is within normal gestation time; therefore, the nurse would not need to assess this baby first.

CLINICAL JUDGMENT GUIDE: When deciding which client to assess first, the test taker should determine whether the signs and symptoms the client is exhibiting are normal for the client's situation. After eliminating the expected options, the test taker should determine which situation is more life threatening.

11. 1. This client is preterm but is stable according to the data in the option. Terbutaline (Brethine) is a uterine relaxant and the client should be on strict bedrest.
    2. A Biophysical Profile is used to determine if the fetus is ready to make the trip down the vaginal canal. Up to two points each are given for fetal breathing movements, gross body movements, fetal tone (flexion), amniotic fluid volume, and reactive (or not) non-stress test, with a score of 10 being the best.
    3. This client is ready to deliver the fetus; therefore, the most experienced nurse would not need to be assigned to this client.
    4. **This client is postmature and the fetus is at risk for meconium aspiration; therefore, this client should be assigned to the most experienced nurse.**

CLINICAL JUDGMENT GUIDE: The test taker must determine which client is least stable and assign this client to the most experienced nurse.

12. 1. This client needs to urinate because the number one reason for a displaced fundus is a full bladder. Because a medical nurse may not know how to palpate a fundus, this client should be assigned to a more experienced nurse.
    2. This client may be hemorrhaging and should be assigned to a more experienced nurse.
    3. **This client is still at risk for a seizure, but a medical nurse should be able to care for a client who has a seizure. This client should be assigned to the medical nurse.**
    4. This nurse must evaluate the mother's ability to care for the new infant or complete discharge teaching; therefore, a more experienced nurse should be assigned to this client.

CLINICAL JUDGMENT GUIDE: The test taker must determine which client is most stable or which client may be at risk for a complication a medical nurse could care for safely.

13. 1. The client should be in the fetal position, but the possibility of anesthesia ascending the spinal cord is the priority.
    2. **If the anesthesia ascends the spinal cord, the client will quit breathing; therefore, this is the priority intervention.**
    3. The client should be prehydrated, but it is not a priority over the airway.
    4. Clients are made NPO to prevent aspiration pneumonia secondary to vomiting if the client is undergoing general anesthesia, not epidural anesthesia.

CLINICAL JUDGMENT GUIDE: The test taker should apply Maslow's Hierarchy of Needs. Airway is the priority. Remember that priority intervention means all the options are something the RN can implement, but there is only one correct option.

14. 1. There is nothing in the stem of the question that suggests the client has an infant. It is a question the nurse could ask the female client, but it is not a priority.
    2. This is a question the nurse could ask the client, but because the question states the client is a 28-year-old female, age and gender are pertinent to which option the test taker should select.
    3. This is a question all clients should be asked, but the adjectives describing the client as "a

28-year-old" and "female" should identify the fourth option as the most priority question.

4. Because the client will have to have anesthesia for the surgery and the client is within childbearing age, the nurse should determine whether the client is pregnant.

CLINICAL JUDGMENT GUIDE: The test taker must acknowledge adjectives in questions when determining the correct answer. When the stem gives the client a gender and an age, it is pertinent to the correct answer.

15. 1. Normal fetal heart rate is 110 to 160 beats a minute, so this client is stable.
    2. Nonreassuring fetal heart rate patterns indicate the fetus is in danger, which requires a more experienced nurse.
    3. A scheduled C-section is a stable client, so a less experienced nurse could care for this client.
    4. Pushing for 1 hour before a vaginal birth is normal; therefore, a less experienced nurse could care for this client.

CLINICAL JUDGMENT GUIDE: The most experienced nurse should be assigned to the most critical client. Nonreassuring fetal heart patterns indicate the infant is in distress.

16. 1. The RN should first assess the client to determine whether the UAP was negligent in reporting before talking to the UAP.
    2. This client may or may not be experiencing excessive bleeding, but the nurse's first intervention is to assess the client.
    3. Excessive bleeding could indicate the uterus is boggy, which would require the RN to massage the uterus. This assessment and intervention cannot be delegated to a UAP.
    4. The nurse should not document any information before verifying the client's situation.

CLINICAL JUDGMENT GUIDE: Any time the nurse receives information from another staff member about a client who may be experiencing a complication, the nurse must assess the client. The nurse should not make decisions about the client's needs based on another staff member's information.

17. 1. The infant should be securely swaddled in a blanket to maintain body heat.
    2. The UAP should wear nonsterile gloves when being exposed to blood or body fluids.
    3. When bathing a newborn, soap is not necessary. Soap can be very drying to the skin; therefore, this action warrants intervention by the nurse.

4. The UAP should wipe the crib with disinfectant to decrease the potential for contamination.

CLINICAL JUDGMENT GUIDE: When the question asks, "Which warrants immediate intervention?" it is an "except" question. Three of the actions are appropriate for the UAP, and one is incorrect.

18. 1. Braxton Hicks contractions are irregular contractions of the uterus throughout the pregnancy and are not true labor. This client would not need to be assigned to the most experienced nurse.
    2. The client having triplets on bedrest is not in imminent danger; therefore, this client would not need the most experienced nurse.
    3. This client is progressing normally and would not require the most experienced nurse.
    4. Late decelerations on the fetal monitor indicate fetal distress; this is a life-threatening situation, and an emergency C-section may be necessary. The charge nurse should assign the most experienced nurse to this client.

CLINICAL JUDGMENT GUIDE: The test taker must determine which client is the most unstable and assign this client to the most experienced nurse.

19. Correct answers are 1 and 5.
    1. The UAP can provide hygiene care to the client. A sitz bath requires the UAP to check the temperature of the water and does not require nursing judgment.
    2. The UAP's primary responsibility is direct client care. The unit secretary, not the UAP, should call the laboratory.
    3. The RN cannot delegate teaching to the UAP.
    4. The RN cannot delegate assessment; therefore, the UAP cannot check the client's fundus.
    5. The UAP can take the meal tray to the client.

CLINICAL JUDGMENT GUIDE: This is an alternate type of question included in the NCLEX-RN®. The RN must be able to select all the options that answer the question correctly. There are no partially correct answers. Remember, the nurse cannot delegate assessment, evaluation, teaching, administration of medications, or care of an unstable client to a UAP.

20. 1. A client diagnosed with mastitis who is trying to breastfeed requires a nurse experienced in the postpartum unit who can teach the

client about breastfeeding and assess for complications.

2. **This is a routine surgical procedure that would not require the nurse to have any specialized postpartum experience. This client would be most appropriate to assign the float nurse who has experience on the medical-surgical unit.**

3. A client who is having difficulty bonding would require a nurse with experience in the postpartum unit to care for the client as well as document pertinent information if bonding does not occur.

4. There are many legal issues surrounding an adoption as well as caring for the mother who is giving up her child; this client should be assigned a nurse more experienced in postpartum care.

CLINICAL JUDGMENT GUIDE: The test taker must determine which client requires the least amount of specialized knowledge and assign the float nurse to that client. Remember, legal issues, teaching, and psychosocial concepts require the more experienced nurse.

21. 1. An experienced nurse, a chaplain, or social worker should be assigned to sit with the family during this crisis.

2. Even though the UAP is not administering the medication, the UAP should not be handling the RN medication in a crisis situation.

3. The UAP cannot assist with intubation; this must be assigned to a registered nurse or respiratory therapist.

4. **The UAP can stand by and be ready to obtain any supplies needed for the code. This would be a most appropriate task to delegate in an emergency situation.**

CLINICAL JUDGMENT GUIDE: The RN cannot delegate assessment, teaching, evaluation, medications, or an unstable client to a UAP. Tasks that cannot be delegated are nursing interventions that require nursing judgment.

22. 1. Volunteers are often asked to rock irritable infants so that the nurse can have more time to perform higher-level nursing care for the infants. This action would not warrant immediate intervention by the charge nurse.

2. The nurse is using palpation to determine whether the newborn has a cleft palate. This assessment is within the scope of practice for the newborn nursery nurse.

3. **The Ortolani maneuver is performed to assess developmental hip dysplasia. Only**

a pediatrician or a nurse practitioner should perform this maneuver because it can cause further damage if it is done incorrectly.

4. The LPN can bathe a newborn infant; therefore, this would not warrant immediate intervention by the RN charge nurse.

CLINICAL JUDGMENT GUIDE: When the question asks, "Which warrants immediate intervention?" it is an "except" question. Three of the actions are appropriate, whereas one action is not.

23. 1. This client is unable to urinate, which may or may not be a complication of the delivery and anesthesia. Catheterization is a sterile procedure, and many facilities do not allow the UAP to perform sterile procedures. The RN should not delegate this task.

2. This is teaching, and the RN cannot delegate teaching to the UAP.

3. **The infant must be transported in a car safety seat. The UAP can determine whether there is a car seat and take the appropriate action if there is not one.**

4. Anesthetic foam is a topical medication, and the RN cannot delegate medication administration to the UAP.

CLINICAL JUDGMENT GUIDE: The RN cannot delegate assessment, evaluation, teaching, medications, or an unstable client to a UAP.

24. 1. The more pregnancies the client has had, the more likely it will be that the uterus will not contract to prevent bleeding. The RN should be assigned to this client.

2. A client diagnosed with a fever and a surgical incision may be experiencing a complication and should be assigned to an RN.

3. Foul-smelling lochia indicates the client has an infection; therefore, this client should not be assigned to the LPN.

4. **The client who is ambulating is stable and not exhibiting any complications; therefore, this client should be assigned to the LPN.**

CLINICAL JUDGMENT GUIDE: The test taker must determine which client is the most stable, which makes this an "except" question. Three clients are either unstable or have potentially life-threatening conditions.

25. 1. **The Joint Commission and safety standards mandate that all hospital personnel must check the parent's ID band with the infant's ID band before releasing the infant to the care of the mother or father.**

2. The UAP can bring diapers to the mother; therefore, this would not warrant immediate intervention.
3. The UAP can put lotion on the infant while the mother is watching because this is not teaching.
4. This may be teaching, but the UAP is making sure the newborn is safe; therefore, this action would not warrant immediate intervention.

CLINICAL JUDGMENT GUIDE: When the question asks, "Which warrants immediate intervention?" it is an "except" question. Three of the actions are appropriate, whereas one action is not.

26. Correct answers are 1, 2, and 4.
    1. **The UAP can take vital signs on a stable client.**
    2. **The UAP can pass out breakfast trays.**
    3. Rho(D) immune globulin (RhoGAM) is a medication that cannot be delegated to the UAP.
    4. **The UAP can remove an indwelling urinary catheter. It is not a medication.**
    5. The UAP should not assist with breastfeeding. The RN must perform teaching and evaluate the breastfeeding.

CLINICAL JUDGMENT GUIDE: The RN cannot delegate assessment, teaching, evaluation, medication, or an unstable client to a UAP.

27. 1. Ice packs are applied to acute injuries, so this intervention is appropriate for the UAP.
    2. **Only the client pushes the PCA pump; therefore, this action requires immediate intervention by the nurse.**
    3. Using nonsterile gloves is appropriate when handling blood and body fluids, so this is an appropriate intervention for the UAP.
    4. The UAP can encourage a client to eat the food on the breakfast tray; therefore, this behavior does not warrant immediate intervention.

CLINICAL JUDGMENT GUIDE: The phrase "warrants immediate intervention" means one of the options is inappropriate for the UAP to perform or the UAP is performing the task inappropriately.

28. 1. The UAP cannot assess, teach, evaluate, administer medications, or care for an unstable client.
    2. The sharps container can be changed by a housekeeper, UAP, or an LPN, so this is not an appropriate task to assign to the RN.

3. **The LPN can administer medications, and ibuprofen has an antiprostaglandin effect that is appropriate for a client experiencing afterbirth pains.**
4. The RN charge nurse should not assign a LPN to an unstable client. This client may have another seizure and should be monitored closely for at least 24 to 48 hours post-delivery.

CLINICAL JUDGMENT GUIDE: The RN must know what can be delegated and assigned to the UAP and LPN. There will be numerous questions on the NCLEX-RN® concerning delegation and assignment. Remember that the nurse may not delegate the following to the UAP: assessment, teaching, evaluation, administering medications, or the care of an unstable client.

29. 1. The RN should document the sitz bath, but it is not a priority over making sure the UAP gave the sitz bath.
    2. **The most important intervention for the nurse to do when delegating a task is to follow-up to ensure it was done.**
    3. The RN should assess the client, but the priority intervention is to ensure the UAP completed the assigned task.
    4. The nurse should ensure the client does not get constipated, but the test taker must read the stem of the question to determine how to answer it correctly.

CLINICAL JUDGMENT GUIDE: When the question asks which option is the priority intervention, it means one or more of the options are something a nurse can implement. The test taker must determine what the question is asking in order to select the right answer. There is always something in the stem of the question that will help the test taker determine the correct option.

30. 1. This newborn is postmature and may have complications, so she should be assigned to an RN.
    2. The newborn is experiencing hypoglycemia and should be assigned to an RN.
    3. The newborn is at risk for going through heroin withdrawals and should be assigned to an RN.
    4. **The newborn born vaginally after 2 hours' labor is stable and should be assigned to the LPN.**

CLINICAL JUDGMENT GUIDE: The test taker must decide which newborn is the most stable and which is the more critical newborn. Once the test taker makes this decision, the newborn who is most stable should be selected to be assigned to the LPN.

31. **1. This requirement is violating the client's autonomy, which is a client's right to self-determination without outside control. This approach has been used as a condition of probation, to allow women accused of child abuse or neglect to get out of a jail term.**
    2. Justice is the duty to treat all clients fairly, without regard to age, socioeconomic status, and other variables.
    3. Fidelity is the duty to be faithful to commitments.
    4. Beneficence is the duty to do good actively for the clients.

CLINICAL JUDGMENT GUIDE: The nurse must be cognizant of ethical principles that guide nursing and health-care practices. The judge is acting under legal guidelines that can supersede the client's rights.

32. Correct answers are 1, 3, and 5.
    1. Magnesium sulfate, a uterine relaxant, is the drug of choice to help prevent seizures. The medication relaxes smooth muscles and reduces vasoconstriction, thus promoting circulation to the vital organs of the mother and increasing placental circulation to the fetus.
    2. The mother is not placed on telemetry, but continuous electronic fetal monitoring is required to identify fetal heart rate patterns that suggest fetal compromise.
    3. The deep tendon reflexes are monitored to evaluate for magnesium sulfate toxicity.
    4. After delivery, the mother will excrete large volumes of fluid, a sign of recovery from preeclampsia. However, the loop diuretic furosemide (Lasix) would not be given before delivery because it may lead to hypovolemia.
    5. The nursery should be notified of the delivery so it will be prepared for the neonate. Because the client is in labor, the baby will be born within a reasonable timeframe.

CLINICAL JUDGMENT GUIDE: This is an alternate format type of question included in the NCLEX-RN® examination. The nurse must be able to select all the options that answer the question correctly. There are no partially correct answers.

33. 1. The nurse should encourage the father to remain calm for his wife in this crisis situation, but this is not the first intervention.
    2. Assigning staff members is part of the Code Pink protocol, but it is not the nurse's first intervention.
    3. The nurse's first intervention is to call a Code Pink. Then, the nurse should institute all other nursing interventions. The infant's safety is the priority.
    4. The nurse should question the father for exact details, but the nurse should first call the Code Pink so that the person who took the infant can be found.

CLINICAL JUDGMENT GUIDE: The nurse is responsible for knowing and complying with hospital protocols as well as the local, state, and federal standards of care.

34. 1. This pain is normal and does not require seeing the HCP today.
    2. During the first few days after delivery, hormone levels and the ligaments and cartilage of the pelvis return to their pre-pregnancy position. These changes cause hip and joint pain that interfere with ambulation. The mother should understand that the pain is temporary and does not indicate a problem.
    3. Kegel exercises tone up the client's peritoneal muscles after a pregnancy. These exercises would not help hip and joint pain.
    4. Emptying the bladder will not help the client's joint and hip pain.

CLINICAL JUDGMENT GUIDE: The test taker should be knowledgeable of the physiological process of pregnancy and postpartum and provide factual information to the client.

35. 1. SIDS occurs among infants who are living, not fetuses in utero.
    2. The case manager is responsible for coordinating care between disciplines for clients diagnosed with chronic illnesses. This client has lost a baby and would not need a referral to a case manager.
    3. According to the NCLEX-RN® test plan, management of care includes appropriate use of referrals. The chaplain is responsible for intervening in a case where there is spiritual distress. The loss of a child is devastating.
    4. Child Protective Services (CPS) are notified only if the child is being abused. This baby died in utero; therefore, CPS would

not be notified, except in states where the mother is a drug abuser or has chronic alcoholism.

CLINICAL JUDGMENT GUIDE: The nurse must be knowledgeable about referrals and implement the referral to the most appropriate person or agency.

36. 1. This statement is making the assumption the client is being abused—which is probably true—but the nurse should not put words in the client's mouth. Because this is a legal issue, the nurse cannot suggest in any manner to the client that verbal or physical abuse is occurring. If the client is being abused and decides to file charges, then the accused can use the defense that indeed this is not abuse and that the client decided to consider the actions as abuse only after the nurse suggested it.
   2. This is a true statement, but it is judgmental and would not encourage a therapeutic relationship with the client.
   3. Research indicates that abusive situations escalate during pregnancy, particularly with the woman being hit in the abdominal area; therefore, this question is not necessary. These bruises indicate that abuse is occurring.
   4. **The nurse's best intervention is to assess the safety of the client and infant and provide information to the client about a safe haven.**

CLINICAL JUDGMENT GUIDE: The nurse is responsible for knowing and complying with local, state, and federal standards of care.

37. 1. The nurse should not upset the client by telling her that her boyfriend is creating problems.
   2. The nurse should not allow a person displaying this behavior to remain on the unit.
   3. **The nurse should first contact hospital security to intervene and escort the boyfriend off the unit.**
   4. Confronting a drunken individual could escalate the situation. The nurse should contact security to take care of this situation.

CLINICAL JUDGMENT GUIDE: There will be legal and management questions on the NCLEX-RN®. In many instances, there is no test taking strategy; the nurse should protect the safety of the client.

38. 1. **Jehovah's Witnesses do not believe in accepting blood products, but it is the**

individual's choice. The nurse is a client advocate and should make sure the client is aware that without the injection her next pregnancy could result in erythroblastosis fetalis. However, with the injection her religious belief may be compromised because Rho(D) immune globulin (RhoGAM) is a blood product.
   2. The father of the baby must be Rh-positive; otherwise, the baby would not be Rh-positive and the mother would not require the Rho(D) immune globulin (RhoGAM) injection. The baby's blood type determines whether the mother needs the RhoGAM injection.
   3. When administering RhoGAM to the client, this question is not pertinent. Rho(D) immune globulin (RhoGAM) is prescribed only for Rh-negative mothers who have Rh-positive babies, or within 72 hours of a miscarriage.
   4. The client's insurance status is not pertinent information for the nurse caring for the client.

CLINICAL JUDGMENT GUIDE: Any time there is a cultural or religious factor in the question, the test taker should be aware that this will affect the correct answer.

39. 1. The nurse would not question administering this medication because a negative titer means the client is not immune to rubella (German measles). This vaccine prevents rubella infection and possible severe congenital defects in a fetus in a subsequent pregnancy.
   2. **The flu vaccine is made using egg-based technology; therefore, the nurse should question the administration of this vaccine to a client who is allergic to eggs.**
   3. A positive PPD test determines whether the client was exposed to tuberculosis.
   4. The nurse would not question administering the hepatitis B vaccine to a mother who is breastfeeding because 1-day-old infants receive the vaccine.

CLINICAL JUDGMENT GUIDE: The nurse must be aware of the indications for certain medications, appropriate interventions when administering medications, and adverse side effects that can occur from medications. This is a knowledge-based question.

40. 1. A chignon is newborn scalp edema created by vacuum extraction and will resolve within a few days of delivery. This infant would not need to be assessed first.

2. Caput succedaneum appears over the vertex of the newborn's head because of pressure against the mother's cervix during labor. The edematous area crosses suture lines, is soft, and varies in size. It resolves quickly and disappears within 12 hours to several days after birth. This newborn would not need to be seen first.

3. A cephalohematoma results when there is bleeding between the periosteum and the skull from pressure during birth. The firm swelling is not present at birth but develops within the first 24 to 48 hours. Any time a client is bleeding, it warrants intervention by the nurse.

4. A port-wine stain, nevus flammeus, is a permanent, flat, reddish purple mark that varies in size and location and does not blanch with pressure. This would not require immediate intervention from the nurse.

CLINICAL JUDGMENT GUIDE: When deciding which client to assess first, the test taker should determine which conditions or signs and symptoms the client is exhibiting are normal or expected for the client's situation. After eliminating the expected option, the test taker should determine which situation is more life threatening.

41. 1. Refusal of two or more feedings indicates the infant has a problem that requires the mother to notify the health-care provider. This indicates the mother understands the discharge teaching.

2. Green liquid stools indicate a problem and require the mother to notify the health-care provider.

3. Vitamin K is administered intramuscularly to the infant in the newborn nursery to prevent the infant from bleeding. The gastrointestinal tract is sterile when the infant is born and requires bacteria to synthesize vitamin K from the food eaten by the infant.

4. The infant will have meconium stool for a few days after being born, so the mother should not notify the health-care provider.

CLINICAL JUDGMENT GUIDE: When the question asks, "Which statement indicates the teaching is effective?" the test taker must select the option with correct information.

42. 1. Nausea and vomiting are normal for a 12-week gestation client.

2. Ankle edema is expected in a 24-week gestation client.

3. Facial edema is a sign of gestational hypertension, which requires the clinic nurse to contact the certified nurse midwife.

4. The increasing size of the uterus compresses on the bladder, leading to increased frequency of urination, so this is an expected finding.

CLINICAL JUDGMENT GUIDE: The test taker should ask, "Is it normal for this client?" For example, "Is it normal for the 12-week gestation client to have nausea and vomiting?" If this is normal, then the nurse would not need to notify anyone of this finding.

43. 1. The "taking in" phase is the first phase the mother goes through after the delivery. The mother is not ready to learn or be taught anything in this phase.

2. This is a nursing intervention but is not part of the "taking in" phase.

3. The client during the "taking in" phase is self-absorbed and needs to be cared for, so allowing the client to talk about her own experience is the most appropriate intervention.

4. The client in the "taking in" phase is not ready to learn or be taught anything.

CLINICAL JUDGMENT GUIDE: The test taker must be knowledgeable of the "taking in" phase and be able to appropriately apply the knowledge. Remembering information is not the same as being able to apply the information.

44. Correct answers are 1 and 2.

1. The breasts should be palpated to assess for fullness or engorgement.

2. The nurse should check for the amount, color, and consistency of vaginal discharge.

3. The nurse should assess for deep vein thrombosis (DVT), but this does not include assessing pedal pulses.

4. The client following a vaginal delivery will not have a surgical incision.

5. The nurse does not need to check pupillary response for a postpartum client; this would be appropriate for a client diagnosed with a neurological disorder.

CLINICAL JUDGMENT GUIDE: This is an alternate type of question included in the NCLEX-RN®. The nurse must be able to select all the options that answer the question correctly. There are no partially correct answers. The key to the assessment data is a "postpartum" client.

45. Correct answers are 2 and 4.
1. Soap will dry out the nipples, which can cause cracking and openings in the skin for possible bacterial entry.
2. **Mastitis is a result of bacterial invasion of the breast tissue from cracks or fissures in the nipples, overdistention of the breasts, or milk stasis. These issues can be avoided by frequent breastfeeding with the proper technique.**
3. Nipple shields are used for inverted nipples, not prevention of mastitis.
4. **Hands can carry bacteria such as *Staphylococcus aureus* and *Escherichia coli* that can cause mastitis; therefore, hand washing should be performed to reduce the risks.**
5. A breast binder is utilized for lactation suppression, not to reduce the risk of mastitis.

CLINICAL JUDGMENT GUIDE: This is an alternate type of question included in the NCLEX-RN®. The nurse must be able to select all the options that answer the question correctly. There are no partially correct answers.

46.
1. The HCP in a free clinic would not be able to refer this client to an infertility clinic because of cost. The nurse can discuss this with the client.
2. **If the couple has not been able to conceive in 6 years, then a referral to an infertility clinic would be appropriate, but the tests and treatment for infertility are very expensive. The client is being seen in a free clinic, which indicates a lack of funds. The nurse has a relationship with this client over the time period of "several weeks." The nurse should answer the client's question.**
3. This is a therapeutic response, which does not answer the client's question, "What can we do?"
4. If the client has not conceived in 6 years, this is not a probable solution to the client's concern.

CLINICAL JUDGMENT GUIDE: The test taker should be knowledgeable of the physiological process of pregnancy and infertility and provide factual information to the client.

47. The correct order is 1, 2, 3, 5, 4.
1. **The client who is 10 cm dilated, 100% effaced, and "needing to push" is ready to deliver the fetus; therefore, the nurse should assess this client first.**
2. **Early decelerations are not associated with fetal compromise but indicate head compression. The nurse should assess this client second to determine if delivery is imminent.**
3. **This client does not have an immediate need, although epidurals are offered to clients in active labor; therefore, the nurse should assess this client third.**
5. **The latent phase of labor is early labor when cervical dilation is 3 cm or less. This client is stable and ambulating but should be assessed fourth.**
4. **Although this information is causing distress to the mother, there is nothing the nurse can do about this situation. The on-call obstetrician or certified nurse midwife will have to deliver the fetus. This client should be assessed fifth.**

CLINICAL JUDGMENT GUIDE: This is an alternate type of question included in the NCLEX-RN®. The nurse must be able to determine the order to assess clients.

48.
1. The pregnant client has an increased circulating blood volume, which results in a slight decrease of the hemoglobin and hematocrit; therefore, this client would not warrant intervention.
2. The normal fasting blood glucose level is lower than 100 mg/dL; therefore, this client does not warrant intervention by the nurse.
3. **Protein in the urine indicates the client is at risk for gestational hypertension; therefore, this client warrants intervention and further assessment by the nurse.**
4. The white blood cell count increases during pregnancy; the normal range is 5 to 12×10^3/microL and rises during labor. This client does not warrant intervention.

CLINICAL JUDGMENT GUIDE: The nurse must be knowledgeable of normal laboratory values. These values must be memorized and the nurse must be able to determine if the laboratory value is normal for the client's disease process or medications the client is taking.

49.
1. If the client is unable to urinate, then the nurse will have to perform an in-and-out catheterization to empty the bladder. However, the nurse should implement the least invasive intervention.
2. The nurse could use a bladder scanner to determine whether the bladder is full, but

the first intervention is to ask the client to urinate.

3. Massaging the fundus will not put the fundus in a midline position until the bladder is empty.

4. **The most common reason for a displaced fundus is a full bladder. The nurse should always do the least invasive procedure first, which is to ask the client to attempt to void. The emptying of the bladder should allow the fundus to return to the midline position.**

CLINICAL JUDGMENT GUIDE: The nurse must be knowledgeable of expected medical treatment for a client. This is a knowledge-based question.

50. Correct answers are 1, 3, and 4.
    1. **The charge nurse should notify the unit manager and information technology to ensure automatic locks are set on workstations. Typically, the workstations should be set to lock after 10 minutes of inactivity.**
    2. The charge nurse should immediately secure the EHR, leaving it inaccessible to unauthorized viewing.
    3. **The staff should be informed that this could be a violation of HIPAA if an unauthorized person read the client's personal health information contained in the EHR.**
    4. **Protection of the workstation from unauthorized viewing is a priority. The charge nurse should lock the screen or remain with the workstation.**
    5. The Health and Human Services Office for Civil Rights is responsible for enforcing Privacy and Security rules but a breach of personal health information is not indicated in the question.

CLINICAL JUDGMENT GUIDE: This is an alternate format type of question included in the NCLEX-RN® examination. The nurse must be able to select all the options that answer the question correctly. There are no partially correct answers.

51. 1. The nurse really does not need to know when the client had her last chest x-ray when scheduling this chest x-ray.
    2. **The nurse should ask whether the client may be pregnant because if there is a chance of pregnancy, the client should not have an x-ray. Any time a female client is of childbearing age and is having any type of x-ray, this question should be asked.**

3. The date of the client's last period would not affect the client's having a chest x-ray.

4. This question would be asked if the client was receiving some type of contrast or dye.

CLINICAL JUDGMENT GUIDE: The test taker must be knowledgeable of diagnostic tests and client screening before the procedure. This is a knowledge-based question.

52. 1. The clinical manager should first talk to the nurse to determine what is causing the medication error.
    2. Three medication errors in a short period of time require the clinical manager to investigate the cause.
    3. **This should be the clinical manager's first intervention, to assess whether the system is responsible for the medication errors or whether it is a nursing error problem. For example, a system error problem would be when the medication is not available at the prescribed time.**
    4. This may be needed, but it is not the nurse's first intervention. If the clinical manager determines the nurse is at fault, then this is a possible action.

CLINICAL JUDGMENT GUIDE: The nurse needs to be knowledgeable of management issues for the NCLEX-RN® and appropriate interventions.

53. 1. **When the infant is placed in the supine position, the infant should extend the arm and leg on the side to which the head is turned and then flex the extremities on the other. This is known as the tonic-neck reflex or fencing reflex, which is normal for the newborn. The newborn remaining in a fetal position when supine warrants further intervention to assess for neurological problems.**
    2. The Babinski reflex is elicited by stroking the lateral sole of the foot from the heel forward. Normal reflexes are the toes flare outward and the big toe dorsiflexes. This is a normal response for an infant but is abnormal in an adult, indicating neurological deficit in the adult. Therefore, this does not warrant immediate intervention.
    3. This is the rooting reflex, which is normal for a newborn. This would not warrant immediate intervention.
    4. The Moro reflex or the startle reflex is a sharp extension and abduction of the arm with thumbs and forefingers in a C-position followed by flexion and adduction to embrace

position. This response occurs with loud noise or when the newborn is startled. This would not warrant immediate intervention.

CLINICAL JUDGMENT GUIDE: When the question asks which client warrants "immediate intervention" it is an "except" question. Three of the clients are exhibiting normal responses, whereas one is not.

54. 1. This is the ethical principle of veracity, which is truth telling.
   2. **Nonmaleficence is the duty to do no harm. Many ethicists think that the principle of nonmaleficence has priority over other ethical principles except for autonomy. Nonmaleficence allows the nurse to answer a question or make a decision that does not create further complications for the client.**
   3. This is paternalism, which is giving advice and telling the client what is best for her.
   4. This is an assessment question that could guide the nurse in helping the client make a decision, but it does not demonstrate the ethical principle of nonmaleficence.

CLINICAL JUDGMENT GUIDE: The NCLEX-RN® test plan describes nursing care that addresses ethical principles including autonomy, beneficence, justice, veracity, and others.

55. 1. This statement describes primary care, which is a type of nursing care delivery.
   2. **Modular nursing is frequently called care pairs, in which nurses are paired with lesser-trained caregivers to provide nursing care to a group of clients.**
   3. This statement describes team nursing, which is a type of nursing care delivery.
   4. This statement describes functional nursing, in which there is a charge nurse, a medication nurse, and a treatment nurse.

CLINICAL JUDGMENT GUIDE: There will be management and research questions on the NCLEX-RN®. In many instances, there is no test-taking strategy for these questions.

56. 1. Threatening and attempting to manipulate the staff will create distrust and anger, which will not facilitate a smooth transition for the medication delivery system.
   2. This action is not fair because the new system is being implemented whether the staff members vote for it or not. There are situations, resulting from financial or other constraints, which require the clinical

manager to implement a change without the input of the staff.
   3. **To be an effective change agent, the manager needs to develop a sense of trust, establish common goals, and facilitate effective communication.**
   4. Sending the documentation by hospital e-mail is pertinent to ensure all staff members receive the information, but it is not effective in producing a smooth transition and reducing resistance to change.

CLINICAL JUDGMENT GUIDE: There will be management and research questions on the NCLEX-RN®. In many instances, there is no test-taking strategy for these questions.

57. 1. This behavior may be normal for some individuals and may not be detrimental to the infant or mother, but the nurse must investigate the situation first before making this statement.
   2. Clay and dirt in the gut may decrease the absorption of nutrients such as iron. Therefore, asking this question is appropriate, but the first intervention should be to determine whether there are complications related to pica.
   3. **Pica, ingesting substances not normally considered food, may decrease the intake of food and therefore essential nutrients. Iron deficiency was once thought to be a cause of pica but is now considered a result. The nurse must first assess to determine whether the behavior is detrimental to the mother or infant before further action is taken.**
   4. Pica may be related to cultural beliefs about materials that will ensure a healthy mother and infant. This should not be the nurse's first intervention. The safety of the mother and fetus is the priority. If the H&H is within normal limits, the nurse should support the cultural belief.

CLINICAL JUDGMENT GUIDE: The test taker should apply the nursing process when the question asks, "Which action should the nurse implement first?" If the client is in distress, do something. In this case, the test taker should select an option that directly assesses the client's condition.

58. 1. **Insurance companies contract with certain providers to provide care to the client at a reduced rate. Using this doctor, who**

is not a preferred provider of care, will result in a greater out-of-pocket expense for the client.

2. This is not a true statement, and the nurse should not give the client false information, especially about money.

3. This therapeutic response is to encourage the client to vent feelings. This client needs factual information.

4. Some insurance companies will not cover a preexisting condition for 1 year after the policy is initiated; therefore, this pregnancy may not be covered.

CLINICAL JUDGMENT GUIDE: The nurse should be aware of insurance guidelines in order to provide factual information to the client.

59. 1. The 16-year-old client must sign for her child's care. The grandmother does not have the authority to sign informed consent for the procedure.

2. The cost of the procedure should not be a factor for the nurse when discussing a medical procedure with the client.

3. The client is not requesting assistance to pay the medical bills; therefore, this intervention is not appropriate.

4. **A 16-year-old mother has the right to make decisions for her child; therefore, the mother must sign the informed consent for the procedure.**

CLINICAL JUDGMENT GUIDE: The test taker should be aware of legal rights and responsibilities, and understand best practices for obtaining informed consent.

60. 1. The UAPs may or may not cross the picket line, and the managers will not be able to provide care to all the clients. This is not the best response.

2. Abandonment is leaving the shift without notifying the supervisor after accepting the assignment. Going on strike with a 10-day notice is not abandonment.

3. This may or may not be a true statement; therefore, it is not the best response.

4. **Federal law requires that there must be a 10-day notice before going on strike. This gives the hospital a chance to prepare for the strike and make changes to ensure client safety.**

CLINICAL JUDGMENT GUIDE: The NCLEX-RN® test plan describes nursing care that is ruled by legal requirements. The nurse must be knowledgeable of these issues.

61. 1. Anencephaly is a congenital abnormality that entails an absence of all or a major part of the brain. The infant has no chance of life outside of a health-care institution. The health-care team refers situations to the ethics committee to help resolve dilemmas when caring for clients.

2. This is not an ethical dilemma because the 16-year-old client has a right to place her infant up for adoption. This would not need to be referred to an ethics committee.

3. If the nurse wants to take the child away from the mother, then this must be reported to Child Protective Services. Therefore, this is not an ethical dilemma. The nurse has a law that directs the decision. This would not need to be referred to an ethics committee.

4. This is a legal issue, not an ethical issue. The health-care team can request the hospital attorney to take these parents to court and request a court order to administer blood. The parents do not have the right to refuse life-sustaining treatment for their child.

CLINICAL JUDGMENT GUIDE: The NCLEX-RN® test plan identifies that the nurse must be knowledgeable of ethical practices, recognize ethical dilemmas, and take appropriate actions.

62. Correct answers are 1, 2, and 3.

1. **The mother should be encouraged to hold and cuddle the infant to help with the grieving process.**

2. **The mother should not be required to stay on a unit where she can hear crying infants and happy families. The nurse should transfer the client to another unit.**

3. **The nurse should remember the father has lost the baby, too. Acknowledging and encouraging the father to talk about the loss will help with the grieving process.**

4. The nurse's beliefs about funerals should not be imposed on the client. This is a boundary-crossing violation.

5. Grief support groups recommend giving the infant a name because it acknowledges the infant's existence.

CLINICAL JUDGMENT GUIDE: This is an alternate format type of question included in the NCLEX-RN® examination. The nurse must be able to select all the options that answer the question correctly. There are no partially correct answers.

63. 1. The clinical manager could ask the primary nurse why she provides such excellent care, but it is not the most important action. Excellence in care should be documented in writing in the nurse's personnel file to support merit raises, transfers, and promotions.

2. **The clinical manager should recognize the comments of clients and families during the performance evaluation. Excellence in care should be documented in writing in the nurse's personnel file to support merit raises, transfers, and promotions. Many health-care facilities have employee recognition programs.**

3. This is a possible action, but this could single out the nurse and cause dissension among the other staff. Parties on the unit should celebrate the unit's accomplishments, not a single individual.

4. Excellent care is the expectation of all clinical managers, but when multiple clients and families recognize the nurse's care, then there should be documentation in the nurse's personnel file.

CLINICAL JUDGMENT GUIDE: There will be management and research questions on the NCLEX-RN®. In many instances, there is no test-taking strategy for these questions.

64. **Correct answers are 2, 4, and 5.**
    1. The client should decrease the amount of caffeine, which includes coffee, tea, cola, and chocolate, because caffeine increases irritability, insomnia, anxiety, and nervousness.
    2. **Avoiding simple sugars will prevent rebound hypoglycemia and exacerbation of the signs and symptoms of PMS.**
    3. Alcohol is a central nervous system depressant and aggravates the depression associated with PMS. This is not an appropriate intervention.
    4. **Decreasing the intake of salt will decrease fluid retention, thereby decreasing edema.**
    5. **Insomnia is a symptom of PMS, and a regular schedule for sleep will help decrease the severity of PMS.**

CLINICAL JUDGMENT GUIDE: This is an alternate format type of question included in the NCLEX-RN® examination. The nurse must be able to select all the options that answer the question correctly. There are no partially correct answers.

65. 1. **Vegans are individuals who avoid animal proteins, which are complete proteins that contain all the essential amino acids the** body cannot synthesize from other sources. Vegetable proteins lack one or more of the essential amino acids, so the vegan must combine different plant proteins, grains, legumes, and nuts to allow for intake of all essential amino acids. Vegans avoid all animal products and have difficulty meeting adequate nutritional protein needs.

2. Vegans avoid animal products. If she does not drink milk, she will not eat eggs.

3. The nurse should assist the client in adhering to cultural, spiritual, or personal beliefs. The nurse should not try to convince the client to change her beliefs unless it is a danger to the fetus or the mother.

4. A vegan diet requires extra iron supplements; iron in the vegetarian diet is poorly absorbed because of the lack of heme iron that comes from meat.

CLINICAL JUDGMENT GUIDE: The nurse must attempt to support a client's cultural beliefs. This is a knowledge-based question and the nurse must be knowledgeable of cultural beliefs.

66. **Correct answers are 1 and 4.**
    1. **This client has delivered her infant and has pain. The medical-surgical nurse can care for this client.**
    2. This client requires teaching, a knowledge base the medical-surgical nurse should not be assumed to have encountered on a medical-surgical unit.
    3. HELLP syndrome stands for H—hemolysis (the breakdown of red blood cells), EL—elevated liver enzymes, LP—low platelet count. HELLP syndrome is a group of symptoms that occur in pregnant women who have preeclampsia or eclampsia. Symptoms include fatigue or feeling unwell, fluid retention and excess weight gain, headache, nausea and vomiting that continues to get worse, pain in the upper right part of the abdomen, blurry vision, nosebleed or other bleeding that won't stop easily (rare), and seizures or convulsions (rare). A medical-surgical nurse does not have the expertise required to care for this client.
    4. **This is a preterm client who is on a monitor. The medical-surgical nurse can care for this client. If something occurs on the monitor or the client goes into labor, the nurse can get help.**
    5. Pitocin is a medication that stimulates uterine contraction; it is used to induce labor or

administered postpartum to help a boggy uterus contract. It must be administered by a nurse familiar with the medication and its potential adverse effects.

CLINICAL JUDGMENT GUIDE: The test taker must decide on each option individually. Would the medical-surgical nurse have the knowledge and skill to care for the client or should the client be cared for by a nurse familiar with the specialized area of antepartum and postpartum care?

67. 1. This is a semi-Fowler's position, useful for increasing ease of breathing, and so on, but it does not provide access to the epidural space.
    2. This is the Sims position used for administering an enema.
    3. **This position allows for a space to be created between the vertebrae and allow the anesthetist to insert the catheter into the epidural space.**
    4. The laboring client would not be able to lie on her stomach.

CLINICAL JUDGMENT GUIDE: The test taker should assess which position would allow access to the anatomical area needed to insert the catheter. Remember that the epidural space is part of the central nervous system.

68. 1. The nurse should notify the health-care practitioner (HCP) after making sure no more magnesium is administered to the client.
    2. Documenting the data is important but does not come before safety of the client or notifying the HCP.
    3. It is not necessary for the nurse to have the finding verified before protecting the client.
    4. **The adverse effects of parenterally administered magnesium sulfate, an anticonvulsant, usually are the result of magnesium intoxication. These include flushing, sweating, hypotension, depressed reflexes, flaccid paralysis, hypothermia, circulatory collapse, and cardiac and central nervous system depression proceeding to respiratory paralysis. This client is demonstrating magnesium toxicity. The nurse should immediately discontinue the magnesium and administer the antidote, calcium gluconate.**

CLINICAL JUDGMENT GUIDE: The test taker should read all graphs, charts, or legends very

carefully when choosing an option. Absent reflexes should indicate a need for an action on the part of the nurse. Documentation, although important, is not directly taking care of the client and should only be chosen first when the data supplied is normal.

69. Correct order is 4, 5, 3, 1, 2.
    4. **The client came to the clinic for treatment and it should be the first intervention.**
    5. **All sexual partners of the client should be notified of possible exposure to an STD. This is the responsibility of the public health nurse.**
    3. **The nurse's only opportunity to teach the client about safe sex practices may be this clinic visit.**
    1. **The nurse should attempt to notify the sexual partners of the client to prevent spreading of the disease to other unsuspecting individuals.**
    2. **The report is filed monthly or quarterly.**

CLINICAL JUDGMENT GUIDE: The test taker must logically deduce the steps for the nurse to implement. Care of the client is first. Next, the nurse must consider other clients who may be affected and get the names and contact information of the sexual partners; this must be done in order to contact the individuals. Reports and documentation are last.

70. 1. At the scene of an accident, it is not important how far along the driver is.
    2. **The driver must be assessed for signs of trauma before anything else can be done. If the client dies, then the fetus will die, too.**
    3. Whether or not the driver was wearing a seat belt is a legal matter, and possible assessment data for the labor and delivery nurse to determine potential trauma to the fetus, but not at the scene of the accident.
    4. This might be done if the nurse has a stethoscope, but the mother's status is first because the fetus's life depends on her.

CLINICAL JUDGMENT GUIDE: The nurse has two clients in this scenario, the mother and the fetus, but one life definitely depends on the status of the other. All the options in this question have words that can be used to indicate assessment, so the test taker must choose the first assessment to make.

The correct answer number and rationale for why it is the correct answer are given in **boldface type.** Rationales for why the other possible answer options are incorrect also are given, but they are not in boldface type.

1. 1. **This pain needs to be assessed and pain medication administered. A new graduate would be able to care for this client safely.**
   2. Saturating multiple peri-pads indicates heavy bleeding, which may indicate hemorrhaging. A more experienced nurse should be assigned to this client.
   3. The nurse needs to assess this client for possible maternal and infant bonding problems and would require a nurse who has experience with psychosocial problems. This client should be assigned to a more experienced nurse.
   4. This client requires a nurse who is knowledgeable and experienced in breastfeeding; therefore, a more experienced nurse should be assigned to this client.

2. 1. These are called milia and look similar to pimples; they will fade within a few days and do not warrant immediate intervention.
   2. **The normal respiratory rate for a newborn is 30 to 60; therefore, this information warrants immediate intervention.**
   3. The newborn who is turning red when crying is not in distress; therefore, this would not warrant immediate intervention.
   4. The newborn should pass meconium within 24 hours of birth. It is viscous, sticky (similar to tar), and has no odor. This would not warrant intervention by the nursery nurse.

3. 1. **The fetus is in distress; after increasing blood supply by placing the client in the left lateral position, the labor and delivery nurse needs to contact the obstetrician for immediate C-section.**
   2. Panting during contractions will help prevent the client from pushing, but it is not the first intervention. This client needs immediate evaluation by an obstetrician.
   3. Oxytocin (Pitocin) is a uterine stimulant; this fetus is in distress and does not need uterine contractions. This is an inappropriate intervention.
   4. The nurse needs to prepare for immediate delivery of the fetus but not before

contacting the obstetrician. The nurse cannot perform a C-section.

4. 1. The white blood cell count rises normally during labor and postpartum—up to 25×10^3 microL; therefore, this does not warrant intervention.
   2. The serum potassium level is within normal limits, 3.5 to 5.3 mEq/L, so this client does not warrant immediate intervention by the charge nurse.
   3. **HELLP syndrome is a group of symptoms that occur in pregnant women who have hemolysis (H), elevated liver enzymes (EL), and low platelet count (LP), which occurs in women who are severely preeclamptic and eclamptic. Normal platelet count is 140 to 400×103/microL, so this client's platelet count requires immediate intervention.**
   4. This glucose level is elevated, but because the client had gestational diabetes this blood glucose level does not require immediate intervention.

5. 1. Braxton Hicks contractions are irregular contractions of the uterus throughout the pregnancy and are not true labor. This client would not need to be assigned to the most experienced nurse.
   2. The client having twins on bedrest is not in imminent danger; therefore, this client would not be assigned to the most experienced nurse.
   3. **This client is ready to deliver; therefore, the most experienced nurse should be assigned to this client because the other three clients are not experiencing any life-threatening complications.**
   4. Early decelerations on the fetal monitor do not indicate fetal distress; therefore, this client does not need to be assigned to the most experienced nurse.

6. 1. **The UAP can assist the client to the bathroom to urinate. The UAP cannot assess the client's fundus. The most common reason for a non-midline fundus is a full bladder. The RN cannot delegate assessment, teaching, evaluation, medication administration, or an unstable client to the UAP.**
   2. The client diagnosed with HELLP syndrome is unstable; therefore, the RN should not delegate these vital signs to the UAP.

3. The RN cannot delegate teaching to the UAP.
4. The RN cannot delegate medication administration to the UAP.

7. 1. **The float nurse should be able to address the psychosocial concerns of the mother and family. The client has no physiological problems, so the float nurse could care for this client. Often, following a fetal demise, the mother is transferred to a medical-surgical unit so she does not have to hear babies crying.**
   2. A boggy uterus indicates a potentially life-threatening situation and requires an experienced postpartum nurse to care for this client.
   3. This client is potentially hemorrhaging and requires a more experienced nurse to care for her.
   4. There are many legal issues surrounding an adoption as well as caring for the mother who is giving up her child; this client should be assigned a nurse more experienced in postpartum care.

8. 1. The flu vaccine is made using duck eggs; therefore, the nurse should question the administration of this vaccine to a client who is allergic to eggs, not tomatoes.
   2. The nurse would not question administering the hepatitis B vaccine to a mother who is breastfeeding because 1-day-old infants receive the vaccine.
   3. Rho(D) immune globulin (RhoGAM) should be administered to the client because the baby is Rh-positive. This will help prevent erythroblastosis fetalis in the woman's next pregnancy.
   4. **The nurse would question administering this medication because a positive titer means the client is immune to rubella (German measles).**

9. 1. Mongolian spots are blue- or purple-colored splotches on the baby's lower back and buttocks. The spots are caused by a concentration of pigmented cells that usually disappear in the first 4 years of life. This newborn does not need to be assessed first.
   2. A port-wine stain is a flat pink-, red-, or purple-colored birthmark. These are caused by a concentration of dilated tiny blood vessels called capillaries. The most effective way of treating port-wine stains is with a special type of laser done when the baby is older. This newborn does not need to be assessed first.
   3. Erythema toxicum is a red rash on newborns that is often described as "flea bites." The rash is common on the chest and back, but may be found all over. It does not require any treatment and disappears by itself in a few days; therefore, the nurse does not need to assess this newborn first.
   4. **A cephalohematoma results when there is bleeding between the periosteum and the skull from pressure during birth. The firm swelling, edema, is not present at birth but develops within the first 24 to 48 hours. Any time a client is bleeding, it warrants intervention by the nurse.**

10. 1. **When the infant is placed in the supine position, the infant should extend the arm and leg on the side to which the head is turned and then flex the extremities on the other. This is known as the tonic-neck reflex or fencing reflex, which is normal for the newborn. The newborn remaining in a fetal position when supine warrants further intervention to assess for neurological problems.**
    2. The Babinski reflex is elicited by stroking the lateral sole of the foot from the heel forward. Normal reflexes are toes flared outward and the big toe dorsiflexes. This is a normal response for an infant but is abnormal in an adult, indicating neurological deficit in the adult. Therefore, this does not warrant immediate intervention.
    3. The stepping reflex is intact when the nurse places the baby on a flat surface. The baby will "walk" by placing one foot in front of the other. This is expected and does not warrant intervention by the nurse.
    4. The grasp reflex is elicited by placing a finger on the infant's open palm. The hand will close around the finger. Newborn infants have strong grasps and can almost be lifted from the examination table if both hands are used. This would not warrant intervention.

Pediatric Health Management 12

People are like stained-glass windows. They sparkle and shine when the sun is out but when the darkness sets in, their true beauty is revealed only if there is light from within.

—Elisabeth Kübler-Ross

QUESTIONS

1. The nurse is working in the emergency department (ED) of a children's medical center. Which client should the nurse assess **first?**
   1. The 1-month-old infant who has developed colic and is crying
   2. The 2-year-old toddler who was bitten by another child at the day-care center
   3. The 6-year-old school-age child who was hit by a car while riding a bicycle
   4. The 14-year-old adolescent whose mother suspects her child is sexually active

2. The 8-year-old client diagnosed with a vaso-occlusive sickle cell crisis is reporting a severe headache. Which intervention should the nurse implement **first?**
   1. Administer 6 L of oxygen via nasal cannula.
   2. Assess the client's neurological status.
   3. Administer a narcotic analgesic by intravenous push (IVP).
   4. Increase the client's intravenous (IV) rate.

3. The 6-year-old client who has undergone abdominal surgery is attempting to make a pinwheel spin by blowing on it with the nurse's assistance. The child starts crying because the pinwheel won't spin. Which action should the nurse implement **first?**
   1. Praise the child for the attempt to make the pinwheel spin.
   2. Notify the respiratory therapist to implement incentive spirometry.
   3. Encourage the child to turn from side to side and cough.
   4. Demonstrate how to make the pinwheel spin by blowing on it.

4. The nurse is caring for clients on the pediatric medical unit. Which client should the nurse assess **first?**
   1. The child diagnosed with type 1 diabetes who has a blood glucose level of 180 mg/dL
   2. The child diagnosed with pneumonia who is coughing and has a temperature of 100°F
   3. The child diagnosed with gastroenteritis who has a potassium (K+) level of 3.9 mEq/L
   4. The child diagnosed with cystic fibrosis who has a pulse oximeter reading of 90%

5. The nurse has received the a.m. shift report for clients on a pediatric unit. Which medication should the nurse administer **first?**
   1. The third dose of antibiotic to the child diagnosed with methicillin-resistant *Staphylococcus aureus* (MRSA)
   2. The IVP methylprednisolone to the child diagnosed with asthma
   3. The sliding scale insulin to the child diagnosed with type 1 diabetes mellitus
   4. The methylphenidate to a child diagnosed with attention deficit-hyperactivity disorder (ADHD)

6. The nurse enters the client's room and realizes the 9-month-old infant is not breathing. Which interventions should the nurse implement? **Rank in order of priority.**
   1. Perform cardiac compression 30:2.
   2. Check the infant's brachial pulse.
   3. Administer two puffs to the infant.
   4. Determine unresponsiveness.
   5. Open the infant's airway.

7. The 3-year-old client has been admitted to the pediatric unit. Which task should the RN instruct the unlicensed assistive personnel (UAP) to perform **first?**
   1. Orient the parents and child to the room.
   2. Obtain an admission kit for the child.
   3. Post the child's height and weight at the HOB.
   4. Provide the child with a meal tray.

8. The clinic nurse is preparing to administer an intramuscular (IM) injection to the 2-year-old toddler. Which intervention should the nurse implement **first?**
   1. Immobilize the child's leg.
   2. Explain the procedure to the child.
   3. Cleanse the area with an alcohol swab.
   4. Administer the medication in the thigh.

9. The nurse is writing a care plan for the 5-year-old child diagnosed with gastroenteritis. Which client problem is the **priority?**
   1. Imbalanced nutrition
   2. Fluid volume deficit
   3. Knowledge deficit
   4. Risk for infection

10. Which data would **warrant immediate** intervention from the pediatric nurse?
    1. Proteinuria for the child diagnosed with nephrotic syndrome
    2. Petechiae for the child diagnosed with leukemia
    3. Drooling for a child diagnosed with acute epiglottitis
    4. Elevated temperature in a child diagnosed with otitis media

11. Which client should the pediatric nurse assess **first** after receiving the a.m. shift report?
    1. The 6-month-old child diagnosed with bacterial meningitis who is irritable and crying
    2. The 9-month-old child diagnosed with tetralogy of Fallot (TOF) who has edema of the face
    3. The 11-month-old child diagnosed with Reye syndrome who is lethargic and vomiting
    4. The 13-month-old child diagnosed with diarrhea who has sunken eyeballs and decreased urine output

12. The pediatric clinic nurse is triaging telephone calls. Which client's parent should the nurse call **first?**
    1. The 4-month-old child who had immunizations yesterday and the parent is reporting a high-pitched cry and a 103°F fever
    2. The 8-month-old whose parent is reporting the child is pulling on the right ear and has a fever
    3. The 2-year-old child who has patent ductus arteriosis whose parent reports running out of digoxin
    4. The 3-year-old child whose mother called and reported her daughter may have chickenpox

13. The parent of a 12-year-old male child with a left below-the-knee cast calls the pediatric clinic nurse and tells the nurse, "My son's foot is cold and he told me it feels as if his foot is asleep." Which action should the nurse implement **first?**
    1. Prepare to bifurcate the left below-the-knee cast.
    2. Tell the parent to bring the child to the office.
    3. Instruct the parent to elevate the left leg on two pillows.
    4. Notify the child's orthopedist of the situation.

14. Which child requires the nurse to notify the health-care provider?
    1. The 1-year-old child diagnosed with iron deficiency anemia who has dark-colored stool
    2. The 3-year-old child diagnosed with phenylketonuria (PKU) whose parent does not feed the child any meat or milk products
    3. The 5-year-old child diagnosed with rheumatic heart fever who is having difficulty breathing
    4. The 7-year-old child diagnosed with acute glomerulonephritis who has dark "tea"-colored urine

15. The pediatric nurse on the surgical unit has just received the a.m. shift report. Which client should the nurse assess **first?**
    1. The 3-week-old child 1-day postoperative with surgical repair of a myelomeningocele who has bulging fontanels
    2. The 3-month-old child 2 days postoperative temporary colostomy secondary to Hirschsprung's disease who has a moist, pink stoma
    3. The 9-month-old child with a cleft palate repair who is spitting up formula and refusing to eat
    4. The 4-year-old child 1-day postoperative for repair of hypospadias who has clear amber urine draining from an indwelling catheter

16. The charge nurse has assigned a staff nurse to care for an 8-year-old client diagnosed with cerebral palsy. Which nursing action by the staff nurse would **warrant immediate** intervention by the charge nurse?
    1. The staff nurse performs gentle range-of-motion (ROM) exercises to extremities.
    2. The staff nurse puts the client's bed in the lowest position possible.
    3. The staff nurse takes the client in a wheelchair to the activity room.
    4. The staff nurse places the child in the semi-Fowler's position to eat lunch.

17. The RN and the unlicensed assistive personnel (UAP) are caring for clients on the pediatric unit. Which action by the nurse indicates appropriate delegation?
    1. The nurse requests the UAP to check the circulation on the child with a cast.
    2. The nurse asks the UAP to feed an infant who has just had a cleft palate repair.
    3. The nurse has the UAP demonstrate a catheterization for a child diagnosed with a neurogenic bladder.
    4. The nurse checks to make sure the UAP's delegated tasks have been completed.

18. The RN on a pediatric unit has received the a.m. shift report and tells the unlicensed assistive personnel (UAP) to keep the 2-year-old child NPO for a procedure. At 0830, the nurse observes the mother feeding the child. Which action should the nurse implement **first?**
    1. Determine if the UAP did not understand the instructions.
    2. Tell the HCP the UAP did not follow the nurse's direction.
    3. Ask the mother why she was feeding her child if the child was NPO.
    4. Notify the dietary department to hold the child's meal trays.

19. The charge nurse on the six-bed pediatric burn unit is making shift assignments and has one registered nurse (RN), one scrub technician, one unlicensed assistive personnel (UAP), and a unit secretary. Which client care assignment indicates the **best** use of the hospital personnel?
    1. The RN performs daily whirlpool dressing changes.
    2. The unit secretary prints the discharge instructions for a client.
    3. The scrub technician medicates the client before dressing changes.
    4. The UAP evaluates the current laboratory results for the client.

20. The RN and the UAP are caring for clients on a pediatric surgical unit. Which tasks would be **most** appropriate to delegate to the UAP? **Select all that apply.**
    1. Pass dietary trays to the clients.
    2. Obtain routine vital signs on the clients.
    3. Complete the preoperative checklist.
    4. Change linens on the clients' beds.
    5. Document the clients' intake and output.

21. Which client should the charge nurse on the pediatric unit assign to the **most** experienced nurse?
    1. The 4-year-old child diagnosed with hemophilia receiving factor VIII
    2. The 8-year-old child diagnosed with headaches who is scheduled for a CT scan
    3. The 6-year-old child recovering from a sickle cell crisis
    4. The 11-year-old child newly diagnosed with rheumatoid arthritis

22. The RN charge nurse is making shift assignments on a pediatric oncology unit. Which delegation or assignment would be **most** appropriate?
    1. Delegate the unlicensed assistive personnel (UAP) to obtain routine blood work from the central line.
    2. Instruct the licensed practical nurse (LPN) to contact the leukemia support group.
    3. Assign the chemotherapy-certified RN to administer chemotherapeutic medication.
    4. Have the dietitian check the meal trays for the amount eaten.

23. The RN observes the unlicensed assistive personnel (UAP) bringing a cartoon video to a 6-year-old female child on bedrest so that she can watch it on the television. Which action should the nurse take?
    1. Tell the UAP that the child should not be watching videos.
    2. Explain that this is the responsibility of the child life therapist.
    3. Praise the UAP for providing the child with an appropriate activity.
    4. Notify the charge nurse that the UAP gave the child videos to watch.

24. Which newborn should the RN in the neonatal intensive care unit (NICU) assign to a new graduate (GN) who has just completed a NICU internship?
    1. The 1-day-old infant diagnosed with a myelomeningocele
    2. The 2-week-old infant who was born 6 weeks premature
    3. The 3-hour-old infant who is being evaluated for esophageal atresia
    4. The 1-week-old infant diagnosed with tetralogy of Fallot

25. The newly hired RN is working on a pediatric unit and needs the unlicensed assistive personnel (UAP) to obtain a urine specimen on an 11-month-old infant. Which statement made to the UAP indicates the nurse **understands** the delegation process?
    1. "Be sure to weigh the diaper when obtaining the urine specimen."
    2. "Do you know how to apply the urine collection bag?"
    3. "Use a small indwelling catheter when obtaining the urine specimen."
    4. "I need for you to get a urine specimen on the infant."

26. Which task is **most** appropriate for the RN pediatric nurse to delegate to the unlicensed assistive personnel (UAP)?
    1. Ask the UAP to orient the parents and child to the room.
    2. Tell the UAP to prepare the child for an endoscopy.
    3. Request the UAP to log roll the client who had a spinal surgery.
    4. Instruct the UAP to assess the child's developmental level.

27. Which behavior by the unlicensed assistive personnel (UAP) **warrants** intervention by the RN?
    1. The UAP weighs the child's diaper on a scale and records the urine output on the intake & output (I&O) sheet.
    2. The UAP sits with the child while the parent goes down to the cafeteria to get something to eat.
    3. The UAP bathes the child diagnosed with congenital dislocated hip with the Pavlik harness on the child.
    4. The UAP applies wrist restraints on the 7-month-old who is 1-day postoperative cleft palate repair.

28. The RN is caring for pediatric clients. Which tasks are **most** appropriate to assign to an unlicensed assistive personnel (UAP) or a licensed vocational nurse (LPN)? **Select all that apply.**
    1. Instruct the LPN to teach the parent of a child newly diagnosed with type 1 diabetes.
    2. Tell the UAP to apply an ice collar to the child who is 1-day postoperative tonsillectomy.
    3. Ask the UAP to place ointment on a child's diaper rash around the anal area.
    4. Request the LPN to double-check the medication dose for the child receiving an antibiotic.
    5. Tell the LPN to enter the HCP's orders into the EHR for the child diagnosed with cystic fibrosis.

29. The nurse is discharging a 4-month-old child with a temporary colostomy. Which intervention should the RN implement?
    1. Request the UAP to complete the discharge written documentation.
    2. Tell the LPN to show the parent how to irrigate the colostomy.
    3. Ask the UAP to remove the child's intravenous catheter.
    4. Request the UAP to escort the parent and child to the car.

30. The unlicensed assistive personnel (UAP) tells the RN the child diagnosed with Down syndrome who is 2 days postoperative appendectomy is having pain. Which intervention should the nurse implement **first?**
    1. Tell the UAP to check the child's vital signs.
    2. Assess the child's abdominal dressing and pain level.
    3. Notify the health-care provider immediately.
    4. Check the MAR for the last time pain medication was administered.

31. The 8-year-old male child in the pediatric unit is refusing to ambulate postoperatively. Which intervention would be **most** appropriate?
    1. Give the child the option to ambulate now or after lunch.
    2. Ask the parents to insist the child ambulate in the hall.
    3. Refer the child to the child developmental therapist.
    4. Tell the child he can play a video game if he cooperates.

32. The clinic nurse overhears a mother in the waiting room tell her 6-year-old son, "If you don't sit down and be quiet, I am going to get the nurse to give you a shot." Which action should the nurse implement?
    1. Do not take any action because the mother is attempting to discipline her son.
    2. Tell the child the nurse would not give him a shot because the mother said to.
    3. Report this verbally abusive behavior to Child Protective Services.
    4. Tell the mother this behavior will cause her son to be afraid of the nurses.

33. The parents of an infant born with Down syndrome are holding their infant and crying. The father asks, "I have heard children who are this way are hard to take care of at home." Which referral would be **most** appropriate for the parents?
    1. The National Down Syndrome Society Web site
    2. The hospital chaplain
    3. A Down syndrome support group
    4. A geneticist

34. The charge nurse on the pediatric unit hears the overhead announcement of Code Pink (infant abduction), newborn nursery. Which action should the charge nurse implement?
    1. Send a staff member to the newborn nursery.
    2. Explain the situation to the clients and visitors.
    3. Continue with the charge nurse's responsibilities.
    4. Station a staff member at all the unit exits.

35. The mother of a 4-year-old child diagnosed with Duchenne's muscular dystrophy is overwhelmed and asks the nurse, "I have been told a case manager will come and talk to me. What will they do for me?" Which statement indicates the nurse **understands** the role of the case manager?
    1. "You will have a case manager so that the hospital can save money."
    2. "She will make sure your child gets the right medication for muscular dystrophy."
    3. "She will help you find the resources you need to care for your child."
    4. "The case manager helps your child to have a normal life expectancy."

36. The nurse is assigned to the pediatric unit performance improvement committee. The unit is concerned with IV infection rates. Which action should the nurse implement **first** when investigating the problem?
    1. Contact central supply for samples of IV start kits.
    2. Obtain research to determine the best length for IV dwell time.
    3. Identify how many IV infections have occurred in the last year.
    4. Audit the EHR to determine if hospital policy is being followed.

37. The clinic nurse is discussing a tubal ligation with a 17-year-old adolescent diagnosed with Down syndrome. The adolescent does not want the surgery, but her parents (who are also in the room) are telling her she must have it. Which statement by the nurse would be an example of the ethical principle of justice?
    1. "I think this requires further discussion before scheduling this procedure."
    2. "You will not be able to have children after you have this procedure."
    3. "You should have this procedure because you could not care for a child."
    4. "You can refuse this procedure and your parents can't make you have it."

38. The school nurse has referred an 8-year-old student for further evaluation of vision. The single mother has told the school nurse she does not have the money for the evaluation or glasses. Which action by the nurse would be an example of client advocacy?
    1. Tell the mother the child cannot read the board.
    2. Refer the mother to a local service organization.
    3. Ask the mother if the family is on Medicaid.
    4. Loan the mother money for the examination.

39. The emergency department (ED) nurse is scheduling the 16-year-old client for an emergency appendectomy. Which intervention should the nurse implement when obtaining permission for the surgery?
    1. Withhold the narcotic pain medication until the client signs the permit.
    2. Have the client's parent or legal guardian sign the operative permit.
    3. Explain the procedure to the client and the parents in simple terms.
    4. Get a visitor from the ED waiting area to witness the parent's signature.

40. The unit manager has been notified by central supply that many client items are missing from stock and have not been charged to the client. Which action should the nurse manager implement regarding the lost charges?
    1. Send out a memo telling the staff to follow the charge procedures.
    2. Form a performance improvement committee to study the problem.
    3. Determine whether the items in question are being restocked daily.
    4. Schedule a staff meeting to discuss how to prevent further lost charges.

41. Which child's behavior **warrants** notifying the child developmental specialist?
    1. The 1-year-old child who cries when the parent leaves the room
    2. The 2-year-old child who can talk in two- or three-word sentences
    3. The 3-year-old child who is toilet trained for bowel and bladder
    4. The 4-year-old child who throws frequent temper tantrums

42. Which child should the RN pediatric nurse assign to the new graduate nurse (GN) who has just completed orientation to the pediatric unit?
    1. The 5-year-old child admitted in a sickle cell crisis whose patient-controlled analgesia (PCA) pump is not controlling the child's pain
    2. The 6-year-old child in Russell's traction for a fractured femur who has insertion pin sites that are inflamed and infected
    3. The 12-year-old child who is newly diagnosed with type 1 diabetes who needs medication teaching
    4. The 16-year-old female diagnosed with scoliosis who is being admitted for insertion of a spinal rod in the morning

43. Which action by the emergency department (ED) nurse **warrants** intervention by the charge nurse?
    1. The nurse is elevating the right arm of a child who appears to have fractured the wrist.
    2. The nurse is notifying Child Protective Services for a child who is suspected of being sexually abused.
    3. The nurse is assessing the tonsils on a 4-year-old child who has a sore throat and is drooling.
    4. The nurse is obtaining a midstream urine specimen for the child who is reporting burning upon urination.

44. The day shift nurse is preparing to administer 0730 medications to the 12-year-old child diagnosed with type 1 diabetes. The child's 0730 blood glucose level is 252. Which insulin coverage should the nurse administer?

Client's Name: A.B.	Account Number: 134567	
Allergies: NKA	Date:	
Medication	**0701–1900**	**1901–0700**
Sliding scale regular insulin ac & hs		
Less than 150 no insulin		
151–200 4 units		
201–250 6 units		
251–300 8 units		
301 notify HCP		
10 units regular insulin	0730	
20 units isophane insulin		
Signature/Initials	Day Nurse RN/DN	Night Nurse RN/NN

    1. Regular insulin 6 units
    2. Regular insulin 18 units and isophane insulin 20 units
    3. Regular insulin 10 units and isophane insulin 20 units
    4. Regular insulin 8 units

45. Which interventions should the nurse implement to help establish a nurse and parent relationship? **Select all that apply.**
    1. Include the parents when developing the plan of care for their child.
    2. Encourage the parents to hold their child as much as possible.
    3. Allow the parents to verbalize their feelings of fear and anxiety.
    4. Tell the parents to never leave while the child is hospitalized.
    5. Request the parents to bring toys from home the child will enjoy.

46. The nurse is caring for clients on the pediatric unit. Which child would **warrant** a referral to the early childhood development specialist?
    1. The 9-month-old child who says only "mama" or "dada"
    2. The 11-month-old child who walks hanging onto furniture
    3. The 8-month-old child who sits by leaning forward on both hands
    4. The 4-month-old infant who turns from the abdomen to the back

47. The 10-year-old child diagnosed with leukemia is scheduled for a bone marrow aspiration. Which intervention is **most** important when obtaining informed consent for the procedure?
    1. Obtain assent from the child.
    2. Have the parent sign the permit.
    3. Refer any questions to the HCP.
    4. Witness the signature on the permit.

48. The 13-year-old client has just delivered a 4-pound baby boy. The stepfather of the client becomes verbally abusive to the nurse when he is asked to leave the room. The client is withdrawn and silent. Which legal action should the nurse implement?
    1. Call hospital security to come to the room.
    2. Contact Child Protective Services.
    3. Refer the child to the social worker.
    4. Ask the client whether she feels safe at home.

49. The fire alarm on the pediatric unit has just started sounding. Which action should the charge nurse implement **first**?
    1. Call the hospital operator to find out the location of the fire.
    2. Ensure that all visitors and clients are in the room with the door closed.
    3. Prepare to evacuate the clients and visitors down the stairs.
    4. Make a list of which clients are not currently on the unit.

50. A nurse overhears two other nurses talking about a client in the hospital dining room. Which action should the nurse implement **first**?
    1. Notify the HIPAA officer about the breach of confidentiality.
    2. Immediately report the two nurses to their clinical manager.
    3. Document the situation in writing and submit to the chief nursing officer (CNO).
    4. Tell the two nurses they are violating the client's confidentiality.

51. The nurse is caring for newborns in the nursery. Which newborn **warrants immediate** intervention by the nurse?
    1. The 8-hour-old newborn who has not passed meconium
    2. The 15-hour-old newborn who is slightly jaundiced
    3. The 4-hour-old newborn who is jittery and irritable
    4. The 10-hour-old newborn who will not stop crying

52. At 1300, the nurse is assessing a 12-year-old child who is reporting abdominal pain and rating it as a 5 on a scale of 1 to 10. Which intervention should the nurse implement?

Client's Name: R.J.	Account Number: 1023456		Allergies: NKDA
Height: 60 inches	Date:		Weight: 98 pounds
Medication	**1901–0700**		**0701–1900**
Aluminum hydroxide; magnesium hydroxide 30 mL q 1 hour PRN			
Acetaminophen 650 mg PO q 6 hours PRN			
Hydrocodone 5 mg PO PRN pain q 4–6 hours	0600 NN		
Morphine 2 mg IVP PRN pain q 4 hours			
Signature/Initials	Night Nurse RN/NN		Day Nurse RN/DN

1. Administer 30 mL of aluminum hydroxide; magnesium hydroxide PO.
2. Administer 650 mg of acetaminophen PO.
3. Administer 5 mg of hydrocodone PO.
4. Administer 2 mg of morphine IVP.

53. The nurse who has never worked on the maternity ward has been pulled from the surgical unit to work in the newborn nursery. Which assignment would be **most** appropriate for the nurse to accept?
    1. Perform an assessment on the newborn.
    2. Assist the pediatrician with a circumcision.
    3. Gavage feed a newborn who is 8 hours old.
    4. Transport newborns to the mothers' room.

54. The nurse is instructing the unlicensed assistive personnel (UAP) on gross motor skill activity that is appropriate for a developmentally delayed 9-month-old infant. Which activity should the RN delegate to the UAP?
    1. Help the child to sit without support.
    2. Teach the child to catch the beach ball.
    3. Reward the child with food for sitting up.
    4. Teach the child to blow a kiss.

55. Which incident should the primary nurse report to the clinical manager concerning a violation of information technology guidelines?
    1. The nurse keeps the computer screen turned away from public view.
    2. The nurse researches medications using the online formulary.
    3. The nurse shares the computer access code with another nurse.
    4. The nurse logs off the computer when leaving the terminal.

56. The nurse is caring for clients in a pediatric emergency department (ED). Which client should the nurse assess **first?**
    1. The child diagnosed with a dog bite on the left hand who is bleeding
    2. The child who has a laceration on the right side of the forehead
    3. The child diagnosed with a fractured tibia who will not move the foot
    4. The child who has ingested a bottle of prenatal vitamins

57. The nurse is caring for a client in a children's medical center. Which behavior indicates the nurse **understands** the pediatric client's rights?
    1. The nurse administers an injection without talking to the child.
    2. The nurse covers the 5-year-old child's genitalia during a code.
    3. The nurse discusses the child's condition with the grandparents.
    4. The nurse leaves an uncapped needle at the client's bedside.

58. The home health nurse is planning the care of a 14-year-old client diagnosed with leukemia who is receiving chemotherapy. Which psychosocial problem is the **priority** for this client?
    1. Diversional activity deficit
    2. High risk for infection
    3. Social isolation
    4. Hopelessness

59. The nurse is administering IV fluids to a 3-year-old client. Which action by the nurse would **warrant** intervention by the charge nurse?
    1. The nurse places the IV on an infusion pump.
    2. The nurse does not use a volume-controlled device.
    3. The nurse checks the child's IV site every hour.
    4. The nurse labels the IV tubing with date and time.

60. The nurse is caring for clients on a psychiatric pediatric unit. Which action by the nurse is reportable to the state board of nursing?
    1. The nurse leaves for lunch and does not return to complete the shift.
    2. The nurse fails to check the ID band when administering medications.
    3. The nurse has had three documented medication errors in the last 3 months.
    4. The nurse has admitted to having an affair with another staff member.

61. The nurse is working in a free health-care clinic. Which client situation **warrants** further investigation?
    1. The child diagnosed with rheumatoid arthritis who is wearing a copper bracelet
    2. The mother of a child diagnosed with a sunburn who is using juice from an aloe vera plant on the burn
    3. The grandmother who reports rubbing mentholated topical ointment on the child's chest for a cold
    4. The father who tells the nurse that the child receives a variety of herbs every day

62. The unlicensed assistive personnel (UAP) tells the RN primary nurse that the 4-year-old child is alone in the room because the mother went to the cafeteria to get something to eat. Which action should the nurse implement **first?**
    1. Arrange for the mother to have a tray sent to the room.
    2. Go to the cafeteria and ask the mother to return to the room.
    3. Tell the UAP to stay with the child until the mother returns.
    4. Notify social services that the mother left the child alone.

63. The nurse is evaluating an 18-month-old child in the pediatric clinic. Which data would indicate to the nurse that the child is meeting tasks according to Erikson's Stages of Psychosocial Development? **Select all that apply.**
    1. The child stamps his or her foot and says "no" frequently.
    2. The child does not interact with the mother.
    3. The child cries when the mother leaves the room.
    4. The child responds when called by name.
    5. The child smiles when successful at toilet training.

64. Which statement by the RN charge nurse indicates she has an autocratic leadership style?
    1. "You must complete all the a.m. care before you take your morning break."
    2. "I don't care how the work is done as long as it is completed on time."
    3. "I want to talk to you about your ideas on a new staffing mix."
    4. "I think we should have a potluck lunch tomorrow because it is Saturday."

65. The nurse is evaluating the care of a 5-year-old client diagnosed with a cyanotic congenital heart defect. Which outcome would support that discharge teaching has been **effective?**
    1. The mother makes the child get up when squatting.
    2. The child is playing in the dayroom without oxygen.
    3. The father buys the child a baseball and a bat.
    4. The nurse finds unopened packs of salt on the meal tray.

66. The nurse is administering morning medications on a pediatric unit. Which action should the nurse take **first** when preparing to administer medication to the client?

Client Name: T.R.	Account Number: 5948726	Allergies: Milk and dairy products
Height: 21 inches	Date: Today	Weight in pounds: 15
Weight in kg: 6.82	Date of Birth: 2 weeks ago	
Medication	**1901–0700**	**0701–1900**
Digoxin 0.125 mg/5 mL q day PO		0900
250 mL 0.33% dextrose IV @ 10 mL/hour	0215 NN via buretrol setup and IV pump	
Signature/Initials	Night Nurse RN/NN	Day Nurse RN/DN

1. Check the client's apical pulse rate.
2. Ask the parent for the baby's date of birth.
3. Look to see if a digoxin level has been drawn.
4. Call the health-care provider to discuss the digoxin.

67. The nurse working in a pediatrician's office is preparing to administer the initial Haemophilus influenzae type B (HIB) vaccination to a 2-month-old infant. Which is the preferred site for the injection?

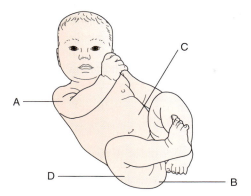

   1. A
   2. B
   3. C
   4. D

68. The nurse is preparing to administer an intravenous piggyback to an 8-year-old child. The child has an IV running at 45 mL per hour. The medication comes prepared in 50 mL of NS. At which rate should the nurse set the IV pump?

   [   ]

69. The unconscious 4-year-old child is brought to the emergency department by paramedics; the child has bruises covering the torso in varying stages of healing. The nurse notes small burn marks on the child's genitalia. Which actions should the nurse implement? **Select all that apply.**
   1. Notify Child Protective Services.
   2. Ask the parent how the child was injured.
   3. Perform a thorough examination for more injuries.
   4. Tell the parents that the police have been called.
   5. Prepare the child for skull x-rays and a CT scan.

70. The 24-month-old toddler is admitted to the pediatric unit diagnosed with vomiting and diarrhea. Which interventions should the nurse implement? **Rank in order of performance.**
   1. Teach the parent about weighing diapers to determine output status.
   2. Show the parent the call light and explain safety regimens.
   3. Assess the toddler's tissue turgor.
   4. Place the appropriate size diapers in the room.
   5. Take the toddler's vital signs.

PEDIATRIC CLINICAL SCENARIO

The RN charge nurse on a 7 a.m.–7 p.m. shift is in the pediatric emergency department (ED) of a level II trauma adult and child county hospital in a mixed suburban and rural setting. There are three registered nurses, two unlicensed assistive personnel (UAP), and a unit secretary. The pediatric clients are multicultural and economically diverse.

1. Which child should the charge nurse assess **first?**
    1. The 1-month-old infant who is crying, is inconsolable, and has inspiratory retractions
    2. The 4-year-old toddler diagnosed with cystic fibrosis who has a pulse oximeter reading of 93%
    3. The 6-year-old child diagnosed with gastroenteritis who has a potassium level of 3.6 mEq/L
    4. The 14-year-old child diagnosed with type 2 diabetes with a blood glucose level of 210 mg/dL

2. Which task should the RN charge nurse delegate to the UAP?
    1. Take the vital signs of an African American child who is having a sickle cell crisis.
    2. Place oxygen via nasal cannula on a teenage child diagnosed with cystic fibrosis.
    3. Obtain the weight of the restless child who is diagnosed with nephrotic syndrome.
    4. Escort the 9-year-old child diagnosed with traumatic brain injury (TBI) to the ICU.

3. The charge nurse is observing the RN administer an intramuscular (IM) injection to a 2-year-old toddler. Which action by the nurse **warrants** intervention by the charge nurse?
    1. The pediatric nurse immobilizes the child's leg.
    2. The nurse explains the procedure to the child.
    3. The pediatric nurse places the syringe in the sharps container.
    4. The nurse recaps the needle after administering the medication.

4. Which tasks should the RN delegate to the UAP? **Select all that apply.**
    1. Document the intake and output (I&O) on the 15-year-old child diagnosed with congestive heart failure (CHF).
    2. Feed the 9-year-old child who is experiencing an acute exacerbation of inflammatory bowel disease (IBD).
    3. Elevate the child's leg who just had a cast applied for a fractured right ankle.
    4. Take the incapacitated child's catheterized urine specimen to the laboratory.
    5. Assess the vital signs of a 7-year-old child reporting ear pain.

5. Which client should the charge nurse assign to the **most** experienced pediatric emergency department nurse?
    1. The 1-year-old child who is tugging at the right ear and has a temperature of 100.4°F
    2. The 6-year-old child who is wheezing and reporting chest tightness
    3. The 8-year-old female child who is reporting burning when she urinates
    4. The 11-year-old child diagnosed with bilateral crackles and a productive cough

6. The 13-year-old child is admitted to the emergency department with nucal rigidity, a positive Kernig's sign, a positive Brudzinki's sign, and an elevated temperature. Which intervention should the charge nurse implement **first?**
    1. Administer acetaminophen (Tylenol) PO with water.
    2. Place the young teenage child in droplet isolation.
    3. Prepare the teenager for a lumbar puncture.
    4. Notify the hospital infection control nurse about this client.

7. The RN answers the phone and a distraught woman says, "My daughter just drank a bottle of cleaning solution." Which intervention should the nurse implement **first?**
   1. Instruct the mother to bring her daughter to the emergency department immediately.
   2. Request of the mother how old the child is and how much the child weighs.
   3. Inquire if the mother has syrup of ipecac that could be given to the child.
   4. Ask the charge nurse to call poison control immediately.

8. The 9-year-old child is brought to the emergency department by his parents with a pencil penetrating the right eye. Which intervention should the charge nurse implement **first?**
   1. Remove the harmful object with a lightly moistened gauze pad.
   2. Ask the parents about the child's medical history and any known allergies.
   3. Stabilize the pencil penetrating the right eye in place and patch the left eye.
   4. Assess the 9-year-old child's vital signs and pulse oximeter reading.

9. The RN is caring for a 7-year-old child who was hit in the head with a baseball. One hour ago, the child had a 15 on the Glasgow Coma Scale and now has a 12. Which intervention should the pediatric nurse implement **first?**
   1. Notify the hospital neurologist immediately.
   2. Document the findings in the EHR.
   3. Complete a Glasgow Coma Scale in 2 hours.
   4. Place the child in the high-Fowler's position.

10. Which client should the charge nurse assign to the **least** experienced nurse in the pediatric emergency department?
    1. The child whose parents report the child had a sore throat and is now drooling
    2. The 4-year-old child who has a distended abdomen and absent bowel sounds
    3. The 13-year-old child who has an edematous and contused right ankle
    4. The child whose parents report the child has blood in his urine

The correct answer number and rationale for why it is the correct answer are given in **boldface type.** Rationales for why the other possible answer options are incorrect also are given, but they are not in boldface type.

1. 1. The main sign of colic is intense crying; therefore, this is expected and would not warrant the nurse's assessing the child first.
2. A human bite is dangerous, but it is not life threatening.
3. **The child hit by a car should be assessed first because he or she may have life-threatening injuries that must be assessed and treated promptly.**
4. This client is not a priority over a client diagnosed with a physiological problem.

CLINICAL JUDGMENT GUIDE: When deciding which client to assess first, the test taker should determine whether the signs and symptoms the client is exhibiting are normal or expected for the client's situation. After eliminating the expected option, the test taker should determine which situation is more life threatening.

2. 1. Administering oxygen may help decrease the sickling of the cells, but this should not be the first intervention to address the client's headache.
2. **Because the client is reporting a headache, the nurse should first rule out cerebrovascular accident (CVA) by assessing the client's neurological status and then determine whether it is a headache that can be treated with medication.**
3. Before administering any pain medication to a client, the nurse must first assess the client to determine whether the pain is what is expected with the disease process or whether it is a complication that requires further nursing intervention.
4. Only after CVA has been ruled out should the nurse medicate the client. Adequate hydration will help decrease sickling of the cells, but this is not the first intervention to address the client's pain.

CLINICAL JUDGMENT GUIDE: Assessment is the first step of the nursing process, and the test taker should use the nursing process or some other systematic process to assist in determining priorities.

3. 1. **The nurse should always praise the child for attempts at cooperation even if the child did not accomplish what the nurse asked.**

2. This action can be taken by the nurse after praising the child for the attempt.
3. This action is appropriate and should be implemented, but not before the nurse praises the child for the attempt.
4. The nurse can demonstrate the correct technique for the child, but not before praising the child for the attempt.

CLINICAL JUDGMENT GUIDE: All options are plausible in questions that ask the test taker to identify an intervention to implement first. The test taker must identify the most important intervention.

4. 1. A 180 mg/dL glucose level for a child diagnosed with type 1 diabetes is not life threatening, and the nurse would not assess this child first.
2. The nurse would expect the child diagnosed with pneumonia to have these signs and symptoms; therefore, the nurse would not assess this child first.
3. This is a normal potassium level; therefore, the nurse would not assess this child first.
4. **A pulse oximeter reading of lower than 93% is significant and indicates hypoxia, which is life threatening; therefore, this child should be assessed first.**

CLINICAL JUDGMENT GUIDE: When deciding which client to assess first, the test taker should determine whether the signs and symptoms the client is exhibiting are normal or expected for the client's situation. After eliminating the expected options, the test taker should determine which situation is more life threatening.

5. 1. The third dose of an aminoglycoside antibiotic would not be a priority over sliding scale insulin because insulin must be administered before the breakfast meal.
2. Routine medications have a 1-hour leeway before and after the scheduled time; therefore, the steroid methylprednisolone (Solu-Medrol) does not have to be administered first.
3. **Sliding scale insulin is ordered ac, which is before meals; therefore, this medication must be administered first after receiving the a.m. shift report.**
4. Routine medications have a 1-hour leeway before and after the scheduled time; therefore, the stimulant methylphenidate (Ritalin) does not have to be administered first.

CLINICAL JUDGMENT GUIDE: The test taker should know which medications are a priority, such as insulin, mucolytics, and so on. These medications should be administered first by the nurse.

6. Correct order is 4, 5, 3, 2, 1.
   4. The nurse must first determine the infant's responsiveness by flicking the baby's feet.
   5. The nurse should then open the child's airway using the head-tilt chin-lift technique, with care taken not to hyperextend the neck. Then the nurse should look, listen, and feel for respirations.
   3. The nurse then administers quick puffs of air while covering the child's mouth and nose, preferably with a rescue mask.
   2. The nurse should determine whether the infant has a pulse by checking the brachial artery.
   1. If the infant has no pulse, the nurse should begin chest compressions using two fingers at a rate of 30:2.

CLINICAL JUDGMENT GUIDE: This is an alternate type of question included in the NCLEX-RN® test plan. The nurse must be able to perform skills in the correct order.

7. 1. **The first intervention after the child is admitted to the unit is to orient the parents and child to the room, the call system, and the hospital rules, such as not leaving the child alone in the room.**
   2. This task is within the scope of the UAP, but it is not a priority over orienting the child and parents to the room.
   3. The height and weight should be posted in case the client codes, but this can be done after the child and parents are oriented to the room.
   4. The child should receive a meal tray, but not before orientation to the room.

CLINICAL JUDGMENT GUIDE: All options are plausible in questions that ask the test taker to identify an intervention to implement first. The test taker must identify the most important intervention.

8. 1. The nurse should immobilize the child's leg, but it is not the first intervention.
   2. **The nurse must explain any procedure in words the child can understand. It does not matter how old the child is.**
   3. This is an appropriate intervention, but it is not the first intervention.
   4. This is an appropriate intervention, but it is not the first intervention.

CLINICAL JUDGMENT GUIDE: All options are plausible in questions that ask the test taker

to identify an intervention to implement first. The test taker must identify the most important intervention.

9. 1. This is not the priority problem because lack of fluids is more life threatening to a child than lack of food.
   2. **The child diagnosed with gastroenteritis is at high risk for hypovolemic shock resulting from vomiting and diarrhea; therefore, maintaining fluid and electrolyte homeostasis is the priority.**
   3. Knowledge deficit is a psychosocial diagnosis, and although it is important to teach the parents and child, it is not a priority over a physiological problem.
   4. The child already has an infection; thus, there is no risk.

CLINICAL JUDGMENT GUIDE: The test taker should use Maslow's Hierarchy of Needs to determine the client's priority problem. Physiological problems are the priority.

10. 1. The child diagnosed with nephrotic syndrome would be expected to have proteinuria.
    2. The child diagnosed with leukemia would be expected to have petechiae.
    3. **Drooling indicates the child is having trouble swallowing, and the epiglottis is at risk of completely occluding the airway. This warrants immediate intervention. The nurse should notify the HCP and obtain an emergency tracheostomy tray for the bedside.**
    4. A child diagnosed with an ear infection would be expected to have an elevated temperature.

CLINICAL JUDGMENT GUIDE: When deciding which client to assess first, the test taker should determine whether the signs and symptoms the client is exhibiting are normal or expected for the client's situation. After eliminating the expected options, the test taker should determine which situation is more life threatening.

11. 1. Irritability and crying are expected signs and symptoms for a child diagnosed with bacterial meningitis; therefore, this child does not need to be assessed first.
    2. The child diagnosed with tetralogy of Fallot (TOF) would be expected to have signs of congestive heart failure, so this child would not be assessed first.
    3. The child diagnosed with Reye syndrome would present with lethargy and vomiting, so this child would not be assessed first.

4. **Sunken eyeballs and decreased urine output are signs of dehydration, which is a life-threatening complication of diarrhea; therefore, this child should be assessed first.**

CLINICAL JUDGMENT GUIDE: The test taker must determine if the signs and symptoms are normal for the disease process; if the signs and symptoms are normal, then the nurse should not assess the child first. If two or more are not expected, then the nurse must determine which is more life threatening, needs further assessment, or needs notification of the health-care provider.

12. 1. **A high fever and high-pitched crying may indicate a reaction to the immunizations; therefore, this parent needs to be called first to bring the child to the clinic.**
    2. This child probably has an ear infection, which needs to be seen but is not a priority over a reaction to immunizations.
    3. The nurse needs to call in a prescription for the digoxin but not before calling the parent whose child is having a reaction to an immunization.
    4. The child may need to be seen but primarily kept in isolation, so this parent does not need to be called first.

CLINICAL JUDGMENT GUIDE: The test taker must determine if the signs and symptoms are normal for the disease process; if the signs and symptoms are not normal, then the nurse should call this parent first.

13. 1. These are signs and symptoms of neurovascular compromise and the cast may need to be cut (bifurcated), but it is not the first intervention.
    2. The child should be brought to the office, but the parent should first attempt to decrease edema by elevating the extremity.
    3. **The nurse should first take care of the client's body by having the parent elevate the left leg.**
    4. The orthopedist should be notified, but it is not the first intervention.

CLINICAL JUDGMENT GUIDE: When the question asks the nurse which intervention should be implemented first, it means all the interventions are possible. The nurse should implement an action that will help the client's situation first.

14. 1. The child diagnosed with iron deficiency anemia would be taking an iron elixir, which causes the stool to be black.

2. The child diagnosed with phenylketonuria (PKU) should not eat any meats, milk, dairy, and eggs because the child lacks the enzyme that breaks down phenylalanine.
3. **A complication of rheumatic heart disease is valvular disorders that may be manifested by respiratory problems; therefore, the nurse should notify the child's health-care provider.**
4. The child diagnosed with acute glomerulonephritis would be expected to have dark urine.

CLINICAL JUDGMENT GUIDE: The nurse should notify the health-care provider of any signs and symptoms that are not expected with the disease process or are signs of a complication.

15. 1. **Bulging fontanels is a sign of increased intracranial pressure, which is a complication of neurological surgery; therefore, this child should be assessed first.**
    2. A moist, pink stoma is normal; therefore, this child does not need to be assessed first.
    3. This child needs to be assessed but is not a priority over a child with a surgical, possibly life-threatening, complication.
    4. The child will have an indwelling urinary catheter and clear amber urine is normal, so this child does not need to be assessed first.

CLINICAL JUDGMENT GUIDE: The test taker must determine if the signs and symptoms are expected for the surgical procedure. If the signs and symptoms are not expected, this child should be assessed first. If two clients have signs and symptoms that are not expected, then the child diagnosed with a life-threatening complication should be assessed first.

16. 1. It is appropriate for the nurse to perform ROM exercises to help prevent contractures, specifically scissoring of the legs. This action would not require intervention.
    2. Safety issues should always be addressed, and keeping the bed in the lowest position may prevent injury to the child.
    3. Taking the child to the activity room is being a client advocate and would not warrant intervention.
    4. **The child should be positioned upright to prevent aspiration during meals; therefore, this action would require the charge nurse to intervene.**

CLINICAL JUDGMENT GUIDE: When the question asks, "Which nursing action warrants immediate intervention?" it is an "except" question. Three of the actions are appropriate, whereas one is not.

17. 1. The UAP cannot assess a client; therefore, this is an inappropriate delegation.
    2. The child with a cleft palate repair is at risk for choking or damaging the incision site; therefore, this task should not be delegated to a UAP.
    3. Demonstrating is teaching, and the UAP cannot teach a client.
    4. **The last step of delegating to a UAP is for the RN to evaluate and determine whether the delegated tasks have been completed and performed correctly. This indicates the nurse has delegated appropriately.**

CLINICAL JUDGMENT GUIDE: When delegating to a UAP, the RN must follow the four rights of clinical delegation: the right task, to the right person, using the right communication, and providing the right feedback. The right feedback includes determining whether the delegated tasks were performed correctly.

18. 1. **Communication to the UAP must be clear, concise, correct, and complete. The RN must determine why there was a lack of communication, which resulted in the child receiving food; therefore, this action should be implemented first.**
    2. The RN retains ultimate accountability for any delegated tasks and cannot blame the UAP for the child being fed by the mother. The HCP needs to be notified to cancel the procedure.
    3. The RN should talk to the mother about why the child was being fed, but the nurse must first determine whether the UAP told the mother not to feed the child and that the child was to be given nothing by mouth.
    4. This action is too late to take care of the situation.

CLINICAL JUDGMENT GUIDE: There will be communication and management questions on the NCLEX-RN®. The nurse should first assess the situation and determine if there was a misunderstanding of the communication between the RN and the UAP.

19. 1. The scrub technician is assigned to perform daily whirlpool dressing changes, which is a lengthy procedure. Therefore, assigning the one RN to this task would be inappropriate

because he or she cannot be unavailable for an extended period of time.
    2. **One of the responsibilities of the unit secretary is to perform clerical duties to support the nurses. The unit secretary can print the discharge instructions for the RN but the RN retains total responsibility for the correctness and accuracy of the information.**
    3. The scrub technician cannot administer medications.
    4. The UAP is not responsible for the evaluation of laboratory data for the clients. The UAP should be on the unit taking care of the clients.

CLINICAL JUDGMENT GUIDE: The test taker must be knowledgeable of the role and scope of practice for each member of the health-care team. The nurse should not delegate tasks that are not appropriate for the level of licensure.

20. Correct answers are 1, 2, 4, and 5.
    1. **The UAP can pass the dietary trays to the clients because it does not require judgment.**
    2. **One of the responsibilities of the UAP is taking routine vital signs on clients.**
    3. The RN must complete the preoperative checklist because it requires nursing judgment to determine whether the client is ready for surgery.
    4. **One of the responsibilities of the UAP is changing bed linens.**
    5. **The UAP can document the client's intake and output, but the UAP cannot evaluate the numbers.**

CLINICAL JUDGMENT GUIDE: This is an alternative type of question included in the NCLEX-RN® examination. The nurse must be able to select all the options that answer the question correctly. There are no partially correct answers.

21. 1. The administration of blood products does not require the most experienced nurse.
    2. Preparing a child for a routine procedure does not require the most experienced nurse.
    3. The child recovering from a sickle cell crisis would not require the most experienced nurse.
    4. **The child newly diagnosed with a chronic disease, which will have acute exacerbations, requires extensive teaching; therefore, the most experienced nurse should be assigned to this child and family.**

CLINICAL JUDGMENT GUIDE: The test taker must determine which client is the most unstable and would require the most experienced nurse, thus making this type of question an "except" question. Three clients are either stable or have non-life-threatening conditions.

22. 1. Only the RN can withdraw blood from a central line.
    2. The social worker or case manager is responsible for referring clients to support groups. This is not an expected responsibility of a floor nurse or LPN.
    3. **Only chemotherapy-certified RNs can administer antineoplastic, chemotherapeutic medications. This is a national minimal standard of care according to the Oncology Nursing Society.**
    4. The dietitian is responsible for ensuring that the proper food is provided along with evaluating the child's nutritional intake, not checking the amount of food eaten—this is the responsibility of the nursing staff.

CLINICAL JUDGMENT GUIDE: The test taker must be knowledgeable of the role and scope of practice for each member of the health-care team. The nurse should not delegate tasks that are not appropriate for the level of licensure or required experience.

23. 1. A 6-year-old child on bedrest needs an appropriate activity to help with distraction; a cartoon video would be an age-appropriate activity.
    2. The child life therapist is responsible for recreational and developmental activity for the hospitalized child, but any staff member should address the child's psychosocial needs.
    3. **Part of the delegation process is to evaluate the UAP's performance of duties, and the RN should praise any initiative on the part of the UAP in being a client advocate.**
    4. Videos are one of the few age-appropriate activities to occupy a 6-year-old on bedrest; therefore, there is no reason to notify the charge nurse.

CLINICAL JUDGMENT GUIDE: This is an "except" question. The test taker should ask which task is appropriate to delegate to the UAP. The RN is responsible for evaluating the UAP's actions.

24. 1. The newborn diagnosed with the myelomeningocele has a portion of the spinal cord and membranes protruding through the back and is at risk for hydrocephalus and meningitis; this client should be assigned to a more experienced nurse.

2. The new graduate who has completed the NICU internship should be able to care for a premature infant because care is primarily supportive.
3. Esophageal atresia, a congenital anomaly in which the esophagus does not completely develop, is a clinical and surgical emergency. It puts the newborn at risk for aspiration because the upper esophagus ends in a blind pouch with the lower part of the esophagus connected to the trachea. This newborn should be assigned to a more experienced nurse.
4. Tetralogy of Fallot is a cyanotic, congenital anomaly. It includes a combination of four defects of the heart, all of which result in unoxygenated blood being pumped into the systemic circulation. This newborn must be assigned to an experienced nurse.

CLINICAL JUDGMENT GUIDE: The test taker must determine which client is the most stable, which makes this an "except" question. Three clients are either unstable or have potentially life-threatening conditions.

25. 1. Weighing the diaper is the procedure for determining the infant's urinary output and is not part of the procedure for obtaining a urine specimen.
    2. **The NCSBN defined *delegation* as transferring to a competent individual the authority to perform a selected nursing task in a selected situation. The RN retains the accountability for the delegation. The nurse must determine whether the UAP has the ability and knowledge to perform a task. This question clarifies whether the UAP has the ability to obtain a urine specimen.**
    3. Obtaining a urine specimen with an indwelling catheter on an 11-month-old infant would require more expertise than a UAP would have on the pediatric unit. Furthermore, it does not determine whether the UAP understands how to do the procedure.
    4. This statement does not determine whether the UAP understands how to perform the procedure of obtaining a urine specimen from an 11-month-old infant.

CLINICAL JUDGMENT GUIDE: The nurse cannot delegate any task in which the UAP admits to not being able to perform. Delegation means the nurse is responsible for the UAP's actions; therefore, the nurse should confirm the UAP is knowledgeable of the appropriate procedure.

26. 1. **The UAP can orient the parents and child to the room, and demonstrate how to use the call light, how the bed works, or how the television works.**
    2. The UAP cannot prepare a child for endoscopy; this requires assessment and evaluation to determine if the child is ready for the procedure.
    3. There must be at least two people to log roll a child, and the UAP cannot do this procedure alone.
    4. The RN cannot delegate assessment to the UAP.

CLINICAL JUDGMENT GUIDE: The RN cannot delegate assessment, teaching, evaluation, medications, or an unstable client to a UAP.

27. 1. The UAP can weigh the diapers and obtain urine output. The RN must evaluate the output.
    2. A child under 12 years of age cannot be left alone in the room, and the UAP could stay with the child while the parent gets something to eat.
    3. The Pavlik harness should not be removed, so bathing the child in the harness is appropriate and does not warrant intervention.
    4. **The 7-month-old should have elbow restraints, not wrist restraints. Elbow restraints prevent the child from putting fingers into the mouth, but allow the child to move the arms.**

CLINICAL JUDGMENT GUIDE: The RN is responsible for supervising and evaluating the care the UAP provides to any clients. The nurse must intervene and correct the UAP's behavior.

28. Correct answers are 2, 3, 4, and 5.
    1. The RN cannot assign teaching to the LPN.
    2. **The UAP can apply an ice collar because the client is stable.**
    3. **The UAP can apply ointment to a diaper rash—it is a medication but it can be applied by the UAP.**
    4. **The LPN can double-check a dose of medication. The RN can assign medication administration to an LPN.**
    5. **The LPN can enter a health-care provider's orders into the EHR.**

CLINICAL JUDGMENT GUIDE: This is an alternative type of question included in the NCLEX-RN® examination. The nurse must be able to select all the options that answer the question correctly. There are no partially correct answers. Additionally, the RN cannot delegate assessment, teaching, evaluation, medications, or an unstable client to a UAP. The RN cannot assign assessment, teaching, evaluation, or an unstable client to an LPN.

29. 1. The RN cannot delegate teaching to the UAP.
    2. The LPN could teach a client how to irrigate a colostomy, but a 4-month-old is incontinent of stool; therefore, irrigating the colostomy is not done.
    3. The LPN or RN should remove the IV catheter of a 4-month-old child, not the UAP.
    4. **The UAP can escort the child and parents to the car.**

CLINICAL JUDGMENT GUIDE: The RN cannot delegate assessment, teaching, evaluation, medications, or an unstable client to a UAP. The RN cannot assign assessment, teaching, evaluation, or an unstable client to an LPN. Many questions on the NCLEX-RN® are evaluating the test taker's knowledge of the disease process or surgical procedure, as well as delegation and assignments.

30. 1. The UAP can take vital signs but the RN should assess the child to determine whether this is routine postoperative pain (expected), or whether a complication is occurring.
    2. **A rule of thumb—if anyone else gives the RN information about a client, the nurse should first assess the client before taking any further action.**
    3. The nurse may need to notify the HCP, but not before assessing the child.
    4. The nurse may need to administer pain medication but not before assessing the child.

CLINICAL JUDGMENT GUIDE: When the question asks, "Which intervention should the nurse implement first?" it means all or at least more than one option is plausible. Remember: If another person, a machine, or laboratory datum provides information about the client, the RN should assess the client first.

31. 1. **The nurse should offer the child choices that ensure cooperation with the therapeutic regimen. The choices are when the child will ambulate, not whether the child will ambulate.**
    2. The nurse could ask the parents for help in making sure the client ambulates, but this may cause a rift in the nurse, parent, and child relationship. This is not the most appropriate intervention.
    3. The child development therapist could assist with activities that would encourage the

client to ambulate, but the nurse should take control of the situation and ensure the client ambulates. This is not the most appropriate intervention.

4. This is bribery, and the nurse should not use this technique to ensure cooperation with the therapeutic regimen.

CLINICAL JUDGMENT GUIDE: The test taker should be familiar with communication techniques appropriate to a child's developmental stages.

32. 1. The nurse must take action or the child will be afraid of the nurse.
2. The nurse should discuss the inappropriate comment with the mother, not with the child.
3. If every nurse who overheard this type of comment reported it to Child Protective Services, it would only unnecessarily increase the workload in an already overloaded system. Furthermore, reporting perceived potential abuse to Child Protective Services is a very serious accusation.
4. **The nurse should explain to the mother that threatening the child with a shot will cause the child to be frightened of health-care professionals. This type of comment is inappropriate and should not be used to discipline a child.**

CLINICAL JUDGMENT GUIDE: The test taker should be familiar with communication techniques and tactfully discuss this statement with the parent.

33. 1. There is a Web site to obtain information about Down syndrome, but this type of referral would not be the most appropriate for parents who need to deal with emotional aspects of having a child with special needs.
2. The hospital chaplain is an important part of the multidisciplinary health-care team but would not have specialized knowledge regarding caring for a special needs child.
3. **According to the NCLEX-RN® test plan, referrals are included in management of care. The most appropriate referral would be to a support group where other parents who have children with special needs can share their feelings and provide advice on how to care for their child in the home.**
4. Although Down syndrome results from a trisomy chromosome 21, it is primarily associated with maternal age of more than 35 years. Furthermore, a geneticist would not have specialized knowledge regarding caring for a child with special needs.

CLINICAL JUDGMENT GUIDE: The test taker must be knowledgeable of the role of each member of the multidisciplinary health-care team and be prepared to make referrals for clients. These topics will be tested on the NCLEX-RN® examination.

34. 1. The newborn nursery does not need any more people in the area. Personnel are needed to monitor any and all exits.
2. The purpose of using code names to alert hospital personnel of emergency situations is to avoid panic among the clients and visitors; therefore, the nurse should not explain the situation to the clients and visitors.
3. Any time there is an overhead emergency announcement, the charge nurse is responsible for following the hospital emergency plan.
4. **Code Pink means an infant has been abducted from the newborn nursery. The priority intervention is to prevent the abductor from taking the child from the hospital, which can be prevented by placing a staff member at all the unit exits.**

CLINICAL JUDGMENT GUIDE: The nurse must be knowledgeable of hospital emergency preparedness. Students as well as new employees receive this information in hospital orientations and are responsible for implementing procedures correctly. The NCLEX-RN® test plan includes questions on the safe and effective care environment.

35. 1. Even though case management is a strategy to ensure coordination of care while reducing costs, the nurse should not share this with the mother.
2. The case manager is not responsible for ensuring that the client receives the correct medication; it is the responsibility of the HCP.
3. **According to the NCLEX-RN® test plan, questions on case management are included. The case manager will coordinate the care for a client diagnosed with a chronic illness with other members of the multidisciplinary health-care team. This attempts to prevent duplication of services and allows the mother to have a specific individual to coordinate services to meet the child's needs.**
4. The life expectancy of a child diagnosed with Duchenne's muscular dystrophy is approximately 25 years. The case manager is not responsible for helping the child have a normal life expectancy.

CLINICAL JUDGMENT GUIDE: The test taker must be knowledgeable of the role of all members of the multidisciplinary health-care team. These will be tested on the NCLEX-RN® examination.

36. 1. Although this would not be the first step in investigating a problem, this action may be initiated if it is determined to be the cause for the increase in infection rates.
2. The nurse should utilize evidence-based practice research when proposing changes because it is part of the performance improvement process, but it is not the first intervention when investigating the problem.
3. **The first intervention is to determine the extent of the problem and who owns the problem. The NCLEX-RN® test plan includes performance improvement (quality improvement) in the management of care content.**
4. This action may need to be implemented once it is determined whether there is a problem with IV infection rates. However, this would be the second step in the process.

CLINICAL JUDGMENT GUIDE: Performance improvement (quality improvement) activities are tested under the Management of Care section of the NCLEX-RN® test plan.

37. 1. **The ethical principle of justice is to treat all clients fairly, without regard to age, socioeconomic status, or any other variable, including clients with special needs. This statement supports the adolescent's right to her opinion even though she has Down syndrome.**
2. If the adolescent needs clarification of the procedure, this would be an appropriate response, which is an example of the ethical principle of veracity or truth telling.
3. This statement is an example of the ethical principle of paternalism, in which the nurse knows what is best for the client.
4. This is an example of autonomy, in which the client has the right to self-determination. The Nuremburg Code of Ethics specifically supports the rights of individuals with special needs against being forced to participate in procedures they do not want.

CLINICAL JUDGMENT GUIDE: The NCLEX-RN® test plan includes nursing care that addresses ethical principles, including autonomy, beneficence, justice, and veracity, to name a few.

38. 1. Although this may be the case, this is not client advocacy, and doing so may make the mother feel guilty about not being able to afford glasses for her child.
2. **This is an example of client advocacy because many local service organizations, such as the Lions Club or the Rotary Club, will subsidize the cost of the vision test and glasses.**
3. Medicaid does not pay for glasses, and it is not the school nurse's business whether the family is on Medicaid.
4. The nurse should not loan the mother money because this crosses professional boundaries.

CLINICAL JUDGMENT GUIDE: Advocating for a client's rights and needs is a responsibility of the RN and is tested under the Management of Care section of the NCLEX-RN® test plan. A client advocate acts as a liaison between clients and health-care providers to help improve or maintain a high quality of health care.

39. 1. The 16-year-old client is not old enough to sign the permit; therefore, pain medication would not be withheld.
2. **Legally, a child under the age of 18 must have a parent or legal guardian sign for informed consent. The nurse should determine whether the child is aware of the situation and assents to the procedure.**
3. The surgeon is responsible for explaining the procedure; the nurse is responsible for witnessing the signature on the operative permit.
4. The nurse is responsible for witnessing the signature. Having a visitor sign the operative permit is a violation of HIPAA.

CLINICAL JUDGMENT GUIDE: The test taker should be knowledgeable of legal guidelines and informed consent. This is included in the NCLEX-RN® test plan.

40. 1. A written memo does not allow the staff to have input into how to correct the problem. This memo might lead to blaming and arguments among the staff.
2. The performance improvement committee is designed to improve client care, not to address management issues.
3. This is implying that the unit manager does not believe the central supply lost charges. If the unit manager has this concern, it should be addressed directly with the central supply supervisor.
4. **Because the staff is responsible for following the hospital procedure for charging for items used in client care,**

the unit manager should discuss this with staff to determine what should be done to correct the problem.

CLINICAL JUDGMENT GUIDE: There will be management questions on the NCLEX-RN® examination. In many instances, there is no test-taking strategy; the nurse must be knowledgeable of management issues.

41. 1. A 1-year-old child who cries when the parent leaves the room is developmentally on target.
2. The 2-year-old who can speak in two- or three-word sentences is developmentally on target.
3. The 3-year-old should be toilet trained by this age.
4. **The toddler (age 1–3) is expected to throw temper tantrums, but a 4-year-old child should not be doing this; therefore, the child is not developmentally on target and the child developmental specialist should be notified.**

CLINICAL JUDGMENT GUIDE: The pediatric nurse must be knowledgeable of the normal developmental tasks for each age. The Joint Commission (TJC) mandates all children in a pediatric unit must have a developmental assessment and intervention if the child is not on task.

42. 1. The child diagnosed with uncontrolled pain would require a more experienced nurse.
2. Infected skeletal pin sites can lead to osteomyelitis, which would require a more experienced nurse.
3. This child and parents require extensive teaching and should be assigned to a more experienced nurse.
4. **The new graduate should be able to complete preoperative teaching and prepare the young client for surgery. This client is stable.**

CLINICAL JUDGMENT GUIDE: An inexperienced nurse should be assigned the most stable client.

43. 1. Elevating the arm to help decrease edema is an appropriate intervention and does not warrant intervention.
2. The nurse is legally obligated to notify CPS for any suspected child abuse.
3. **A child who is drooling may have epiglottitis and opening the mouth may lead to respiratory distress. This action warrants intervention by the charge nurse.**
4. The nurse needs to confirm a urinary tract infection by obtaining a urine specimen.

CLINICAL JUDGMENT GUIDE: The test taker must be able to apply assessment data and interventions to determine if the action is appropriate. This is an NCLEX-RN® style application question.

44. 1. The nurse must administer the scheduled insulin dose along with the sliding scale coverage; therefore, this is the incorrect dose.
2. **The nurse must administer the scheduled dose along with an additional 8 units, so the total dose is 18 units regular insulin and insulin isophane (NPH) 20 units. The nurse should not administer two injections to the child.**
3. This is the scheduled dose and does not include the sliding scale coverage.
4. This covers the sliding scale coverage but not the scheduled dose.

CLINICAL JUDGMENT GUIDE: This is an alternate type question included in the NCLEX-RN® test plan. The test taker must be able to read a medication administration record (MAR), be knowledgeable of medications, and be able to decide the most appropriate intervention.

45. Correct answers are 1 and 3.
1. **Including the parents in developing the plan of care will help establish a positive relationship.**
2. Holding their child will help with the child and parent relationship, but not with the nurse and parent relationship.
3. **Allowing the parents to vent their feelings will help form a positive nurse and parent relationship.**
4. The nurse must not make the parents feel guilty if they have to work while the child is hospitalized. A relative can stay with the child if parents have to work.
5. This will help the child and parent relationship, not the nurse and parent relationship.

CLINICAL JUDGMENT GUIDE: "Select all that apply" questions require the test taker to select all options that answer the question correctly. There are no partially correct answers.

46. 1. The 9-month-old infant's language and cognitive skills include imitating sounds, saying single syllables, and beginning to put syllables together. Using "mama" and "dada" indicates this child is developmentally on target.
2. The 10- to 12-month-old infant can walk with one hand held by another or with one hand holding onto the furniture, but will usually crawl to get places more

rapidly. This behavior indicates the child is developmentally on target.

3. **The 8-month-old infant should be able to sit steadily unsupported; therefore, this child is developmentally delayed and warrants a referral to the early childhood development specialist. Leaning forward on both hands to sit is normal for a 6-month-old.**

4. The 4-month-old infant should be able to turn from the abdomen to back; therefore, this child is developmentally on target.

CLINICAL JUDGMENT GUIDE: The pediatric nurse must be knowledgeable of the normal developmental tasks for each age. The Joint Commission (TJC) mandates all children in a pediatric unit must have a developmental assessment and intervention if the child is not on task.

47. 1. **The most important intervention for this child is to make sure the child has some control and input into the decision making. It is customary to obtain assent from children 7 years of age and older. Assent means the child has been fully informed about the procedure and concurs with those giving the informed consent.**

2. The parents must sign the permit because the child is under age 18, but the most important intervention is to make sure the child is included and aware of decisions being made about the child's body.

3. The nurse may be able to clarify some of the child's or parent's questions and does not need to refer all questions to the HCP.

4. Witnessing the signature on the permit is required before the child has surgery, but it is not the most important intervention.

CLINICAL JUDGMENT GUIDE: The test taker should be knowledgeable of legal guidelines and informed consent. This is included in the NCLEX-RN® test plan.

48. 1. The nurse should call hospital security when a client or visitor is being abusive, but this is not a legal action.

2. **Legally, the nurse is required to report any suspected child abuse. A 13-year-old child who is having a baby and is withdrawn and silent along with a potential abuser who is trying to control access to the child should make the nurse suspect child abuse.**

3. Referring the client to a social worker is not a legal action.

4. Asking the client whether she feels safe at home is an appropriate assessment question, but it is not a legal action.

CLINICAL JUDGMENT GUIDE: The test taker should be knowledgeable of legal guidelines and requirements. This is included in the NCLEX-RN® test plan.

49. 1. The charge nurse must first make sure that clients and visitors are safe. Someone will notify the charge nurse about the location of the fire.

2. **Safety of the clients and visitors is the priority; therefore, ensuring that they are in a room with the door closed is the first intervention.**

3. The charge nurse may need to prepare for evacuation, but it is not the first intervention.

4. Although making a list of clients not currently on the unit is an appropriate intervention, the charge nurse must first ensure the safety of the clients and visitors who are on the pediatric unit.

CLINICAL JUDGMENT GUIDE: The nurse must be knowledgeable of hospital emergency preparedness. Students as well as new employees receive this information in hospital orientation and are responsible for implementing procedures correctly. The NCLEX-RN® test plan includes questions on the safe and effective care environment.

50. 1. The HIPAA officer can be notified of the breach of confidentiality, but the nurse must first confront the two nurses and correct the behavior.

2. The nurses can be reported to their clinical manager, but the nurse must first confront the two nurses and correct the behavior.

3. The situation can be documented in writing and turned into the HIPAA officer (not the CNO), but the nurse must first confront the two nurses and correct the behavior.

4. **This is a violation of HIPAA; therefore, the nurse must first confront the two nurses and correct the behavior.**

CLINICAL JUDGMENT GUIDE: There will be management questions on the NCLEX-RN®. In many instances, there is no test-taking strategy; the nurse must be knowledgeable of management issues. The Health Insurance Portability and Accountability Act (HIPAA) was passed in 1996 to standardize the exchange of information between health-care providers and to ensure client record confidentiality.

ANSWERS

51. 1. The nurse would not be concerned about not passing meconium until at least 24 hours after delivery.

2. The nurse would not be concerned about a newborn who is slightly jaundiced until after 24 hours after delivery, at which point the HCP would investigate to determine whether the jaundice is pathological.

3. **A newborn who is jittery and irritable needs to be assessed first for possible hypoglycemia. The nurse could feed the newborn glucose water or provide more frequent, regular feedings.**

4. Although the nurse should determine why the newborn will not stop crying, the newborn who is showing signs of hypoglycemia warrants immediate intervention.

CLINICAL JUDGMENT GUIDE: When the question asks, "Which warrants immediate intervention?" it is an "except" question.

52. 1. Aluminum hydroxide; magnesium hydroxide (Maalox), an antacid, is administered to neutralize gastric acidity and help with heartburn, not abdominal pain.

2. A nonnarcotic analgesic, acetaminophen (Tylenol), is used to treat mild pain, a 2 to 4 on a pain scale.

3. **The narcotic analgesic, hydrocodone (Vicodin), is used for moderate-to-severe pain; a 5 is considered moderate pain. The child received a dose at 0600, which relieved the pain for 7 hours; therefore, this would be the most appropriate medication.**

4. An IVP narcotic analgesic should be administered for severe pain, that is, pain greater than 7 on a pain scale of 1 to 10.

CLINICAL JUDGMENT GUIDE: This is an alternate type question included in the NCLEX-RN® test plan. The test taker must be able to read a medication administration record (MAR), be knowledgeable of medications, and be able to decide the nurse's most appropriate intervention.

53. 1. The nurse should not accept any assignment for which he or she is unqualified. A newborn assessment requires specialized knowledge and skills to detect potential complications.

2. The nurse who is not familiar with the procedure or the unit should not be assigned to assist a pediatrician to perform a procedure.

3. This is a dangerous procedure because the nurse must insert a tube into the newborn's stomach. A nurse who is not familiar with this procedure should refuse the assignment.

4. **Any nurse can take an infant to the mother's room and check the bands to ensure the right infant is with the right mother. This is an appropriate task for a nurse who has never worked in the nursery.**

CLINICAL JUDGMENT GUIDE: The nurse should not accept any assignments that require knowledge, skills, or abilities beyond the nurse's expertise.

54. 1. **The 9-month-old infant should be able to sit without support. Therefore, the RN should instruct the UAP to perform the developmental task of helping the child sit without support.**

2. Teaching a child to catch a beach ball would be appropriate for a 15- to 18-month-old child, so the RN should not instruct the UAP to perform this task.

3. The UAP should not use food as a reward or comfort measure because it may lead to childhood obesity.

4. Teaching a child how to blow a kiss is a language or cognitive activity and will not help the child's gross motor development.

CLINICAL JUDGMENT GUIDE: An RN cannot delegate assessment, teaching, evaluation, medications, or an unstable client to a UAP. Tasks that cannot be delegated are interventions requiring nursing clinical judgment.

55. 1. Making sure no one can view the screen is an appropriate information technology guideline.

2. Researching medication online is ensuring safe and effective nursing care and shows that the nurse is keeping abreast of new medications.

3. **According to the NCLEX-RN® test plan, the nurse must be knowledgeable of information technology. Giving another nurse his or her access code is a very serious violation of information technology guidelines and should be reported.**

4. Logging off the computer is an appropriate information technology guideline.

CLINICAL JUDGMENT GUIDE: The test taker must be knowledgeable of information technology security and confidentiality. These topics will be tested on the NCLEX-RN® examination.

56. 1. A dog bite is an emergency, but it is not life threatening; therefore, this child would not be assessed first.
2. The child diagnosed with a head laceration must be assessed, but not before a child who might die of medication poisoning.
3. The child diagnosed with a fractured tibia would not be expected to move the foot.
4. **A child who ingested a bottle of prenatal vitamins presents a medication poisoning that is a potentially life-threatening situation. This child must be assessed first to determine how many vitamins were taken, how long ago they were taken, and whether or not the vitamins contained iron. The child's neurological status must also be assessed.**

CLINICAL JUDGMENT GUIDE: When deciding which client to assess first, the test taker should determine whether the signs and symptoms the client is exhibiting are normal or expected for the client's situation. After eliminating the expected option, the test taker should determine which situation is more life threatening.

57. 1. The pediatric client has the right to an explanation of procedures being done to his or her body.
2. **The pediatric client has a right to be treated with dignity and respect. Just because the child is being coded does not mean the nurse should allow the child's body to be exposed to everyone in the room.**
3. The pediatric client has a right to confidentiality, and the parents or legal guardians are the only individuals who have a right to the child's health information. Talking to the grandparents is a violation of HIPAA unless the parents have approved.
4. The nurse is responsible and accountable to protect the health, safety, and rights of the pediatric client. Leaving an uncapped needle at the bedside could cause serious harm to the child.

CLINICAL JUDGMENT GUIDE: There will be management questions on the NCLEX-RN® addressing client advocacy. A client advocate acts as a liaison between clients and health-care providers to help improve or maintain a high quality of care.

58. 1. Diversional activity deficit would be appropriate if the client did not have sufficient activities to keep him or her occupied. Most children of this age will watch television, play video games, or read books.

2. The client has leukemia and is receiving chemotherapy, which leads to an increased risk of infection; however, this is a physiological problem, not a psychosocial problem.
3. **The client will be isolated from peers and schools because of the high risk of infection resulting from the immunosuppression secondary to chemotherapy and the disease process. At this stage, the child needs to be developing peer relationships and independence from parents. Therefore, social isolation is the priority psychosocial problem for this client.**
4. The nurse should not identify hopelessness because childhood leukemia has a good prognosis.

CLINICAL JUDGMENT GUIDE: The NCLEX-RN® integrates the nursing process throughout the Client Needs categories and subcategories. The nursing process is a scientific, clinical reasoning approach to client care that includes assessment, analysis, planning, implementation, and evaluation. The nurse will be responsible for identifying nursing diagnosis for clients.

59. 1. Placing the IV line on an infusion pump helps to make sure the client does not receive an overload of IV fluid. Most facilities require an IV pump and volume-controlled chamber when administering fluids in a pediatric clinic.
2. **A volume-controlled device (Buretrol) is an infusion device that is used with children when administering IV fluids. The chamber is filled with 1 hour's amount of fluid so that the child will not inadvertently receive an overload of fluid. Fluid volume overload is a potentially life-threatening situation in children.**
3. The site should be checked frequently to ensure that the IV does not infiltrate; therefore, this does not warrant intervention.
4. The IV tubing should not be used longer than 72 hours; therefore, labeling the tubing with the date and time would not warrant intervention.

CLINICAL JUDGMENT GUIDE: When the question asks, "Which warrants immediate intervention?" it is an "except" question. Three of the statements indicate an appropriate intervention, whereas one does not.

60. 1. **Abandonment is a reportable offense to the state board of nursing in every**

state. Reportable offenses could result in stipulations made to the nurse's license.

2. This is failure to follow the five rights of medication administration, but it is not a reportable offense.

3. Multiple medication errors are a management issue, not a reportable offense.

4. Having an affair with a fellow employee is not a reportable offense.

CLINICAL JUDGMENT GUIDE: The NCLEX-RN® test plan includes nursing care that is ruled by legal requirements and scope of practice. The nurse must be knowledgeable of these issues. The nurse's actions should be documented, then reported as necessary.

61. 1. A copper bracelet may or may not help the child diagnosed with rheumatoid arthritis, but because it will not hurt the child, it does not warrant further investigation.

2. Aloe vera is used in many topical burn preparations; therefore, this practice would not warrant further investigation.

3. Mentholated topical ointment (Vick's VapoRub) may or may not help the child's cold, but, because it will not hurt the child, it does not warrant further investigation.

4. **Herbal products are not regulated by the Food and Drug Administration, and there is very little (if any) research on herbal use with children. The nurse should investigate which herbs the child is receiving before taking further action.**

CLINICAL JUDGMENT GUIDE: The test taker should be knowledgeable of Complementary and Alternative Medicine (CAM).

62. 1. This is an appropriate nursing intervention so that the mother will not have to leave her child, but it is not the first intervention. The child's safety is the priority.

2. The RN could go to the cafeteria and tell the mother to return to the room, but during this time the UAP should stay with the child.

3. **The child's safety is the priority; therefore, the RN should have the UAP stay with the child until the mother returns.**

4. Social services would not need to be notified at this time. If the mother continually leaves the child alone, then this would be an appropriate action.

CLINICAL JUDGMENT GUIDE: The test taker should apply the nursing process when the question asks the nurse, "Which intervention

should be implemented first?" In this case, the safety of the client is the priority intervention.

63. Correct answers are 1, 3, 4, and 5.

1. **An 18-month-old child should be throwing temper tantrums. This indicates the child is developing a sense of autonomy.**

2. An 18-month-old child should cling to the mother and interact continuously with the primary caregiver. A child not interacting with the mother is not meeting the task of developing a sense of autonomy.

3. **The child has met the task of trust when he or she cries if the mother leaves the room.**

4. **When a child responds to his or her name, it indicates a sense of identity; therefore, the task is met.**

5. **When a child is smiling and happy with successful toilet training, it indicates development of autonomy and independence.**

CLINICAL JUDGMENT GUIDE: The pediatric nurse must be knowledgeable of the normal developmental tasks for each age. The Joint Commission (TJC) mandates all children in a pediatric unit must have a developmental assessment and intervention if the child is not on task.

64. 1. **An autocratic manager uses an authoritarian approach to direct the activities of others. This individual makes most of the decisions alone without input from other staff members.**

2. A laissez-faire manager maintains a permissive climate with little direction or control.

3. A democratic manager is people oriented and emphasizes efficient group functioning. The environment is open, and communication flows both ways.

4. A democratic manager is people oriented and emphasizes efficient group functioning.

CLINICAL JUDGMENT GUIDE: There will be management questions on the NCLEX-RN®. In many instances, there is no test-taking strategy; the nurse must be knowledgeable of management issues.

65. 1. Squatting relieves the hypoxic episodes, and the child should be able to remain in the squatting position.

2. The child diagnosed with a cyanotic, congenital heart defect should have oxygen when being active.

3. This indicates the father does not understand that the child will not be able to participate

in active sports because of the stress that is placed on the heart.

4. **This behavior indicates the child understands the importance of salt restriction because of potential congestive heart failure.**

CLINICAL JUDGMENT GUIDE: When the question asks, "Which outcome would support the teaching has been effective?" it is an "except" question. Three of the comments indicate the client or family does not understand the teaching and one indicates the client or family does understand the teaching.

66. 1. This is appropriate once the dose has been adjusted for a neonate.
2. This is appropriate once the dose has been adjusted for a neonate.
3. At 2 weeks old there probably will not be a level yet.
4. **Digoxin can be administered to neonates but this is an adult dose: The neonate maintenance dose is 4–8 mcg/kg; 0.125 mg equals 125 mcg. The dose for a 6.82 kg infant would be 27–54 mcg per day.**

CLINICAL JUDGMENT GUIDE: This is an alternate type question included in the NCLEX-RN® test plan. The test taker must be able to read a medication administration record (MAR), be knowledgeable of medications, and be able to decide the nurse's most appropriate intervention.

67. 1. The infant's arm does not have enough tissue for an injection.
2. The infant has a poorly developed dorsogluteal muscle and the sciatic nerve is in this area of the body. Injecting a needle into the nerve could cause permanent damage.
3. Vaccines are not administered into the abdomen.
4. **The anterior lateral thigh muscle (vastus lateralis) is the preferred site for an infant to receive an injection. It is the largest muscle the infant has and is far away from nerves.**

CLINICAL JUDGMENT GUIDE: The nurse must be aware of the appropriate location to administer medications based on the type of medication and the age or body size of the client.

68. **Answer: 45 mL per hour.**
The IV pump is set at an hourly rate. Pediatric clients receive medications at the rate per hour prescribed by the health-care provider. Increasing the rate to a higher rate is not within the realm of nursing judgment.

The medication should be administered at the rate determined by the health-care provider to be a safe volume.

CLINICAL JUDGMENT GUIDE: This is an alternate type of question included in the NCLEX-RN® examination. The nurse must know how to solve math questions.

69. **Correct answers are 1, 3, and 5.**
1. **This child has injuries consistent with child abuse. Child Protective Services and the police should be notified.**
2. This could result in not being able to prosecute the perpetrator if the nurse is not trained in forensic medicine.
3. **The nurse should determine the full extent of the child's injuries.**
4. The nurse should not notify the parents of the potential involvement. The police are fully capable of doing this for themselves. The nurse could instigate an inflammatory situation with this action.
5. **The child needs x-ray studies to determine the extent of internal injuries.**

CLINICAL JUDGMENT GUIDE: This is an alternative type of question included in the NCLEX-RN® examination. The nurse must be able to select all the options that answer the question correctly. There are no partially correct answers.

70. **Correct order is 5, 3, 2, 4, 1.**
5. **Taking the vital signs is part of the assessment and a beginning point for the nurse.**
3. **Because the child has been losing fluids, the nurse should assess tissue turgor to try and determine whether fluid replacement by the parents has been effective.**
2. **The nurse should make sure that the parents do not leave the child alone in the room and make sure the parents are aware of any safety measures used to protect the toddler from abduction and how to call the nurse in case of need.**
4. **The parents will need to change diapers so the child will not develop skin irritation problems.**
1. **When the nurse provides diapers it is a good opportunity to teach the parents about weighing the diapers before and after the child soils them.**

CLINICAL JUDGMENT GUIDE: This is an alternate type of question included in the NCLEX-RN® test plan. The nurse must be able to perform skills in the correct order.

CLINICAL SCENARIO ANSWERS AND RATIONALES

The correct answer number and rationale for why it is the correct answer are given in **boldface type.** Rationales for why the other possible answer options are incorrect also are given, but they are not in boldface type.

1. 1. **The child who is having respiratory difficulty, inspiratory retractions, should be assessed first. Remember Maslow's Hierarchy of Needs.**
   2. A pulse oximeter reading of 93% is within normal limits (93%–100%). It is on the low side because CF causes chronic hypoxia and a low arterial oxygen level is expected.
   3. This is a normal potassium level; therefore, the nurse would not assess this child first.
   4. A 210 mg/dL glucose level for a child diagnosed with type 2 diabetes is not life threatening, and the nurse would not assess this child first.

2. 1. The child in a sickle cell crisis is not stable; therefore, the RN charge nurse should not delegate this task to a UAP.
   2. Oxygen is considered a medication and the RN cannot delegate medication administration to a UAP.
   3. **The child diagnosed with nephrotic syndrome experiences weight gain secondary to edema, which is expected with this disease process. This child is stable, and the UAP can obtain weights; therefore, the RN charge nurse can delegate this task to the UAP.**
   4. The child diagnosed with a traumatic brain injury (TBI) is not stable; therefore, the UAP should not transfer this client to the ICU.

3. 1. Immobilizing the child's leg is appropriate for the RN; therefore, this would not warrant intervention by the charge nurse.
   2. The RN should explain the procedure to the 2-year-old using age-appropriate terms; therefore, this would not warrant intervention by the charge nurse.
   3. The needle and syringe should be disposed of in the sharps container; therefore, this action does not warrant intervention.
   4. **The RN should not recap the needle after administering the medication, so this warrants intervention by the charge nurse. The syringe and needle should be disposed of in the sharps container.**

4. 1. The UAP can document intake and output, and the child has a chronic illness; therefore, the child is stable. This task could be delegated safely.
   2. **The child diagnosed with an acute exacerbation of IBD must be NPO; therefore, this task should not be delegated to the UAP. This cannot be delegated by the RN.**
   3. The UAP can elevate this child's leg and it is appropriate to elevate the leg to help decrease edema. This task could be delegated safely.
   4. The UAP can take laboratory specimens to the laboratory.
   5. The UAP can take the vital signs of a child reporting ear pain.

5. 1. The charge nurse should suspect this child has otitis media and would not have to assign the most experienced nurse to this child. A less experienced emergency department nurse could care for this client.
   2. **The charge nurse should suspect this child is experiencing an acute exacerbation of reactive airway disease and assign the most experienced nurse to this child. This child is in a potentially life-threatening situation.**
   3. The charge nurse should suspect this child has a urinary tract infection, which is not a life-threatening situation. The charge nurse should think about possible sexual abuse, but the most experienced nurse would not need to care for this child.
   4. The charge nurse should suspect the child has pneumonia, which is not a life-threatening situation; therefore, the most experienced nurse does not need to be assigned to this child.

6. 1. The child's temperature should be reduced by receiving an antipyretic medication such as acetaminophen (Tylenol), but it is not the first intervention the charge nurse should implement.
   2. **The charge nurse should suspect bacterial meningitis and place the young teenage child in isolation until definitive diagnosis is made. The nurse must protect the child but also all the other clients, visitors, and staff in the emergency department. This intervention must be implemented first.**

3. The child will need to receive a lumbar puncture for definitive diagnosis of bacterial meningitis, but it is not the first intervention. Protecting others from this very contagious disease by placing the child in isolation is the priority.

4. Notifying the infection control nurse is an important intervention, but not a priority over protecting other individuals in the emergency department.

7. 1. The mother should call 911 so that immediate medical treatment can be given to the child.

2. This is an appropriate question to ask to determine appropriate treatment, but the first thing the nurse should do is to have direct contact with Poison Control to determine the medical treatment for the child.

3. Syrup of ipecac is no longer recommended because vomiting may cause more damage to the child, or lead to aspiration pneumonia.

4. **Contacting Poison Control is the first intervention. Poison Control will be able to provide the nurse with the correct instructions for the mother to help dilute this poison and remove it from her daughter's body.**

8. 1. The object should not be removed until surgery. Removing the object can cause more damage and possible hemorrhaging.

2. The child's medical history and allergies should be determined, but it is not the charge nurse's first intervention.

3. **The charge nurse should first stabilize the pencil in place so further damage will not take place. The left eye should be patched to prevent eye movement. If the uninjured eye moves, the injured eye will**

also move involuntarily, possibly causing more damage.

4. The child's vital signs and pulse oximeter reading should be assessed, but not before stabilizing the injury.

9. 1. **The best response on the Glasgow Coma Scale is 15, so a score of 12 indicates neurological deterioration and requires notifying the neurologist first. The nurse cannot implement any independent nursing interventions to help the child.**

2. The nurse should document the findings in the EHR, but first should notify the neurologist because this indicates a deteriorating condition. To select this option, the data in the stem must be expected or normal for the client.

3. The nurse should continue to assess the client's Glasgow Coma Scale, but not before notifying the neurologist.

4. Placing the child in the high-Fowler's position will not help increased intracranial pressure; therefore, the nurse should not implement this intervention.

10. 1. The charge nurse should suspect acute epiglottis, which is a potential medical emergency and should not be assigned to an inexperienced nurse.

2. The charge nurse should suspect this child will be having emergency abdominal surgery and should not assign the child to an inexperienced nurse.

3. **This child is stable and will need an x-ray; therefore, an inexperienced nurse could care for this client.**

4. The charge nurse should realize this child may be hospitalized and should assign this child to a more experienced nurse.

Learn from yesterday, live for today, hope for tomorrow.

—Albert Einstein

QUESTIONS

1. The nurse in the outpatient psychiatric unit is returning phone calls. Which client should the psychiatric nurse call **first?**
   1. The female client diagnosed with histrionic personality disorder who needs to talk to the nurse about something very important
   2. The male client diagnosed with schizophrenia who is hearing voices telling him to hurt his mother
   3. The male client diagnosed with major depression whose wife called and said he was talking about killing himself
   4. The client diagnosed with bipolar disorder who is manic and has not slept for the last 2 days

2. The RN is caring for children in a psychiatric unit. Which client requires **immediate** intervention by the psychiatric nurse?
   1. The 10-year-old child diagnosed with oppositional defiant disorder who refuses to follow the directions of the mental health worker (MHW)
   2. The 5-year-old child diagnosed with pervasive developmental disorder who refuses to talk to the nurse and will not make eye contact
   3. The 7-year-old child diagnosed with conduct disorder who is throwing furniture against the wall in the day room
   4. The 8-year-old intellectually disabled child who is sitting on the playground and eating dirt and sand

3. The male client diagnosed with major depression is returning to the psychiatric unit from a weekend pass with his family. Which intervention should the nurse implement **first?**
   1. Ask the wife for her opinion of how the visit went.
   2. Determine whether the client took his medication.
   3. Ask the client for his opinion of how the visit went.
   4. Check the client for sharps or dangerous objects.

4. The client on the psychiatric unit is yelling at other clients, throwing furniture, and threatening the staff members. The charge nurse determines the client is at imminent risk for harming the staff and clients and instructs the staff to place the client in seclusion. Which intervention should the RN charge nurse implement **first?**
   1. Document the client's behavior in the nurse's notes.
   2. Instruct the MHWs to clean up the day room area.
   3. Obtain a restraint or seclusion order from the HCP.
   4. Ensure that none of the other clients were injured.

5. A woman comes to the emergency department (ED) and tells the triage nurse she was raped by two men. The woman is crying and disheveled, and has bruises on her face. Which action should the triage nurse implement **first?**
   1. Ask the client whether she wants the police department notified.
   2. Notify a Sexual Assault Nurse Examiner (SANE) to see the client.
   3. Request an ED nurse to take the client to a room and assess for injuries.
   4. Assist the client to complete the emergency department admission form.

6. The nurse is working in an outpatient mental health clinic and returning phone calls. Which client should the psychiatric nurse call **first?**
   1. The client diagnosed with agoraphobia who is calling to cancel the clinic appointment
   2. The client diagnosed with a somatoform disorder who has numbness in both legs
   3. The client diagnosed with hypochondriasis who is afraid she may have breast cancer
   4. The client diagnosed with post-traumatic stress disorder (PTSD) who is threatening his wife

7. The psychiatric nurse is working in an outpatient mental health clinic. Which client should the nurse intervene with **first?**
   1. The client who had a baby 2 months ago and who is sitting alone and looks dejected
   2. The client whose wife just died and who wants to go to heaven to be with her
   3. The client whose mother brought her to the clinic because the mother thinks the client is anorexic
   4. The client who is rocking compulsively back and forth in a chair by the window

8. The emergency department nurse is assessing a female client who has a laceration on the forehead and a black eye. The nurse asks the man who is with the client to please leave the room. The man refuses to leave the room. Which action should the nurse take **first?**
   1. Tell the man the client needs to go to the x-ray department.
   2. Notify hospital security and have the man removed from the room.
   3. Explain that the man must leave the room while the nurse checks the client.
   4. Give the client a brochure with information about a woman's shelter.

9. The charge nurse received laboratory data for clients in the psychiatric unit. Which client data **warrants** notifying the psychiatric health-care provider?
   1. The client on lithium whose serum lithium level is 1.0 mEq/L
   2. The client on clozapine whose white blood cell count is 13,000
   3. The client on alprazolam whose potassium level is 3.7 mEq/L
   4. The client on quetiapine whose glucose level is 128 mg/dL

10. The client diagnosed with a panic attack disorder in the busy day room of a psychiatric unit becomes anxious, starts to hyperventilate and tremble, and is diaphoretic. Which intervention should the RN psychiatric nurse implement **first?**
    1. Administer alprazolam.
    2. Discuss what caused the client to have a panic attack.
    3. Escort the client from the day room to a quiet area.
    4. Instruct the UAP to take the client's vital signs.

11. The client diagnosed with a somatization disorder is reporting vomiting, diarrhea, and having a fever. Which intervention should the nurse implement **first?**
    1. Assess the client's anxiety level on a scale of 1 to 10.
    2. Check the client's vital signs.
    3. Discuss problem-solving techniques.
    4. Notify the client's health-care provider.

12. Which nursing intervention is a **priority** for the client diagnosed with anorexia who is admitted to an inpatient psychiatric unit?
    1. Obtain the client's weight.
    2. Assess the client's laboratory values.
    3. Discuss family issues and health concerns.
    4. Teach the client about selective serotonin reuptake inhibitors.

13. Which client should the psychiatric clinic nurse assess **first**?
    1. The client diagnosed with long-term alcoholism who wants to stop drinking
    2. The client who is a cocaine abuser who is having chest discomfort
    3. The client diagnosed with obsessive-compulsive disorder who won't quit washing his hands
    4. The client who thinks she was given "the date rape drug" and was raped last night

14. The client diagnosed with schizophrenia is being seen by the psychiatric clinic nurse for the initial visit. Which intervention should the nurse implement **first**?
    1. Develop a trusting nurse and client relationship.
    2. Determine the client's knowledge of medication.
    3. Assess the client's support systems.
    4. Allow the client to vent his or her feelings.

15. The client diagnosed with hypochondriasis is angry and yells at the psychiatric clinic nurse, "No one believes I am sick! Not my family, not my doctor, and not you!" Which statement is the nurse's **best** response?
    1. "Have you discussed your feelings with your family?"
    2. "I am sure your doctor believes you are sick."
    3. "I can see you are upset. Sit down and let's talk."
    4. "We cannot find any physiological reason for your illness."

16. The clinical manager assigned the psychiatric nurse a client diagnosed with major depression who attempted suicide and is being discharged tomorrow. Which discharge instruction by the psychiatric nurse would **warrant** intervention by the clinical manager?
    1. The nurse provides the client with phone numbers to call if needing assistance.
    2. The nurse makes the client a follow-up appointment in the psychiatric clinic.
    3. The nurse gives the client a prescription for a 1-month supply of antidepressants.
    4. The nurse tells the client not to take any over-the-counter medications.

17. The charge nurse is caring for clients in an acute care psychiatric unit. Which client would be **most** appropriate for the charge nurse to assign to the licensed practical nurse (LPN)?
    1. The client diagnosed with dementia who is confused and disoriented
    2. The client diagnosed with schizophrenia who is experiencing tardive dyskinesia
    3. The client diagnosed with bipolar disorder who has a lithium level of 2.0 mEq/L
    4. The client diagnosed with chronic alcoholism who is experiencing delirium tremens

18. Which task would be **inappropriate** for the RN psychiatric charge nurse to delegate to the mental health worker (MHW)?
    1. Instruct the MHW to escort the client to the multidisciplinary team meeting.
    2. Ask the MHW to stay in the day room and watch the clients.
    3. Tell the MHW to take care of the client on a 1-to-1 suicide watch.
    4. Request the MHW to draw blood for a serum carbamazepine level.

19. The male client in the psychiatric unit asks the MHW to mail a letter to his family for him. Which action would **warrant** intervention by the RN psychiatric nurse?
    1. The MHW tells the client to place the letter in the mailbox.
    2. The MHW informs the client he cannot send mail to his family.
    3. The MHW takes the letter and places it in the unit mailbox.
    4. The MHW reports the client mailed a letter at the team meeting.

20. The male client admitted to the medical unit after a motor vehicle accident (MVA) admits using heroin. The unlicensed assistive personnel (UAP) tells the RN the client is really agitated and anxious, and has slurred speech. Which intervention should the nurse implement **first?**
   1. Assess the client for heroin withdrawal.
   2. Ask the UAP to take the client's vital signs.
   3. Notify the client's health-care provider.
   4. Administer chlordiazepoxide.

21. Which task would be **most** appropriate for the RN psychiatric nurse to delegate to the mental health worker (MHW)?
   1. Request the MHW to take the client diagnosed with lithium toxicity to the emergency room.
   2. Have the MHW sit with a client diagnosed with bulimia for 1 hour after the meal.
   3. Encourage the MHW to teach the client how to express his or her anger in a positive way.
   4. Ask the MHW to sit with the client while the client talks to his mother on the telephone.

22. The RN psychiatric charge nurse is making shift assignments for the admission unit. The staff includes one registered nurse (RN), two licensed practical nurses (LPNs), four mental health workers (MHWs), and a unit secretary. Which task would be **most** appropriate to assign to the LPNs?
   1. Update the clients' individualized care plans.
   2. Stay in the lobby area and watch the clients.
   3. Administer routine medications to the clients.
   4. Enter a laboratory order into the EHR for a client.

23. The mental health worker (MHW) has tried to calm down the client on the psychiatric unit who is angry and attempting to fight with another client. The RN observes the MHW "taking down" the client to the floor. Which intervention should the nurse implement?
   1. Assist the MHW with the "take down" of the client.
   2. Call the hospital security to come and assist the MHW.
   3. Document the client "take down" in the nurse's notes.
   4. Remove the other clients from the day room area.

24. The mental health worker (MHW) reports to the RN psychiatric nurse that two clients were kissing each other while watching the movie in the lobby area. Which action should the nurse implement?
   1. Tell the MHW to tell the clients not to kiss each other again.
   2. Discuss the inappropriate behavior at the weekly team meeting.
   3. Transfer one of the clients to another psychiatric unit.
   4. Talk to the clients about kissing each other in the lobby area.

25. The nurse is caring for clients in the psychiatric unit. Which task would be **most** appropriate for the RN to delegate to the mental health worker (MHW)?
   1. Instruct the MHW to walk with the client who is agitated and anxious.
   2. Ask the MHW to clean up the floor where the client has urinated.
   3. Tell the MHW to phone the HCP to obtain a PRN medication order.
   4. Request the MHW to explain seizure precautions to another staff member.

26. Which behavior by the mental health worker (MHW) is an example of assault requiring **immediate** intervention by the RN psychiatric nurse?
   1. The MHW injures a client who is forcibly being put in the "quiet" room.
   2. The MHW refuses to let the client come into the day room until putting on socks.
   3. The MHW escorts the client to the anger management class in another building.
   4. The MHW threatened to forcibly remove the client who is refusing to get out of bed.

27. The RN charge nurse has assigned the licensed practical nurse (LPN) to administer medications to the clients on an inpatient psychiatric unit. Which client should the LPN force to take the prescribed medications?
    1. The client diagnosed with bipolar disorder who has been declared incompetent in a court of law
    2. The client diagnosed with major depression who voluntarily admitted herself to the unit
    3. The client diagnosed with paranoid schizophrenia who was involuntarily admitted to the unit
    4. The client diagnosed with a borderline personality who has legal charges pending in the court

28. Which client should the psychiatric charge nurse assign to the nurse from the surgical unit who was assigned to the psychiatric unit for the shift?
    1. The client diagnosed with schizophrenia who is hallucinating and delusional
    2. The client diagnosed with bipolar disorder who is manic and aggressive toward staff and clients
    3. The client who is diagnosed with chronic depression and will not talk to anyone
    4. The client diagnosed with antisocial personality disorder who is angry

29. The psychiatric nurse assigned the mental health worker (MHW) to stay with a client 1-to-1 because of the high risk for suicide. Which behavior by the MHW **warrants** intervention by the RN?
    1. The MHW stays with the client while in the bathroom.
    2. The MHW provides the client with plastic utensils for breakfast.
    3. The MHW stays outside the room during the client's group therapy.
    4. The MHW watches the client walking outside from the porch area.

30. Which statement by the mental health worker (MHW) **warrants** intervention by the RN psychiatric nurse?
    1. "I assisted the client with dressing and hygiene this morning."
    2. "I am going to the team meeting for the next hour."
    3. "I gave the client diagnosed with heartburn some Maalox."
    4. "I am going to play cards with some clients in the day room."

31. The nurse on the substance abuse unit is administering medications. For which client would the nurse **question** administering the medication?
    1. The client admitted for alcohol detoxification who is receiving lorazepam and has an apical pulse of 110
    2. The client admitted for heroin addiction who is receiving methadone and has a respiratory rate of 22
    3. The client admitted for opioid withdrawal who is receiving clonidine and has a blood pressure (BP) of 88/60
    4. The client diagnosed with Wernicke-Korsakoff syndrome receiving IV thiamine who has an oral temperature of 96.8°F

32. The psychiatric nurse overhears a mental health worker (MHW) telling a client diagnosed with schizophrenia, "You cannot use the phone while you are here on the unit." Which action should the RN psychiatric nurse take?
    1. Praise the MHW for providing correct information to the client.
    2. Tell the MHW this is not correct information in front of the client.
    3. Explain to the MHW that the client does not lose any rights.
    4. Discuss this situation at the weekly multidisciplinary team meeting.

33. The client diagnosed with bipolar disorder is admitted to the psychiatric unit in an acute manic state. The nurse needs to complete the admission assessment, but the client is restless, very energetic, and agitated. Which intervention should the nurse implement?
    1. In a very firm voice, ask the client to sit down.
    2. Administer lithium.
    3. Ask questions while walking and pacing with the client.
    4. Do not complete the admission assessment at this time.

34. The client in the psychiatric setting tells the nurse, "There were so many people at the team meeting; I am not sure what the psychiatric social worker is supposed to do for me." Which statement is the psychiatric nurse's **best** response?
    1. "The social worker evaluates the effectiveness of the client's medication."
    2. "This person provides activities that promote constructive use of leisure time."
    3. "The social worker will assist you in keeping your job or help you find a new one."
    4. "This person works with your family and community and makes referrals if needed."

35. The male client diagnosed with paranoid schizophrenia is yelling, talking to himself, and blocking the view of the television. The other clients in the day room are becoming angry. Which action should the RN take **first?**
    1. Obtain a restraint order from the HCP.
    2. Escort the other clients from the day room.
    3. Administer an intramuscular (IM) antipsychotic medication.
    4. Approach the client calmly along with a mental health worker (MHW).

36. A young boy was admitted to the pediatric unit diagnosed with a fractured jaw, bruises, and multiple cigarette burns to the arms. The mother reported the father hurt the child. A man comes to the nurse's station saying, "I am the boy's father; can you tell me how he is doing?" Which statement is the nurse's **best** response?
    1. "Your son has a fractured jaw and some bruises but he is doing fine."
    2. "I am sorry I cannot give you any information about your son."
    3. "You should go talk to your wife about your son's condition."
    4. "The social worker can discuss your son's condition with you."

37. During an interview, the client tells the psychiatric nurse in a mental health clinic, "Sometimes I feel as if life is not worth living. I am going to kill myself." Which interventions should the nurse implement? **Select all that apply.**
    1. Make a no-suicide contract with the client.
    2. Place the client on a 1-to-1 supervision.
    3. Ask the client whether she has a plan.
    4. Commit the client to the psychiatric unit.
    5. Assess the client's support system.

38. The psychiatric nurse is caring for clients on a closed unit. Which client would warrant **immediate** intervention by the nurse?
    1. The client who refuses to attend the anger management class
    2. The client who is requesting to go outside to smoke a cigarette
    3. The client who is nauseated and has vomited twice
    4. The client who has her menses and has abdominal cramping

39. The clinical manager wants to reward the staff on the psychiatric unit for having no tardies or absences for 1 month. Which action would be **most** appropriate for the clinical manager?
    1. Provide pizza, drinks, and dessert for all the shifts.
    2. Post a thank-you note on the board in the employee lounge.
    3. Individually acknowledge this accomplishment with the staff.
    4. Place official documentation in each staff's employee file.

40. The nurse is working in an outpatient psychiatric clinic. The male client tells the nurse, "I am going to kill my wife if she files for divorce. I know I can't live without her." Which action should the nurse implement?
    1. Take no action because this is confidential information.
    2. Document the statement in the client's nurse's notes.
    3. Inform the client's psychiatric health-care provider (HCP) of the comment.
    4. Encourage the client to talk to his wife about the divorce.

41. Which interventions should the inpatient RN psychiatric nurse implement for the client experiencing sleepwalking? **Select all that apply.**
    1. Encourage the client to exercise before going to bed.
    2. Place the client on elopement precautions.
    3. Instruct to client to drink decaffeinated beverages.
    4. Place an alarm on the bed activated when the client gets up.
    5. Tell the MHW to be on a 1-to-1 watch during the night.

42. The nurse is discussing the grieving process with the client. Which of the following stages make up Kübler-Ross's stages of grief? **Rank in the correct order.**
    1. Acceptance
    2. Bargaining
    3. Denial
    4. Anger
    5. Depression

43. The nurse is in the middle or working phase of the nurse and client relationship. Which statement is a task in the middle or working phase?
    1. Identify the client's strengths and weaknesses.
    2. Help the client identify problem-solving techniques.
    3. Evaluate the client's experience while in the group.
    4. Establish the rules for how the meetings will be conducted.

44. Which situation requires **priority** intervention on an inpatient psychiatric unit?
    1. A client is threatening to throw the television at another client.
    2. A male client wants to use the phone to call his spouse.
    3. A client sitting in a chair is delusional and hallucinating.
    4. A client has refused to eat anything for the last 2 days.

45. The client diagnosed with long-term alcoholism asks the nurse, "How does Alcoholics Anonymous help me quit drinking?" Which statements are the nurse's **best** responses? **Select all that apply.**
    1. "AA has sponsors whom you can contact if you want to take a drink."
    2. "AA discusses medications used to help prevent drinking alcohol."
    3. "AA is a support group of alcoholics who have successfully quit drinking."
    4. "AA helps you realize the power you have over your addiction to alcohol."
    5. "AA has professional guest speakers to address addictive personalities."

46. The client diagnosed with bipolar disorder is prescribed lithium and admitted to the psychiatric unit in an acute manic state. Which intervention should the nurse implement **first?**
    1. Have the laboratory draw a STAT serum lithium level.
    2. Evaluate what behavior prompted the psychiatric admission.
    3. Assess and treat the client's physiological needs.
    4. Administer a STAT dose of lithium to the client.

47. The psychiatric unit staff is upset about the new female charge nurse who just sits in her office all day. One of the staff members informs the clinical manager about the situation. Which statement by the clinical manager indicates a laissez-faire leadership style?
    1. "I will schedule a meeting to discuss the concerns of the charge nurse."
    2. "I hired the new charge nurse and she is doing what I told her to do."
    3. "You and the staff really should take care of this situation on your own."
    4. "I will talk to the charge nurse about your concerns and get back to you."

48. The mental health worker (MHW) reports that one of the registered nurses threatened to force-feed the male client diagnosed with schizophrenia if the client did not eat the meal on the lunch tray. Which action should the RN charge nurse take **first?**
1. Tell the MHW that this intervention is part of the client's care plan.
2. Request the nurse to come to the office and discuss the MHW's allegation.
3. Ask the client what happened between him and the nurse during lunch.
4. Ask the MHW to write down the situation to submit to the head nurse.

49. The client diagnosed with paranoid schizophrenia is imminently aggressive and is dangerous to himself, the other clients, and the psychiatric staff members. The client is placed in a seclusion room. Which interventions should the RN psychiatric nurse implement? **Select all that apply.**
1. Assess the client every 2 hours for side effects of medication.
2. Tell the client what behavior will prompt the release from seclusion.
3. Do not notify the client's family of the initiation of seclusion.
4. Explain that the client will be in the seclusion room for 24 hours.
5. Instruct the MHW to check the client every 10 to 15 minutes.

50. The psychiatric nurse overhears a mental health worker (MHW) arguing with a client diagnosed with paranoid schizophrenia. Which action should the RN implement?
1. Ask the MHW to go to the nurse's station.
2. Tell the MHW to quit arguing with the client.
3. Notify the clinical manager of the psychiatric unit.
4. Report this behavior to the client abuse committee.

51. Which client should the psychiatric nurse working in a mental health clinic refer to the psychiatric social worker?
1. The client who was raped and wants help to be able to get on with her life
2. The client who is scheduled for the first electroconvulsive therapy treatment
3. The client who reports having difficulty going to work every day
4. The client who is unable to buy the prescribed antipsychotic medications

52. The psychiatric nurse has taken 15 minutes extra for the lunch break two times in the last week. Which action should the clinical manager implement?
1. Take no action and continue to watch the nurse's behavior.
2. Document the behavior in writing and place in the nurse's file.
3. Tell the nurse to check in and out with the manager when taking lunch.
4. Talk to the nurse informally about taking 45 minutes for lunch.

53. The client diagnosed with Alzheimer's disease is on a special unit for clients diagnosed with cognitive disorders. Which assessment data would warrant **immediate** intervention by the psychiatric nurse?
1. The client does not know his or her name, date, or place.
2. The client is unable to dress himself or herself without assistance.
3. The client is difficult to arouse from sleep.
4. The client needs assistance when eating a meal.

54. The mother of a client recently diagnosed with schizophrenia says to the nurse, "I was afraid of my son. Will he be all right?" Which response by the psychiatric nurse supports the ethical principle of veracity?
1. "I can see your fear; you are concerned your son will not be all right."
2. "If your son takes medication, the symptoms can be controlled."
3. "Why were you afraid of your son? Did you think he would hurt you?"
4. "Schizophrenia is a mental illness and your son will not be all right."

55. The nurse is caring for clients in an outpatient psychiatric clinic. Which client would the nurse discuss with the health-care provider?
1. The client diagnosed with bipolar disorder who is receiving carbamazepine
2. The client diagnosed with schizophrenia who reports taking aluminum hydroxide and magnesium hydroxide daily for heartburn
3. The client diagnosed with major depression who is receiving isoniazid
4. The client diagnosed with anorexia nervosa who is receiving amitriptyline

56. The client in the psychiatric unit tells the nurse, "Someone just put a bomb under the couch in the lobby." Which action should the nurse implement **first?**
1. Look under the couch for a bomb.
2. Implement the bomb scare protocol.
3. Have the staff evacuate the unit.
4. Tell the client there is no bomb.

57. The new nurse on the psychiatric unit tells the charge nurse, "I don't like how the shift report is given." Which statement is the charge nurse's **best** response?
1. "Because you're new I think you should try it our way before making any comments."
2. "We have been doing the shift report this way since I started working here more than 5 years ago."
3. "Have you discussed your concerns about the shift report with the other nurses?"
4. "I would be happy to listen to any ideas you have on how to give the shift report."

58. The client on the psychiatric unit tells the nurse, "I am so bored. I hate just sitting on the unit doing nothing." Which intervention should the nurse implement?
1. Explain that with time the client will be able to go to the activity area.
2. Allow the client to vent feelings of being bored on the unit.
3. Notify the psychiatric recreational therapist about the client's concerns.
4. Tell the client that there is nothing that can be done about being bored.

59. The head nurse in a psychiatric unit in the county emergency department is assigning clients to the staff nurses. Which client should be assigned to the **most** experienced nurse?
1. The client who is crying and upset because she was raped
2. The client diagnosed with bipolar disorder who is agitated
3. The client who was found wandering the streets in a daze
4. The client diagnosed with schizophrenia who is hallucinating

60. The client diagnosed with anorexia is refusing to eat and is lower than 20% of ideal body weight (IBW) for her height and structure. The client has not eaten anything since admission 2 days ago. Which action should the nurse implement?
1. Notify the psychiatrist to request a court order to feed the client.
2. Take no action because the client has the right to refuse treatment.
3. Discharge the client because she is not complying with the treatment.
4. Physically restrain the client and insert a nasogastric tube for feeding.

61. The client on a psychiatric involuntary admission is threatening to run away from the unit. Which intervention should the nurse implement **first?**
1. Notify the police department of the client's threats.
2. Place the unit on high alert for unauthorized departure.
3. Talk to the client about the threat of running away.
4. Have the client sign out against medical advice (AMA).

62. The nurse answers the client's phone in the lobby area and the person asks, "May I speak to Mr. Jones?" Which action should the nurse implement?
1. Ask the caller who is asking for Mr. Jones.
2. Tell the caller Mr. Jones cannot have phone calls.
3. Request the caller to give the access code for information.
4. Find Mr. Jones and tell him he has a phone call.

63. The client seeing the psychiatric nurse in the mental health clinic tells the nurse, "If I tell you something very important, will you promise not to tell anyone?" Which statement is the nurse's **best** response?
    1. "I promise I will not tell anyone if you don't want me to."
    2. "If it affects your care I will have to tell someone who can help."
    3. "If you don't want me to tell anyone, then please don't tell me."
    4. "Why do you not want me to tell anyone if it is so important?"

64. Which situation would warrant **immediate** intervention by the RN charge nurse on the psychiatric unit after receiving the a.m. shift report?
    1. The client diagnosed with paranoid schizophrenia is delusional.
    2. The p.m. shift licensed practical nurse (LPN) called in to say he or she would not be able to work today.
    3. The male mental health worker (MHW) reports losing his unit key card and identification badge.
    4. The unit secretary has a supply order to be approved by the charge nurse before it can be sent to materials management.

65. The client enters a mental health clinic with a gun and is threatening to kill the nurse who told his wife to leave him. Which action should the nurse implement **first?**
    1. Instruct a staff member to call the local police department.
    2. Evacuate the clients and staff to a safe and secure place.
    3. Encourage the client to talk about his feelings of anger.
    4. Calmly and firmly ask the man to put the gun down on the floor.

66. The charge nurse of the psychiatric unit is making assignments. Which clients should be assigned to the medical-surgical nurse who is working in the psychiatric unit for the day? **Select all that apply.**
    1. The client diagnosed with depression who has attempted suicide four times and now is refusing to go to therapy
    2. The client diagnosed with bipolar disease who has diabetes and requires blood glucose monitoring
    3. The female client diagnosed with dissociative identity disorder (DID) who is reporting that she is being falsely imprisoned
    4. The client diagnosed with schizophrenia who is blocking the screen of the television and refuses to move so other clients can watch the television
    5. The client diagnosed with major depression who started taking antidepressant medication 2 days ago and who wants to remain in bed

67. The outpatient clinic psychiatric nurse is preparing to assist the health-care provider to perform electroconvulsive therapy. **Rank in order of performance.**
    1. Attach the electrodes to the client.
    2. Check the client's name and date of birth against the EHR or orders.
    3. Start an intravenous line and run at a keep open rate.
    4. Determine that the client has not eaten or had any liquids since midnight.
    5. Notify the health-care provider to begin the procedure.

68. The psychiatric nurse is reviewing client laboratory values. Which data requires **immediate** intervention by the nurse?
   1. Mr. A.N., who is diagnosed with bipolar disease

Client: A. N.	Allergies: None
Diagnosis: Bipolar Disease	Medical Records Number: 123456

Laboratory Report		
Laboratory Test	**Client Value**	**Normal Value**
Lithium level	1.2	0.5 to 1.2 mEq/L

   2. Ms. D.C., who is diagnosed with mania

Client: D.C.	Allergies: Dilantin
Diagnosis: Mania	Medical Records Number: 109875

Laboratory Report		
Laboratory Test	**Client Value**	**Normal Value**
Valproic acid level	98	50 to 125 mcg/L

   3. Mr. J.M., who is diagnosed with schizophrenia

Client: J.M.	Allergies: NKDA
Diagnosis: Schizophrenia	Medical Records Number: 245689

Laboratory Report		
Laboratory Test	**Client Value**	**Normal Value**
White blood cell count	2.68	4.5 to 11.1 x 10^3/microL

   4. Ms. S.R., who is diagnosed with acute psychosis

Client: S.R.	Allergies: Penicillin
Diagnosis: Acute Psychosis	Medical Records Number: 874521

Laboratory Report		
Laboratory Test	**Client Value**	**Normal Value**
Potassium	4.68	3.5 to 5.3 mEq/L
Sodium	139	135 to 145 mEq/L
Chloride	102	97 to 107 mEq/L

69. The charge nurse responds to an emergency situation on the psychiatric unit in which the male client is angry, yelling, and attempting to hit other clients and the staff. Which interventions should the nurse implement? **Select all that apply.**
   1. Notify the operator to initiate a call for emergency responders to assist.
   2. Tell the client to sit down and be quiet or he will lose privileges.
   3. Have the mental health worker escort the other clients to their rooms.
   4. Make sure that the staff speaks loudly and directly to the client.
   5. Request the unit secretary to stand by the locked doors to allow emergency responders on the unit.

70. The psychiatric nurse is assessing the Abnormal Involuntary Movement Scale (AIMS) for clients on antipsychotic medications. Which client's scores require **immediate** intervention?

Abnormal Involuntary Movement Scale (AIMS)

Adapted		
PT Initials: _____ Gender: _____ Date: _____ Interviewer: _____ **MOVEMENT RATINGS: (Circle One)** 0 = None 1 = Minimal, may be extreme of normal 2 = Mild 3 = Moderate 4 = Severe **Note: #10** 0 = no awareness 1 = aware, no distress 2 = aware, mild distress 3 = aware, moderate distress 4 = aware, severe distress		
Facial & Oral Movements	1. **Muscles of facial expression** (e.g., movement of forehead, eyebrows, periorbital area, cheeks; include frowning, blinking, smiling, grimacing)	0 1 2 3 4
	2. **Lips and perioral area** (e.g., puckering, pouting, smacking)	0 1 2 3 4
	3. **Jaw** (e.g., biting, clenching, chewing, mouth opening, lateral movement)	0 1 2 3 4
	4. **Tongue** (rate only increase in movement both in and out of mouth, NOT inability to sustain movement)	0 1 2 3 4
Extremity Movements	5. **Upper body** (arms, wrists, hands, fingers) (e.g., include **choreic movements** [rapid, objectively purposeless, irregular, spontaneous], **athetoid movements** [slow irregular, complex, serpentine]). Do NOT include tremor (repetitive, regular, and rhythmic).	0 1 2 3 4
	6. **Lower body** (legs, knees, ankles, toes) (e.g., lateral knee movement, foot tapping, and heel dropping, foot squirming, inversion and eversion of foot)	0 1 2 3 4
Trunk Movements	7. **Neck, shoulders, hips**	0 1 2 3 4
Global Judgments	8. **Severity of abnormal movements**	0 1 2 3 4
	9. **Incapacitation due to abnormal movements**	0 1 2 3 4
	10. **Client's awareness of abnormal movements** (rate only client's report; see previous note)	0 1 2 3 4
Dental Status	11. **Current problem with teeth or dentures**	Yes = 1 No = 0
	12. **Does client usually wear dentures?**	Yes = 1 No = 0
	SCORE	

1. The client who scored a 6 on the scale
2. The client who scored a 10 on the scale
3. The client who scored a 15 on the scale
4. The client who scored a 24 on the scale

MENTAL HEALTH CLINICAL SCENARIO

The RN psychiatric nurse manager in a demographically diverse, urban outpatient mental health clinic has two RNs along with two LPNs and two mental health workers (MHWs) who are unlicensed assistive personnel. There are two receptionists at the front desk. The multiethnic, mostly adult clients have a wide variety of diagnosed and treatable psychiatric conditions. Some of the clients are potentially dangerous to themselves and to others. Most of the clients are currently addicts or have a history of alcohol and drug abuse.

1. The nurse manager is triaging and returning phone calls. Which client should the mental health nurse call **first?**
   1. The client diagnosed with a narcissistic personality disorder who needs to see the psychiatrist today
   2. The client diagnosed with schizophrenia who is hearing voices telling him to hurt his wife
   3. The client diagnosed with major depression who is refusing to get out of bed and go to work
   4. The client diagnosed with bipolar disorder who is manic and has sold the family car for cash

2. The psychiatric nurse is working at the triage desk. Which client should the nurse intervene with **first?**
   1. The client who had a baby 2 months ago and thinks she has postpartum depression
   2. The client who told the receptionist he wants to kill himself and has a gun in the car
   3. The woman who thinks her mother has Alzheimer's disease because her mother is confused
   4. The client who has been washing his hands in the bathroom for almost 20 minutes

3. The mental health clinic nurse manager is reviewing laboratory data for clients seen in the clinic. Which client data **warrants** notifying the psychiatric health-care provider?
   1. The client on lithium whose serum lithium level is 2.0 mEq/L
   2. The client on clozapine whose white blood cell count is 10,000
   3. The client on alprazolam whose potassium level is 3.7 mEq/L
   4. The client on divalproex sodium who has a depakote serum level of 60 μg/mL

4. The nurse manager is working in the mental health clinic and returns a telephone call to a male client who says that "voices are telling me to hurt myself, now." Which intervention should the psychiatric nurse implement **first?**
   1. Call 911 and tell the paramedics the client is a danger to himself or others.
   2. Ask the client if he has taken his medication this morning.
   3. Notify the health-care provider of the client's statement.
   4. Keep the client on the telephone to discuss the voices he is hearing.

5. The client diagnosed with a panic attack disorder in the clinic waiting room becomes anxious, starts to hyperventilate and tremble, and is diaphoretic. After removing the client from the day room, which intervention should the RN mental health nurse implement next?
   1. Administer alprazolam.
   2. Allow the client to verbalize feelings of anxiety.
   3. Encourage the client to take slow, deep breaths.
   4. Instruct the MHW to obtain the client's pulse oximeter reading.

6. Which client would be **most** appropriate for the RN nurse manager to assign to the LPN in the outpatient psychiatric clinic?
   1. The client diagnosed with dementia who is confused and disoriented
   2. The client diagnosed with schizophrenia who is experiencing extrapyramidal side effects
   3. The client diagnosed with bipolar disorder who is pacing up and down the hallway
   4. The client diagnosed with anorexia nervosa who is hypotensive and reporting dizziness

7. Which task is inappropriate for the RN psychiatric nurse manager to delegate to the MHW?
   1. Instruct the MHW to observe the client who is exhibiting compulsive behavior.
   2. Ask the MHW to stay in the waiting room and watch the clients.
   3. Tell the MHW to sit with the client who reports being suicidal.
   4. Request the MHW to draw blood for a serum lithium level.

8. The client diagnosed with paranoid schizophrenia is yelling, talking to himself, and blocking the view of the television. The other clients in the waiting room are becoming angry. Which action should the RN nurse manager implement **first?**
   1. Place the client in a quiet room.
   2. Escort the other clients from the day room.
   3. Request the receptionist to call 911.
   4. Approach the client calmly along with the LPN.

9. The RN mental health nurse manager observes the MHW arguing with a client in the waiting room. The nurse manager requests the MHW to go to his office **immediately.** Which action should the nurse manager implement **first?**
   1. Ask the client what caused the argument.
   2. Discuss the behavior with the MHW.
   3. Document the MHW's behavior in writing.
   4. Terminate the MHW immediately.

10. The nurse has been late to work three times in the last week. The nurse manager talks to the nurse and finds out she has to take the bus to work until her car is fixed, which should be completed in 1 week. Which action should the RN nurse manager implement?
    1. Ask another nurse to give the chronically late nurse a ride to work until the car is fixed.
    2. Document the behavior in writing and place in the nurse's file.
    3. Tell the nurse if she is late again she will be placed on administrative leave.
    4. Do not take any action at this time because the nurse has an excellent attendance record.

The correct answer number and rationale for why it is the correct answer are given in **boldface type.** Rationales for why the other possible answer options are incorrect also are given, but they are not in boldface type.

1. 1. The client diagnosed with a histrionic personality has excessive emotionality and seeks attention. Her saying "something important" must be understood within this context and would not warrant calling this client first.

2. **The nurse should contact this client first because the client realizes the voices are telling him to hurt his mother. The nurse should inform this client to come to the clinic immediately, and he should be admitted to a psychiatric unit.**

3. Because the wife called the clinic, the client is being watched and should be safe from killing himself. The nurse should call this client immediately but not before a client who made the phone call himself and who may be alone and hearing voices.

4. The nurse should expect the client who is manic not to be sleeping; therefore, this is expected behavior. The nurse should call this client immediately but not before the client who is hearing voices telling him to hurt his mother.

CLINICAL JUDGMENT GUIDE: When answering questions in mental health nursing, the test taker should identify safety as a priority intervention in any situation. All these situations require intervention by the nurse but safety is the priority.

2. 1. Oppositional defiant disorder consists of a pattern of uncooperative, defiant, and hostile behavior toward authority figures. Not following the MHW's directions would be expected behavior in a child diagnosed with this disorder and would not require immediate intervention by the RN.

2. Refusal to talk or make eye contact is a sign of autism, the best known of the pervasive developmental disorders; therefore, this client would not require immediate intervention by the nurse.

3. **The child diagnosed with conduct disorder is aggressive to people and animals, bullies and threatens others, destroys property, and sets fires. Throwing furniture could endanger the child or other clients. This behavior warrants immediate intervention.**

4. Eating dirt and sand is pica, or the ingestion of non-nutritive substances such as paint, hair, cloth, leaves, sand, clay, or soil. It is commonly seen in intellectually disabled children, but it is not life threatening unless a medical complication such as a bowel obstruction, infection, or a toxic condition (e.g., lead poisoning) occurs. This behavior would not require immediate intervention.

CLINICAL JUDGMENT GUIDE: When deciding which client to assess first, the test taker should determine whether the signs and symptoms the client is exhibiting are normal for the client's situation. After eliminating the expected options, the test taker should determine which situation is more life threatening.

3. 1. The nurse should discuss how the visit went, but it is not the first intervention.

2. The nurse should make sure the client took his medications during the weekend pass, but it is not the first intervention.

3. The client should discuss how the visit went, but it is not the first intervention.

4. **The nurse's first intervention should be to provide for the client's safety by ensuring the client has no sharps or dangerous objects that he could use to hurt himself, because he is diagnosed with major depression.**

CLINICAL JUDGMENT GUIDE: When answering questions in mental health nursing, the test taker should identify safety as a priority intervention in any situation.

4. 1. The nurse must document the client's behavior that prompted the need for seclusion, but it is not the first intervention.

2. The day room area should be cleaned up, but it is not the nurse's first intervention.

3. **The use of restraints and seclusion requires an HCP's order every 4 hours for adults and more frequently for children. Additionally, an evaluation must be performed by the HCP within 1 hour of initiation of restraints or seclusion. The nurse must obtain this order first after placing the client in the seclusion room. The nurse can place the client in seclusion for the safety of the client, staff, and other clients, but the nurse must then immediately obtain a HCP's order.**

4. The charge nurse should make sure the other clients are not injured, but the first intervention is to put the client who is acting out into seclusion, safely and legally.

ANSWERS

CLINICAL JUDGMENT GUIDE: The NCLEX-RN® test plan includes nursing care that is ruled by legal requirements. The nurse must be knowledgeable of these issues. The nurse may have to respond first then follow-up with another action.

5. 1. The client may or may not want the police notified, but this is not the triage nurse's first intervention. The triage nurse should first care for the client.
   2. The SANE nurse is a nurse who is specialized in caring for clients who have been raped. The SANE nurse is able to spend time with the client, is knowledgeable of legal issues, and would be an appropriate intervention, but it is not the triage nurse's first intervention.
   3. **The triage nurse's first intervention is to address the client's physiological needs, which means to assess for any type of trauma or injury.**
   4. The client can complete the admission form while in the room; the triage nurse's first intervention should be to care for the client, not paperwork.

CLINICAL JUDGMENT GUIDE: When the question asks which intervention to implement first, the test taker should determine whether any of the options concern the physiological needs of the client and then apply Maslow's Hierarchy of Needs to find the correct answer. Remember: Physiological needs take priority over all other needs.

6. 1. The client diagnosed with agoraphobia is afraid to leave the house; therefore, canceling a clinic appointment would be expected of this client. The nurse would not need to return this client's phone call first.
   2. The client diagnosed with a somatoform disorder has physical symptoms without a physiological cause; therefore, reporting numbness in the legs is expected behavior. The nurse would not need to return this client's phone call first.
   3. The client diagnosed with hypochondriasis is preoccupied with the fear that one has or will get a serious disease; fearing breast cancer is then expected behavior. The nurse would not need to return this client's phone call first.
   4. **Post-traumatic stress disorder (PTSD) is an illness that occurs to someone who has experienced a traumatic event. The client feels a numbing of general responsiveness but has outbursts of anger. The nurse should return this call first and assess the**

situation to determine whether the client should be seen in the clinic.

CLINICAL JUDGMENT GUIDE: When deciding which client to assess first, the test taker should determine whether the signs and symptoms the client is exhibiting are normal or expected for the client situation. After eliminating the expected options, the test taker should determine which situation is more life threatening.

7. 1. The client who is depressed would be expected to look dejected; therefore, the nurse would not need to assess this client first.
   2. **This client who says he wants to go to heaven to be with his wife may be suicidal and should be assessed first to see whether he has a plan.**
   3. This client needs to be assessed for anorexia but not before a client who may be suicidal.
   4. The nurse should not interrupt a client who is acting compulsively. The nurse should wait until the client finishes the behavior before talking to the client.

CLINICAL JUDGMENT GUIDE: When deciding which client to assess first, the test taker should determine whether the signs and symptoms the client is exhibiting are normal or expected for the client situation. After eliminating the expected options, the test taker should determine which situation is more life threatening.

8. 1. **The nurse needs to remove the man from the room so that the nurse can talk to the client and discuss probable abuse. Taking the client to the x-ray department may not arouse suspicion in the man and may allow the client to discuss the situation.**
   2. This may be needed, but it is not the first intervention. This action may cause the man to get angrier in the emergency department, or it may cause more problems for the woman if she goes home with him.
   3. The nurse could demand the man leave the room, but this action may cause the man's anger to escalate; therefore, the first intervention is to remove the client from the room.
   4. The nurse should not allow the man to see the nurse discussing a woman's shelter with the client or providing a client with a brochure. This could cause further anger in the man, especially if the woman goes home with the man.

CLINICAL JUDGMENT GUIDE: The nurse should address the client's needs first and follow the nursing process. Assessment is the first step in the nursing process. The nurse should protect the client's safety to perform an assessment.

9. 1. The therapeutic serum level for lithium is 0.6 to 1.2 mEq/L. Because the client's 1.0 mEq/L level is within normal limits, the charge nurse would not need to notify the psychiatric HCP about the lithium (Eskalith) medication.
   2. **The WBC count is elevated, which may indicate that the client is experiencing agranulocytosis, a life-threatening complication of clozapine (Clozaril). This laboratory data would warrant notifying the psychiatric health-care provider.**
   3. The client's serum potassium level is within normal limits; therefore, this laboratory information does not warrant notifying the psychiatric health-care provider.
   4. This glucose level is slightly elevated for a fasting reading but would not warrant notifying the psychiatric health-care provider.

CLINICAL JUDGMENT GUIDE: The nurse must be knowledgeable of normal laboratory values. These values must be memorized and the nurse must be able to determine if the laboratory value is normal for the client's disease process or medications the client is taking.

10. 1. The benzodiazepine, alprazolam (Xanax), is an appropriate medication for an anxiety attack, but it will take at least 15 to 30 minutes for the medication to treat the physiological signs and symptoms. Therefore, this is not the first intervention.
   2. The nurse should discuss the panic attack and what prompted it, but it is not the nurse's first intervention.
   3. **The first intervention is to remove the client from the busy day room to a quiet area to help decrease the anxiety attack.**
   4. The client's vital signs should be taken, but this is not the nurse's first intervention.

CLINICAL JUDGMENT GUIDE: The nurse should remember that if a client is in distress and the nurse can do something to relieve the distress, that action should be done first, before assessment. The test taker should select an option that directly helps the client's condition.

11. 1. The nurse should assess the client's anxiety level but not before ruling out a physiological reason for the client's reports.
   2. **The nurse should first determine if the client's vital signs are abnormal, which rules out any physiological reason for the client's symptoms.**
   3. The nurse should discuss techniques to address increased anxiety level, but a

physiological cause of these symptoms should be ruled out first.
   4. The client's HCP will need to be notified if the reports are secondary to a physiological reason, but would not if the vital signs are within normal limits.

CLINICAL JUDGMENT GUIDE: If the question asks the nurse, "Which intervention to implement first?" then the test taker should apply the nursing process. The psychiatric nurse must first assess to determine if the client has a physiological problem; because option A and B are assessment interventions, the test taker should then select physiological assessment over psychosocial assessment.

12. 1. The nurse should assess the client's weight, but it is not a priority over assessing laboratory values, which may be indicative of a life-threatening disease process, especially potassium level.
   2. **The client's laboratory values are the priority, especially potassium, because these reflect long-term effects of anorexia and possible life-threatening disease processes that must be corrected immediately.**
   3. This is an appropriate intervention, but physiological needs are a priority over problem-solving.
   4. A teaching intervention is not a priority over a physiological need.

CLINICAL JUDGMENT GUIDE: When a question asks, "Which intervention should the nurse implement first?" the test taker should use the nursing process to determine the correct answer. If the client is not in distress, then the nurse should assess. If two options address assessment, select the intervention that addresses a life-threatening complication.

13. 1. This client needs to be assessed but not before the client diagnosed with chest discomfort. If the client exhibited signs of alcohol withdrawal, then this client would have a physiological need.
   2. **Cocaine causes vasoconstriction of the coronary arteries and can lead to life-threatening cardiovascular problems; therefore, this client should be seen first.**
   3. The client who is performing compulsive behavior should not be interrupted but should be allowed to finish the behavior.
   4. This client is not exhibiting physiological complications; therefore, this client should not be assessed first.

ANSWERS

CLINICAL JUDGMENT GUIDE: The test taker should first determine if the signs or symptoms are normal or expected for the client situation. If there are two or more clients exhibiting unexpected signs or symptoms, then select the client who is exhibiting life-threatening signs or symptoms, needs more assessment, or would warrant notifying the health-care provider.

14. 1. **If the nurse does not establish the foundation for a trusting nurse and client relationship, then the nurse will not be effective in caring for this client. This is the first nursing intervention.**
2. Medication is a vital part of the treatment for schizophrenia, but on the initial visit a trusting relationship is the priority.
3. Support systems are an important part of the client's treatment in the community, but the client must be able to trust the nurse when sharing information.
4. Venting feelings about disease, the current situation, and life is vital to the treatment of a client diagnosed with schizophrenia, but the client must be able to trust the nurse when sharing feelings.

CLINICAL JUDGMENT GUIDE: In mental health nursing, the foundation for all nursing care is having a trusting nurse and client relationship. All the options are possible or plausible for the nurse to implement, but there is only one correct answer.

15. 1. The psychiatric nurse should address the client's feelings, not the feelings of family members.
2. This comment does not address the client's feelings, and the nurse should not talk about what the doctor believes or doesn't believe.
3. **The nurse must first calm the client, assess the situation, and ensure a therapeutic nurse and client relationship. This response addresses all these issues.**
4. This response will more than likely further antagonize the client and is not a therapeutic response.

CLINICAL JUDGMENT GUIDE: The psychiatric nurse's responsibility is to deescalate the client's anger. Being empathetic and allowing the client to verbalize feelings is the nurse's priority intervention.

16. 1. Providing phone numbers for the client and family is an intervention that the nurse should discuss with the client and would not warrant intervention by the clinical manager.
2. Follow-up appointments are important for the client after being discharged from a psychiatric facility; therefore, this instruction would not warrant intervention by the clinical manager.
3. **The client should be given a 7-day supply of antidepressants because safety of the client is the priority. As antidepressant medications become more effective, the client is at a higher risk for suicide; therefore, the nurse should ensure that the client cannot take an overdose of medication. This instruction warrants intervention by the clinical manager.**
4. The client should not take any OTC medications without talking to the HCP or pharmacist. This instruction would not warrant intervention by the clinical manager.

CLINICAL JUDGMENT GUIDE: When the question asks, "Which warrants immediate intervention?" it is an "except" question. Three of the actions are correct interventions, whereas one is not.

17. 1. **The client diagnosed with dementia would be expected to have confusion and disorientation; therefore, the LPN could be assigned this client. This client is not experiencing any potentially life-threatening complication of dementia.**
2. The client is experiencing tardive dyskinesia, a potentially life-threatening complication of antipsychotic medication. An experienced RN should be assigned to this client.
3. The therapeutic serum level for lithium is 0.6 to 1.2 mEq/L. The client's level is toxic, and an experienced RN should care for the client.
4. This client is experiencing a potentially life-threatening complication of alcohol withdrawal. An experienced RN should be assigned to this client.

CLINICAL JUDGMENT GUIDE: The test taker must determine which client is the most stable, which makes this an "except" question. Three clients are either unstable or have potentially life-threatening conditions.

18. 1. Clients are allowed, encouraged, and expected to participate in the multidisciplinary team meeting. This is an appropriate task to delegate to the MHW.
2. One of the MHW's primary responsibilities is to watch clients in the day room area. This is an appropriate task to delegate.
3. The MHW can remain with a client who is on 1-to-1 suicide watch. This is an appropriate nursing task to delegate.

4. The MHW does not draw blood, and this would be an inappropriate task to delegate. The laboratory technician draws the client's blood work.

CLINICAL JUDGMENT GUIDE: The nurse is responsible for knowing the scope of practice for the health-care team members who are subordinates.

19. 1. Telling the client to place the letter in the mailbox is empowering the client to take responsibility. This action would not warrant intervention by the nurse.
    2. **The RN should explain to the MHW that mental health clients retain all the civil rights afforded to all persons, except the right to leave the hospital in the case of involuntary commitments. The client has the right to mail and receive letters.**
    3. Mailing the client's letter is an appropriate action to take; therefore, this would not warrant intervention by the nurse.
    4. Reporting the client mailed a letter to his family at the team meeting may or may not be pertinent to the client's care, but this action would not warrant intervention by the nurse.

CLINICAL JUDGMENT GUIDE: The NCLEX-RN® test plan includes nursing care that is ruled by legal requirements. The nurse must be knowledgeable of these issues.

20. 1. **Whenever the nurse is given information that indicates a complication or is potentially life threatening, the nurse must first assess the client.**
    2. The client is unstable; therefore, the RN should not instruct the UAP to take the client's vital signs.
    3. The nurse should not notify the health-care provider before assessing the client.
    4. Chlordiazepoxide (Librium) is an antianxiety medication used for alcohol withdrawal, not for heroin withdrawal.

CLINICAL JUDGMENT GUIDE: If the test taker wants to select "notify the HCP" as the correct answer, the test taker must examine the other three options. If information in any of the other options is data the HCP would need to make a decision, then the test taker should eliminate the "notify the HCP" option.

21. 1. The client diagnosed with lithium toxicity is unstable, and the RN should not delegate this task to an MHW.

2. **Having someone stay with the client after a meal will prevent the client from inducing vomiting and could be delegated to an MHW. The client diagnosed with bulimia needs someone there to prevent vomiting, which is a sign of this mental health problem.**
3. The RN should not delegate teaching. Helping the client with anger management would be the responsibility of the nurse or possibly the therapy department.
4. The client has a right to talk to his mother on the phone without someone listening.

CLINICAL JUDGMENT GUIDE: An RN cannot delegate assessment, teaching, evaluation, medications, or an unstable client to a UAP or MHW. Tasks that cannot be delegated are nursing interventions requiring nursing clinical judgment.

22. 1. The RN should be assigned to update the individualized care plans.
    2. The MHWs should be assigned to watch the clients in the day area.
    3. **The LPNs' scope of practice allows the administration of medication. This is an appropriate assignment.**
    4. The LPNs can enter a laboratory order into the EHR, but the unit secretary can also perform this duty. This would not be the most appropriate assignment for the LPNs.

CLINICAL JUDGMENT GUIDE: The nurse is responsible for knowing the scope of practice for the health-care team members who are subordinates.

23. 1. **All psychiatric staff members are taught how to "take down" a client physically if the client is a danger to self or to others. The RN should assist the MHW in subduing the client so that no one is injured.**
    2. The psychiatric staff members are trained to deal with clients who are angry and aggressive; there is no need to contact hospital security.
    3. The nurse can document the occurrence, but because the nurse observed the "take down," the nurse should assist the MHW. The psychiatric staff members have to be able to depend on each other no matter what the situation.
    4. The nurse can have other staff members remove clients from the day room area; the RN psychiatric nurse should help the MHW with the "take down."

CLINICAL JUDGMENT GUIDE: When answering questions in mental health nursing, the test taker should identify safety as a priority intervention

in any situation. The nurse should assist the MHW to promote the safety of the client and the MHW.

24. 1. The nurse should address the behavior with the clients and not delegate this task to the MHW. This inappropriate behavior needs further investigation to determine whether it is consensual or under duress.
    2. The inappropriate behavior should be addressed immediately with both clients.
    3. If the behavior does not stop, one of the clients may need to be transferred to another unit, but this is not the appropriate action at this time.
    4. **The nurse needs to talk to the clients to determine whether the kissing was consensual or under duress. Either way, the behavior is inappropriate, and the clients should be told there is no kissing or sexual activity allowed between clients while they are hospitalized on the psychiatric unit.**

CLINICAL JUDGMENT GUIDE: The nurse should assess the situation to gather information and reinforce the rules of the psychiatric unit.

25. 1. **The MHW could walk with the client who is agitated. This may help decrease the client's agitation and anxiety.**
    2. The nurse should not assign a task that is the responsibility of another staff member. The housekeeping or custodial department should be assigned to clean the floor.
    3. The MHW cannot take telephone orders from a HCP. This must be done by a licensed nurse.
    4. The RN cannot delegate teaching to an MHW. The nurse should explain seizure precautions to staff members.

CLINICAL JUDGMENT GUIDE: The RN cannot delegate assessment, evaluation, teaching, administering medications, or the care of an unstable client to a UAP.

26. 1. This is an example of battery, which is the touching of a client without consent.
    2. This is an example of false imprisonment, which is the deliberate and unauthorized confinement of a person within fixed limits by the use of verbal or physical means.
    3. This is an appropriate action by the MHW, which would not require immediate intervention.
    4. **This is an example of assault, which is an act that results in a person's genuine**

fear and apprehension of being touched without consent.

CLINICAL JUDGMENT GUIDE: The nurse is responsible to ensure all clients' legal rights are maintained, even when on a locked psychiatric unit.

27. 1. **When an individual is declared incompetent in a court, a guardian makes decisions for the client. The client loses the right to refuse medication.**
    2. Unless a mental health court orders the client to receive medication, the LPN cannot force the client to take the medication. This client voluntarily admitted herself to the unit.
    3. Unless a mental health court orders the client to receive the medication, the LPN cannot force a client to take it, even if the client was involuntarily admitted to the unit.
    4. Charges pending in court do not remove the client's right to refuse medication.

CLINICAL JUDGMENT GUIDE: The charge nurse must be knowledgeable of the client's rights in the mental health–nursing arena. The two options addressing a court of law should be included as possible correct options because the word "force" is in the stem of the question.

28. 1. The more experienced psychiatric nurse should be assigned the client who is actively hallucinating and delusional.
    2. The client who is aggressive should be assigned to a more experienced psychiatric nurse because this is a safety issue.
    3. **The client who is chronically depressed should be assigned to the surgical nurse who is being floated to the psychiatric unit. The client is not identified as suicidal in the option.**
    4. The client diagnosed with antisocial personality disorder who is angry is manipulative and tends to split staff, so this client should be assigned to a more experienced psychiatric nurse.

CLINICAL JUDGMENT GUIDE: The test taker should select the client who is most stable and would require the least amount of psychiatric nursing knowledge. The primary concern on the psychiatric unit is safety, for which client assignments must be based.

29. 1. A client on a 1-to-1 watch must not be left alone for any reason and the MHW should be within arm's length at all times.
    2. The client should not be allowed steel utensils while on suicide watch, so plastic utensils are appropriate.

3. As long as the client is with a member of the staff, the client can attend group therapy.
4. **The MHW should remain in constant presence of the client, not observing the client from the porch.**

CLINICAL JUDGMENT GUIDE: The RN is responsible for supervising any task delegated to an MHW, who is an unlicensed assistive personnel in mental health nursing.

30. 1. The MHW can assist the client with activities of daily living.
2. The MHW is a vital part of the mental health team and is included in team meetings to discuss the client's psychiatric care.
3. **The MHW cannot administer medication; therefore, this comment warrants intervention.**
4. The MHW should stay in the day room to maintain safety for the clients, so this comment does not warrant intervention.

CLINICAL JUDGMENT GUIDE: The MHW is an unlicensed assistive personnel. The RN cannot delegate assessment, teaching, evaluation, medication administration, or an unstable client to a UAP.

31. 1. Lorazepam (Ativan) is used to prevent delirium tremens, and an elevated pulse would not warrant questioning the administration of this medication.
2. Methadone (Methadose) is prescribed to prevent withdrawal symptoms from heroin addiction, and an increased respiratory rate would not warrant questioning the administration of this medication.
3. **Clonidine (Catapres) is administered primarily to treat hypertension but is also used to reduce the symptoms of withdrawal from opioids, nicotine, and alcohol. The nurse would question administering this medication because of the client's low blood pressure, no matter why it is being prescribed.**
4. Thiamine (vitamin B_1) is used to diminish Wernicke-Korsakoff encephalopathy, which is characterized by confusion, memory loss, and loss of cranial nerve function resulting from chronic alcohol abuse. The nurse would not question giving this medication to a client diagnosed with Wernicke-Korsakoff syndrome, and a subnormal temperature would not warrant questioning the administration of this medication.

CLINICAL JUDGMENT GUIDE: The nurse must be aware of expected actions of medications. The nurse must be aware of assessment data indicating if the medication should be administered or held. Also, the nurse should be able to determine if the medication is effective or causing a side effect or an adverse event.

32. 1. This is not correct information; therefore, the RN should not praise the MHW.
2. The psychiatric nurse should not correct the MHW in front of the client because it will compromise the MHW's authority with the client.
3. **The RN should explain to the MHW that the mental health client retains all the civil rights afforded to all persons, except the right to leave the hospital in the case of involuntary commitments. The client may have phone calls restricted if that is included in the care plan—for example, if the client is calling and threatening the president.**
4. This situation does not need to be discussed at the weekly team meeting. The RN psychiatric nurse can discuss this on a one-on-one basis with the MHW.

CLINICAL JUDGMENT GUIDE: The nurse is responsible to ensure client legal rights are maintained, even when on a locked psychiatric unit.

33. 1. The client has a chemical imbalance in the brain, and a firm voice will not be effective in getting the client to sit down. The client cannot sit still.
2. The mood stabilizer medication lithium (Eskalith) is the medication of choice, but it takes up to 3 weeks to become therapeutic; therefore, this intervention would not help the nurse complete the admission assessment.
3. **Walking or pacing with the client will allow the client to work off energy and may decrease restlessness and agitation. The nurse should implement this intervention to obtain information for the admission assessment.**
4. The nurse must obtain an admission assessment; therefore, the nurse should walk and pace with the client while attempting to obtain the priority admission assessment.

CLINICAL JUDGMENT GUIDE: In mental health nursing, the foundation for all nursing care is having a trusting nurse and client relationship. The nurse can choose an intervention that supports client needs.

34. 1. Evaluating the effectiveness of a client's medication is primarily the role of the psychiatric nurse, psychologist, and psychiatrist, not the social worker.
2. The recreational therapist helps the client to balance work and play, then provides activities that promote constructive use of leisure or unstructured time.
3. The vocational therapist helps the client with job-seeking or job-retention skills and with the pursuit of further education if needed and desired.
4. **According to the NCSBN referrals area content on the NCLEX-RN® test plan, the psychiatric social worker may conduct therapy and often has the primary responsibility for working with families, for community support, and for referrals.**

CLINICAL JUDGMENT GUIDE: The test taker must be knowledgeable of the role of all members of the multidisciplinary health-care team as well as appropriate referrals. The nurse must implement a referral to the most appropriate person or agency.

35. 1. The first intervention should be to talk to the client and remove him from the day room to the least restrictive environment. Restraining the client is the most restrictive environment.
2. The nurse should first attempt to talk to the client and remove the client from the day room area, not try to remove all the other clients.
3. The client will probably need a PRN medication to calm the behavior, but it is not the nurse's first intervention. An intramuscular medication takes at least 30 minutes to become effective.
4. **The first intervention is to approach the client calmly and attempt to remove him from the day room. Staff members should not approach the agitated client alone, but should be accompanied by other personnel.**

CLINICAL JUDGMENT GUIDE: When answering questions in mental health nursing, the test taker should identify safety as a priority intervention in any situation.

36. 1. This child has been abused, and until Child Protective Services has been notified, the nurse should not share any information with the child's father.
2. **The Health Insurance Portability and Accountability Act (HIPAA) considers parents the "personal representative" of the minor child with the right to information. However, there are exceptions to this rule, including when the provider reasonably believes that the minor may be a victim of abuse or neglect by the parent or guardian. This statement is the nurse's best response.**
3. Because the mother is accusing the father of the abuse, this is not an appropriate response.
4. The social worker must adhere to HIPAA regulations; therefore, referring the father to the social worker will not help the father find out how his son is doing.

CLINICAL JUDGMENT GUIDE: The nurse is responsible for knowing and complying with local, state, and federal standards of care.

37. Correct answers are 1, 3, and 5.
1. **A no-suicide contract is one of the first interventions the nurse implements with the client. It states that if the client feels suicidal, then the client must talk to someone and will not take action on the thoughts.**
2. This is the most stringent form of supervision in which one staff person per shift is assigned to be in close proximity to the client. This would be implemented in an inpatient psychiatric unit, not an outpatient clinic.
3. **The nurse should ask the client whether she has a plan. The more specific the plan is, the more seriously the statement should be taken.**
4. The nurse cannot commit every client reporting thoughts of suicide to a psychiatric unit. The nurse must assess the lethality, the absolute possibility, and the available support systems before committing a client to the psychiatric unit. After the nurse requests an emergency commitment, the client must be evaluated by a psychiatrist.
5. **The nurse should assess the client's support system and the type of help each person or group can give the client, such as hotlines, church groups, and self-help groups, as well as family members.**

CLINICAL JUDGMENT GUIDE: This is an alternate type of question included in the NCLEX-RN®. The nurse must be able to select all the options that answer the question correctly. There are no partially correct answers.

38. 1. This client should be instructed to go to the anger management class, but this does not warrant immediate intervention.
2. The mental health worker (MHW) could escort the client outside to smoke, but this does not warrant immediate intervention by the RN.
3. **This client who is nauseated and has vomited has a physiological problem that should be assessed by the nurse immediately. This client warrants immediate intervention.**
4. A client who has her menses, or "period," may experience abdominal cramping and would need to be assessed, but not before the client who has vomited twice.

CLINICAL JUDGMENT GUIDE: When the question asks, "Which warrants immediate intervention?" it is an "except" question. Physiological problems have the highest priority when deciding on a course of action. If the client is in distress, then the nurse must intervene with a nursing action that attempts to alleviate or control the problem.

39. 1. **Because the clinical manager wants to reward the unit for no absences or tardies, the manager must reward all shifts, so providing a thank-you meal to all shifts would be most appropriate. This allows all the staff members to celebrate the unit accomplishment.**
2. A thank-you note is a nice action, but knowing the clinical manager took the time to arrange for the meal means a lot to staff members. The meal could encourage the staff to try and do the same the next month.
3. Individually telling the staff "job well done" is a possible action to take, but for the clinical manager to take the time to arrange for the meal on all shifts is above and beyond just saying thank you to each individual staff member.
4. Having no absences or tardies for 1 month for an individual employee is the expected behavior. The fact the entire unit had no absences or tardies is what is being acknowledged.

CLINICAL JUDGMENT GUIDE: All options are plausible in this question. The test taker must identify the most important intervention. There will be management questions on the NCLEX-RN®. In many instances, there is no test taking strategy for these questions. The nurse must be knowledgeable of management issues.

40. 1. The nurse must take action to protect the wife.
2. The statement can be documented, but this is not the appropriate action for the nurse to implement.
3. **Mental health clinicians have a duty to warn identifiable third parties of threats made by a person even if these threats were discussed during a therapy session (*Tarasoff v. Regents of the University of California*, 1976). The nurse should notify the client's psychiatric HCP so that the wife can be notified of the threat.**
4. The nurse should not encourage this behavior because it could cause serious harm to the wife.

CLINICAL JUDGMENT GUIDE: The NCLEX-RN® test plan includes nursing care that is ruled by legal requirements. The nurse must be knowledgeable of these issues.

41. **Correct answers are 3 and 4.**
1. Exercise often causes the client to have trouble sleeping. This intervention is not appropriate.
2. Elopement precautions are implemented for clients who are at risk for leaving the facility; therefore, this is not appropriate.
3. **Caffeinated beverages are stimulants; therefore, this is an appropriate intervention.**
4. **An alarm on the bed would help ensure safety for the client because the nurse will know immediately when the client leaves the bed.**
5. The 1-to-1 watches are for clients who are suicidal; therefore, this is not an appropriate intervention.

CLINICAL JUDGMENT GUIDE: The test taker must select all the correct interventions for "select all that apply" questions. The test taker should read each option and determine if it is an appropriate intervention.

42. **Correct order is 3, 4, 2, 5, 1.**
3. **Denial**
4. **Anger**
2. **Bargaining**
5. **Depression**
1. **Acceptance**

CLINICAL JUDGMENT GUIDE: This is a knowledge-based question, but the test taker is required to remember many facts that must be applied when taking the NCLEX-RN®

examination. This information is the basis for many questions addressing the grieving process. The nurse must know these in the correct order, and the appropriate interventions for each stage of grief.

43. 1. Identifying strengths and weaknesses is included in the orientation phase.
    2. **Identifying problem-solving techniques is part of the working phase.**
    3. Evaluating the client's experience is part of the termination phase.
    4. Establishing the rules for the meetings is part of the orientation phase.

CLINICAL JUDGMENT GUIDE: If the test taker is not familiar with the phases of group dynamics, then the word "middle" may give the test taker an idea of what may be the goals of this part of group dynamics. Evaluation is usually done at the end.

44. 1. **On the inpatient psychiatric unit, the priority is maintaining safety for the clients and staff.**
    2. Contacting family members is not priority over safety.
    3. **Safety is the priority over a client who is exhibiting behavior common in an inpatient psychiatric unit.**
    4. This client needs to be assessed, but fasting for 2 days is not a safety issue for the inpatient psychiatric unit.

CLINICAL JUDGMENT GUIDE: When answering questions in mental health nursing, the test taker should identify safety as a priority intervention in any situation. All these situations require intervention but safety is the priority.

45. Correct answers are 1 and 3.
    1. **Each member of AA has a sponsor who has successfully quit drinking and is a support for a new member trying to stop drinking.**
    2. AA does not discuss medications used to help prevent drinking alcohol.
    3. **AA is a support group made up of recovering alcoholics who help others to stop drinking based on the 12-step approach.**
    4. AA helps alcoholics realize they are helpless over the addiction. They have no power over the addiction.
    5. Recovering alcoholics speak at the meetings, not professional guest speakers.

CLINICAL JUDGMENT GUIDE: "Select all that apply" questions require the test taker to select more than one option. The test taker must select

all correct options to get the question correct. This is an alternate type of question on the NCLEX-RN®.

46. 1. The nurse should determine the lithium level, but it is not the first intervention the nurse should implement.
    2. The nurse should assess the behavior that prompted the admission, but this is not the first intervention.
    3. **The nurse should first assess the client's physiological needs because the client in the manic state may not have slept, bathed, or had anything to eat for days. The client's physiological needs are the priority.**
    4. Lithium, a mood stabilizer medication, takes 2 to 3 weeks to become therapeutic; therefore, a STAT dose of lithium orally will not help the client's manic state. This is not the nurse's first intervention.

CLINICAL JUDGMENT GUIDE: Assessment is the first step of the nursing process, and the test taker should use the nursing process or some other systematic process to assist in determining priorities.

47. 1. A democratic manager is people oriented and emphasizes efficient group functioning. The environment is open and communication flows both ways, which includes having meetings to discuss concerns.
    2. This statement is that of an autocratic manager who uses an authoritarian approach to direct the activities of others.
    3. **This statement is that of a laissez-faire manager who maintains a permissive climate with little direction or control. Instructing the staff to handle the situation on their own does not support the staff.**
    4. This statement is taking control of the situation; therefore, this is not a statement indicating a laissez-faire manager.

CLINICAL JUDGMENT GUIDE: There will be management questions on the NCLEX-RN®. In many instances, there is no test taking strategy for these questions. The nurse must be knowledgeable of management issues.

48. 1. Unless the client is anorexic and there is a court order, the nurse cannot force-feed a client.
    2. **This is client abuse, and the charge nurse must investigate the allegation immediately with the nurse. If the allegations**

are true, they should be documented in writing and reported to the client abuse committee.

3. The charge nurse should not ask the client about the situation first. The RN and MHW should be involved in the investigation of the allegation. Then, if needed, the client can be asked about the situation.

4. The RN charge nurse should investigate the allegations first and then, if needed, have the MHW document details of the situation.

CLINICAL JUDGMENT GUIDE: There will be management questions on the NCLEX-RN®. In many instances, there is no test taking strategy for these questions. The nurse must be knowledgeable of management issues.

49. Correct answers are 1, 2, and 5.
1. **The nurse should assess the client for any injury, side effects of medication, and general well-being every 2 to 4 hours.**
2. **As soon as possible, the nurse must inform the client of what behavior will allow the client to be released from the seclusion room.**
3. According to the Joint Commission Restraint and Seclusion Standards for Behavioral Health, the client's family is notified promptly of the initiation of restraint or seclusion.
4. The nurse's goal is to release the client as soon as possible from the seclusion room. When the client has calmed down and is able to verbalize feelings and concerns in a rational manner, the client should be released. The seclusion order must be renewed every 24 hours, but the client should not be secluded for 24 hours unless absolutely necessary.
5. **Clients must be checked at least every 10 to 15 minutes in person and may be continuously monitored on video cameras.**

CLINICAL JUDGMENT GUIDE: This is an alternate type of question included in the NCLEX-RN®. The nurse must be able to select all the options that answer the question correctly. There are no partially correct answers.

50. 1. **The RN should first separate the MHW from the client; therefore, asking the MHW to go to the nurse's station would be the first intervention.**
2. The nurse should not correct the MHW in front of the client and should not use the

word "arguing"; therefore, this would not be an appropriate action.

3. The psychiatric nurse should handle this situation immediately. If this is a pattern of behavior of the MHW, then the RN clinical manager should be notified.

4. This behavior may or may not need to be reported to the client abuse committee, but if the RN overhears the MHW and client arguing, the nurse should stop the behavior.

CLINICAL JUDGMENT GUIDE: In any business, including a health-care facility, arguments or discussions of confidential information should not occur between staff or clients. In this case, the MHW should be removed from the situation to stop the behavior.

51. 1. The psychiatric social worker can refer clients, but the nurse should assess the client to see what type of help she wants.
2. The psychiatric social worker does not perform or participate in ECT treatment; therefore, this client should not be referred.
3. The nurse needs to assess the client to determine why the client is having difficulty going to work. For example, is it sedation secondary to medications?
4. **The psychiatric social worker can assist with financial arrangements, referrals, and nonphysiological concerns.**

CLINICAL JUDGMENT GUIDE: The test taker must be knowledgeable of the role of all members of the multidisciplinary health-care team as well as appropriate referrals. The nurse must implement a referral to the most appropriate person or agency.

52. 1. Two times in 1 week is becoming a pattern of behavior. The clinical manager should talk informally to the nurse to find out what is going on.
2. This is only the second time the nurse has taken 45 minutes for lunch and does not warrant formal counseling. The clinical manager should assess the situation before formally documenting the behavior.
3. This is very punitive behavior for the psychiatric nurse. The clinical manager should talk to the nurse before taking this type of action.
4. **The clinical manager should talk to the nurse informally and find out what is going on. This behavior cannot continue, but it is not behavior that requires anything more than informally finding out why the nurse has been late.**

ANSWERS

CLINICAL JUDGMENT GUIDE: There will be management questions on the NCLEX-RN®. In many instances, there is no test taking strategy for these questions. The nurse must be knowledgeable of management issues.

53. 1. The client diagnosed with Alzheimer's disease would be expected to be confused; therefore, this would not warrant immediate intervention.
   2. The client diagnosed with Alzheimer's disease has difficulty completing simple routine activities of daily living. This would not warrant immediate intervention.
   3. **The client diagnosed with Alzheimer's disease should not be difficult to arouse from sleep. This is not a typical symptom of this disease and would warrant immediate intervention from the nurse.**
   4. The client diagnosed with Alzheimer's disease has difficulty completing simple routine activities of daily living. This would not warrant immediate intervention.

CLINICAL JUDGMENT GUIDE: When the question asks, "Which warrants immediate intervention?" it is an "except" question. Three of the clients are exhibiting symptoms which are normal or expected for the client situation. After eliminating the expected options, the test taker should select the one remaining.

54. 1. This is a therapeutic response that helps the client to vent feelings, but this statement does not support the ethical principle of veracity.
   2. **Veracity is the ethical principle "to tell the truth." The truth is that schizophrenia is a thought disorder caused by a chemical imbalance of the brain. Antipsychotic medication can control the client's hallucinations and delusions.**
   3. This is interviewing the client, and this statement does not support the ethical principle of veracity.
   4. Schizophrenia is a mental illness, but if the client takes the antipsychotic medication, the client may be able to work, get married, and live a productive life. This is a false statement.

CLINICAL JUDGMENT GUIDE: The NCLEX-RN® test plan includes nursing care that addresses ethical principles including autonomy, beneficence, justice, and veracity, to name a few.

55. 1. Carbamazepine (Tegretol), an anticonvulsant, is a medication that is often prescribed for clients diagnosed with bipolar disorder even though it is classified as an anticonvulsant. Many times, a medication with a different classification is prescribed for another disease process.
   2. **Antacids such as aluminum hydroxide; magnesium hydroxide (Maalox) neutralize gastric acid and may reduce the effects of antipsychotic medications and lead to medication failure. The client diagnosed with schizophrenia would be on an antipsychotic medication; therefore, the nurse should discuss this client with the psychiatric HCP.**
   3. The client receiving isoniazid (INH), an antituberculosis medication, must receive it to prevent resistant strains of tuberculosis and protect the community. The nurse would not need to discuss this client with the HCP.
   4. Amitriptyline (Elavil), a tricyclic antidepressant, has shown efficacy in promoting weight gain in clients diagnosed with anorexia nervosa; therefore, the nurse would not discuss this medication with the HCP.

CLINICAL JUDGMENT GUIDE: The nurse should be aware of expected actions and side effects of medications.

56. 1. **The nurse must know the bomb scare policy of the facility, and in many cases the nurse looks for the bomb but does not touch it if it is found. In some instances, the nurse should not attempt to look for a bomb, but because the client is on a psychiatric unit, the nurse should look for a suspicious-looking object before notifying the bomb squad and evacuating the clients.**
   2. The nurse would implement the bomb scare protocol if there was a bomb or suspicious-looking bag, but the nurse should first investigate the comment because the client is on a psychiatric unit.
   3. The nurse would evacuate the clients if a bomb or suspicious-looking bag was under the couch. The nurse should have the clients leave the lobby area, but not the unit.
   4. Just because the client is in a psychiatric unit does not mean that someone did or did not put a bomb under the couch. The nurse should look under the couch and take appropriate action.

CLINICAL JUDGMENT GUIDE: The nurse must be knowledgeable of emergency preparedness. Employees receive this information in employee orientation and are responsible for implementing procedures correctly. The NCLEX-RN® includes questions on a safe and effective care environment. The protocol may be different in the mental health setting; therefore, the nurse should follow policy.

57. 1. The response is closed and does not allow the new nurse to voice her opinion and be part of the team.
    2. The charge nurse should be open to change. Just because something has been done the same way for years does not mean it can't be done another way.
    3. The charge nurse should not make the new nurse talk to the other nurses just because the shift report is not done the way she wants.
    4. **The best response is to allow the new nurse to share any new ideas with the charge nurse. The charge nurse could then talk to the other staff members and take the change to the clinical manager to determine whether the change should be instituted.**

CLINICAL JUDGMENT GUIDE: There will be management questions on the NCLEX-RN®. In many instances, there is no test taking strategy for these questions. The nurse must be knowledgeable of management issues.

58. 1. The client may eventually be able to go to the activity area, but while the client is confined to the unit, the nurse should refer the client to a recreational therapist to be provided with activities to alleviate boredom.
    2. Allowing the client to vent feelings will not help alleviate the client's boredom on the unit.
    3. **According to the NCLEX-RN® test plan, the nurse must be knowledgeable of the multidisciplinary team. The recreational therapist helps the client to balance work and play, then provides activities that promote constructive use of leisure or unstructured time.**
    4. The nurse should acknowledge the client's concern and contact the recreational therapist.

CLINICAL JUDGMENT GUIDE: The test taker must be knowledgeable of the role of all members of the multidisciplinary health-care team as well as appropriate referrals. The nurse must implement a referral to the most appropriate person or agency.

59. 1. A client who was raped would be expected to be upset and crying. This client would not require the most experienced nurse.
    2. The client who is diagnosed with bipolar disorder would be agitated in the manic state. This client would not require the most experienced nurse.
    3. **The client who was found wandering in a daze and has no diagnosis requires an in-depth assessment. This client should be assigned to the most experienced nurse.**
    4. The client diagnosed with schizophrenia would have hallucinations if not taking anti-psychotic medication. The client would not require the most experienced nurse.

CLINICAL JUDGMENT GUIDE: The test taker must determine which client is the most unstable and would require the most experienced nurse, thus making this type of question an "except" question. Three clients are either stable or have non-life-threatening conditions.

60. 1. **When a person is admitted to a psychiatric unit, the client does not lose any rights. The client has a right to refuse treatment, but if the client is a danger to herself, then the psychiatric team must go to court and obtain an order to force-feed the client. This could be with naso-gastric tube feedings or total parenteral nutrition.**
    2. The client has a right to refuse treatment, but if the client is a danger to herself, then the psychiatric team must intervene. If the client does not eat, the client will die.
    3. If the client is discharged and dies, the psychiatric team will be responsible. If a person is mentally ill, the psychiatric team must protect the client.
    4. This is against the client's rights. The nurse cannot restrain a client without a court order.

CLINICAL JUDGMENT GUIDE: The NCLEX-RN® test plan includes nursing care that is ruled by legal requirements. The nurse must be knowledgeable of these issues.

61. 1. The nurse would notify the police department if the client ran away from the unit.

    2. The nurse's first intervention is to place the unit on high alert, which includes putting signs on the exit doors warning all people coming in and out that there is a client threatening to leave the unit.

    3. The nurse should talk to the client, but the first intervention is to prevent the client from making good on the threat of running away.

    4. The client who is on an involuntary admission loses the right to sign out of the psychiatric unit against medical advice (AMA).

CLINICAL JUDGMENT GUIDE: When answering questions in mental health nursing, the test taker should identify safety as a priority intervention in any situation.

62. 1. The nurse does not have a right to ask the caller for his or her name. Mr. Jones has a right to telephone calls.

    2. Mr. Jones retains all his civil rights when admitted to a psychiatric unit unless phone restriction is part of the individualized care plan.

    3. The access code for client information is requested when the caller is asking questions about the client. It is not used when the caller wants to talk directly to the client.

    4. The nurse should find Mr. Jones and tell him he has a phone call. The client cannot have rights restricted unless it is a part of the client's individualized care plan. For example, the client may not be able to use the phone if he or she is calling 911 and making false reports.

CLINICAL JUDGMENT GUIDE: The NCLEX-RN® test plan includes nursing care that is ruled by legal requirements. The nurse must be knowledgeable of these issues.

63. 1. The psychiatric nurse should not make promises he or she cannot keep. If the information must be shared with the health-care team, then the nurse will have to break a promise to the client. This will compromise the nurse-client relationship.

    2. This is the nurse's best response. The nurse is being honest with the client but will keep the information confidential if it does not affect the client's care.

    3. The client may need to share information that is pertinent to the client's care and should be encouraged to communicate with the nurse.

    4. Asking the client "Why?" may put the client on the defensive, thereby being less inclined to share the information.

CLINICAL JUDGMENT GUIDE: In mental health nursing, the foundation for all nursing care is having a trusting nurse and client relationship. The nurse should be honest with the client about the information the nurse can keep confidential and which information must be shared with the health-care team.

64. 1. The client diagnosed with schizophrenia would be expected to be delusional; therefore, this situation would not warrant immediate intervention.

    2. The charge nurse has the entire shift to arrange for another nurse to cover the LPN; therefore, this situation does not warrant immediate intervention.

    3. The loss of a unit key card is a priority because the RN must determine when the MHW last had the key card and determine whether it may be lost on the psychiatric unit. If a client finds the key card, then the unit is no longer secure.

    4. The signing of the supply order is important, but it does not warrant immediate intervention.

CLINICAL JUDGMENT GUIDE: When answering questions in mental health nursing, the test taker should identify safety as a priority intervention in any situation. The loss of a key card could put the safety of all the clients on the unit at risk.

65. 1. The local police department needs to be called, but the nurse must first talk to the man and attempt to diffuse the situation. This action tries to ensure safety for the man, the other clients, and the staff.

    2. Ensuring safety of the other clients and staff is important, but the nurse should first attempt to make contact with the man.

    3. The nurse should not encourage the client to talk about his feelings until the gun is removed. The anger may cause the client to shoot an innocent person accidentally or on purpose.

    4. The nurse should first try to talk to the client and diffuse the situation. This action is attempting to ensure the safety of the man, the other clients, and the staff.

CLINICAL JUDGMENT GUIDE: When answering questions in mental health nursing, the test taker should identify safety as a priority intervention in any situation. All these actions could be performed by the nurse, but safety is the priority.

66. **Correct answers are 2 and 5.**
    1. This client requires the care of a nurse who can make attempts to get the client to participate in therapy.
    2. **The client diagnosed with diabetes can be monitored by the medical-surgical nurse. The option does not state that any unusual situations are occurring with the client's diagnosed illness. The client wishes to remain in bed and the medications have not had enough time in the client's body to cause concern for suicide risk.**
    3. Dissociative identity disorder (DID) is formerly known as multiple personality disorder (MPD). This client may be experiencing a different personality; an experienced psychiatric nurse should assess this situation.
    4. This client is creating a disturbance in the day room by blocking the television and may be at risk from the other clients. This client needs intervention by an experienced psychiatric nurse to diffuse the situation.
    5. **A client diagnosed with major depression who has started antidepressant medications 2 days ago could be cared for by the medical-surgical nurse. It is expected that this client has not received medication therapy long enough to make a difference in the depression. The medication requires 2 to 3 weeks of administration before showing effectiveness.**

CLINICAL JUDGMENT GUIDE: The test taker must evaluate each option individually and make a determination based solely on the facts included in the option to select correctly in a "select all that apply" question. One option does not rule out another option. The test taker must decide if the medical-surgical nurse has the knowledge required to care for the client.

67. **Correct order is 2, 4, 3, 1, 5.**
    2. **Part of the National Patient Safety Goals is implementing two identifiers when the client is to receive a procedure. The nurse must do this to determine that it is the correct client and the correct procedure.**
    4. **The client should have been NPO for several hours before the procedure for safety reasons. If the client were to vomit during the procedure, then aspiration might occur.**
    3. **The client will require an intravenous line for medication administration and emergency reasons.**
    1. **The electric impulses will be administered via electrodes.**
    5. **The health-care provider is not notified to begin the procedure until the nurse is sure that all the required pre-procedure steps are complete.**

CLINICAL JUDGMENT GUIDE: The test taker should mentally visualize the procedure area and identify which steps would be required to complete. Some steps such as identifying the correct client should be first after washing the nurse's hands.

68. 1. This laboratory value is within normal range.
    2. This laboratory value is within normal range.
    3. **This client has schizophrenia and also has a low white blood cell count. Many clients diagnosed with schizophrenia are placed on atypical antipsychotic agents such as clozapine (Clozaril); these medications can cause agranulocytosis. This places the client at risk for a life-threatening infection. The nurse should hold the dose of any atypical antipsychotic medication and notify the health-care provider of the result.**
    4. This laboratory value is within normal range.

CLINICAL JUDGMENT GUIDE: The test taker must be aware of complications that occur because of treatments for particular diseases. However, the laboratory data in this question have only one abnormal result. If the test taker is unsure, then the abnormal result should be chosen.

69. **Correct answers are 1, 3, and 5.**
    1. **Psychiatric units have emergency codes to request assistance for a "take down" procedure when a client is deemed uncontrollable; the charge nurse should request this assistance.**
    2. The client is in an excited state, so telling him that he will lose privileges is useless at this time.
    3. **The other clients should be removed from possible harm.**
    4. The staff should speak in a calm, soft tone to assist the client in regaining composure.

5. **The psychiatric unit is a locked unit. When the notification is made for assistance, someone must open the door so the emergency responders can enter the unit.**

CLINICAL JUDGMENT GUIDE: The test taker must decide on each option individually and cannot make a decision based on any other option in "select all that apply" questions. A "take down" procedure requires that safety is a major consideration for the client and staff.

70. 1. This client has some beginnings of tardive dyskinesia but can continue the antipsychotic medications.
    2. This client has some moderate signs of tardive dyskinesia but can continue the antipsychotic medications.

3. This client has some tardive dyskinesia but can continue the antipsychotic medications with frequent monitoring of the AIMS test. At a score of 20 or above the medications must be discontinued.
4. **This client is exhibiting severe abnormal behavior and the antipsychotic medication should be discontinued. The AIMS test was devised to detect extrapyramidal symptoms. If continued, the client will have permanent tardive dyskinesia from the medication.**

CLINICAL JUDGMENT GUIDE: This question can be answered from the chart by recognizing that the higher the number, the more serious the side effects of the medications will be.

CLINICAL SCENARIO ANSWERS AND RATIONALES

The correct answer number and rationale for why it is the correct answer are given in **boldface type.** Rationales for why the other possible answer options are incorrect also are given, but they are not in boldface type.

1. 1. Narcissistic personality disorder (NPD) is a personality disorder in which the client is described as being excessively preoccupied with issues of personal adequacy, power, prestige, and vanity.
   2. **The nurse should contact this client first because the client realizes the voices are telling him to hurt his wife. The nurse should inform this client to come to the clinic immediately, and he should be admitted to a psychiatric unit.**
   3. The nurse should call this client, but refusing to get out of the bed is not a priority over the client who is hearing voices and may hurt his wife.
   4. The nurse should expect the client who is manic to make poor decisions such as selling a car. The nurse should call this client, but the client is not a danger to self or others so the phone call does not need to be returned first.

2. 1. This client needs to be assessed but not before a client who is suicidal.

2. **This client who is suicidal and has a gun in the car should be assessed first to see whether he has a plan to use the gun. This client needs to be assessed first.**
3. This client needs to be assessed for Alzheimer's disease, but not before a client who may be suicidal.
4. The nurse should not interrupt a client who is acting compulsively. The nurse should wait until the client finishes the behavior before talking to the client.

3. 1. **The therapeutic serum level for lithium is 0.6 to 1.2 mEq/L. Because the client's level is 2.0 mEq/L, the nurse manager should notify the client's psychiatric health-care provider about the lithium (Eskalith).**
   2. The WBC count is within normal limits (4,500 to 11,100), so the nurse manager would not need to notify the psychiatric HCP. An elevated WBC count may indicate the client is experiencing agranulocytosis, a life-threatening complication of clozapine (Clozaril).
   3. The client's serum potassium level is within normal limits; therefore, this laboratory information does not warrant notifying the psychiatric health-care provider.

4. A serum divalproex sodium (Depakote) level between 50 and 125 mcg/mL is within normal limits, so the nurse manager does not need to notify the client's psychiatric health-care provider.

4. 1. **The client is a risk to himself and the EMS should be notified to go to the client and make sure that no harm comes to the client. The client is not in the outpatient clinic with the nurse; therefore, the EMS should be notified to go to the client before the client harms himself.**

   2. This is an assessment question, but not the first intervention. The first intervention is to arrange for help to get to the client as soon as possible.

   3. The HCP will be notified, but it is not the first intervention.

   4. The nurse manager should remain on the telephone to try to keep the client occupied until the paramedics arrive on the scene.

5. 1. The benzodiazepine, alprazolam (Xanax), is an appropriate medication for an anxiety attack, but it will take at least 15 to 30 minutes for the medication to treat the physiological signs and symptoms. Therefore, this is not the first intervention.

   2. Allowing the client to vent feelings is an appropriate intervention, but not the first intervention because the client is hyperventilating.

   3. **The first intervention is to address the client's physical discomfort, which is hyperventilating; therefore, encouraging the client to take slow, deep breaths is the next intervention for the nurse.**

   4. The client's pulse oximeter reading can be obtained, but it will not address the client's hyperventilating; therefore, it is not the nurse's first intervention.

6. 1. **The client diagnosed with dementia would be expected to have confusion and disorientation; therefore, the LPN could be assigned this client. This client is not experiencing any potentially life-threatening complication of dementia.**

   2. Extrapyramidal side effects are a complication of antipsychotic medication. A more experienced RN should be assigned to this client.

   3. The client who is pacing up and down the hallway is exhibiting the manic behavior of bipolar disorder. This client needs further

assessment and should be assigned to a registered nurse.

   4. This client is experiencing potentially life-threatening complications of anorexia and needs further assessment, so he should be assigned to a registered nurse.

7. 1. The client who is exhibiting compulsive behavior should be observed, but the MHW should not attempt to stop the client's behavior. This is an appropriate task to delegate to the MHW.

   2. An MHW can sit in the waiting room and watch the clients. This is an appropriate nursing task to delegate.

   3. The MHW can sit with a client who is suicidal even though the client may be unstable. The MHW should be in close proximity to the suicidal client. This is an appropriate nursing task to delegate.

   4. **The MHW does not draw blood, and this would be an inappropriate task to delegate. The laboratory technician draws the client's blood work.**

8. 1. The first intervention should be to approach the client calmly. Placing the client in a quiet room may be appropriate depending on the behavior of the client, but it is not the first intervention.

   2. The nurse should first attempt to talk to the client and remove the client from the day room area, not try to remove all the other clients.

   3. Calling 911 may be an appropriate intervention, but it is not the first intervention the nurse manager should implement. Talking to the client is the first intervention.

   4. **The first intervention is to approach the client calmly and attempt to remove him from the day room. Staff members should not approach the agitated client alone, but should be accompanied by other personnel.**

9. 1. The nurse manager should talk to the client but not to discuss the argument. The RN should diffuse the situation and calm the client, not interview the client to determine what happened. That should be discussed with the MHW.

   2. **The RN mental health nurse manager should discuss the behavior with the MHW and then take appropriate disciplinary action. Psychiatric staff members cannot argue with clients.**

   3. The RN manager needs to document the MHW's behavior, but the nurse manager

should discuss the situation with the MHW before taking any other action.

4. The MHW's behavior may warrant termination, but the first action of the RN psychiatric nurse manager is to discuss the behavior with the mental health worker.

10. 1. The nurse manager should not involve other employees in the nurse's situation. A clinical manager should allow the nurse to resolve the problem.

2. Because the nurse has a reason for being late and the car will be fixed in a week, the behavior does not need to be documented and placed in her file.

3. This is very punitive behavior for the nurse manager to take, because she is having car trouble and riding the bus to get to work.

4. **The nurse manager needs to work with the employees, and being understanding of situations is an attribute of an effective clinical manager. The nurse has a valid reason for being late and because she has an excellent attendance record, the nurse manager should be understanding and work with the nurse.**

Case Studies: Care of Clients in Various Settings

14

The ultimate measure of a man is not where he stands in moments of comfort, but where he stands at times of challenge and controversy.

– Martin Luther King, Jr.

MEDICAL NURSING CASE STUDY #1: MULTIPLE CLIENTS

The RN staff nurse on the medical unit is assigned to care for clients on the 7 a.m. to 7 p.m. shift. The primary RN staff nurse's assignments include:

- Mr. K.B., a 42-year-old African American male who is diagnosed with abdominal pain of unknown etiology
- Ms. M.W., a 50-year-old Asian female who is diagnosed with cellulitis of the left leg
- Ms. A.S., a 24-year-old Caucasian female who is diagnosed with diabetic ketoacidosis
- Mr. G.D., a 38-year-old Caucasian male, diagnosed with renal calculi

1. The primary RN has received the morning shift report and is preparing to make rounds on the clients. Which client should the nurse see **first?**
   1. Mr. K.B.
   2. Ms. M.W.
   3. Ms. A.S.
   4. Mr. G.D.

2. The nurse has delegated a.m. care for Ms. A.S. Which nursing tasks can the UAP implement for Ms. A.S.? **Select all that apply.**
   1. Assist Ms. A.S. to the shower.
   2. Change the linens on the bed.
   3. Trim Ms. A.S.'s toenails.
   4. Feed Ms. A.S. the breakfast meal.
   5. Massage Ms. A.S.'s lower back.

3. The UAP reports to the primary nurse that Ms. A.S. is reporting feeling nervous, jittery, and having a headache. Which interventions should the primary RN perform? **Select all that apply.**
   1. Assess Ms. A.S.'s blood glucose with a glucometer.
   2. Give Ms. A.S. a glass of orange juice.
   3. Give Ms. A.S. a complex carbohydrate if she is feeling better.
   4. Administer the scheduled regular insulin immediately.
   5. Encourage the client to ambulate in the hallway.

4. Mr. K.B. is scheduled for an endoscopy this morning. He is scheduled to receive an intravenous proton-pump inhibitor and an oral ACE inhibitor. Which interventions should the primary nurse implement when preparing Mr. K.B. for this diagnostic test? **Select all that apply.**
   1. Ensure the client is NPO.
   2. Confirm with the HCP to hold the oral medication.
   3. Administer the IV medication.
   4. Confirm the informed consent is signed.
   5. Insert the indwelling urinary catheter.

5. Mr. K.B. has just returned from the endoscopy procedure. Which **priority** intervention should the nurse perform?
   1. Assess Mr. K.B.'s gag reflex.
   2. Administer Mr. K.B.'s a.m. medications.
   3. Give Mr. K.B. water to gargle for his sore throat.
   4. Determine if Mr. K.B. is hungry for his breakfast.

6. Mr. K.B has a nasogastric (N/G) tube. Which interventions can the nurse delegate to the UAP? **Select all that apply.**
   1. Determine the amount of N/G tube output.
   2. Examine the nares for irritation.
   3. Palpate the abdomen for firmness and tenderness.
   4. Listen to bowel sounds in all four quadrants.
   5. Provide mouth care.

7. Mr. G.D., who was diagnosed with a renal calculus, is reporting severe pain. Which interventions should the nurse perform **before** administering intravenous narcotic pain medication? **Select all that apply.**
   1. Assess the urine for blood and strain for particulates.
   2. Check the MAR to determine the last time pain medicine was given.
   3. Determine if the medication is compatible with the primary IV solution.
   4. Document the medication administration in the EHR.
   5. Compare the MAR with the client's ID band.

8. Mr. G.D. just passed a renal stone. Which action should the nurse implement **first?**
   1. Obtain a urine sample for urinalysis.
   2. Send the calculi to the laboratory.
   3. Assess the client with a bladder scanner.
   4. Administer a urinary analgesic.

9. The laboratory determined that Mr. G.D. had an oxalate renal calculus. The HCP has ordered a low oxalate diet. Which interventions should the nurse include in the teaching plan for Mr. G.D.? **Select all that apply.**
   1. Drink 8 to 12 cups of fluid a day.
   2. Avoid high doses of vitamin C supplements.
   3. Avoid foods such as nuts, soy, and whole wheat bread.
   4. Limit oxalate intake to 100 mg per day.
   5. Increase consumption of berries such as blueberries.

10. Ms. M.W., who is diagnosed with left leg cellulitis, is being discharged today. Which information should the nurse include in the discharge instructions? **Select all that apply.**
   1. Elevate your left leg on two pillows.
   2. Eat meals high in protein, vitamins, and minerals.
   3. Apply a topical corticosteroid ointment to the affected area daily.
   4. Take all prescription oral antibiotics as ordered.
   5. Apply warm compresses to the reddened area.

MEDICAL NURSING CASE STUDY #2: SYMPTOMATIC BRADYCARDIA

Mr. L.B., a 75-year-old male client, presents to the emergency department reporting dizziness, activity intolerance, and chronic fatigue for the last month. The client's daughter describes her father as "almost fainting" during ambulation to the bathroom. The initial vital signs are:

Blood Pressure	94/56 mm Hg
Heart Rate	48
Respirations	20
O₂ Saturation	94%
Temperature	98.4°F (36.9°C)
Pain	4 on a 1 to 10 scale

1. Which **priority** questions should the nurse ask the client? **Select all that apply.**
   1. "When did you last eat anything?"
   2. "Do you have a history of heart problems?"
   3. "Can you describe the location of your pain?"
   4. "Are you on any medications?"
   5. "Do you feel safe in your home?"

2. The nurse is using the PQRST pain assessment tool to evaluate Mr. L.B.'s pain. Which factors are included in the tool? **Select all that apply.**
   1. Precipitating or Provoking factors
   2. Quality or intensity of the pain
   3. Risk factors for the pain
   4. Severity of symptoms of the pain
   5. Timing and duration of the pain

During the assessment of Mr. L.B., the triage nurse notices the client is slow to answer the questions and appears confused. With assistance from his daughter, Mr. L.B. relates a history of hyperlipidemia and GERD. The client's current medications include omeprazole (Prilosec), atorvastatin (Lipitor), and a daily multivitamin.

3. The nurse places the client on continuous cardiac monitoring and records the following telemetry strip. Which **priority** test should the nurse expect to be performed at this time?

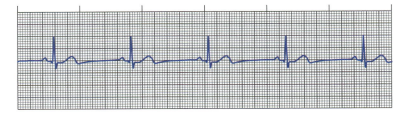

   1. Arterial blood gas
   2. 12-lead EKG
   3. Stress echocardiogram
   4. Blood glucose

4. The client is diagnosed with symptomatic bradycardia. Which medication should the nurse prepare to administer to the client?
   1. Atropine
   2. Adenosine
   3. Digoxin
   4. Nitroglycerin

The client remains unresponsive to medication administered to treat the symptomatic bradycardia. After further evaluation, the physician determines the client is a candidate for a leadless pacemaker. Mr. L.B. and his daughter consent to the leadless pacemaker and the client is admitted to the medical unit for preparation to undergo the procedure.

5. The daughter asks the medical nurse, "How long will my father be under general anesthesia?" Which response by the nurse is **most** appropriate?
   1. "Your father will only be under general anesthesia for 1 hour."
   2. "Your father will have an epidural placed for the procedure."
   3. "The procedure only involves a local anesthetic injected at the insertion site."
   4. "The procedure will be done without anesthesia to avoid complications."

6. Mr. L.B. returns to the medical floor from the procedure and a 2-hour recovery in the PACU. Which interventions should the nurse perform? **Select all that apply.**
   1. Assist the client to ambulate to the bathroom to measure urine output.
   2. Remove the groin dressing to assess the incision site.
   3. Palpate the pedal pulses distal to the incision site.
   4. Ensure the client remains on continuous cardiac monitoring.
   5. Assess vital signs every 30 minutes for 24 hours after the procedure.

7. Mr. L.B. has recovered from the procedure and the nurse is preparing him for discharge. Which instructions should the nurse include in the discharge teaching? **Select all that apply.**
   1. Avoid heavy lifting for 1 week.
   2. Expect symptoms of dizziness to last for 2 to 3 days.
   3. Keep all follow-up appointments with your HCP.
   4. Do not carry your cell phone in your shirt pocket.
   5. Assess your radial pulse daily.

8. Two months after the procedure, Mr. L.B. tells the office nurse he is planning to fly to another state to visit his son. Which teaching interventions should the office nurse implement? **Select all that apply.**
   1. Remind the client to carry his pacemaker identification card.
   2. Instruct the client to avoid all airport security screenings.
   3. Teach the client to report any syncope or dizziness.
   4. Advise the client to avoid ambulating long distances.
   5. Explain to the client he cannot travel without an examination by the HCP.

MEDICAL NURSING CASE STUDY #3: COMMUNITY-ACQUIRED BACTERIAL PNEUMONIA

Ms. B.W., a 65-year-old female client, presents to the emergency department reporting a productive cough, shortness of breath, and fatigue for the last week. The client exhibits labored breathing and the nurse detects the odor of cigarettes. The client reports smoking 1 pack a day of cigarettes for 40 years. The initial vital signs are:

Blood Pressure	128/76 mm Hg
Heart Rate	89
Respirations	24
O₂ Saturation	90%
Temperature	102.9°F (39°C)
Pain	4 on a 1 to 10 scale

1. In addition to the previous information, which **priority** assessment data should the nurse report to the HCP?
   1. Sputum, thick and yellow tinged
   2. Bilateral crackles in lower lung lobes
   3. Capillary refill in fewer than 3 seconds
   4. Loose brown stool x one

2. Ms. B.W. is experiencing shortness of breath and feeling anxious. Which interventions should the nurse implement? **Select all that apply.**
   1. Elevate the head of the bed.
   2. Administer oxygen via nasal cannula.
   3. Encourage fluid intake.
   4. Stay with the client to attempt to calm her.
   5. Request the client take slow, deep breaths.

3. The health-care provider has ordered a sputum culture for Ms. B.W. Which interventions should the nurse implement? **Rank in order of performance.**
   1. Teach the client to expectorate directly into the specimen container.
   2. Instruct the client to rinse her mouth with water.
   3. Have the client take several deep breaths.
   4. Label the specimen container and send to the laboratory.
   5. Position the client sitting or in a high Fowler's position.

Ms. B.W. has a chest x-ray performed and is diagnosed with community acquired bacterial pneumonia. The emergency department is extremely busy, so Ms. B.W. is immediately transferred to the medical unit.

4. Ms. B.W. is admitted to the medical unit. Which interventions are required to be performed within the **first 24 hours** according to CMS and TJC Pneumonia Core Measures? **Select all that apply.**
   1. Refer to substance abuse counseling.
   2. Administer a broad-spectrum antibiotic.
   3. Provide smoking cessation counseling.
   4. Perform influenza vaccination.
   5. Obtain blood cultures.

5. Ms. B.W. remains on the medical unit. Which interventions should the nurse include in Ms. B.W.'s daily care? **Select all that apply.**
   1. Restrict the client's smoking to 3 cigarettes per day.
   2. Place the client on oxygen via nasal cannula.
   3. Allow for periods of rest during activities of daily living.
   4. Implement fluid restrictions of 1,000 mL/day.
   5. Monitor the client's oxygen saturation with a pulse oximeter.

CASE STUDIES

6. The LPN is assisting Ms. B.W. to use her incentive spirometer. Which action by the LPN **warrants intervention** by the RN?
   1. The LPN assists the client to an upright position in the bed.
   2. The LPN instructs the client to blow into the incentive spirometer.
   3. The LPN encourages the client to cough after using the spirometer.
   4. The LPN tells the client to repeat the procedure frequently throughout the day.

7. Ms. B.W. has continued to improve and is being discharged. Which interventions should the nurse perform before sending Ms. B.W. home? **Select all that apply.**
   1. Provide smoking cessation information to the client.
   2. Administer the influenza and pneumonia vaccine.
   3. Arrange for continuous at-home oxygen therapy.
   4. Teach the client to perform frequent hand hygiene.
   5. Tell the client to use a warm steam vaporizer at home.

INTENSIVE CARE NURSING CASE STUDY: MULTIPLE CLIENTS

The nurses are caring for multiple clients in the intensive care unit (ICU) of a community hospital.

- Ms. J.C., a 32-year-old female diagnosed with acute respiratory distress syndrome and smoke inhalation from a house fire
- Mr. A.W., a 20-year-old male diagnosed with a C-6 spinal cord injury after diving into a shallow pool
- Ms. T.G., a 42-year-old female diagnosed with a traumatic brain injury following a motor vehicle accident (MVA)
- Mr. D.N., a 67-year-old male diagnosed with disseminated intravascular coagulation (DIC) and pancreatitis

1. The primary nurse caring for Ms. J.C. assesses tachypnea, intercostal and suprasternal retractions, and a change in mental status in the client. Which **priority** interventions should the nurse perform? **Select all that apply.**
   1. Prepare to place the client on a ventilator.
   2. Administer oxygen using a high-flow system.
   3. Place the client in the supine position.
   4. Address nutritional needs.
   5. Continuously monitor oxygen saturation.

2. The primary nurse assists the provider in endotracheal intubation of Ms. J.C. Which **priority** interventions should be performed to determine correct placement of the endotracheal (ET) tube? **Select all that apply.**
   1. Obtain arterial blood gas readings.
   2. Auscultate the lungs bilaterally.
   3. Perform a chest x-ray.
   4. Check capillary refill.
   5. Suction secretions from the ET tube.

3. The nurse is preparing to perform endotracheal suctioning on Ms. J.C. Which interventions should the nurse implement? **Rank in order of performance.**
   1. Provide mouth care to the client.
   2. Apply suction while withdrawing the catheter.
   3. Hyperoxygenate the client as needed.
   4. Determine measurement of length to suction.
   5. Lubricate the catheter tip with saline solution.

4. Which alternate methods should the nurse use to communicate with the client intubated with an ET tube and on a ventilator? **Select all that apply.**
   1. Usage of an electrolarynx
   2. Communication boards
   3. Hand gestures
   4. Eye blinks for yes or no questions
   5. Augmented communication device

5. Which interventions should the nurse implement when caring for Ms. J.C., who is on the ventilator? **Select all that apply.**
   1. Collaborate with the respiratory therapist.
   2. Continuously monitor the pulse oximeter reading.
   3. Ensure a manual resuscitation bag is at the bedside.
   4. Assess the ventilator settings throughout the shift.
   5. Confirm ventilator alarms are set to silence.

6. The nurse is performing an assessment on Mr. A.W. Which set of assessment findings indicate Mr. A.W. is experiencing spinal shock?
   1. Decreased reflexes and flaccid paralysis
   2. Hypotension and bradycardia
   3. Dyspnea and constricted airway
   4. Tachycardia and confusion

7. After 5 days in the intensive care unit (ICU), Mr. A.W. becomes agitated, very disoriented, and reports "hearing voices." Which interventions should the nurse perform? **Select all that apply.**
   1. Use clocks and calendars to orient the client to time.
   2. Dim lights at night and open window blinds during the day.
   3. Schedule activities frequently throughout the day and night.
   4. Have the family bring familiar objects from home.
   5. Minimize noise from shift change and monitoring equipment.

8. The nurse is assessing Ms. T.G. The nurse notes Ms. T.G. opens her eyes when the nurse calls her name but only moans when questioned. When the nurse applies pressure to the nail bed of the finger, Ms. T.G. slowly pulls her hand away from the nurse. Which rating on the Glasgow Coma Scale should the nurse document?

Glasgow Coma Scale

Appropriate Stimulus Response Score		
Eyes Open		
Approach to bedside	Spontaneous response	4
Verbal command	Opens eyes to name on command	3
Pain	Lack of opening of eyes to previous stimuli but opens to pain	2
	Lack of opening of eyes to any stimulus	1
	Untestable	0
Best Verbal Response		
Verbal questioning with maximum arousal	Oriented to person, place, time, and events	5
	Confusion, conversant but disoriented	4
	Disorganized use of words	3
	Incomprehensible words, groaning	2
	Lack of sound even with painful stimuli	1
	Untestable	0
Best Motor Response		
Verbal command	Follows verbal command	6
Pain (pressure on proximal nail bed)	Localizes pain, attempts to remove offending stimulus	5
	Flexion withdrawal of arm in response to pain without abnormal posturing	4
	Abnormal flexion, flexing of arm at elbow and pronation, making a fist	3
	Abnormal extension, extension of arm at elbow with adduction, and internal rotation of arm at shoulder	2
	Lack of response	1
	Untestable	0

1. Glasgow Coma Scale rating of 14
2. Glasgow Coma Scale rating of 12
3. Glasgow Coma Scale rating of 9
4. Glasgow Coma Scale rating of 7

9. Which interventions should the nurse include in Ms. T.G.'s plan of care? **Select all that apply.**
   1. Keep the head of the bed elevated 30 degrees.
   2. Perform active range of motion exercises every 4 hours.
   3. Explain all procedures to the client.
   4. Turn the client every 4 hours.
   5. Maintain normal body temperature.

10. Mr. D.N. is diagnosed with disseminated intravascular coagulation (DIC). Which findings by the nurse support the diagnosis of DIC?
    1. Sudden onset of chest pain and frothy sputum
    2. Foul-smelling, concentrated urine
    3. Oozing of blood from the IV site
    4. Fever of unknown origin

OUTPATIENT CLINIC NURSING CASE STUDY: MULTIPLE CLIENTS

The RN is caring for clients in a free outpatient clinic located in a suburban area. The clinic provides a variety of laboratory and diagnostic tests for the clients. Additionally, the clinic provides informational sessions on many subjects including health promotion screenings.

1. The health-care provider has ordered an endoscopy for a client. Which teaching interventions should the nurse include when explaining the procedure to the client? **Select all that apply.**
   1. Explain that the client cannot eat or drink anything 8 hours before the procedure.
   2. Tell the client he will have an IV and be sedated during the procedure.
   3. Inform the client he will have his vital signs taken frequently after the procedure.
   4. Instruct the client that he will be given narcotics after the procedure for the pain.
   5. Teach the client to contact the HCP if he has any bleeding or vomiting.

2. The HCP has ordered a colonoscopy for a client. Which teaching interventions should the nurse include when explaining the procedure to the client? **Select all that apply.**
   1. Explain the bowel preparation necessary before the procedure.
   2. Teach the client not to eat or drink anything 8 hours before the procedure.
   3. Instruct the client to remain on a clear liquid diet for 24 hours after the procedure.
   4. Inform the client that she will need to stay overnight in the hospital.
   5. Tell the client to report any rectal bleeding, dizziness, or abdominal pain to the HCP.

3. The clinic nurse must obtain a throat culture from a client who has possible strep throat. Which interventions should the nurse perform? **Rank in order of performance.**
   1. Instruct the client to tilt his head back and open his mouth.
   2. Insert the applicator stick into the specimen tube until the swab is in the culture medium.
   3. Remove the sterile applicator from the culture tube by rotating the cap to break the seal.
   4. Label the specimen tube and send to the laboratory.
   5. Swab the back of the throat along the tonsillar area from left to right.

4. The clinic nurse is caring for a client with a sprained right ankle. Which interventions should the nurse include in the discharge teaching for the client? **Select all that apply.**
   1. Instruct the client to rest and avoid stress on the right ankle.
   2. Tell the client to apply warm compresses to the injury.
   3. Show the client how to apply an elastic bandage to the ankle.
   4. Recommend the client elevate the right foot above the level of the heart.
   5. Teach the client to alternate acetaminophen and ibuprofen for pain.

5. The clinic nurse is caring for a client who is diagnosed with a common cold. The client asks the nurse, "Why won't the doctor give me some antibiotics when I feel so bad?" Which response by the nurse is **most** appropriate?
   1. "Over-the-counter medications are cheaper than antibiotics for the common cold."
   2. "The doctor will know which antibiotics to give you based on your nasal culture."
   3. "The common cold is caused by a virus; antibiotics only treat bacterial infections."
   4. "You should go to a different doctor so you will get proper treatment."

CASE STUDIES

6. The client diagnosed with the common cold asks the nurse about interventions to help with cold symptoms. Which interventions should the nurse teach the client? **Select all that apply.**
   1. Avoid alcohol, coffee, and caffeinated sodas.
   2. Recommend intranasal zinc for symptoms.
   3. Encourage intake of chicken noodle soup.
   4. Suggest a warm, saltwater gargle.
   5. Avoid saline nasal sprays and drops.

Refer to the Electronic Health Record Order Screen to answer the next set of questions:

Laboratory and Diagnostic Services

Chemistry	Hematology/COAG	Micro/Cultures
• Albumin	• Platelet count	• Blood
• Calcium	• White blood count	• Sputum
• Cholesterol, total	• Prothrombin, PT with INR	• Strep screen
• Creatinine	• PTT, activated	• Stool
• Folic acid	**Toxicology**	• Urinalysis
• Glucose	• Blood alcohol	• Wound, deep
• Glucose tolerance, OB	• Digoxin	• Wound, superficial
• HCG	• Lithium	**Diagnostic Tests**
• Hemoglobin A1C	• Valproic acid	• Audiometry
• Hepatitis panel	**Serology**	• Electromyography, EMG
• HIV screen	• Influenza	• Endoscopy, upper GI
• Iron, total	• Mono screen	• Mammogram
• Potassium	• Rapid plasma reagin, RPR	• Scratch test
• PSA, screening		• Tensilon test
• Rubella		• X-ray, chest
• TSH, thyroid panel		

7. The clinic nurse is assessing the client who is taking prescribed diuretics and reports leg cramps in the calf. Which laboratory or diagnostic test should the nurse expect to be ordered for this client?

[   ]

8. The client tells the clinic nurse, "I am having burning upon urination." Which laboratory or diagnostic test should the nurse expect to be ordered for this client?

[   ]

9. The client states, "I am having pain in my right lower abdomen and I have a low-grade fever."

Which laboratory or diagnostic test should the nurse expect to be ordered for this client?

[   ]

10. The client states, "I am taking warfarin every day." Which laboratory or diagnostic test should the nurse expect to be ordered for this client?

[   ]

11. The client states, "I am having burning in my chest after I eat, especially if I lie down after I eat." Which laboratory or diagnostic test should the nurse expect to be ordered for this client?

[   ]

12. The client states, "I have type 2 diabetes and have been taking my medication as directed for the last 3 months." Which laboratory or diagnostic test should the nurse expect to be ordered for this client?

13. The client states, "The last doctor I saw told me I might have a peripheral nerve disease and needed a test but I can't remember the name of the test." Which laboratory or diagnostic test should the nurse expect to be ordered for this client?

14. The client states, "I am weak all the time since I became a vegetarian. My family tells me I am pale and I don't have any energy." Which laboratory or diagnostic test should the nurse expect to be ordered for this client?

15. The client states, "I have been a type 2 diabetic for 20 years and I think I may have diabetic nephropathy." Which laboratory or diagnostic test should the nurse expect to be ordered for this client?

16. The client states, "I think I have myasthenia gravis, similar to my sister. Could you please give me the test to diagnose myasthenia gravis?" Which laboratory or diagnostic test should the nurse expect to be ordered for this client?

17. The client states, "I am hot all the time, I have problems holding my pen when I write, and I am breathing faster." Which laboratory or diagnostic test should the nurse expect to be ordered for this client?

18. The client states, "I think I may have been exposed to syphilis." Which laboratory or diagnostic test should the nurse expect to be ordered for this client?

19. The client states, "I am receiving chemotherapy and have noticed bleeding after I brush my teeth and when I blow my nose." Which laboratory or diagnostic test should the nurse expect to be ordered for this client?

20. The client states, "I have been on a heart healthy diet for more than 6 months since my heart attack." Which laboratory or diagnostic test should the nurse expect to be ordered for this client?

21. The client states, "My wife says I am having trouble hearing but I don't think so." Which laboratory or diagnostic test should the nurse expect to be ordered for this client?

22. The client states, "I think I am allergic to dust or mold because my nose gets stuffy, I sneeze all the time, and sometimes I break out in a rash." Which laboratory or diagnostic test should the nurse expect to be ordered for this client?

    ┌─────────────────────┐
    │   │
    └─────────────────────┘

The clinic nurse is teaching adult clients at the local community center about the American Cancer Society (ACS) early detection of cancer guidelines. Men and women of various ages have come to ask questions about health promotion screenings.

23. The female client asks the nurse how often she should get a breast cancer screening with a mammogram. Which information should the nurse provide to the community group? **Select all that apply.**
    1. Women 45 to 54 years old should get a mammogram yearly.
    2. Women 55 years old and older should get a mammogram every 2 years.
    3. Women under 45 years old do not need mammograms.
    4. Women should perform formal breast self-examinations monthly.
    5. Women with a high-risk factor should get MRIs with mammograms.

24. The male client asks the clinic nurse at what age colorectal cancer screenings should start. Which information should the nurse provide to the community group? **Select all that apply.**
    1. Regular colorectal screenings should begin at 45 years old.
    2. Continue with regular colorectal screenings until age 75.
    3. People older than 55 years old should no longer get colorectal screenings.
    4. Colorectal screenings can be done in your own home.
    5. Colonoscopy is recommended for abnormal results of any colorectal screening test.

25. The female client in the community group asks the clinic nurse, "What are the recommendations for detecting cervical cancer?" Which information should the nurse provide to the community group? **Select all that apply.**
    1. All women should follow the same schedule for cervical cancer screening.
    2. Cervical cancer screening should begin at 21 years old.
    3. Women 21 to 29 years old should have a Pap test with HPV testing every year.
    4. Women 30 to 65 years old should have a Pap test with HPV testing every 5 years.
    5. Women older than 65, with no abnormal cervical test for 10 years, can stop cervical cancer screenings.

26. The male client in the community group asks about the current recommendations for detecting prostate cancer. Which information should the nurse provide to the community group?
    1. Prostate cancer screening should begin at age 50.
    2. African Americans are at a low risk for prostate cancer.
    3. Testing can be with a PSA blood test with or without a rectal examination.
    4. Harm caused by prostate cancer testing outweighs the benefits.

HOME HEALTH NURSING CASE STUDY: MULTIPLE CLIENTS

The nurse is caring for clients in the Angel Home Healthcare Agency. The home health agency is located in a rural setting and provides skilled nursing care, physical therapy, occupational therapy, and speech therapy to a variety of clients from different socioeconomic and culturally diverse backgrounds.

1. The home health nurse is caring for a female client who needs her indwelling urinary catheter changed. After explaining the procedure to the client and performing hand hygiene, which interventions should the nurse implement? **Rank in order of performance.**
   1. Don sterile gloves.
   2. Insert the lubricated urinary catheter.
   3. Spread the labia and cleanse the urinary meatus.
   4. Inflate the catheter balloon using a prefilled syringe.
   5. Open the sterile catheter set.

2. The home health nurse is caring for a client with a central venous access device in the subclavian vein. The nurse must perform a central line dressing change. Which interventions should the nurse implement? **Rank in order of performance.**
   1. Don sterile gloves and arrange sterile field.
   2. Remove old dressing and assess needle insertion site.
   3. Allow area to dry and cover with transparent dressing.
   4. Scrub insertion site using a back and forth motion.
   5. Document date and time of the dressing change.

3. The home health nurse is teaching the home health aide how to perform a colostomy irrigation for the client with a sigmoid colostomy. After explaining the procedure to the client and performing hand hygiene, which interventions should the nurse implement? **Rank in order of performance.**
   1. Lubricate cone tip of tubing, insert into the stoma opening, begin inflow of water.
   2. Fill the irrigation bag with 1,000 mL of warm tap water and hang at shoulder height.
   3. Put irrigation sleeve over the stoma and place outflow into toilet above the water line.
   4. Cleanse stoma site and apply a new colostomy pouch over the stoma.
   5. Allow evacuation of feces and water; may take 30 minutes to 1 hour.

4. The home health nurse must draw an International Normalized Ratio (INR) for a client who is taking warfarin daily. Which interventions should the nurse implement? **Rank in order of performance.**
   1. Hold skin taut and insert needle with bevel up at 30° angle.
   2. Place tourniquet 4 to 6 inches above the client's elbow.
   3. With vacutainer system, insert blood collection tube into plastic adapter.
   4. Remove needle from vein, cover site with gauze, and apply pressure.
   5. Cleanse antecubital fossa with antimicrobial wipe.

5. The home health nurse must insert a nasogastric (N/G) tube for a client receiving tube feedings for 1 month. Which interventions should the nurse implement? **Rank in order of performance.**
   1. Elevate the head of the bed and assess the nares for patency.
   2. Have the client swallow or sip water while inserting tube to predetermined mark.
   3. Measure the N/G tube from tip of client's nose to earlobe to xiphoid process.
   4. Have client extend head, then insert tube through nostril to back of throat.
   5. Lubricate the end of the tube with water-soluble lubricant.

6. The home health nurse is teaching the male client how to perform a midstream urine specimen collection. Which instructions should the nurse provide? **Rank in order of performance.**
   1. Urinate into the toilet then place sterile container under urine stream.
   2. Replace cap on the specimen container.
   3. Fill cup with 30 to 60 mL of urine then remove before stopping urine stream.
   4. Open specimen cup, place cap inside surface up, do not touch inside of container.
   5. Cleanse penis with antiseptic wipe using a circular motion from center out.

7. The home health nurse must administer a cleansing enema to a client. Which interventions should the nurse implement? **Rank in order of performance.**
   1. Assist the client to the toilet or bedpan to expel the total volume of the enema.
   2. Fill the container with 750 to 1,000 mL of lukewarm water and soap as ordered.
   3. Lubricate the tip, gently spread the client's buttocks, and insert tubing 3 to 4 inches.
   4. Instruct the client to hold fluid for at least 10 to 15 minutes or longer.
   5. Hold the tubing in place and infuse the solution slowly.

8. The home health nurse is teaching the client's spouse how to transfer the client from the bed to the chair. Which instructions should the nurse provide? **Rank in order of performance.**
   1. Assist the client to dangle at the side of the bed and apply the gait belt.
   2. Instruct the client to move back in chair until client's back is flush with chair back.
   3. Have the client reach for the arms of the chair, flex hips and knees, and lower slowly.
   4. Position a chair at the side of the bed and apply nonslip footwear on the client.
   5. Have the spouse stand facing the client; client stands and pivots with back to chair.

9. The home health nurse is teaching the client how to administer 20 units of 70% insulin isophane and 30% regular insulin mixture in a bottle. Which instructions should the nurse provide? **Rank in order of performance.**
   1. Expose the abdomen and identify an area 2 inches from the umbilicus.
   2. Insert 20 units of air into the bottle in upright position, invert, and withdraw 20 units.
   3. Discard needle safely and do not reuse.
   4. Holding the syringe similar to a dart, insert needle at 45° or 90° angle.
   5. Slowly administer the insulin, then remove needle from skin.

10. The home health nurse must apply a hydrocolloid dressing to a client's wound. Which interventions should the nurse implement? **Rank in order of performance.**
    1. With the backing in place, cut the hydrocolloid dressing to desired shape.
    2. Cleanse the wound as directed and allow to dry completely.
    3. Peel the backing from one edge of the dressing and apply to the skin with a rolling motion.
    4. Apply skin prep to area around the wound bed, approximately 1 to 2 inches.
    5. Smooth the dressing and hold in place for several seconds.

MENTAL HEALTH NURSING CASE STUDY: MULTIPLE CLIENTS

The charge nurse of an inpatient psychiatric unit is orienting new nurses to the unit, the client admission process, nursing documentation, and the care of the client with a mental illness. The charge nurse explains the importance of identifying defense mechanisms and asks the new nurses to select the defense mechanism each client is displaying.

1. The client has been arrested several times for drunk driving but does not believe he has a problem with alcohol. Which defense mechanism is the client exhibiting?
   1. Isolation
   2. Denial
   3. Projection
   4. Sublimation

2. The client experiences an intense rage but redirects it into playing sports such as boxing and football. Which defense mechanism is the client exhibiting?
   1. Isolation
   2. Rationalization
   3. Projection
   4. Sublimation

3. The client believes it is acceptable to cheat on his final examination because she studied for all previous examinations in the course. Which defense mechanism is the client exhibiting?
   1. Rationalization
   2. Altruism
   3. Projection
   4. Displacement

4. The client gets mad at her husband and stomps off into another room and pouts. Which defense mechanism is the client exhibiting?
   1. Humor
   2. Isolation
   3. Regression
   4. Suppression

5. The client has an intense feeling of dislike for someone but buys that person a gift. Which defense mechanism is the client exhibiting?
   1. Undoing
   2. Repression
   3. Altruism
   4. Regression

6. The nurse is caring for a client who is angry at his sister but says nothing and goes outside and kicks the dog. Which defense mechanism is the client exhibiting?
   1. Displacement
   2. Splitting
   3. Undoing
   4. Isolation

7. The client is very mad at her doctor but screams that her husband is the person mad at the doctor. Which defense mechanism is the client exhibiting?
   1. Splitting
   2. Humor
   3. Projection
   4. Denial

8. The nurse is caring for a client who chooses not to discuss the details of her father's funeral. Which defense mechanism is the client exhibiting?
   1. Regression
   2. Suppression
   3. Denial
   4. Rationalization

The charge nurse continues the orientation by discussing the responsibilities for leading groups on the unit. The groups will discuss medications, symptom management, anger management, and self-care interventions. The charge nurse questions the new nurses about their knowledge of groups.

CASE STUDIES

9. Which are the phases of group work the clients progress through? **Select all that apply.**
   1. Denial phase
   2. Initial phase
   3. Working phase
   4. Recovery phase
   5. Termination phase

10. The charge nurse is discussing leadership styles for groups. Which leadership style encourages group members to participate and give input?
    1. Autocratic style
    2. Democratic style
    3. Laissez-faire style
    4. Situational style

The charge nurse invites the new nurses in orientation to the multidisciplinary team meeting. The goal of the meeting is to collaboratively design and implement treatment plans for each client in the inpatient psychiatric unit. The focus today is on the following clients:

- Mr. W.C., a 27-year-old male client diagnosed with schizophrenia who is experiencing an active phase
- Ms. A.S., a 33-year-old female client diagnosed with bipolar disorder who is experiencing a manic episode
- Ms. D.J., a 44-year-old female client diagnosed with major depression who is saying, "Life is not worth living"
- Mr. B.R., a 56-year-old male client diagnosed with depression who is reporting anxiety and shakiness

11. Which signs and symptoms should the nurse expect Mr. W.C., who is diagnosed with schizophrenia, to exhibit? **Select all that apply.**
    1. Auditory and visual hallucinations
    2. Delusions
    3. Amplified emotional expression
    4. Disorganized speech
    5. Disorganized behavior

12. The primary nurse caring for Mr. W.C. reports the client is currently having active hallucinations and thinks he is God. Which interventions should the nurse perform? **Select all that apply.**
    1. Ask the client what the hallucinations are saying.
    2. Pretend to accept what the client is saying about the hallucinations.
    3. Attempt to distract the client from the hallucination.
    4. Pat the client on the hand to show a personal connection.
    5. Provide short, simple directions displaying a supportive, accepting attitude.

13. Which signs and symptoms should the nurse expect Ms. A.S., who is diagnosed with bipolar disorder and severe mania, to exhibit? **Select all that apply.**
    1. Increased need for sleep
    2. Flight of ideas
    3. Talkative, pressured speech
    4. Easily distracted
    5. Low self-esteem

14. Which interventions can the primary nurse implement when caring for Ms. A.S.? **Select all that apply.**
    1. Encourage the client to play ping-pong in the recreation room.
    2. Provide the client with protein bars or peanut butter crackers to eat.
    3. Administer a mood stabilizer or antipsychotic medication as ordered.
    4. Remove glass and smoking materials from the client's surroundings.
    5. Set firm limits on intrusive, manipulative behaviors.

15. The primary nurse caring for Ms. D.J., a 44-year-old female client diagnosed with major depression, reports to the team meeting that Ms. D.J. is saying, "I am tired of living, I just need to die and everyone will be better off." Which interventions should the nurse perform to assess the client's suicide risk? **Select all that apply.**
    1. Ask the client directly if she is thinking about suicide.
    2. Determine if the client has a specific suicide plan.
    3. Discover if the client has access to lethal methods to commit suicide.
    4. Question the client about any previous suicide attempts.
    5. Check if the client has had other family members commit suicide.

16. Ms. D.J. is placed on a 1-on-1 high risk suicide protocol. Which tasks can the nurse delegate to the mental health worker (MHW)? **Select all that apply.**
    1. Evaluate the client's support system.
    2. Provide the client with plastic utensils for meals.
    3. Stay with the client in the day room.
    4. Escort the client to the bathroom.
    5. Give the client the ordered medications.

17. The charge nurse is teaching the new nurses about the signs and symptoms exhibited by clients diagnosed with major depression. Which findings should the charge nurse include in the teaching? **Select all that apply.**
    1. Change in appetite resulting in weight loss or gain
    2. Grandiose behavior and beliefs
    3. Loss of pleasure in life and usual pursuits
    4. Attentiveness and concentration in activities
    5. Insomnia or excessive sleepiness

18. The health-care provider determines Mr. B.R. is having alcohol withdrawal and arranges for him to be transferred to the acute care hospital. Which interventions should the nurse implement for the client experiencing alcohol withdrawal? **Select all that apply.**
    1. Assess the client for delirium tremens (DTs).
    2. Administer benzodiazepines.
    3. Monitor IV fluids.
    4. Reduce environmental stimuli.
    5. Refer to Alcoholics Anonymous.

MATERNAL/CHILD NURSING CASE STUDY

Ms. K.S., a 25-year-old gravida 1, Para 0 client, presents to the Childbirth Center at 39 weeks gestation. Ms. K.S. began regular prenatal care at 8 weeks gestation. She states her uterine contractions started about 4 hours ago and are 5 minutes apart. A sterile vaginal examination indicates the client is 4 centimeters dilated, 100% effaced, and −1 station. The amniotic sac is intact.

1. Ms. K.S. asks the labor and delivery nurse, "What stage of labor am I in?" Which response by the nurse is **most** appropriate?
    1. "You are in the first stage of labor, in the latent phase."
    2. "You are in the first stage of labor, in the active phase."
    3. "You are in the second stage of labor."
    4. "You are in the third stage of labor."

CASE STUDIES

2. Ms. K.S. is having regular contractions and her amniotic membranes rupture spontaneously. Which **priority** action should the nurse implement?
   1. Elevate the head of the bed.
   2. Assess the fetal heart rate.
   3. Administer a tocolytic medication.
   4. Document the color and amount of fluid.

3. Ms. K.S. has received epidural anesthesia. Which **priority** assessment should the labor and delivery nurse perform?
   1. Assess for paresthesia in the feet and legs.
   2. Assess for a drop in maternal blood pressure.
   3. Assess for an increase in maternal temperature.
   4. Assess for presence of fetal heart rate accelerations.

4. The labor and delivery nurse is evaluating Ms. K.S.'s fetal monitor strip, which follows. Which intervention should the labor and delivery nurse perform **first?**

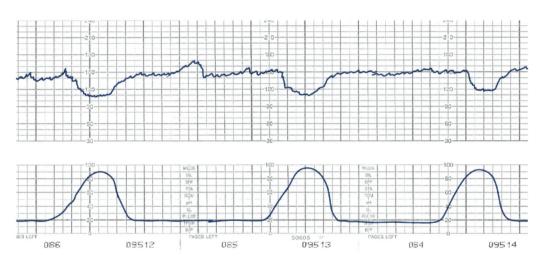

   1. Reposition the client on her left side.
   2. Perform a sterile vaginal examination.
   3. Notify the health-care provider.
   4. Prepare to administer IV oxytocin.

Ms. K.S. is completely dilated. The health-care provider arrives and spontaneously delivers a viable, male newborn. The HCP hands the newborn to the nursery nurse who places the newborn on a prewarmed infant warmer, dries the newborn, and removes the wet linens. The nurse performs the initial assessment:

Assessment	Newborn Finding
Heart rate	110 bpm
Respirations	Slow, weak cry
Muscle tone	Minimal flexion of extremities
Reflex irritability	Grimace with stimulation
Color	Acrocyanosis

5. Which Apgar score should the nurse assign the neonate?
   1. Apgar score of 8
   2. Apgar score of 7
   3. Apgar score of 6
   4. Apgar score of 5

6. Based on the initial assessment, which interventions should the nurse perform? **Select all that apply.**
   1. Suction the mouth and nose.
   2. Provide oxygen via face mask.
   3. Administer epinephrine endotracheally.
   4. Initiate an IV line of normal saline.
   5. Assess the need to administer naloxone.

Following interventions provided by the nurse, the newborn has an Apgar score of 10 at 5 minutes. After breastfeeding and bonding with Ms. K.S., couplet care is assigned. The baby boy and postpartum client are assessed by the nurse and teaching is provided to the mother.

7. The nurse lifts the newborn baby up from the bed, releases the infant briefly, but quickly supports again. The baby responds by extending his head and legs; his arms extend with palms facing upward, thumbs flex, and he cries briefly. Which newborn reflex should the nurse document the newborn is exhibiting?
   1. Walking (stepping) reflex
   2. Tonic-neck (fencing) reflex
   3. Moro (startle) reflex
   4. Palmar grasp reflex

8. The nurse is assessing Ms. K.S.'s uterine fundus and finds it firm, 2 centimeters above the umbilicus, and displaced to the right of midline. Which **priority** intervention should the nurse implement?
   1. Massage the fundus until firm.
   2. Assist the client to void.
   3. Notify the health-care provider.
   4. Start a perineal pad count.

9. The nurse is teaching Ms. K.S. about care of the newborn's umbilical cord. Which assessment indicates to the nurse that Ms. K.S. **understands** proper cord care?
   1. Ms. K.S. views a video on newborn hygiene and umbilical cord care.
   2. Ms. K.S. reads a pamphlet on newborn umbilical cord care.
   3. Ms. K.S. verbalizes she will apply antibiotic ointment to the cord stump daily.
   4. Ms. K.S. folds down the top of the diaper below the cord stump.

10. The nurse is preparing to discharge Ms. K.S. Which teaching interventions should the nurse include in the discharge instructions for this client? **Select all that apply.**
   1. Avoid sexual activity or tampons until your postpartum visit.
   2. Take a daily laxative to avoid straining and constipation.
   3. Cleanse perineal area with warm water after urination.
   4. Notify the health-care provider if you experience heavy bleeding.
   5. Take frequent rest periods, especially when the baby is sleeping.

CASE STUDIES

ANSWERS TO CASE STUDIES

The correct answer number and rationale for why it is the correct answer are given in **boldface type.** Rationales for why the other possible answer options are incorrect also are given, but they are not in boldface type.

MEDICAL NURSING CASE STUDY #1: MULTIPLE CLIENTS ANSWERS

1. 1. Mr. K.B., diagnosed with abdominal pain with unknown etiology, should be seen to evaluate his current pain level and assess the abdomen, but the priority is the client diagnosed with diabetic ketoacidosis.
   2. Ms. M.W., diagnosed with cellulitis of the left leg, should be seen, but not before the client diagnosed with diabetic ketoacidosis.
   3. **Ms. A.S., diagnosed with diabetic ketoacidosis, should be assessed first to determine blood glucose levels and whether insulin replacement therapy is needed.**
   4. Mr. G.D., diagnosed with renal calculi, should be seen to determine his current pain level, but not before the client diagnosed with diabetic ketoacidosis.

2. Correct answers are 1, 2, and 5.
   1. **The UAP can assist Ms. A.S. to the shower.**
   2. **The UAP can change the linens on Ms. A.S.'s bed.**
   3. The UAP should not cut a client's toenails, especially a client who has diabetes. This presents an opportunity for the client to develop an infection and possibly lose the foot.
   4. The UAP should not feed a client who is 24 and can feed herself. The client should be encouraged to be independent.
   5. **The UAP can massage Ms. A.S.'s lower back as a comfort measure.**

3. Correct answers are 1, 2, and 3.
   1. **The client is experiencing signs of hypoglycemia including shakiness or jitteriness, headache, and anxiety. The nurse should assess the client's blood glucose.**
   2. **The nurse should give Ms. A.S. a glass of orange juice. It has a high glycemic index, meaning it rapidly affects blood sugar levels.**

   3. **After Ms. A.S. is feeling better, the nurse should give her a complex carbohydrate such as graham crackers, peanut butter crackers, or cheese and crackers.**
   4. The client is exhibiting signs of hypoglycemia and the nurse should not administer the scheduled regular insulin at this time.
   5. The client is exhibiting signs of hypoglycemia and should remain in bed until her blood glucose has stabilized to avoid the risk of injury.

4. Correct answers are 1, 2, 3, and 4.
   1. **The client is sedated during an endoscopy and should avoid eating or drinking for 8 hours before the procedure.**
   2. **The client should not take oral medications such as ACE inhibitors, diuretics, or oral hypoglycemics immediately before the endoscopy procedure. The nurse should confirm with the HCP if the oral ACE inhibitor should be administered.**
   3. **The nurse may administer the IV proton-pump inhibitor.**
   4. **The nurse should confirm the consent for the procedure is signed and in the EHR.**
   5. An endoscopy takes about 15 minutes to perform. An indwelling urinary catheter is not indicated.

5. 1. **The nurse should determine the presence or absence of Mr. K.B.'s gag reflex before administering any PO fluids or medications.**
   2. The nurse will give Mr. K.B. his a.m. medications but should assess the gag reflex first.
   3. Mr. K.B. can be given water to gargle for his sore throat, but the nurse should assess the gag reflex first.
   4. The nurse can assess if Mr. K.B. is hungry, but the nurse should assess the gag reflex before giving Mr. K.B. anything by mouth.

6. Correct answers are 1 and 5.
   1. The UAP can record the amount of output from the N/G tube.
   2. This is an assessment. The RN should not delegate assessment to the UAP.
   3. This is an assessment. The RN should not delegate assessment to the UAP.
   4. This is an assessment. The RN should not delegate assessment to the UAP.
   5. Performing mouth care is within the scope of duties for the UAP.

7. Correct answers are 1, 2, 3, and 5.
   1. The nurse should rule out complications before administering narcotic pain medication which, in this case, includes assessment of the client's urine for blood and straining the urine.
   2. The nurse should determine the last time the client received any form of pain medication.
   3. The medication is to be administered intravenously, so the nurse should determine if the narcotic medication is compatible with the existing intravenous solution.
   4. The nurse should not document the administration of the medication in the EHR until it has been given.
   5. The nurse should identify the client and confirm the correct medication, in addition to other safety checks, before giving the medication.

8. 1. A urinalysis is not indicated immediately following the passage of a renal stone.
   2. The nurse should place the calculi in a sterile specimen cup, label it with the client's information, and send it to the laboratory for analysis.
   3. The bladder scanner is used to evaluate for urinary retention and prevent unnecessary urinary catheterization. It is not

indicated immediately following passage of a renal stone.
   4. Urinary analgesics such as phenazopyridine (AZO, Pyridium) relieve symptoms caused by urinary tract infections and irritation of the urinary tract. The nurse should first ensure the calculi is sent to the laboratory for analysis.

9. Correct answers are 1, 2, and 3.
   1. The client should be encouraged to consume 8 to 12 cups of fluid a day.
   2. The body may turn extra vitamin C into oxalate. The client should avoid high doses of vitamin C (more than 2,000 mg of vitamin C a day).
   3. Oxalate is found in many foods. The client should limit foods such as nuts or seeds, soy cheese, soy milk, soy yogurt, cereal (bran or high fiber), fruitcake, pretzels, wheat bran, wheat germ, whole wheat bread, whole wheat flour, dark or "robust" beer, black tea, chocolate milk, cocoa, instant coffee, and hot chocolate.
   4. The client should limit oxalate intake to 40 to 50 mg per day.
   5. Blueberries are high in oxalate and contain more than 10 mg of oxalate per serving. The client should be instructed to limit the consumption of these and other berries.

10. Correct answers are 1, 2, 4, and 5.
   1. The client should be instructed to elevate her affected leg to reduce edema.
   2. Meals high in protein, vitamins, and minerals will promote wound healing.
   3. Cellulitis is not treated with topical ointments; it requires systemic antibiotic therapy.
   4. The client should take all systemic antibiotics ordered by the health-care provider.
   5. Warm compresses to the affected area can help to decrease pain.

MEDICAL NURSING CASE STUDY #2: SYMPTOMATIC BRADYCARDIA

1. Correct answers are 2, 3, and 4.
   1. Assessing the client's last oral intake is important in preparing for a procedure or diagnostic test but will not provide information about the cause of the client's signs and symptoms.

2. The client has hypotension and bradycardia. This is an appropriate question for the nurse to ask.
3. A rating of 4 on a 1 to 10 pain scale is considered moderate pain. The nurse

should assess the pain utilizing the PQRST scale.

4. The nurse should assess the client for any medication usage. Hypotension and bradycardia can be caused by adverse reactions to medications. This is an appropriate question for the nurse to ask.

5. All clients should be assessed for violence or abuse, but this is not indicated by the assessment data; therefore, the nurse should focus on client signs and symptoms.

2. Correct answers are 1, 2, 4, and 5.
   1. The nurse should assess any activities the client was engaging in that he associates with the onset of the pain.
   2. Quality or intensity of pain should be assessed. The client should be asked to describe the pain such as crushing, stabbing, aching, and so on.
   3. Risk factors for cardiac disease are important to assess but are not part of the pain assessment.
   4. Severity should be assessed using a numerical scale of 1 to 10 with 1 representing no pain and 10 representing the worst pain the client can imagine.
   5. Timing and duration should be assessed. How long does the pain last?

3. 1. An arterial blood gas is a more precise reading of the client's oxygenation status, but the telemetry strip reveals bradycardia and a 12-lead EKG will better define the rhythm.
   2. A 12-lead EKG should be performed to better define the cause of the cardiac rhythm. The nurse should expect this test to be ordered next.
   3. A stress echocardiogram can identify coronary artery problems, but the priority diagnostic test would be the 12-lead EKG.
   4. A blood glucose test is not indicated by the telemetry strip.

4. 1. Atropine, an antidysrhythmic medication, decreases vagal stimulation, increases the heart rate, and is the medication of choice to treat symptomatic bradycardia (weakness, dizziness, and light-headedness).
   2. Adenosine (Adenocard) is an antidysrhythmic agent used to treat SVT.
   3. Digoxin (Lanoxin) is a cardiac glycoside that slows the heart rate and increases the

contractility of the cardiac muscle. It is used to treat atrial dysrhythmias or CHF.
   4. Nitroglycerin is a coronary vasodilator that allows increased blood flow to the myocardium. It will cause the blood pressure to decrease.

5. 1. General anesthesia is not used for this procedure.
   2. Epidural anesthesia is not used for this procedure.
   3. The leadless pacemaker is placed with only a local anesthetic injected at the insertion site located in the groin area. The leadless pacemaker is inserted into the femoral vein using a catheter, then advanced and attached to the right ventricle.
   4. A local anesthetic is utilized for this procedure.

6. Correct answers are 3 and 4.
   1. The client should be on complete bedrest for 4 to 6 hours after the procedure.
   2. The nurse should not remove the dressing. It is in place to prevent an infection. The nurse can assess and document in the EHR any drainage noted on the dressing.
   3. The nurse should palpate the pulses in the involved extremity to assess circulation distal to the insertion site.
   4. The client should remain on continuous cardiac monitoring until discharge.
   5. The client does not need his vital signs assessed that frequently. The nurse should follow hospital protocol unless assessment data indicates they should be done more frequently.

7. Correct answers are 1, 3, and 4.
   1. The client should avoid heavy lifting and squatting for 1 week after the procedure to allow the groin incision to heal.
   2. The client should notify the HCP if he experiences dizziness, syncope, or activity intolerance as this could indicate a problem with the pacemaker.
   3. The client should be instructed to keep all follow-up appointments with the HCP.
   4. Although cell phones have a low risk of interfering with the pacemaker, the client should avoid carrying his cell phone close to the pacemaker.
   5. The client is not expected to assess his pulse.

8. Correct answers are 1 and 3.
   1. The client should always carry his pacemaker identification card to inform other health-care providers about his leadless pacemaker.
   2. The client can pass through metal detectors but should avoid the hand-held metal detector wands. The client can show security the ID card and request a different manner of security screening.

3. The client should inform the HCP of any syncope or dizziness as this could indicate pacemaker malfunction.
4. The client has no restrictions on daily activities such as ambulation.
5. The client does not need an examination to fly in an airplane.

MEDICAL NURSING CASE STUDY #3: COMMUNITY-ACQUIRED BACTERIAL PNEUMONIA

1. 1. The sputum color and consistency can vary in color from green, yellow, or blood tinged. This is an important assessment, but the adventitious lung sounds are the priority to report to the health-care provider.
   2. Assessment of the lungs for adventitious sounds is the priority assessment. Adventitious breath sounds vary by different pulmonary conditions such as pneumonia, emphysema, asthma, or acute respiratory distress syndrome. This should be reported to the health-care provider.
   3. Capillary refill in fewer than 3 seconds is a normal finding.
   4. Some clients experience loose stools or diarrhea with pneumonia. This is not the priority to report to the health-care provider.

2. Correct answers are 1, 2, 4, and 5.
   1. The nurse should elevate the head of the client's bed.
   2. The nurse should provide supplemental oxygen.
   3. Fluid intake is important to maintain the hydration status of the client and thin secretions; however, providing oral fluids at a time of respiratory distress can cause aspiration of fluid into the lungs.
   4. The nurse should remain with the client and assist her in remaining calm.
   5. The nurse should encourage the client to take slow, deep breaths.

3. Correct order is 5, 2, 3, 1, 4.
   5. The client should be positioned sitting on the side of the bed or in a high Fowler's position.
   2. The nurse should instruct the client to rinse her mouth with water to avoid contaminating the specimen with bacteria from the mouth.
   3. The nurse should instruct the client to take several deep breaths. This opens the airway and provides force to expel the sputum from the lungs.
   1. The client should cough forcefully and expectorate directly into the middle of the specimen container to avoid contamination from outside organisms. The client should repeat this step until a minimum of 5 mL of sputum is obtained.
   4. The specimen container should be labeled at the bedside then sent to the laboratory for analysis.

4. Correct answers are 2 and 5.
   1. Clients are to be provided access to substance abuse counseling, but this is not required to be performed within the first 24 hours of admission or presentation to the emergency department.
   2. According to the Pneumonia Core Measures for community-acquired pneumonia, clients must have blood cultures performed and appropriate antibiotics administered within 24 hours of admission or presentation to the emergency department.

CASE STUDY ANSWERS

3. Clients are to be provided resources for smoking cessation, but it is not required to be performed within the first 24 hours of admission or presentation to the emergency department.
4. Clients are to be provided the influenza vaccine per the Pneumonia Core Measures, but it is not required to be performed within the first 24 hours of admission or presentation to the emergency department.
5. **According to the Pneumonia Core Measures for community-acquired pneumonia, clients must have blood cultures performed and appropriate antibiotics administered within 24 hours of admission or presentation to the emergency department.**

5. Correct answers are 2, 3, and 5.
1. Cigarette smoking depresses the action of the cilia in the lungs. Any smoking should be prohibited.
2. **The client diagnosed with pneumonia has some degree of deficit in gas exchange. The client should be placed on oxygen.**
3. **Activities of daily living require energy and increased oxygen consumption. The nurse should allow for rest periods between activities to allow the client to rebuild oxygen reserves.**
4. Clients are encouraged to increase fluid intake to thin secretions, not limit intake.
5. **Pulse oximeter assessment provides the nurse with an estimate of the oxygenation level in the client's periphery.**

6. 1. The client should be instructed to sit upright in the bed or in a chair to use the incentive spirometer. This is an appropriate action by the LPN and would not require immediate intervention.
2. **The client should be instructed to take a slow deep breath for lung expansion, not to blow into the incentive spirometer. The RN should teach the appropriate use of the incentive spirometer.**
3. The client should be encouraged to cough after several repetitions of the incentive spirometer. This is an appropriate action by the LPN and would not require immediate intervention.
4. The client should be instructed to use the incentive spirometer frequently throughout the day, while awake. This is an appropriate action by the LPN and would not require immediate intervention.

7. Correct answers are 1, 2, and 4.
1. **CMS and TJC Pneumonia Core Measures recommend smoking cessation information and counseling be provided to clients.**
2. **CMS and TJC Pneumonia Core Measures recommend administration of the influenza and pneumonia vaccine to clients.**
3. There is no indication that the client would need continuous at-home oxygen therapy during pneumonia recovery.
4. **The client should be taught to perform frequent hand hygiene to avoid community acquired pneumonia.**
5. The client should be instructed to use a cool mist humidifier at home to provide moisture to the air. A steam vaporizer can cause burns and should be avoided.

INTENSIVE CARE NURSING CASE STUDY: MULTIPLE CLIENTS

1. **Correct answers are 1, 2, and 5.**
1. **The client's acute respiratory distress is progressing to respiratory failure. The nurse needs to prepare for immediate intubation and mechanical ventilation.**
2. **The client needs a high-flow oxygen delivery system to correct hypoxia.**
3. The upright or prone positions are used to support oxygenation and lung expansion. It can be complicated to utilize the prone position if a client is too sick.
4. Nutritional needs are important but not a priority over respiratory support.
5. **The client should have continuous monitoring of oxygen saturation levels.**

2. Correct answers are 2 and 3.
   1. Arterial blood gas readings are used to assess a client's oxygenation, but will not confirm ET tube placement.
   2. Listening to the breath sounds in both lungs will indicate if both lungs are being ventilated.
   3. A portable chest x-ray will be performed to confirm correct placement of the ET tube.
   4. Capillary refill assesses the blood flow to the periphery; it will not confirm the correct placement of the ET tube.
   5. Suctioning secretions may be necessary but does not confirm correct placement of the ET tube.

3. Correct order is 4, 3, 5, 2, 1.
   4. The nurse should premeasure the length of the suction catheter. Length is determined by using the marking on the ET tube and adding the additional space for the adapter, usually 1 to 1.5 cm.
   3. The nurse should hyperoxygenate the client before suctioning by having the client take three or four deep breaths, manually ventilating with a bag-mask device, or activating the hyperoxygenate button on the ventilator.
   5. The nurse should lubricate the catheter tip with saline solution and insert the catheter to the premeasured length.
   2. Suction should only be applied when withdrawing the catheter.
   1. The nurse should provide mouth care after the procedure is complete for the client's comfort.

4. Correct answers are 2, 3, 4, and 5.
   1. An electrolarynx is an artificial larynx. It can be successfully used for clients with a tracheostomy.
   2. Communication boards with words, pictures, and dry erase components are helpful to facilitate communication with an intubated client on a ventilator.
   3. Hand gestures are helpful to facilitate communication with an intubated client on a ventilator.
   4. Eye blinks for yes or no questions are helpful to facilitate communication with an intubated client on a ventilator.
   5. Augmented and assistive communication devices, similar to a cell phone or tablet, use icons, pictures, and words to facilitate communication.

5. Correct answers are 1, 2, 3, and 4.
   1. The respiratory therapist is a part of the multidisciplinary team and responsible for the ventilator.
   2. The client should be on continuous monitoring of oxygen saturation.
   3. A manual resuscitation bag should be at the bedside in case of ventilator failure.
   4. The nurse should assess the ventilator settings frequently throughout the shift.
   5. The ventilator alarms should not be silenced, but attempts should be made to decrease alarms to avoid ICU psychosis.

6. **1.** Decreased reflexes, loss of sensation, and flaccid paralysis are signs of spinal shock.
   2. Hypotension and bradycardia are signs of neurogenic shock.
   3. Dyspnea and constricted airway are signs of anaphylactic shock.
   4. Tachycardia and confusion are signs of septic shock.

7. Correct answers are 1, 2, 4, and 5.
   1. The client is experiencing ICU psychosis. Clocks and calendars can be used in the ICU to help orient the client to time and date.
   2. The coordination of the day-night pattern, achieved by dimming the lights at night and opening the window blinds at day, can alleviate ICU psychosis.
   3. The nurse should attempt to structure sleep by creating a wake cycle, clustering sleep, and scheduling rest periods.
   4. The client is experiencing ICU psychosis. Familiar objects from home can decrease anxiety for the client.
   5. The client is experiencing ICU psychosis. All attempts should be made to minimize noise from nursing shift changes and from alarms on monitoring equipment.

8. **1.** The client's Glasgow Coma Scale rating would be 9.
   2. The client's Glasgow Coma Scale rating would be 9.
   3. The client receives 3 points for opening her eyes when her name is called, 2 points for moaning but no words used, and 4 points for withdrawing her arm away from the nurse in response to pain. The Glasgow Coma Scale rating would be 9.

CASE STUDY ANSWERS

4. The client's Glasgow Coma Scale rating would be 9.

9. **Correct answers are 1, 3, and 5.**
   1. **The nurse should keep the head of the bed elevated 30 degrees to help the lungs expand and prevent stasis of secretions.**
   2. Active range of motion exercises require the client to participate. Ms. T.G.'s Glasgow Coma Scale rating was 9, indicating moderate severity. She would not be able to participate in this intervention.
   3. **The nurse should always explain procedures to the client even when the nurse does not know how much the client is hearing.**

4. The client should be turned more frequently than every 4 hours to prevent skin breakdown.
5. **Traumatic brain injuries impact temperature regulation in the body. Steps should be taken to maintain normothermia in the client.**

10. 1. Sudden onset of chest pain and frothy sputum may indicate a pulmonary embolus.
    2. Foul-smelling, concentrated urine may indicate a urinary tract infection.
    3. **Disseminated intravascular coagulation symptoms result from clotting and bleeding. Oozing from the IV site would support this diagnosis.**
    4. Fever of unknown origin may indicate an infection.

OUTPATIENT CLINIC NURSING CASE STUDY: MULTIPLE CLIENTS

1. **Correct answers are 1, 2, 3, and 5.**
   1. **The client should be NPO for 8 hours before the procedure.**
   2. **The client will have an IV and be provided with mild sedation or conscious sedation as determined by the HCP.**
   3. **The client should be informed that the nurse will be taking vital signs every 15 to 30 minutes after the procedure.**
   4. The client will only have a mild sore throat and minimal discomfort following the procedure. Saline gargles and OTC medication will be recommended as needed.
   5. **The client should be instructed to contact the HCP if he has any bleeding, vomiting, or severe pain.**

2. **Correct answers are 1, 2, and 5.**
   1. **The nurse should explain the bowel preparation required before the procedure. This could include PEG-3350 and Electrolytes for Oral Solution (GoLYTELY). The bowel must be free of feces before the procedure.**
   2. **The client should be on a clear liquid diet 24 hours before the procedure and NPO 8 hours before the procedure.**
   3. The client will not have diet restriction after the procedure.

4. The client will be able to go home shortly after the procedure if no complications arise.
5. **The client should be instructed to report any rectal bleeding, dizziness or light-headedness (signs of blood loss), and abdominal pain.**

3. **Correct order is 3, 1, 5, 2, 4.**
   3. **After explaining the procedure to the client, gathering equipment, and performing hand hygiene, the nurse should don nonsterile gloves and position the client in the high Fowler's position. The nurse should remove the sterile applicator from the culture tube by rotating the cap to break the seal.**
   1. **The nurse should have the client tilt his head back and open his mouth.**
   5. **Then, using a tongue depressor (if desired) to depress the tongue, the nurse should swab the back of the throat along the tonsillar area from left to right.**
   2. **Return the applicator stick back to the tube, making sure the swab is saturated with culture medium and the cap reaches the black dot.**
   4. **Label the specimen tube and send to the laboratory.**

4. **Correct answers are 1, 3, 4, and 5.**
    1. **The client should be taught the acronym "RICE"—rest, ice, compression, and elevation. Rest prevents further injury and avoids stress on the injured ankle. The client may need to be taught how to use crutches so no weight will be placed on the right ankle.**
    2. The client should be taught to apply ice to the ankle to help decrease pain and edema. Instruct the client not to apply ice directly to the skin; use a towel and apply the ice for 20 minutes at a time, allowing at least 30 minutes to elapse between applications.
    3. **The nurse should apply a compression to support the ankle and help prevent inflammation. An elastic (ACE) bandage should be applied in a figure 8 wrap. It should not be too tight. Toes should not be cold, turn blue, or tingle.**
    4. **The client should be taught to elevate the foot above the level of the heart.**
    5. **Recommend the client use ibuprofen or alternate with acetaminophen for pain and discomfort.**

5. 1. The common cold is caused by a virus; antibiotics only treat bacterial infections. Over-the-counter medications can alleviate some of the discomforts from the common cold.
    2. Nasal cultures are not performed for the common cold. Antibiotics are not effective on the common cold virus.
    3. **The common cold is caused by a virus; antibiotics only treat bacterial infections. This is the correct response.**
    4. The nurse should not tell the client to go to a different doctor. Not prescribing antibiotics for a viral infection is appropriate treatment.

6. **Correct answers are 1, 3, and 4.**
    1. **Alcohol, coffee, and caffeinated sodas will increase the possibility of dehydration in the client and should be avoided.**
    2. Intranasal zinc is not recommended. In 2009, the Federal Drug Administration issued a warning against intranasal zinc because of its association with long-term or permanent loss of smell in clients. Oral zinc, echinacea, and large dose vitamin C have conflicting research about their effectiveness.
    3. **Chicken noodle soup and other warm fluids can help loosen congestion and have mucous thinning effects.**

4. **A saltwater gargle made with ½ teaspoon of salt in 8 ounces of warm water can help relieve a scratchy throat.**
5. Saline nasal drops and sprays can help alleviate nasal stuffiness and congestion. These items are safe for use even in children.

7. **Potassium**

8. **Urinalysis**

9. **White blood count**

10. **Prothrombin, PT with INR**

11. **Endoscopy, upper GI**

12. **Hemoglobin A1C**

13. **Electromyography, EMG**

14. **Iron, total**

15. **Creatinine**

16. **Tensilon test**

17. **TSH, thyroid panel**

18. **Rapid plasma reagin, RPR**

19. **Platelet count**

20. **Cholesterol, total**

21. **Audiometry**

22. **Scratch test**

23. **Correct answers are 1, 2, and 5.**
    1. **Women 45 to 54 years old should get a mammogram yearly.**
    2. **Women 55 years old and older should get a mammogram every 2 years.**
    3. The ACS recommends women be allowed to choose to start annual breast cancer screenings with mammograms if ages 40 to 44 years old.
    4. Women should know how their breasts normally look and feel and report changes to their HCP. Breast self-examination (BSE) is optional for women starting in their 20s.
    5. **Women with a high risk for breast cancer (genetics or family history) may need to be screened with magnetic resonance imaging (MRI) in addition to a mammogram.**

24. **Correct answers are 1, 2, 4, and 5.**
    1. **According to the ACA guidelines (2018), regular colorectal screenings should begin at age 45.**

CASE STUDY ANSWERS

2. Colorectal screenings should continue through age 75, if the client is in good health.

3. It is not recommended for people older than 85 years old to get colorectal screening.

4. Stool tests, such as fecal immunochemical test (FIT), and stool DNA tests, such as Cologuard, can be ordered by the health-care provider and performed in the privacy of the client's home.

5. Colonoscopy is recommended for abnormal results of any colorectal screening test.

25. Correct answers are 2, 4, and 5.

1. Women diagnosed with HIV, DES exposure, or other high-risk history may need a different screening schedule for cervical cancer. Vaccination against HPV does not alter the age group recommendations.

2. Cervical cancer screening should begin at 21 years old.

3. Women 21 to 29 years old should have a Pap test every 3 years without routine HPV testing.

4. Women 30 to 65 years old should have a Pap test with HPV testing every 5 years.

5. Women older than 65, with no abnormal cervical test for 10 years, can stop cervical cancer screenings. A woman who has had her uterus and cervix removed (unrelated to cervical cancer or pre-cancer) does not need to be tested.

26. 1. The American Cancer Society recommends men make an informed decision about testing for prostate cancer by speaking with their HCP at age 50. The ACA does not recommend all men be screened at age 50.

2. African Americans and men who have a father or brother who had prostate cancer before age 65 are at higher risk for prostate cancer and should have the testing discussion with their HCP at age 45.

3. Testing can be done with a Prostate-Specific Antigen (PSA) test with or without a rectal examination.

4. Research has proven that the potential benefits of testing outweigh the harms of testing and treatment. Men should talk with their HCP and make an informed decision.

HOME HEALTH NURSING CASE STUDY: MULTIPLE CLIENTS

1. Correct order is 5, 1, 3, 2, 4.

5. The nurse should open the sterile catheter set and place the sterile absorbent pad under the client's buttocks.

1. The next step is to don sterile gloves and arrange the sterile items from the catheter set on the sterile field.

3. The nurse should use one gloved hand to separate the client's labia and keep separated during the procedure. Using the sterile gloved hand and sterile applicator or forceps, the nurse should cleanse the meatus and surrounding area in a downward stroke and discard used cleaning materials in a nonsterile area, then repeat.

2. Using the sterile gloved hand, the lubricated catheter is inserted approximately 2 to 3 inches until urine enters the tube.

4. The nurse uses the entire contents of the prefilled syringe (10 mL) to inflate the catheter balloon.

2. Correct order is 2, 1, 4, 3, 5.

2. The nurse performs hand hygiene and dons nonsterile gloves and a mask. The old dressing is removed. The needle insertion site and surrounding area are examined for redness, edema, inflammation, tenderness, and exudate.

1. The nurse performs hand hygiene and dons sterile gloves, then arranges the sterile field.

4. The nurse activates the chlorhexidine cleanser and scrubs the insertion site using a back-and-forth motion with friction.

3. Allow the area to dry. A chlorhexidine impregnated dressing (Biopatch) and a transparent dressing are applied.

5. The nurse should document the date and time of the dressing change. A label should be placed near, but not covering, the insertion site.

3. Correct order is 2, 3, 1, 5, 4.
   2. The irrigation bag should be filled with 1,000 mL of warm tap water and the tubing should be primed. Water that is too cold can cause cramping and discomfort.
   3. The irrigation sleeve should be placed over the stoma, allowing the end to be in the toilet but above the water line.
   1. The cone tip of the irrigation tubing should be lubricated with a water-soluble lubricant, inserted into the stoma opening, and held snugly against the skin. The clamp should be opened to allow the water to flow. If cramping starts, the flow can be stopped briefly, then restarted.
   5. Allow 15 minutes for initial evacuation of stool from the colostomy, then the sleeve can be clamped and the client allowed to ambulate.
   4. After evacuation is complete, cleanse the stoma site with water or disposable wipe and apply a new colostomy appliance.

4. Correct order is 2, 5, 1, 3, 4.
   2. Explain the procedure, perform hand hygiene, and don nonsterile gloves. Place the tourniquet 4 to 6 inches above the client's elbow, and instruct the client to open and close the hand.
   5. Cleanse the antecubital fossa with an antimicrobial wipe starting at the vein site and cleanse in circular motions. Let dry.
   1. Hold the skin taut, then insert the needle with bevel up at a 30° angle. Lower the needle toward the skin and thread the needle along the path of the vein.
   3. When blood is obtained, insert the blood collection tube into the plastic holder while holding the vacutainer system steady. Fill to the desired level.
   4. Remove the needle from the vein, cover the site with gauze, and apply pressure to stop bleeding. Cover with an adhesive bandage or pressure dressing.

5. Correct order is 1, 3, 5, 4, 2.
   1. Explain the procedure, perform hand hygiene, and don nonsterile gloves. Elevate the client's head of bed. Ask the client about nose injury or deviated septum. Check the nares for patency.
   3. Measure the N/G tube from tip of the client's nose to earlobe to xiphoid process, then mark tube.
   5. Lubricate the end of the tube with water-soluble lubricant.

4. Have the client slightly extend head, then insert tube through the nostril to the back of the throat.
   2. Ask the client to flex head forward. Have the client sip water or swallow while inserting tube until predetermined mark is reached.

6. Correct order is 4, 5, 1, 3, 2.
   4. Perform hand hygiene, and don nonsterile gloves. Instruct the client to open the specimen container and place the sterile cap with the inside surface up. Ask client not to touch the inside of the container.
   5. Have the client hold the penis with foreskin retracted if applicable. Using a circular motion, cleanse the area with the antiseptic wipe from center out.
   1. Tell the client to urinate into the toilet, then place the sterile container under the urine stream.
   3. Collect 30 to 60 mL of urine in the specimen cup. Remove specimen container before flow of urine stops and before releasing the penis.
   2. Replace the specimen cap on the cup and cleanse urine from the external surface of the container.

7. Correct order is 2, 3, 5, 4, 1.
   2. Explain the procedure, perform hand hygiene, and don nonsterile gloves. Fill the container with 750 to 1,000 mL of lukewarm water. Add soap if ordered. Prime the tubing with solution.
   3. Lubricate the tip of the tubing with water-soluble lubricant. Gently spread the client's buttocks. Insert the tubing 3 to 4 inches.
   5. Hold the tubing in place and have the client take slow, deep breaths while slowly infusing the solution.
   4. Instruct the client to hold the fluid for at least 10 to 15 minutes or as long as possible.
   1. Assist the client to the toilet or bedpan and provide privacy until the client has expelled the total volume of the enema.

8. Correct order is 4, 1, 5, 3, 2.
   4. A chair with arms should be positioned beside the bed and nonslip footwear placed on the client to avoid slipping during the transfer.
   1. The client should sit on the side of the bed with legs dangling while a gait belt or transfer belt is applied.

5. The spouse should stand facing the client with feet closest to the chair and between the client's feet. The client is assisted to a standing position and the spouse uses the gait belt to assist the client to pivot with back to the chair.
3. The client should reach to place hands on the arm of the chair while slowly lowering onto it.
2. Tell the client to move back in the chair so the client's back is flush with the back of the chair.

9. Correct order is 2, 1, 4, 5, 3.
2. The client should pull the plunger down on the syringe to obtain 20 units of air and insert the air into the bottle in the upright position. Then flip the bottle to a downward position and withdraw 20 units of insulin.
1. The client should expose the abdomen and identify an area 2 inches from the umbilicus. The nurse should instruct the client to rotate sides.
4. Have the client hold the syringe similar to a dart between the thumb and forefinger, then insert the needle into the skin at a 45° or 90° angle. The client does not have to cleanse the skin or aspirate for blood.
5. After slowly administering insulin, the client removes the needle and applies a swab to the injection site if needed.
3. Have the client discard the needle safely so no one else can use it.

10. Correct order is 2, 4, 1, 3, 5.
2. The nurse should perform hand hygiene and don nonsterile gloves. The wound should be cleansed as directed. Assess the wound.
4. With clean nonsterile gloves, apply the skin prep to the area covered by tape, approximately 1 to 2 inches from the wound edge.
1. With the backing intact, trim the hydrocolloid dressing to the desired shape extending 1 to 2 inches from the wound edge.
3. Peel the backing from one edge of the dressing and center over the wound. Apply to skin using a rolling motion.
5. Smooth the hydrocolloid dressing and hold in place for several seconds to improve adhesion.

MENTAL HEALTH NURSING CASE STUDY: MULTIPLE CLIENTS

1. 1. Isolation occurs when the client attempts to avoid a painful thought or feeling by objectifying and emotionally detaching oneself from the feeling.
   2. **The client is not accepting reality because it is too painful. The client is exhibiting denial.**
   3. Projection is attributing unacceptable thoughts or feelings to someone or something else.
   4. Sublimation occurs when the client redirects unacceptable, instinctual drives into personally and socially acceptable channels.

2. 1. Isolation occurs when the client attempts to avoid a painful thought or feeling by objectifying and emotionally detaching oneself from the feeling.
   2. Rationalization occurs when the client justifies his behavior and motivation by substituting acceptable reasons and excuses for these motivations.
   3. Projection is attributing unacceptable thoughts or feelings to someone or something else.
   4. **The client is redirecting unacceptable, instinctual drives into personally and socially acceptable channels. This client is exhibiting sublimation.**

3. 1. **The client is justifying her behavior and motivation by substituting acceptable reasons and excuses for these motivations. This defense mechanism is rationalization.**
   2. Altruism is handling and transforming one's own pain and uncomfortable thoughts into helping others.

3. Projection is attributing unacceptable thoughts or feelings to someone or something else.
4. Displacement is channeling a feeling or thought from its actual source to something or someone else.

4. 1. Humor as a defense mechanism is focusing on funny aspects of a painful situation.
2. Isolation occurs when the client attempts to avoid a painful thought or feeling by objectifying and emotionally detaching oneself from the feeling. This client is exhibiting emotion.
3. **The client is exhibiting regression by reverting to an older, less mature way of handling stress and feelings.**
4. Suppression is the voluntary burying of a painful feeling or thought from awareness.

5. 1. **The client is exhibiting undoing. The client is trying to reverse or "undo" a thought or feeling by performing an action that signifies an opposite feeling than originally thought or felt.**
2. Repression is the involuntary blocking of a painful feeling or experience from awareness.
3. Altruism is handling and transforming one's own pain and uncomfortable thoughts into helping others.
4. Regression is reverting to an older, less mature way of handling stress and feelings.

6. 1. **The client is channeling a feeling or thought from its actual source to something or someone else. This defense mechanism is displacement.**
2. Splitting is where the client sees everything in the world as all good or all bad with nothing in between.
3. Undoing is when the client is trying to reverse or "undo" a thought or feeling by performing an action that signifies an opposite feeling than originally thought or felt.
4. Isolation occurs when the client attempts to avoid a painful thought or feeling by objectifying and emotionally detaching oneself from the feeling.

7. 1. Splitting is where the client sees everything in the world as all good or all bad with nothing in between.
2. Humor as a defense mechanism is focusing on funny aspects of a painful situation.

3. **The client is attributing unacceptable thoughts or feelings to someone else. This defense mechanism is projection.**
4. Denial is when the client does not accept reality because it is too painful.

8. 1. Regression is reverting to an older, less mature way of handling stress and feelings.
2. **The client is exhibiting suppression. Suppression is the voluntary burying of a painful feeling or thought from awareness.**
3. Denial is when the client does not accept reality because it is too painful.
4. Rationalization occurs when the client justifies behavior and motivation by substituting acceptable reasons and excuses for these motivations.

9. Correct answers are 2, 3, and 5.
1. The client in denial is not working through a group process. This is not an identified phase.
2. **The initial phase is usually the first one or two meetings of a group in which the client's anxiety is high. During these meetings the nurse leader will address the reason for the group and group rules, then establish a trusting relationship with the clients and implement appropriate interventions with group members.**
3. **The working phase is when problems are identified, clients begin problem-solving, and the group develops a sense of bonding. These meetings allow for the clients to accomplish goals.**
4. The recovery phase is not an identified phase of the group process.
5. **The termination phase occurs in the last one or two meetings. The clients should evaluate the group experience. Some clients may be anxious about ending the group while others may be glad to disband the group.**

10. 1. The autocratic style is led by the leader with set goals. This style often lacks member input.
2. **The democratic leadership style encourages members to participate in problem-solving and is best for facilitating member participation and input.**
3. Laissez-faire leadership provides no direction to group members and can limit productivity.
4. Situational leadership is not suited to this type of group. It does not necessarily promote long-term goals.

CASE STUDY ANSWERS

11. **Correct answers are 1, 2, 4, and 5.**
    1. **Clients diagnosed with schizophrenia often have false perceptions of sound and images.**
    2. **Clients diagnosed with schizophrenia often have delusions. Delusions are irrational or false beliefs about oneself that are not supported by the individual's education, culture, or talents.**
    3. The client diagnosed with schizophrenia often exhibits negative symptoms such as diminished emotional expression and diminished motivation to perform purposeful activities.
    4. **Schizophrenia can be associated with disorganized, incoherent, and illogical speech.**
    5. **Disorganized behavior in the client diagnosed with schizophrenia can include a decline in daily functioning or even a catatonic state.**

12. **Correct answers are 1, 3, and 5.**
    1. **The nurse should determine if the hallucinations are indicating the client could harm himself or others; however, the nurse should not have prolonged discussions about false ideas.**
    2. The nurse should not pretend to accept what the client is saying. The client must understand that the nurse does not view the hallucinations as real.
    3. **The nurse should use distractions and involve the client in reality-based topics.**
    4. The nurse should avoid touching the client without warning as this could lead to fear and aggression in the client.
    5. **The nurse should provide short, simple directions and convey a supportive and accepting attitude toward the client.**

13. **Correct answers are 2, 3, and 4.**
    1. The client experiencing a severe manic episode will display a decreased need for sleep and often exhibits continuous activity.
    2. **The client experiencing a severe manic episode will experience a flight of ideas or racing thoughts.**
    3. **Talkative, pressured speech is commonly noted in the client experiencing a manic episode.**
    4. **The client experiencing a manic episode is often easily distracted by irrelevant external stimuli.**
    5. Delusions of grandeur and inflated self-esteem are noted in a client experiencing a manic episode.

14. **Correct answers are 2, 3, 4, and 5.**
    1. The nurse should encourage the client to participate in physical activity such as walking, throwing a basketball, and so on. The nurse should avoid encouraging competitive sports such as ping-pong or cards to minimize anxiety and agitation in the client.
    2. **High-protein, high-calorie foods the client can carry around and eat "on the go" are appropriate to provide nutrition in the manic phase as clients are unlikely to sit at a table.**
    3. **Mood stabilizers such as lithium are often combined with antipsychotic medications to control mania. This is a correct intervention although it may take 1 to 3 weeks for the medication to begin working.**
    4. **Glass, smoking materials, and all sharp objects should be removed from the client's surroundings to avoid the client using these objects to harm himself or others.**
    5. **The nurse should set firm limits on intrusive and manipulative behaviors by the client and assist the client to respect boundaries.**

15. **Correct answers are 1, 2, 3, and 4.**
    1. **The nurse should ask the client directly if she is thinking about suicide. This assists the nurse in determining if the client is a suicide risk.**
    2. **The client with a specific plan to commit suicide is at high risk. This information will assist the nurse in determining the seriousness of the client's intent.**
    3. **The nurse should discover how easy it would be for the client to access lethal methods, such as guns or pills, to use in a suicide attempt.**
    4. **Previous suicide attempts increase the client's risk of attempting to commit suicide.**
    5. Suicide is not an inherited family trait.

16. **Correct answers are 2, 3, and 4.**
    1. It is the nurse's role to assess and evaluate the client's support system. This would not be an appropriate task to delegate to the MHW.
    2. **This is an appropriate task to delegate to the MHW.**
    3. **This is an appropriate task to delegate to the MHW.**

4. This is an appropriate task to delegate to the MHW.

5. The MHW cannot administer medications; this is the responsibility of the nursing staff.

17. **Correct answers are 1, 3, and 5.**

   1. **The client diagnosed with major depression often exhibits changes in appetite that result in weight loss or weight gain.**

   2. Grandiose behaviors and beliefs are common in bipolar disorder or schizophrenia but not in major depressive disorders.

   3. **Loss of pleasure in life and in usual pursuits is a symptom exhibited by clients diagnosed with major depression.**

   4. Clients diagnosed with major depression often have difficulty concentrating and thinking clearly, not attentiveness.

   5. **Clients diagnosed with major depression often are either unable to sleep or exhibit excessive sleepiness on a daily basis.**

18. **Correct answers are 1, 2, 3, and 4.**

   1. **Delirium tremens (DTs) occurs approximately 3 days after a client stops drinking following heavy alcohol use. The client exhibits anxiety, tremors, disorientation, and hallucinations. The nurse should assess for DTs as this could be life threatening.**

   2. **Benzodiazepines should be given as ordered to prevent seizures and delirium.**

   3. **The nurse should initiate and monitor IV fluids, which normally include vitamins, thiamine, and folic acid, also known as a "banana bag."**

   4. **The nurse should attempt to keep the environmental stimuli to a minimum.**

   5. A referral to Alcoholics Anonymous is appropriate once the client has recovered from the acute symptoms of alcohol withdrawal, but not at this time.

MATERNAL/CHILD NURSING CASE STUDY

1. **1.** The latent phase of the first stage of labor is the longest and least intense. The client is dilated from 0 to 3 centimeters. As this phase progresses, contractions become more frequent, helping the cervix to dilate so the baby can pass through the birth canal.

   2. **The client is in the active phase of the first stage of labor. The cervix is dilated from 4 to 7 centimeters. The client may feel intense pain or pressure in the back or abdomen during each contraction. She may feel the urge to push or bear down but must wait until the cervix is fully dilated and effaced.**

   3. The second stage of labor begins when the client is fully dilated (10 centimeters) and ends with the delivery of the baby. The client will be instructed to push with the force of the contractions to propel the baby through the birth canal.

   4. The third stage of labor begins with the delivery of the baby and ends with the delivery of the placenta.

2. **1.** Elevating the head of the bed is not indicated. The nurse should determine fetal well-being by assessing the fetal heart rate.

   2. **The first action is to assess the fetal heart rate to ensure the fetus is tolerating the labor.**

   3. A tocolytic medication would decrease or stop the uterine contractions. There is no indication this is necessary.

   4. The nurse should document the color and amount of the amniotic fluid, but the priority intervention is to assess the fetal heart rate.

3. **1.** Paresthesia in the feet and legs is an expected occurrence following epidural anesthesia.

   2. **The most common side effect of epidural anesthesia is a decrease in maternal blood pressure. The client normally receives a bolus of IV fluids before administration of the epidural to prevent this from occurring. This is the priority assessment.**

   3. The nurse should perform frequent assessments of maternal temperature, but the maternal blood pressure is the priority assessment.

   4. Fetal heart rate accelerations are a reassuring sign that the fetus has an adequate oxygen supply. This is important but not before the assessment of maternal blood pressure.

4. 1. The client may be positioned on her left side, but the external fetal monitor is not showing fetal distress. The nurse should first perform a sterile vaginal examination to determine if delivery is imminent.
   2. **The external fetal monitor strip is showing early decelerations of the fetal heart rate, indicating head compression. The nurse should first perform a sterile**

vaginal examination to determine if delivery is imminent.
3. The nurse will need to notify the health-care provider if the delivery is imminent. The nurse needs to perform the sterile vaginal examination in order to provide the information to the health-care provider.
4. The nurse will need to determine if the client is ready to deliver. Oxytocin (Pitocin) is often given after delivery, but this is not the first intervention the nurse should perform.

5.

Sign	Score = 0	Score = 1	Score = 2
Heart Rate	Absent	Below 100 per minute	Above 100 per minute
Respiratory Effort	Absent	Weak, irregular, or gasping	Good, crying
Muscle Tone	Flaccid	Some flexion of arms and legs	Well flexed, or active movements of extremities
Reflex/Irritability	No response	Grimace or weak cry	Good cry
Color	Blue all over, or pale	Body pink, hands and feet blue	Pink all over

1. The Apgar score is 6.
2. The Apgar score is 6.
3. **A heart rate above 100 bpm is 2 points; a slow, weak cry is 1 point; minimal flexion of extremities is 1 point; grimace with stimulation is 1 point; and acrocyanosis is 1 point. Total Apgar score is 6 points.**
4. The Apgar score is 6.

6. **Correct answers are 1, 2, and 5.**
   1. **The mouth and nose should be suctioned to ensure patency of the airway.**
   2. **The infant is breathing and has a heart rate greater than 100 bpm, but is experiencing slow respirations and acrocyanosis, so oxygen should be given via face mask or "blow by."**
   3. The newborn has a normal heart rate, so epinephrine should not be administered at this time.
   4. An IV line is not indicated at this time.
   5. **An infant having a normal heart rate and color (acrocyanosis is a normal finding in a newborn), but poor respiratory effort, should be assessed for the need of naloxone. If the mother received opiates within 4 hours of delivery, naloxone may need to be administered to the infant to counteract respiratory depression.**

7. 1. The walking or stepping reflex is elicited when the soles of the feet touch a flat surface. The newborn will attempt to "walk" by placing one foot in front of the other. This reflex disappears at 6 weeks because of an increased ratio of leg weight to strength.
   2. The tonic-neck reflex, also known as the "fencing posture," is initiated when the infant's head is turned to the side. The arm on that side will straighten and the opposite arm will bend. The motion can be very subtle.
   3. **This is the Moro reflex or startle reflex. The reflex disappears by 3 to 4 months of age.**
   4. The Palmar grasp reflex is elicited when an object is placed in the infant's hand and strokes the palm. The infant's finger will close and grasp the object. The grip is strong but unpredictable. Although it may be able to support the infant's weight, he may also release the grip suddenly without warning.

8. 1. The assessment of the uterus indicated it was firm, so massage will not correct the displaced uterus.
   2. **The first intervention is to have the client void. The most likely cause of this uterine displacement is a full bladder.**

3. The priority intervention is for the nurse to assist the client to empty her bladder.

4. A perineal pad count is important for excessive bleeding, but this is not indicated in the question.

9. 1. The client may view a video, but it does not indicate to the nurse that Ms. K.S. understands the proper care.

2. The client may read a pamphlet, but it does not indicate to the nurse that Ms. K.S. understands the proper care of the umbilical cord stump.

3. Antibiotic ointment does not need to be applied to the normal newborn's umbilical cord stump.

4. **Ms. K.S. demonstrating the need to keep the wet diaper away from the umbilical cord indicates that Ms. K.S. understands the umbilical cord care.**

10. Correct answers are 1, 3, 4, and 5.

1. **The client should be instructed to avoid sexual activity, tampons, or douching until her postpartum visit around 6 weeks.**

2. Daily laxatives are not recommended. The client can avoid constipation by eating a well-balanced diet including fruits and vegetables and drinking plenty of fluids. Stool softeners may be ordered.

3. **The client should be instructed to change perineal pads frequently and cleanse with warm water using a "peri" bottle at each change. A sitz bath and perineal wipes can help with discomfort.**

4. **The client should notify the physician for a temperature above 100°F, severe cramping or abdominal pains with chills and fever, heavy bleeding or passage of large clots, foul-smelling vaginal discharge, and pain or burning on urination.**

5. **The client should be instructed to take frequent rest periods, especially when the baby is sleeping. The client should avoid vigorous exercise or heavy lifting for several weeks.**

QUESTIONS

1. The new graduate (GN) working on a medical unit night shift is concerned that the RN charge nurse is drinking alcohol on duty. On more than one occasion, the new graduate has smelled alcohol when the charge nurse returns from a break. Which action should the new graduate nurse implement **first?**
   1. Confront the charge nurse with the suspicions.
   2. Talk with the night supervisor about the concerns.
   3. Ignore the situation unless the nurse cannot do her job.
   4. Ask to speak to the nurse educator about the problem.

2. The charge nurse observes two unlicensed assistive personnel (UAPs) arguing in the hallway. Which action should the RN implement **first** in this situation?
   1. Tell the manager to check on the UAPs.
   2. Instruct the UAPs to stop arguing in the hallway.
   3. Have the UAPs go to a private room to talk.
   4. Mediate the dispute between the UAPs.

3. The graduate nurse (GN) is working with an unlicensed assistive personnel (UAP) who has been an employee of the hospital for 12 years. However, tasks delegated to the UAP by the graduate nurse are frequently not completed. Which action should the GN take **first?**
   1. Tell the RN charge nurse the UAP will not do tasks as delegated by the nurse.
   2. Write up a counseling record with objective data and give it to the manager.
   3. Complete the delegated tasks and do nothing about the insubordination.
   4. Address the UAP to discuss why the tasks are not being done as requested.

4. The RN primary nurse informs the shift manager that one of the unlicensed assistive personnel (UAPs) is falsifying vital signs. Which action should the RN shift manager implement **first?**
   1. Notify the unit manager of the potential situation of falsifying vital signs.
   2. Take the assigned client's vital signs and compare with the UAP's results.
   3. Talk to the UAP about the primary nurse's allegation.
   4. Complete a counseling record and place it in the UAP's file.

5. The nurse hung the wrong intravenous antibiotic for the postoperative client. Which intervention should the nurse implement **first?**
   1. Assess the client for any adverse reactions.
   2. Complete the incident or occurrence report.
   3. Administer the correct intravenous antibiotic medication.
   4. Notify the client's health-care provider.

6. The registered nurse (RN), a licensed practical nurse (LPN), and an unlicensed assistive personnel (UAP) are caring for clients in a critical care unit. Which task would be **most** appropriate for the RN to assign or delegate?
   1. Instruct the UAP to obtain the client's serum glucose level.
   2. Request the LPN to change the central line dressing.
   3. Ask the LPN to bathe the client and change the bed linens.
   4. Tell the UAP to obtain urine output for the 12-hour shift.

7. Which task should the RN critical care nurse delegate to the unlicensed assistive personnel (UAP)?
   1. Check the pulse oximeter reading for the client on a ventilator.
   2. Take the client's sterile urine specimen to the laboratory.
   3. Obtain the vital signs for the client in an Addisonian crisis.
   4. Assist the HCP with performing a paracentesis at the bedside.

8. Which situation would prompt the health-care team to utilize the client's advance directive when needing to make decisions for the client?
   1. The client diagnosed with a head injury who is exhibiting decerebrate posturing
   2. The client diagnosed with a C-6 spinal cord injury (SCI) who is on a ventilator
   3. The client diagnosed with chronic renal disease who is being placed on dialysis
   4. The client diagnosed with terminal cancer who is intellectually disabled

9. The RN is caring for clients on a skilled nursing unit. Which tasks should be delegated to the unlicensed assistive personnel (UAP)? **Select all that apply.**
   1. Instruct the UAP to apply sequential compression devices to the client on strict bedrest.
   2. Ask the UAP to assist the radiology tech to position a client for a STAT portable chest x-ray.
   3. Request the UAP to prepare the client for a wound debridement at the bedside.
   4. Tell the UAP to obtain the intakes and outputs (I&Os) for all the clients on the unit.
   5. Ask the UAP to check a client's blood glucose with the glucometer ac and hs.

10. The nurse is assigned to a quality improvement committee to decide on a quality improvement project for the unit. Which issue should the nurse discuss at the committee meetings?
    1. Systems that make it difficult for the nurses to do their job
    2. How unhappy the nurses are with their current pay scale
    3. Collective bargaining activity at a nearby hospital
    4. The number of medication errors committed by an individual nurse

11. The clinic manager is discussing osteoporosis with the clinic staff. Which activity is an example of a secondary nursing intervention when discussing osteoporosis?
    1. Obtain a bone density evaluation test on a female client older than 50.
    2. Perform a spinal screening examination on all female clients.
    3. Encourage the client to walk 30 minutes daily on a hard surface.
    4. Discuss risk factors for developing osteoporosis.

12. The female home health (HH) aide calls the office and reports pain after feeling a pulling in her back when she was transferring the client from the bed to the wheelchair. Which **priority** action should the RN home health (HH) nurse tell the HH aide?
    1. Explain how to perform isometric exercises.
    2. Instruct her to go to the local emergency room.
    3. Tell her to complete an occurrence report.
    4. Recommend that she apply an ice pack to the back.

13. The client diagnosed with osteoarthritis is 6 weeks postoperative for open reduction and internal fixation (ORIF) of the right hip. The home health (HH) aide tells the RN HH nurse the client will not get in the shower in the morning because she "hurts all over." Which action would be **most** appropriate by the HH nurse?
    1. Tell the HH aide to allow the client to stay in bed until the pain goes away.
    2. Instruct the HH aide to get the client up to a chair and give her a bath.
    3. Explain to the HH aide the client should get up and take a warm shower.
    4. Arrange an appointment for the client to visit her health-care provider.

14. The RN home health (HH) nurse is discussing the care of a client with the HH aide. Which task should the HH nurse delegate to the HH aide?
    1. Instruct the HH aide to assist the client with a shower.
    2. Ask the HH aide to prepare the breakfast meal for the client.
    3. Request the HH aide to take the client to an HCP's appointment.
    4. Tell the HH aide to show the client how to use a glucometer.

15. The unlicensed assistive personnel (UAP) is preparing to provide post-mortem care to a client with a questionable diagnosis of anthrax. Which instruction is the **priority** for the RN to provide to the UAP?
    1. The UAP is not at risk for contracting an illness.
    2. The UAP should wear a mask, gown, and gloves.
    3. The UAP may skip performing post-mortem care.
    4. Ask whether the UAP is pregnant before she enters the client's room.

16. The client on a medical unit died of a communicable disease. Which information should the nurse provide to the mortuary workers?
    1. No information can be released to the mortuary service.
    2. The nurse should tell the funeral home the client's diagnosis.
    3. Ask the family for permission to talk with the mortician.
    4. Refer the funeral home to the HCP for information.

17. The new graduate nurse (GN) is assigned to work with an unlicensed assistive personnel (UAP) to provide care for a group of clients. Which action by the nurse is the **best** method to evaluate whether delegated care is being provided?
    1. Check with the clients to see whether they are satisfied.
    2. Ask the RN charge nurse whether the UAP is qualified.
    3. Make rounds to see that the clients are being turned as delegated.
    4. Watch the UAP perform all the delegated tasks.

18. The RN pediatric charge nurse is making assignments on a pediatric unit. Which client should be assigned to the licensed practical nurse (LPN)?
    1. The 6-year-old client diagnosed with sickle cell crisis
    2. The 8-year-old client diagnosed with biliary atresia
    3. The 10-year-old client diagnosed with anaphylaxis
    4. The 11-year-old client diagnosed with pneumonia

19. The nurse is caring for the following clients on a medical unit. Which client should the nurse assess **first?**
    1. The client diagnosed with disseminated intravascular coagulation (DIC) who has blood oozing from the intravenous site and is having a seizure
    2. The client diagnosed with benign prostatic hypertrophy (BPH) who is reporting terminal dribbling and inability to empty bladder
    3. The client diagnosed with renal calculi who is reporting severe flank pain and has hematuria
    4. The client diagnosed with Addison's disease who has bronze skin pigmentation and hypoglycemia

20. The charge nurse is making assignments in the day surgery center. Which client should be assigned to the **most** experienced nurse?
    1. The client who had surgery for an inguinal hernia and is being prepared for discharge
    2. The client who is in the preoperative area and is scheduled for laparoscopic cholecystectomy
    3. The client who has completed scheduled chemotherapy treatment and is receiving two units of blood
    4. The client who has end-stage renal disease and has had an arteriovenous fistula created

21. The RN charge nurse of a critical care unit is making assignments for the night shift. Which client should be assigned to the graduate nurse (GN) who has just completed an internship?
    1. The client diagnosed with a head injury resulting from a motor vehicle accident (MVA) whose Glasgow Coma Scale score is 13
    2. The client diagnosed with inflammatory bowel disease (IBD) who has severe diarrhea and a serum K^+ level of 3.2 mEq/L
    3. The client diagnosed with Addison's disease who is lethargic and has a BP of 80/45, P of 124, and R rate of 28
    4. The client diagnosed with hyperthyroidism who has undergone a thyroidectomy and has a positive Trousseau's sign

22. The nurse on a medical unit has just received the evening shift report. Which client should the nurse assess **first?**
    1. The client diagnosed with a deep vein thrombosis (DVT) who has a heparin drip infusion and a PTT of 92
    2. The client diagnosed with pneumonia who has an oral temperature of 100.2°F
    3. The client diagnosed with cystitis who reports burning on urination
    4. The client diagnosed with pancreatitis who reports pain that is an 8

23. The 75-year-old client has undergone an open cholecystectomy for cholelithiasis 2 days ago and has a t-tube drain in place. Which intervention should the RN delegate to the unlicensed assistive personnel (UAP)? **Select all that apply.**
    1. Explain the procedure for using the patient-controlled analgesia (PCA) pump.
    2. Check the client's abdominal dressing for drainage.
    3. Take and record the client's vital signs.
    4. Empty the client's indwelling catheter bag at the end of the shift.
    5. Assist the client to ambulate in the hallway three to four times a day.

24. The surgical unit has a low census and is overstaffed. Which staff member should the house supervisor notify **first** and request to stay home?
    1. The nurse who has the most vacation time
    2. The nurse who requested to be off
    3. The nurse who has the least experience on the unit
    4. The nurse who has called in sick the previous 2 days

25. The nurse and the unlicensed assistive personnel (UAP) are caring for residents in a long-term care facility. Which task should the RN delegate to the UAP?
    1. Apply a sterile dressing to a stage IV pressure wound.
    2. Check the blood glucose level of a resident who is weak and shaky.
    3. Document the amount of food the residents ate after a meal.
    4. Teach the residents how to play different types of bingo.

26. The RN director of nurses in a long-term care facility observes the licensed practical nurse (LPN) charge nurse explaining to an unlicensed assistive personnel (UAP) how to calculate the amount of food a resident has eaten from the food tray. Which action should the director of nurses implement?
    1. Ask the charge nurse to teach all the other UAPs.
    2. Encourage the nurse to continue to work with the UAP.
    3. Tell the charge nurse to discuss this in a private area.
    4. Give the UAP a better explanation of the procedure.

27. The RN wound care nurse in a long-term care facility asks the unlicensed assistive personnel (UAP) for assistance. Which tasks should be delegated to the UAP? **Select all that apply.**
    1. Apply the wound debriding paste to the wound.
    2. Keep the resident's heels off the surface of the bed.
    3. Turn the resident at least every 2 hours.
    4. Encourage the resident to drink a high-protein shake.
    5. Assist the resident to put on a clean shirt.

28. The older adult client becomes confused and wanders in the hallways. Which fall precaution intervention should the nurse implement **first?**
    1. Place a Posey vest restraint on the client.
    2. Move the client to a room near the nurse's station.
    3. Ask the HCP for an antipsychotic medication.
    4. Raise all four side rails on the client's bed.

29. The clinic nurse is caring for a client diagnosed with osteoarthritis. The client tells the nurse, "I am having problems getting in and out of my bathtub." Which intervention should the clinic nurse implement **first?**
    1. Determine whether the client has grab bars in the bathroom.
    2. Encourage the client to take a shower instead of a bath.
    3. Initiate a referral to a physical therapist for the client.
    4. Discuss whether the client takes nonsteroidal anti-inflammatory drugs (NSAIDs).

30. The employee health nurse has cared for six clients who have similar symptoms. The clients have a fever, nausea, vomiting, and diarrhea. Which action should the nurse implement **first** after assessing the clients?
    1. Have another employee drive the clients home.
    2. Notify the public health department immediately.
    3. Send the clients to the emergency department.
    4. Obtain stool specimens from the clients.

31. The clinic nurse is caring for clients in a pediatric clinic. Which client should the nurse assess **first?**
    1. The 4-year-old child who fell and is reporting left leg pain
    2. The 3-year-old child who is drooling and does not want to swallow
    3. The 8-year-old child who has reported a headache for 2 days
    4. The 10-year-old child who is thirsty all the time and has lost weight

32. Which statement is an example of community-oriented, population-focused nursing?
    1. The nurse cares for an older adult client who had a kidney transplant and lives in the community.
    2. The nurse develops an educational program for the type 2 diabetics in the community.
    3. The nurse refers a client diagnosed with Cushing's syndrome to the registered dietitian.
    4. The nurse provides the client diagnosed with chronic renal disease a pamphlet.

33. The home health (HH) agency director of nursing is making assignments for the nurses. Which client should be assigned to the nurse **new** to HH nursing?
    1. The client diagnosed with AIDS who is dyspneic and confused
    2. The client who does not have the money to get prescriptions filled
    3. The client diagnosed with full-thickness burns on the arm who needs a dressing change
    4. The client reporting pain who is diagnosed with diabetic neuropathy

34. The RN home health (HH) nurse along with an HH aide is caring for a client who is 3 weeks postoperative for open reduction and internal fixation of a right hip fracture. Which task would be appropriate for the nurse to delegate to the HH aide?
   1. Instruct the HH aide to palpate the right pedal pulse.
   2. Ask the HH aide to change the right hip dressing.
   3. Tell the HH aide to elevate the right leg on two pillows.
   4. Request the HH aide to mop the client's bedroom floor.

35. The charge nurse has received laboratory data for clients in the medical department. Which client would require intervention by the charge nurse?
   1. The client diagnosed with a myocardial infarction (MI) who has an elevated troponin level
   2. The client receiving IV heparin who has a partial thromboplastin time (PTT) of 68 seconds
   3. The client diagnosed with end-stage liver failure who has an elevated ammonia level
   4. The client receiving phenytoin who has levels of 24 mcg/mL

36. Which client would **most** benefit from acupuncture, a traditional Chinese technique considered complementary alternative medicine?
   1. The client diagnosed with deep vein thrombosis
   2. The client diagnosed with Alzheimer's disease
   3. The client diagnosed with reactive airway disease
   4. The client diagnosed with osteoarthritis

37. The home health (HH) nurse notes the 88-year-old female client is unable to cook for herself and mainly eats frozen foods and sandwiches. Which intervention should the RN implement?
   1. Discuss the situation with the client's family.
   2. Refer the client to the HH occupational therapist.
   3. Request the HH aide to cook all the client's meals.
   4. Contact the community's Meals on Wheels.

38. Which legal intervention should the nurse implement on the initial visit when admitting a client to the home health-care agency?
   1. Discuss the professional boundary-crossing policy with the client.
   2. Provide the client with a copy of the NAHC Bill of Rights.
   3. Tell the client how many visits the client will have while on service.
   4. Explain that the client must be homebound to be eligible for home health care.

39. The unlicensed assistive personnel (UAP) accidentally pulled the client's chest tube out while assisting the client to the bedside commode. Which intervention should the RN implement **first?**
   1. Securely tape petroleum gauze over the insertion site.
   2. Instruct the UAP how to move a client with a chest tube.
   3. Assess the client's respirations and lung sounds.
   4. Obtain a chest tube and a chest tube insertion tray.

40. The RN pediatric nurse and licensed practical nurse (LPN) have been assigned to care for clients on a pediatric unit. Which nursing task should be assigned to the LPN?
   1. Administer PO medications to a client diagnosed with gastroenteritis.
   2. Take the routine vital signs for all the clients on the pediatric unit.
   3. Transcribe the HCP's orders into the computer.
   4. Assess the urinary output of a client diagnosed with nephrotic syndrome.

41. The hospital will be implementing a new electronic medication administration record (eMAR) for documenting medication administration. Which action should the clinical manager take **first** when implementing the new eMAR?
    1. Discuss the new eMAR with each nurse individually.
    2. Schedule meetings on all shifts to discuss the new eMAR.
    3. Require the nurse to read a handout explaining the new eMAR.
    4. Ask the nurses to watch a video explaining the new eMAR.

42. Which client warrants **immediate** intervention from the nurse on the medical unit?
    1. The client diagnosed with an abdominal aortic aneurysm who has an audible bruit
    2. The client diagnosed with pneumonia who has bilateral crackles
    3. The client diagnosed with bacterial meningitis who has nucal rigidity and neck pain
    4. The client diagnosed with Crohn's disease who has abdominal pain, vomiting, and diarrhea

43. Which assessment data warrants **immediate** intervention by the nurse for the client diagnosed with chronic kidney disease (CKD) who is on peritoneal dialysis?
    1. The client's serum creatinine level is 2.4 mg/dL.
    2. The client's abdomen is soft to touch and nontender.
    3. The dialysate being removed from the abdomen is cloudy.
    4. The dialysate instilled was 1,500 mL and removed was 2,100 mL.

44. The nurse is taking a history on a client in a women's clinic when the client tells the nurse, "I have been trying to get pregnant for 3 years." Which question is the nurse's **best** response?
    1. "How many attempts have you made to get pregnant?"
    2. "What have you tried to help you get pregnant?"
    3. "Does your insurance cover infertility treatments?"
    4. "Have you considered adoption as an option?"

45. The nurse working at the county hospital is admitting a client who is Rh-negative to the labor and delivery unit. The client is gravida 2, para 0. Which assessment data is **most** important for the nurse to assess?
    1. Why the client did not have a viable baby with the first pregnancy
    2. If the mother received Rho(D) immune globulin after the last pregnancy
    3. The period of time between the client's pregnancies
    4. When the mother terminated the previous pregnancy

46. The unconscious 4-year-old child diagnosed with bruises covering the torso in varying stages of healing is brought to the emergency department by paramedics. The nurse notes small burn marks on the child's genitalia. Which actions should the nurse implement? **Select all that apply.**
    1. Notify Child Protective Services.
    2. Ask the parent how the child was injured.
    3. Perform a thorough examination for more injuries.
    4. Tell the parents that the police have been called.
    5. Prepare the child for skull x-rays or a CT scan.

47. The 24-month-old toddler is admitted to the pediatric unit diagnosed with vomiting and diarrhea. Which interventions should the nurse implement? **Rank in order of performance.**
    1. Teach the parent about weighing diapers to determine output status.
    2. Show the parent the call light and explain safety regimens.
    3. Assess the toddler's tissue turgor.
    4. Place the appropriate size diapers in the room.
    5. Take the toddler's vital signs.

48. The nurse has received the shift report. Which client should the nurse assess **first?**
1. The client diagnosed with a deep vein thrombosis (DVT) who reports a feeling of doom
2. The client diagnosed with gallbladder ulcer disease who refuses to eat the food served
3. The client diagnosed with pancreatitis who wants the nasogastric tube removed
4. The client diagnosed with osteoarthritis who is reporting stiff joints

49. The nurse and the unlicensed assistive personnel (UAP) are caring for clients on a pediatric unit. Which task should the RN delegate to the UAP?
1. Sit with the 6-year-old client while the parent goes outside to smoke.
2. Stay with the 4-year-old client during scheduled play therapy sessions.
3. Position the 2-year-old client for the postural drainage therapy.
4. Weigh the diaper of the 6-month-old client who is on intake and output (I&O).

50. The home health nurse is planning his rounds for the day. Which client should the nurse plan to see **first?**
1. The 56-year-old client diagnosed with multiple sclerosis who is reporting a cough
2. The 78-year-old client diagnosed with congestive heart failure (CHF) who reports losing 3 pounds
3. The 42-year-old client diagnosed with an L-5 spinal cord injury who has developed a stage 4 pressure ulcer
4. The 80-year-old client diagnosed with a cerebrovascular accident (CVA) who has right-sided paralysis

51. The nurse is preparing to perform a sterile dressing change on a client diagnosed with full-thickness burns on the right leg. Which intervention should the nurse implement **first?**
1. Premedicate the client with a narcotic analgesic.
2. Prepare the equipment and bandages at the bedside.
3. Remove the old dressing with nonsterile gloves.
4. Place a sterile glove on the dominant hand.

52. The physical therapist has notified the unit secretary that the client will be ambulated in 45 minutes. After receiving notification from the unit secretary, which task should the RN charge nurse delegate to the unlicensed assistive personnel (UAP)?
1. Administer a pain medication 30 minutes before therapy.
2. Give the client a washcloth to wash his or her face before walking.
3. Check to make sure the client has been offered the use of the bathroom.
4. Find a walker that is the correct height for the client to use.

53. The volunteer on a medical unit tells the nurse that one of the clients on the unit is her neighbor and asks about the client's condition. Which information should the nurse discuss with the volunteer?
1. Determine how well she knows the client before talking with the volunteer.
2. Tell the volunteer the client's condition in layperson's terms.
3. Ask the client if it is all right to talk with the volunteer.
4. Explain that client information is on a need-to-know basis only.

54. The medical unit is governed by a system of shared governance. Which statement **best** describes an advantage of this system?
1. It guarantees that unions will not be able to come into the hospital.
2. It makes the manager responsible for sharing information with the staff.
3. It involves staff nurses in the decision-making process of the unit.
4. It is a system used to represent the nurses in labor disputes.

55. The visitor on a medical unit is shouting and making threats about harming the staff because of perceived poor care his loved one has received. Which statement is the nurse's **best** initial response?
1. "If you don't stop shouting, I will have to call security."
2. "I hear that you are frustrated. Can we discuss the issues calmly?"
3. "Sir, you are disrupting the unit. Calm down or leave the hospital."
4. "This type of behavior is uncalled for and will not resolve anything."

56. The experienced nurse has recently taken a position on a medical unit in a community hospital, but after 1 week on the job, he finds that the staffing is not what was discussed during his employment interview. Which approach would be **most** appropriate for the nurse to take when attempting to resolve the issue?
1. Immediately give a 2-week notice and find a different job.
2. Discuss the situation with the manager who interviewed him.
3. Talk with the other employees about the staffing situation.
4. Tell the charge nurse the staffing is not what was explained to him.

57. The nurse is preparing to administer the client's **first** intravenous antibiotic. **Rank in order of priority.**
1. Check the health-care provider's order in the EHR.
2. Determine if the client has any known allergies.
3. Hang the secondary IV piggyback higher than the primary IV.
4. Set the intravenous pump at the correct rate.
5. Determine if the antibiotic is compatible with the primary IV.

58. At 0830, the day shift nurse is preparing to administer medications to the client. Which action should the nurse take **first?**

Client's Name: R.B. Height: 62 inches	Account Number: 1253456 Weight: 105 pounds	Allergies: NKDA Date:
Medication	**1901–0700**	**0701–1900**
Digoxin 0.125 mg PO every day		0900
Furosemide 40 mg PO BID		0900 1600
Ranitidine 150 mg in 250 mL NS IV continuous infusion every 24 hours	0300 NN@ 11 mL/hr	
Vancomycin 850 mg IVPB every 24 hours		1200 **1800**
Signature/Initials	Night Nurse RN/NN	Day Nurse RN/DN

1. Check the client's armband against the medication administration record (MAR).
2. Assess the client's IV site for redness and patency.
3. Ask for the client's date of birth.
4. Determine the client's last potassium level.

59. A major disaster has been called, and the charge nurse on a medical unit must recommend to the medical discharge officer on rounds which clients to discharge. Which client should not be discharged?
1. The client diagnosed with chronic angina pectoris who has been on new medication for 2 days
2. The client diagnosed with deep vein thrombosis (DVT) who has had heparin discontinued and has been on warfarin for 4 days
3. The client diagnosed with an infected leg wound who is receiving vancomycin IVPB every 24 hours for methicillin-resistant *Staphylococcus aureus* (MRSA) infection
4. The client diagnosed with COPD who has the following arterial blood gas (ABG) levels: pH, 7.34; Pco_2, 55; Hco_3, 28; Pao_2, 89

60. The nurse has been named in a lawsuit concerning the care provided. Which action should the nurse take **first?**
1. Consult with the hospital's attorney.
2. Review the client's EHR.
3. Purchase personal liability insurance.
4. Discuss the case with the supervisor.

61. The nurse has accepted the position of clinical manager for a medical-surgical unit. Which role is an important aspect of this management position?
1. Evaluate the job performance of the staff.
2. Be the sole decision maker for the unit.
3. Take responsibility for the staff nurse's actions.
4. Attend the medical staff meetings.

62. The charge nurse notices that one of the staff takes frequent breaks, has unpredictable mood swings, and often volunteers to care for clients who require narcotics. Which **priority** action should the charge nurse implement regarding this employee?
1. Discuss the nurse's actions with the unit manager.
2. Confront the nurse about the behavior.
3. Do not allow the nurse to take breaks alone.
4. Prepare an occurrence report on the employee.

63. A health-care provider (HCP) frequently tells jokes with sexual overtones at the nursing station. Which action should the RN charge nurse implement?
1. Tell the HCP that the jokes are inappropriate and offensive.
2. Report the behavior to the medical staff committee.
3. Discuss the problem with the chief nursing officer.
4. Call a Code Purple and have the nurses surround the HCP.

64. The night shift nurse is caring for clients on the surgical unit. Which client situation would **warrant immediate** notification of the surgeon?
1. The client who is 2 days postoperative for bowel resection and who refuses to turn, cough, and deep breathe
2. The client who is 5 hours postoperative for abdominal hysterectomy who reported feeling a "pop" and then her pain went away
3. The client who is 2 hours postoperative for TKR and who has 400 mL in the cell-saver collection device
4. The client who is 1 day postoperative for bilateral thyroidectomy and who has a negative Chvostek sign

65. Which client should the nurse in the post-anesthesia care unit (PACU) assess **first?**
1. The client who received general anesthesia who is reporting a sore throat
2. The client who had right knee surgery and has a pulse oximeter reading of 90%
3. The client who received epidural surgery and has a palpable 2+ dorsalis pedal pulse
4. The client who had abdominal surgery and has green bile draining from the N/G tube

66. The client with a below-the-knee amputation (BKA) has a large amount of bright red blood on the residual limb dressing and the nurse suspects an arterial bleed. Which intervention should the nurse implement **first?**
    1. Increase the client's intravenous rate.
    2. Assess the client's vital signs.
    3. Apply a tourniquet above the amputation.
    4. Notify the client's health-care provider.

67. The client who had surgery on the right elbow has no right radial pulse and the fingers are cold. The client reports tingling, and she cannot move the fingers of the right hand. Which intervention should the nurse implement **first?**
    1. Document the findings in the client's EHR.
    2. Elevate the client's right hand.
    3. Assess the radial pulse with the Doppler.
    4. Notify the client's health-care provider.

68. The HCP writes an order for the client diagnosed with a fractured right hip and operative repair to ambulate with a walker four times per day. Which action should the RN implement?
    1. Tell the unlicensed assistive personnel (UAP) to ambulate the client with the walker.
    2. Request a referral to the physical therapy department.
    3. Obtain a walker that is appropriate for the client's height.
    4. Notify the social worker of the HCP's order for a walker.

69. Which task would be **most** appropriate for the RN surgical nurse to delegate to the unlicensed assistive personnel (UAP) working on a surgical unit?
    1. Escort the client to the smoking area outside.
    2. Obtain vital signs on a newly admitted client.
    3. Administer a feeding to the client with a gastrostomy tube.
    4. Check the toes of a client who just had a cast application.

70. The licensed practical nurse (LPN) is working in a surgical rehabilitation unit. Which nursing task would be **most** appropriate for the LPN to implement?
    1. Bathe the client who is incontinent of urine.
    2. Document the amount of food the client eats.
    3. Conduct the afternoon bingo game in the lobby.
    4. Perform routine dressing changes on assigned clients.

71. The unlicensed assistive personnel (UAP) is changing a full sharps container in the client's room. Which action should the RN implement?
    1. Tell the UAP she cannot change the sharps container.
    2. Explain that the housekeeping department changes the sharps container.
    3. Praise the UAP for taking the initiative to change the sharps container.
    4. Report the behavior to the clinical manager on the unit.

72. The unlicensed assistive personnel (UAP) tells the nurse the client who is 5 hours postoperative for an L-3/L-4 laminectomy is reporting numbness in both feet. Which intervention should the RN implement?
    1. Ask the UAP to take the client's vital signs.
    2. Request the UAP to log roll the client to the right side.
    3. Complete the neurovascular assessment on the client's legs.
    4. Contact the physical therapist to check the client.

73. The ED nurse is requesting a bed in the intensive care unit (ICU). The ICU charge nurse must request a transfer of one client from the ICU to the surgical unit to make room for the client coming into the ICU from the ED. Which client should the ICU charge nurse request to transfer to the surgical unit?
1. The client diagnosed with flail chest who has just come from the operating room with a right-sided chest tube
2. The client diagnosed with acute diverticulitis who is 1 day postoperative for creation of a sigmoid colostomy
3. The client who is 1 day postoperative for total hip replacement (THR) whose incisional dressing is dry and intact
4. The client who is 2 days postoperative for repair of a fractured femur and who has had a fat embolism

74. A terrible storm causes the electricity to go out in the hospital and the emergency generator lights come on. Which action should the RN charge nurse implement?
1. Request all family members to leave the hospital as soon as possible.
2. Instruct the staff to plug critical electrical equipment into the red outlets.
3. Have the unlicensed assistive personnel (UAP) place a portable flashlight on each bedside table.
4. Contact the maintenance department to determine how long the electricity will be out.

75. The HCP is angry and yelling in the nurse's station because the client's laboratory data are not available. Which action should the charge nurse implement **first?**
1. Contact the laboratory for the client's results.
2. Ask the HCP to step into the nurse's office.
3. Tell the HCP to discuss the issue with the laboratory.
4. Report the HCP's behavior to the chief nursing officer.

76. The staff nurse is concerned about possible increasing infection rates among clients with peripherally inserted central catheters (PICCs). The nurse has noticed several clients with problems in the last few months. Which action would be appropriate for the staff nurse to implement **first?**
1. Discuss the infections with the chief nursing officer.
2. Contact the infection control nurse to discuss the problem.
3. Assume the employee health nurse is monitoring the situation.
4. Volunteer to be on an ad hoc committee to research the infection rate.

77. The RN surgery charge nurse on the 30-bed surgical unit has been told to send one staff member to the medical unit. The surgical unit is full, with multiple clients who require custodial care. Which staff member would be **most** appropriate to send to the medical unit?
1. Send the unlicensed assistive personnel (UAP) who has worked on the surgical unit for 5 years.
2. Send the RN who has worked in the hospital for 8 years in a variety of areas.
3. Send the licensed practical nurse (LPN) who has 3 years of experience, which includes 6 months on the medical unit.
4. Send the new graduate nurse who is orienting to the surgical unit.

78. The nurse educator is discussing fire safety with new employees. The nurse should teach the following actions to ensure the safety of clients and employees in the case of fire on the unit. **Rank in order of performance.**
1. Extinguish.
2. Rescue.
3. Confine.
4. Alert.
5. Evacuate.

79. The client tells the surgical nurse, "I am having surgery on my right knee." However, the operative permit is for surgery on the left knee. Which action should the nurse implement **first?**
    1. Notify the operating room team.
    2. Initiate the time-out procedure.
    3. Clarify the correct extremity with the client.
    4. Call the surgeon to discuss the discrepancy.

80. The older adult client fell and fractured her left femur. The nurse finds the client crying, and she tells the nurse, "I don't want to go to the nursing home but my son says I have to." Which response would be **most** appropriate by the nurse?
    1. "Let me call a meeting of the health-care team and your son."
    2. "Has the social worker talked to you about this already?"
    3. "Why are you so upset about going to the nursing home?"
    4. "I can see you are upset. Would you want to talk about it?"

81. The client is confused and pulling at the IV and indwelling catheter. Which order from the HCP should the nurse clarify concerning restraining the client?
    1. Restrain the client's wrists, as needed.
    2. Offer the client fluids every 2 hours.
    3. Apply a hand mitt to the arm opposite the IV site for 12 hours.
    4. Check circulation of the restrained limb every 2 hours.

82. The RN surgery charge nurse on a 20-bed surgical unit has one RN, two licensed practical nurses (LPNs), and two unlicensed assistive personnel (UAPs) for a 12-hour shift. Which task would be an **inappropriate** delegation of assignments?
    1. The RN will perform the shift assessments.
    2. The LPN should administer all IVP medications.
    3. The UAP will complete all a.m. care.
    4. The RN will monitor laboratory values.

83. The head nurse is completing the yearly performance evaluation on a nurse. Which data regarding the nurse's performance should be included in the evaluation?
    1. The number of times the nurse has been tardy
    2. The attitude of the nurse at the client's bedside
    3. The thank-you notes the nurse received from clients
    4. The EHR audits of the clients for whom the nurse cared

84. The nurse is discharging the 72-year-old client who is 5 days postoperative for repair of a fractured hip diagnosed with comorbid medical conditions. At this time, which referral would be the **most** appropriate for the nurse to make for this client?
    1. To a home health-care agency
    2. To a senior citizen center
    3. To a rehabilitation facility
    4. To an outpatient physical therapist

85. The nurse is caring for clients on a 12-bed intermediate care surgical unit. Which task should the nurse implement **first?**
    1. Reinsert the nasogastric tube for the client who has pulled it out.
    2. Complete the preoperative checklist for the client scheduled for surgery.
    3. Instruct the client who is being discharged home about colostomy care.
    4. Change the client's surgical dressing that has a 2 cm area of drainage.

86. The nurse is preparing to administer medications to clients on a surgical unit. Which medication should the nurse **question** administering?
    1. The clopidogrel to a client scheduled for surgery
    2. The enoxaparin to a client who had a TKR
    3. The sliding scale regular insulin to a client who had a Whipple procedure
    4. The vancomycin to a client allergic to the antibiotic penicillin

87. The nurse is caring for clients on a surgical intensive care unit. Which client should the nurse assess **first?**
    1. The client who is 4 hours postoperative for abdominal surgery who is reporting abdominal pain and has hypoactive bowel sounds
    2. The client who is 1 day postoperative for total hip replacement who has voided 550 mL of clear amber urine in the last 8 hours
    3. The client who is 8 hours postoperative for open cholecystectomy who has a T-tube draining green bile
    4. The client who is 12 hours postoperative for total knee replacement (TKR) who is reporting numbness and tingling in the foot

88. Which situation should the charge nurse in the intensive care unit address **first** after receiving the shift report?
    1. Talk to the family member who is irate over his loved one's nursing care.
    2. Complete the 90-day probationary evaluation for a new ICU graduate intern.
    3. Call the laboratory concerning the type and crossmatch for a client who needs blood.
    4. Arrange for a client to be transferred to the telemetry step-down unit.

89. The nurse in the intensive care unit of a medical center answers the phone and the person says, "There is a bomb in the hospital kitchen." Which action should the nurse take?
    1. Notify the kitchen that there is a bomb.
    2. Call the operator to trace the phone call.
    3. Notify the hospital security department.
    4. Call the local police department.

90. The critical care unit is having problems with staff members clocking in late and clocking out early from the shift. Which statement by the charge nurse indicates a democratic leadership style?
    1. "You cannot clock out 1 minute before your shift is complete."
    2. "As long as your work is done you can clock out any time you want."
    3. "We are going to have a meeting to discuss the clocking in procedure."
    4. "The clinical manager will take care of anyone who clocks out early."

91. The nurse in the burn unit is preparing to perform a wound dressing change at the bedside. **Rank in order of priority.**
    1. Obtain the needed supplies for the procedure.
    2. Explain the procedure to the client.
    3. Remove the old dressing with nonsterile gloves.
    4. Medicate the client with narcotic analgesics.
    5. Assess the client's burned area.

92. Which client should the charge nurse of a long-term care facility see **first** after receiving shift report?
    1. The client who is unhappy about being placed in a long-term care facility
    2. The client who wants the HCP to order a nightly glass of wine
    3. The client who is upset because the call light was not answered for 30 minutes
    4. The client whose son is being discharged from the hospital after heart surgery

93. The male client in a long-term care facility says that the staff does not listen to his reports of symptoms unless a family member also describes his discomfort. Which action should the director of nurses implement?
    1. Call a staff meeting and tell the staff to listen to the resident when he talks to them.
    2. Determine who neglected to listen to the resident and place the staff member on leave.
    3. Ignore the situation because a resident in long-term care cannot determine his needs.
    4. Talk with the resident about his concerns and then initiate a plan of action.

94. The newly admitted client in a long-term care facility stays in the room and refuses to participate in client activities. Which statement is a **priority** for the nurse to discuss with the client?
    1. "You have to get out of this room or you will never make friends here at the home."
    2. "It is not so bad living here; you are lucky that we care about what happens to you."
    3. "You seem sad; would you want to talk about how you are feeling about being here?"
    4. "The activities director can arrange for someone to come and visit you in your room."

95. The charge nurse overhears two unlicensed assistive personnel (UAPs) discussing a client in the hallway. Which action should the RN charge nurse implement **first?**
    1. Remind the UAPs that clients should not be discussed in a public area.
    2. Tell the unit manager that the UAPs might have been overheard.
    3. Have the UAPs review policies on client confidentiality and HIPAA.
    4. Find some nursing tasks the UAPs can be performing at this time.

96. The family member of a client in a long-term care facility is unhappy with the care being provided for the loved one. Which person would be **most** appropriate to investigate and report the findings during a client care conference?
    1. The ombudsman for the facility
    2. The social worker for the facility
    3. The family member who is unhappy
    4. The director of nurses

97. The 65-year-old client is being discharged from the hospital following major abdominal surgery and is unable to drive. Which referral should the nurse make to ensure continuity of care?
    1. A church that can provide transportation
    2. A home health agency
    3. An outpatient clinic
    4. The health-care provider's office

98. The nurse in an assisted living facility notes that the client has several new bruises on both of his arms and hands. Which intervention should the nurse implement **first?**
    1. File an elder abuse report with the Department of Human Services.
    2. Ask the client whether he has fallen and hurt himself during the night.
    3. Check the medication administration record (MAR) to determine which medications the client is receiving.
    4. Notify the client's family of the bruises so they are not surprised on their visit.

99. The resident in a long-term care facility tells the nurse, "I think my family just put me here to die because they think I am too much trouble." Which statement is the nurse's **best** response?
    1. "Can you tell me more about how you feel since your family placed you here?"
    2. "Your family did what they felt was best for your safety."
    3. "Why would you think that about your family? They care for you."
    4. "Tell me, how much trouble were you when you were at home?"

100. The admitting nurse is subpoenaed to give testimony in a case in which the client fell from the bed and fractured the left hip. The nurse initiated fall precautions on admission but was not on duty when the client fell. Which issue should the nurse be prepared to testify about the incident?
    1. The events preceding the client's fall from the bed
    2. The extent of injuries the client sustained
    3. The client's mental status before the incident
    4. The facility's policy covering fall prevention

101. The RN charge nurse must notify a staff member to stay home because of low census. The unit currently has 35 clients who all have at least one IV and multiple IV medications. The unit is staffed with two RNs, three licensed practical nurses (LPNs), and three unlicensed assistive personnel (UAPs). Which nurse should be notified to stay home?
1. The least experienced RN
2. The most experienced LPN
3. The UAP who asked to be requested off
4. The UAP who was hired 4 weeks ago

102. The charge nurse in an extended care facility notes an elderly male resident holding hands with an elderly female resident. Which intervention should the charge nurse implement?
1. Do nothing, because this is a natural human need.
2. Notify the family of the residents about the situation.
3. Separate the residents for all activities.
4. Call a care plan meeting with other staff members.

103. The chief nursing officer (CNO) of an extended care facility is attending shift report with two charge nurses, and an argument about a resident's care ensues. Which action should the CNO implement **first?**
1. Ask the two charge nurses to stop arguing and go to a private area.
2. Listen to both sides of the argument and then implement a plan of care.
3. Ask the family to join the discussion before deciding how to implement care.
4. Tell the nurses to stop arguing and continue to give report.

104. Which action by the nurse is a violation of The Joint Commission's Patient Safety Goals?
1. The surgery nurse calls a time-out when a discrepancy is noted on the surgical permit.
2. The unit nurse asks the client for his or her date of birth before administering medications.
3. The nurse educator gives the orientee the answers to the quiz covering the IV pumps.
4. The admitting nurse initiates the facility's fall prevention program on an older adult client.

105. The emergency department nurse is triaging victims at a bus accident. Which client would the nurse categorize as red or immediate priority?
1. The client diagnosed with head trauma whose pupils are fixed and dilated
2. The client diagnosed with compound fractures of the tibia and fibula
3. The client diagnosed with a sprained right wrist and a 1-inch laceration
4. The client diagnosed with a piece of metal embedded in the right eye

106. The clinic nurse is reviewing the laboratory data of clients seen in the clinic the previous day. Which client requires **immediate** intervention by the nurse?
1. The client whose white blood cell (WBC) count is 9.5×10^3/microL
2. The client whose cholesterol level is 230 mg/dL
3. The client whose calcium level is 10.1 mg/dL
4. The client whose International Normalized Ratio (INR) is 3.8

107. The community health nurse is triaging victims at the scene of a building collapse. Which intervention should the nurse implement **first?**
1. Discuss the disaster situation with the media.
2. Write the client's name clearly in the disaster log.
3. Place disaster tags securely on the victims.
4. Identify an area for family members to wait.

108. Which statement **best** describes the role of the parish nurse?
    1. The parish nurse practices holistic health care within a faith community.
    2. The parish nurse cares for clients in a religious-based hospital.
    3. The parish nurse practices nursing in a parish clinic.
    4. The parish nurse is a licensed practical nurse (LPN) who cares for clients in the home.

109. The HH aide calls the HH nurse to report that the client has a reddened spot on the sacral area. Which intervention should the RN implement **first?**
    1. Notify the client's health-care provider.
    2. Visit the client to assess the reddened area.
    3. Document the finding in the client's EHR.
    4. Refer the client to the wound care nurse.

110. The 32-year-old male client diagnosed with a traumatic right above-the-elbow amputation tells the home health (HH) nurse he is worried about supporting his family and finding employment because he can't be a mechanic anymore. Which intervention should the nurse implement?
    1. Contact the HH agency's occupational therapist.
    2. Refer the client to the state rehabilitation commission.
    3. Ask the HH agency's social worker about disability.
    4. Suggest he talk to his wife about his concerns.

111. The labor and delivery nurse has assisted in the delivery of a 37-week fetal demise. Which intervention should the nurse implement?
    1. Remove the baby from the delivery area quickly.
    2. Tell the father to arrange to take the infant home.
    3. Wrap the infant in a towel and place it aside.
    4. Obtain a lock of the infant's hair for the parents.

112. The newborn nursery nurse has received report. Which client should the nurse assess **first?**
    1. The 2-hour-old infant who has nasal flaring and is grunting
    2. The 6-hour-old infant who has not passed meconium stool
    3. The 12-hour-old infant who refuses to latch onto the breast
    4. The 24-hour-old infant who has a positive startle reflex

113. The psychiatric clinic nurse is returning telephone calls. Which telephone call should the nurse return **first?**
    1. The female client who reports being slapped by her husband when he got drunk last night
    2. The male client who reports he is tired of living, because his wife just left him after he lost his job
    3. The female client diagnosed with anorexia who reports she does not think she can stand to eat today
    4. The male client diagnosed with Parkinson's disease who reports his hands are shaking more than yesterday

114. The psychiatric nurse and mental health worker (MHW) on a psychiatric unit are caring for a group of clients. Which nursing task should the RN delegate to the MHW?
    1. Take the school-aged children to the on-campus classroom.
    2. Lead a group therapy session on behavior control.
    3. Explain the purpose of recreation therapy to the client.
    4. Give a bipolar client a bed bath and shampoo the hair.

115. The 36-year-old client in the women's health clinic is being prescribed birth control pills. Which information is important for the nurse to teach the client? **Select all that apply.**
    1. Do not smoke while taking birth control pills.
    2. Take one pill at the same time every day.
    3. If a birth control pill is missed, do not double up.
    4. Stop taking the pill if breakthrough bleeding occurs.
    5. There can be interactions with other medications.

116. The nurse is caring for a female client 3 days post–knee replacement surgery when the client reports vaginal itching. The medication administration report (MAR) indicates the client has been receiving calcium carbonate, ceftriaxone, and enoxaparin. Which **priority** intervention should the nurse implement?
    1. Request the dietary department to send yogurt on each tray.
    2. Explain to the client this is the result of the antibiotic therapy.
    3. Notify the HCP on rounds of the client's vaginal itching.
    4. Ask the client whether she is having unprotected sexual activity.

117. The nurse manager of the maternal-child department is developing the budget for the next fiscal year. Which statement **best** explains the **first** step of the budgetary process?
    1. Ask the staff for input about needed equipment.
    2. Assess any new department project for costs.
    3. Review the department's current year budget.
    4. Explain the new budget requirements to the staff.

118. The nurse on the psychiatric unit observes one client shove another client. Which intervention should the nurse implement **first**?
    1. Discuss the aggressive behavior with the client.
    2. Document the occurrence in the client's EHR.
    3. Approach the client with another staff member.
    4. Instruct the client to go to the unit's quiet room.

119. The client in the operating room states, "I don't think I will have this surgery after all." Which intervention should the nurse implement **first**?
    1. Have the surgeon speak with the client.
    2. Ask the client to discuss the concerns.
    3. Continue to prep the client for surgery.
    4. Immediately stop the surgical procedure.

120. Which data indicates therapy has been **effective** for the client diagnosed with bipolar disorder?
    1. The client only has four episodes of mania in 6 months.
    2. The client goes to work every day for 9 months.
    3. The client wears a nightgown to the day room for therapy.
    4. The client has had three motor vehicle accidents.

121. A new graduate nurse (GN) is assigned to work with an unlicensed assistive personnel (UAP) to provide care for a group of clients. Which action by the graduate nurse is the **best** method to evaluate whether delegated care is being provided?
    1. Check with the clients to see whether they are satisfied.
    2. Ask the RN charge nurse whether the UAP is qualified.
    3. Make rounds to see that the clients are being turned.
    4. Watch the UAP perform all the delegated tasks.

122. The RN pediatric charge nurse is making assignments on a pediatric unit. Which client should be assigned to the licensed practical nurse (LPN)?
    1. The 6-year-old client diagnosed with sickle cell crisis
    2. The 8-year-old client diagnosed with biliary atresia
    3. The 10-year-old client diagnosed with anaphylaxis
    4. The 11-year-old client diagnosed with pneumonia

123. The nurse administered erythropoietin alpha to a client diagnosed with anemia. Which data indicates the client may be experiencing an adverse reaction?
1. BP 200/124
2. Apical pulse 54
3. Hematocrit 38%
4. Long bone pain

124. The client diagnosed with sickle cell disease reports joint pain rated 10 on a pain scale of 1 to 10. Which intervention should the nurse implement **first?**
1. Administer a narcotic analgesic to the client.
2. Check the ID before administering the medication.
3. Assess the client to rule out (R/O) complications.
4. Obtain the medication from the medication administration system.

125. The nurse is caring for a 34-year-old female client who tells the nurse, "I have been diagnosed with a human papillomavirus (HPV) infection in my mouth. I don't **understand.** I get cervical smears for that." Which is the nurse's **best** response?
1. "You must have had oral sex to get the HPV infection in your mouth."
2. "You should have a smear made of your mouth every 6 months from now on."
3. "I would have the test repeated; it is not possible to have an HPV infection in the mouth."
4. "This infection is on the rise from oral contact with a person who has the infection."

126. The nurse is teaching a health class for 14- to 18-year-old females. Which information regarding sexually transmitted infections (STIs) should the nurse include in the discussion?
1. The acquired immunodeficiency syndrome (AIDS) virus is only transmitted through multiple exposures.
2. The use of a condom during intercourse ensures that a sexually transmitted disease is not passed from one partner to the other.
3. The more sexual contacts an individual has both for oral sex and intercourse, the greater the probability that individual has of contracting an STI.
4. Syphilis and gonorrhea are easily treatable and no lasting effects will be experienced with either of these infections.

127. Which nursing task should the experienced pediatric RN delegate to the UAP?
1. Escort the child who is being discharged via wheelchair out to the parent's car.
2. Determine if a young child's growth and developmental level are on target.
3. Explain how to care for the teen's below-the-knee cast to the parents.
4. Assist the health-care provider to suture an older child's leg laceration.

The correct answer number and rationale for why it is the correct answer are given in **boldface type.** Rationales for why the other possible answer options are incorrect also are given, but they are not in boldface type.

1. 1. The new graduate must work under this charge nurse; confronting the nurse would not resolve the issue because the nurse can choose to ignore the new graduate. Someone in authority over the charge nurse must address this situation with the nurse.

    2. The night supervisor or the unit manager has the authority to require the charge nurse to submit to drug screening. In this case, the supervisor on duty should handle the situation.

    3. The new graduate is bound by the nursing practice acts to report potentially unsafe behavior regardless of the position the nurse holds.

    4. The nurse educator would not be in a position of authority over the charge nurse.

2. 1. The nurse should stop the behavior from occurring in a public place. The RN charge nurse can discuss the issue with the UAPs and determine whether the manager should be notified.

    2. The first action is to stop the argument from occurring in a public place. The RN charge nurse should not discuss the UAPs' behavior in public.

    3. The second action is to have the UAPs go to a private area before resuming the conversation.

    4. The charge nurse may need to mediate the disagreement; this would be the third step.

3. 1. The graduate nurse (GN) should handle the situation directly with the UAP first before notifying the RN charge nurse.

    2. This may need to be completed, but not before directly discussing the behavior with the UAP.

    3. The graduate nurse (GN) must address the insubordination with the UAP, not just complete the tasks that are the responsibility of the UAP.

    4. The graduate nurse (GN) must discuss the insubordination directly with the UAP first. The nurse must give objective data as to when and where the UAP did not follow through with the completion of assigned tasks.

4. 1. This should not be implemented until verification of the allegation is complete, and the RN shift manager has discussed the situation with the UAP.

    2. The RN shift manager should have objective data before confronting the UAP about the allegation of falsifying vital signs; therefore, the shift manager should take the client's vital signs and compare them with the UAP's results before taking any other action.

    3. The RN shift manager should not confront the UAP until objective data are obtained to support the allegation.

    4. Written documentation should be the last action when resolving staff issues.

5. **1. The nurse should first assess the client before taking any other action to determine if the client is experiencing any untoward reaction.**

    2. An incident or occurrence report must be completed by the nurse but not before taking care of the client.

    3. The nurse should administer the correct medication but not before assessing the client.

    4. The client's HCP must be notified, but the nurse should be able to provide the HCP with pertinent client information, so this is not the first intervention.

6. 1. The serum blood glucose level requires a venipuncture, which is not within the scope of the UAP's expertise. The laboratory technician would be responsible for obtaining a venipuncture.

    2. This is a sterile dressing change and requires assessing the insertion site for infection; therefore, this would not be the most appropriate task to assign to the LPN.

    3. The RN should ask the UAP to bathe the client and change bed linens because this is a task the UAP can perform. The LPN could be assigned higher-level tasks.

    4. The UAP can add up the urine output for the 12-hour shift; however, the RN is responsible for evaluating whether the urine output is what is expected for the client.

7. 1. The client on the ventilator is unstable; therefore, the RN should not delegate any tasks to the UAP.

    2. The UAP can take specimens to the laboratory; this is within the scope of practice for a UAP.

3. The client in an Addisonian crisis is unstable; therefore, the RN should not delegate any tasks to the UAP.
4. The UAP cannot assist the HCP with an invasive procedure at the bedside.

8. 1. **The client must have lost decision-making capacity because of a condition that is not reversible or must be in a condition that is specified under state law, such as a terminal, persistent vegetative state; irreversible coma; or as specified in the advance directive. A client who is exhibiting decerebrate posturing is unconscious and unable to make decisions.**
2. The client on a ventilator has not lost the ability to make health-care decisions. The nurse can communicate by asking the client to blink his or her eyes to yes or no questions.
3. The client receiving dialysis is alert and does not lose the ability to make decisions; therefore, the advance directive should not be consulted to make decisions for the client.
4. Intellectually disabled does not mean the client cannot make decisions, unless the client has a legal guardian who has a durable power of attorney for health care. If the client has a legal guardian, then the client cannot complete an advance directive.

9. **Correct answers are 1, 2, 4, and 5.**
1. **The UAP can apply sequential compression devices to the client on strict bedrest.**
2. **The UAP can assist to position the client for a portable STAT chest x-ray.**
3. The client will need to be premedicated for a wound debridement; therefore, this task cannot be delegated to the UAP.
4. **The UAP can obtain intake and output for clients.**
5. **The UAP can check the blood glucose level on stable clients. The designation that the checks are to be performed ac (before meals) and hs (at bedtime) indicate a routine order.**

10. 1. **A quality improvement project looks at the way tasks are performed and attempts to see whether the system can be improved. A medication delivery system in which it takes a long time for the nurse to receive a STAT or "now" medication is an example of a system that needs improvement, and should be addressed by a quality improvement committee.**

2. Financial reimbursement of the staff is a management issue, not a quality improvement issue.
3. Collective bargaining is an administrative issue, not a quality improvement issue.
4. The number of medication errors committed by a nurse is a management-to-nurse issue and does not involve a systems issue, unless several nurses have committed the same error because the system is not functioning properly.

11. 1. **A secondary nursing intervention includes screening for early detection. The bone density evaluation will determine the density of the bone and is diagnostic for osteoporosis.**
2. Spinal screening examinations are performed on adolescents to detect scoliosis. This is a secondary nursing intervention, but not to detect osteoporosis.
3. Teaching the client is a primary nursing intervention. This is an appropriate intervention to help prevent osteoporosis, but it is not a secondary intervention.
4. Discussing risk factors is an appropriate intervention, but it is not a secondary nursing intervention.

12. 1. Isometric exercises such as weight lifting increase muscle mass. The RN HH nurse should not instruct the HH aide to do these types of exercises.
2. The HH aide may go to the emergency department, but the RN HH nurse should address the aide's back pain. Many times, the person diagnosed with back pain does not need to be seen in the emergency department.
3. An occurrence report explaining the situation is important documentation and should be completed. It provides the staff member with the required documentation to begin a workers' compensation case for payment of medical bills. However, the HH nurse on the phone should help decrease the HH aide's pain, not worry about paperwork.
4. **The HH aide is in pain, and applying ice to the back will help decrease pain and inflammation. The RN home health (HH) nurse should be concerned about a coworker's pain. Remember: Ice for acute pain and heat for chronic pain.**

13. 1. Allowing the client to stay in bed is inappropriate because a client diagnosed with

osteoarthritis should be encouraged to move, which will decrease the pain.

2. A bath at the bedside does not require as much movement from the client as getting up and walking to the shower. This is not an appropriate action for a client diagnosed with osteoarthritis.

3. Movement and warm or hot water will help decrease the pain; the worst thing the client can do is not to move. The HH aide should encourage the client to get up and take a warm shower or bath.

4. Osteoarthritis is a chronic condition, and the HCP could do nothing to prevent the client from "hurting all over."

14. **1. The HH aide's responsibility is to care for the client's personal needs, which includes assisting with a.m. care.**

2. The HH aide is not responsible for cooking the client's meals.

3. The HH aide is not responsible for taking the client to appointments. This also presents an insurance problem, because the client would be riding in the HH aide's car.

4. Even in the home, the RN home health (HH) nurse should not delegate teaching.

15. 1. The UAP may be at risk of contacting the illness.

2. The UAP should wear appropriate personal protective equipment when providing any type of care.

3. The UAP should not be told to skip performing assigned tasks.

4. The fetus is not affected by anthrax.

16. 1. The mortuary service is considered part of the health-care team in this case. The personnel in the funeral home should be made aware of the client's diagnosis.

2. The mortuary service is considered part of the health-care team. In this case, the personnel in the funeral home should be made aware of the client's diagnosis.

3. The nurse does not need to ask the family for permission to protect the funeral home workers.

4. The nurse, not the HCP, releases the body to the funeral home.

17. 1. The clients would not understand the importance of the specific tasks. Clients will tell the RN whether the UAP is pleasant when in the room but not whether the delegated tasks have been completed.

2. The nurse retains responsibility for the delegated tasks. The charge nurse may be able to tell the RN that the UAP has been checked off as being competent to perform the care but would not know whether the care was actually provided.

3. The nurse retains responsibility for the care. Making rounds to see that the care has been provided is the best method to evaluate the care.

4. The nurse would not have time to complete the nursing duties if the RN watched the UAP perform all the UAP's work.

18. 1. A client in a crisis should be assigned to the registered nurse (RN).

2. Biliary atresia involves liver failure, involving multiple body systems. This client should be assigned to the RN.

3. Anaphylaxis is an emergency situation. The client should be assigned to the RN.

4. The LPN can administer routine medications and care for clients who have no life-threatening conditions.

19. **1. The nurse would expect the client diagnosed with DIC to be oozing blood; however, the presence of a seizure indicates bleeding in the brain. This client should be assessed first.**

2. The nurse would expect the client diagnosed with BPH to have urinary findings such as terminal dribbling, so the nurse should not need to assess this client first.

3. The nurse would expect the client diagnosed with renal calculi to have blood in the urine (hematuria) and to have flank pain; therefore, the nurse does not need to assess this client first.

4. The nurse would expect the client diagnosed with Addison's disease to have a bronze pigmentation and hypoglycemia; therefore, the nurse should not need to assess this client first.

20. **1. The most experienced nurse should be assigned to the client who requires teaching and evaluation of knowledge for home health care, because the client is in the surgery center for less than 1 day.**

2. A routine preoperative client does not require the most experienced nurse.

3. Any nurse can administer and monitor a blood transfusion to the client.

4. Although the creation of an arteriovenous fistula requires assessment and teaching on the

part of the most experienced nurse, this client is not being discharged home at this time.

21. 1. The Glasgow Coma Scale ranges from 0 to 15, with 15 indicating the client's neurological status is intact. A Glasgow Coma Scale score of 13 indicates the client is stable and would be the most appropriate client to assign to the graduate nurse.
   2. This client's K^+ level is low, and the client is at risk for developing cardiac dysrhythmias; therefore, the client should be assigned to a more experienced nurse.
   3. This client has low blood pressure, evidence of tachycardia, and could possibly go into an Addisonian crisis, which is a potentially life-threatening condition. A more experienced nurse should be assigned to this client.
   4. A positive Trousseau sign indicates the client is hypocalcemic and is experiencing a complication of the surgery; therefore, this client should be assigned to a more experienced nurse.

22. 1. The therapeutic PTT level should be $1^1/_2$ to 2 times the control. Most controls average 35 seconds, so the therapeutic levels of heparin would place the control between 52 and 70. With a PTT of 92, the client is at risk for bleeding, and the heparin drip should be held. The nurse should assess this client first.
   2. A client diagnosed with pneumonia would be expected to have a fever. This client can be seen after the client diagnosed with a DVT.
   3. Cystitis is inflammation of the urinary bladder, and burning on urination is an expected symptom.
   4. Pancreatitis is a very painful condition. Pain is a priority but not over the potential for hemorrhage.

23. Correct answers are 3, 4, and 5.
   1. Teaching is the responsibility of the RN and cannot be delegated to a UAP.
   2. The word "check" indicates a step in the assessment process, and the RN cannot delegate assessing to a UAP.
   3. The client is 2 days postoperative and vital signs should be stable, so the UAP can take vital signs. The RN must make sure the UAP knows to immediately report vital signs not within the guidelines the nurse provides to the UAP.
   4. This action does not require judgment on the part of the UAP: It does not require

assessing, teaching, or evaluating. This can be delegated to the UAP.
   5. A client who is 2 days postoperative should be ambulating frequently. The UAP can perform this task.

24. 1. Staff members will not stay if forced to always use their paid time off for the hospital's convenience.
   2. This nurse wants to take time off. Therefore, it is the best option to let the nurse desiring to be off from work to take time off if all other situations are equal.
   3. The nurse will not gain experience if always requested not to come to work, and presumably this nurse would not have benefit time to pay for the time out of work.
   4. This nurse could be allowed to stay home only if the nurse is still ill.

25. 1. An RN, not the UAP, should perform sterile dressing changes.
   2. This client is unstable, and a nurse should perform this task.
   3. The UAP can check to see the amount of food the residents consumed and document the information.
   4. This is the job of the activity director and volunteers working with the activities department. Staffing is limited in any nursing area; the UAP should be assigned a nursing task.

26. 1. The LPN charge nurse is not the nurse educator but is responsible for the subordinate UAPs. This is adding additional duties to the charge nurse.
   2. The director of nurses should encourage responsible behavior on the part of all staff. The LPN charge nurse is performing a part of the responsibility of the charge nurse and should be encouraged to work with the UAP.
   3. Because this is not a private conversation about a client, there is no reason for the charge nurse to be told to go to a private area. The LPN charge nurse is not reprimanding the UAP.
   4. The director of nurses should not interfere with a "better explanation." This could intimidate the charge nurse and make it difficult for the charge nurse to perform duties.

27. Correct answers are 2, 3, 4, and 5.
   1. Wound debriding formulations are medications, and a UAP cannot administer medications.

2. The UAP can position the resident so that pressure is not placed on the resident's heels.
3. The UAP can turn the resident.
4. The UAP can give the resident a protein shake to drink.
5. The UAP can provide assistance to the resident in dressing and changing clothes.

28. 1. The nurse should implement the least restrictive measures to ensure client safety. Restraining a client is one of the last measures implemented.
 2. **Moving the client near the nursing station where the staff can closely observe the client is one of the first measures in most fall prevention policies.**
 3. This is considered medical restraints and is one of the last measures taken to prevent falls.
 4. Four side rails are considered a restraint. Research has shown that having four side rails up does not prevent falls and only gives the client farther to fall when the client climbs over the rails before falling to the floor.

29. 1. **The first intervention is for the nurse to ensure the client is safe in the home. Assessing for grab bars in the bathroom is addressing the safety of the client.**
 2. Taking a shower in a stall shower may be safer than getting in and out of a bathtub, but the nurse should first determine whether the client has grab bars and safety equipment when taking a shower.
 3. According to the NCLEX-RN® test plan for management of care, the nurse must be knowledgeable of referrals. The physical therapist is able to help the client with transferring, ambulation, and other lower extremity difficulties and is an appropriate intervention, but it is not the nurse's first intervention. Safety is the priority.
 4. NSAIDs are used to decrease the pain of osteoarthritis, but this intervention will not address safety issues for the client getting into and out of the bathtub.

30. 1. The employee health nurse should keep the clients at the clinic or send them to the emergency department. The clients should be kept together until the causes of their illnesses are determined. If it is determined that the clients are stable and not contagious, they should be driven home.
 2. **The employee health nurse should be aware that six clients with the same**

symptoms indicate a potential deliberate or accidental dispersal of toxic or infectious agents. The nurse must notify the public health department so that an investigation of the cause can be initiated and appropriate action to contain the cause can be taken.
 3. As long as the clients are stable, the nurse should keep the clients in the employee health clinic. These clients should not be exposed to other clients and emergency department staff. If the clients must be transferred, decontamination procedures may need to be initiated.
 4. The client may need to provide stool specimens, but this would be done at the emergency department. Employee health clinics do not have laboratory facilities to perform tests on stools.

31. 1. This child needs an x-ray to rule out a fractured left leg, but this is not life threatening.
 2. **Drooling and not wanting to swallow are the cardinal signs of epiglottitis, which is potentially life threatening. This child should be assessed first. The nurse should not attempt to visualize the throat area and should allow the HCP to do this in case an emergency tracheostomy is required.**
 3. A child usually does not report a headache and this child should be assessed, but it is not life threatening.
 4. This client may have type 1 diabetes mellitus and should be assessed, but this is not life threatening at this time.

32. 1. This is an example of community-based nursing where nurses care for a client living in the community.
 2. **Community-oriented, population-focused nursing practice involves the engagement of nursing in promoting and protecting the health of populations, not individuals in the community. Therefore, this is an example of community-oriented, population-focused nursing.**
 3. This is an example of community-based nursing where nurses care for a client living in the community.
 4. This is an example of community-based nursing where nurses care for a client living in the community.

33. 1. Dyspnea and confusion are not expected in a client diagnosed with AIDS; therefore, this client would warrant a more

experienced nurse to assess the reason for the complications.

2. The client with financial problems should be assigned to a social worker, not to a nurse.

3. A full-thickness (third-degree) burn is the most serious burn and requires excellent assessment skills to determine whether complications are occurring. This client should be assigned to a more experienced nurse.

4. **The client diagnosed with diabetic neuropathy would be expected to have pain; therefore, this client could be assigned to a nurse new to home health nursing. The client is not exhibiting a complication or an unexpected sign or symptom.**

34. 1. The RN cannot delegate assessment to the HH aide.

2. The HH aide cannot assess the incisional wound, and the wound should be assessed. The RN cannot delegate assessment.

3. **The HH aide can place the right leg on two pillows. This task does not require assessment, teaching, or evaluating, and the client is stable.**

4. Mopping the floor is not part of the HH aide's responsibility. This is not an appropriate task to delegate.

35. 1. The nurse would expect the client diagnosed with a myocardial infarction to have an elevated troponin level; thus, the nurse would not assess this client first.

2. Because the client's PTT of 68 seconds is 1.5 to 2 times the normal range, the anticoagulant heparin is considered therapeutic and would not warrant the nurse's assessing this client first.

3. The nurse would expect a client diagnosed with end-stage liver failure to have an elevated ammonia level.

4. **The therapeutic range for the anticonvulsant phenytoin (Dilantin) is 10 to 20 mcg/mL. This client's higher level warrants intervention because the serum level is above the therapeutic range.**

36. 1. This client would not benefit from acupuncture.

2. Mental health issues are not treated with acupuncture. They may be treated with herbal supplements.

3. The client diagnosed with asthma must be treated with a medical regimen.

4. **Acupuncture, the most common complementary therapy recommended by health-**

care providers, would benefit a client diagnosed with osteoarthritis.

37. 1. The registered nurse should not make the client dependent on family members to prepare meals. If the family were willing to do this, they would probably already be doing it.

2. The occupational therapist would teach the client how to cook, but this client is 88 years old and needs meals provided. Therefore, providing meals through Meals on Wheels is the most appropriate intervention.

3. The HH aide's duties do not include cooking all three meals for the client.

4. **Meals on Wheels delivers a hot, nutritionally balanced meal once a day on weekdays, usually at noon for older people who do not have assistance in the home for food preparation. This intervention would be most helpful to the client.**

38. 1. HH care agency employees are responsible for knowing and adhering to the professional boundary-crossing standards. The nurse should not discuss this with the client.

2. **Home health-care agencies are required by law to address the concepts in the National Association for Home Care (NAHC) Bill of Rights with all home health clients on the initial visit. The agencies may also make additions to the NAHC's original Bill of Rights.**

3. The nurse should discuss this with the client, but it is not a legal intervention.

4. This is a true statement, but it is not a legal intervention. If the client is not homebound, he or she is not eligible for home health care.

39. 1. **Taping petroleum gauze over the chest tube insertion site will prevent air from entering the pleural space. This is the first intervention.**

2. The RN should make sure the UAP knows the correct method to assist a client with a chest tube, but the safety of the client is the first priority.

3. This is the second intervention the nurse should implement. Remember, if the client is in distress and the nurse can do something to relieve that distress, then the nurse should not assess first. The nurse should take action to take care of the client.

4. The nurse should obtain the necessary equipment for the HCP to reinsert the chest tube, but the priority intervention is to prevent air from entering the pleural space.

40. 1. **The LPN can administer routine medications.**
    2. The UAP, not the LPN, should be assigned to take the routine vital signs.
    3. The unit secretary, not an LPN, should be assigned to transcribe the HCP orders.
    4. The RN, not the LPN, should assess the urinary output of the client. The RN should not delegate assessment.

41. 1. The clinical manager may need to discuss the eMAR with some nurses individually, but it is not the clinical manager's first intervention.
    2. **The first intervention should be to arrange meetings to explain the new electronic medication administration record (eMAR) and allow nurses to ask questions to clarify the new policy.**
    3. The clinical manager can provide a written handout explaining the new eMAR, but the first intervention should be small discussion groups.
    4. A video is an excellent tool for explaining new procedures, but the first intervention should be small discussion groups so that all questions can be answered.

42. 1. The nurse would expect the client diagnosed with an abdominal aortic aneurysm to have an audible bruit; therefore, this client does not warrant immediate intervention.
    2. The nurse would expect the client diagnosed with pneumonia to have respiratory symptoms; therefore, this client does not warrant immediate intervention.
    3. One of the findings of bacterial meningitis is nucal rigidity; therefore, this client does not warrant immediate intervention.
    4. **The client diagnosed with Crohn's disease will have pain and diarrhea during an exacerbation. The presence of vomiting, however, could indicate a bowel obstruction, which is a complication of Crohn's disease.**

43. 1. The client diagnosed with chronic kidney disease (CKD) would have an elevated creatinine level. The normal creatinine level is 0.61 to 1.21 mg/dL in males and 0.51 to 1.11 mg/dL in females. The data would not warrant immediate intervention.
    2. Peritonitis, inflammation of the peritoneum, is a serious complication that would result in a hard, rigid abdomen; therefore, a soft abdomen would not warrant immediate intervention.
    3. **The dialysate return should be colorless or straw colored but should never be cloudy, which indicates an infection; therefore, the data warrants immediate intervention.**
    4. Because the client has ESRD, fluid must be removed from the body, so the output should be more than the amount instilled; therefore, this indicates the peritoneal dialysis is effective and does not warrant intervention.

44. 1. The nurse could ask this question, but the client has already told the nurse that 3 years have passed, so the client has tried approximately 36 times.
    2. **This is the best question to assess the client. The nurse would not want to suggest an intervention that has been futile.**
    3. Infertility treatments are very expensive, but the nurse should assess the client's attempts.
    4. This question is not helpful for assessing the client or addressing the client's statement.

45. 1. The reason that the first pregnancy did not yield a viable infant is not relevant at this time. The relevant information is whether the mother received the Rho(D) immune globulin injection.
    2. **The important information to assess is whether the client received the Rho(D) immune globulin (RhoGAM) injection within 72 hours of the loss of the first pregnancy. If the client did not receive the injection, the fetus is at risk for erythroblastosis fetalis.**
    3. This is not important information at this time.
    4. This is not important information at this time.

46. Correct answers are 1, 3, and 5.
    1. **This child has injuries consistent with child abuse. Child Protective Services and the police should be notified.**
    2. This could result in not being able to prosecute the perpetrator if the nurse is not trained in forensic medicine.
    3. **The nurse should determine the full extent of the child's injuries.**
    4. The nurse should not notify the parent of the potential involvement. The police are fully capable of doing this for themselves. The nurse could instigate an inflammatory situation with this action.
    5. **The child needs x-ray studies to determine the extent of internal injuries.**

47. Correct order is 5, 3, 2, 4, 1.

  5. Taking the vital signs is part of the assessment and a beginning point for the nurse.

  3. Because the child has been losing fluids, the nurse should assess tissue turgor to try and determine if fluid replacement by the parents has been effective.

  2. The nurse should make sure that the parents do not leave the child alone in the room; the nurse should make sure the parents are aware of any safety measures used to protect the toddler from abduction, as well as how to call the nurse in case of need.

  4. The client will need diapers. They should be available to the parents so the diaper can be changed and the child will not develop skin irritation problems.

  1. When the nurse provides the diapers, it is a good opportunity for the nurse to teach the parents about weighing the diapers before and after the child soils them.

48. 1. **This client is exhibiting symptoms of a potentially fatal complication of DVT—pulmonary embolism. The nurse should assess this client first.**

  2. Refusing to eat hospital food should be discussed with the client, but the nurse could ask the unit secretary to have the dietitian see the client.

  3. Clients diagnosed with pancreatitis have nasogastric tubes to rest the bowel. However, these tubes are typically uncomfortable. Regardless, the nurse should see this client after the client diagnosed with DVT has been assessed and appropriate interventions initiated. The nurse should discuss the importance of maintaining the tube with the client.

  4. This is an expected symptom of osteoarthritis. This client does not need to be assessed first.

49. 1. This is not an appropriate delegation. Taking the UAP from the floor to stay with a child so the parent can smoke is supporting a bad health habit.

  2. The play therapist will stay with the client during the therapy.

  3. The respiratory therapist will position the client for postural therapy.

  4. **The UAP is capable of completing intake and output on clients. Weighing a diaper is the method of obtaining the output in an infant.**

50. 1. **This client may be developing a complication of immobility, one of which is**
pneumonia. **The nurse should assess this client first.**

  2. Loss of weight in a client diagnosed with CHF indicates the client is responding to therapy. This client does not need to be assessed first.

  3. Pressure ulcers are a chronic problem, which frequently occur in clients who are paralyzed. This client does not need to be assessed first.

  4. Paralysis is expected for a CVA. This client does not need to be assessed first.

51. 1. **The nurse should first medicate the client because this procedure is very painful for the client.**

  2. The nurse should prepare the equipment, but not before medicating the client. This should be done 30 minutes before the procedure starts.

  3. The nurse should use nonsterile gloves to remove the old dressing but not before medicating the client.

  4. The nurse should don sterile gloves (can put one on the dominant hand), but not before medicating the client.

52. 1. Administering pain medication is the RN's responsibility, not that of the UAP.

  2. A washcloth should be provided to the client before a meal, but not before ambulating with the physical therapist.

  3. **The client should be ready to work on therapy when the physical therapist arrives. The UAP should make sure the client has used the bathroom or has not been incontinent before the therapist arrives, thus making the most efficient use of the therapist's time.**

  4. Obtaining a walker that is the correct height for the client is the physical therapist's responsibility, not that of the UAP.

53. 1. The fact that the client is a neighbor of the volunteer has no bearing on whether or not the nurse can discuss a client's condition with the volunteer. The nurse should inform the volunteer that information obtained inadvertently is still confidential.

  2. The nurse cannot release the client's information in layperson's or medical terms; this is a violation of the Health Insurance Portability and Accountability Act (HIPAA). In many facilities, the client can give a "password" to individuals who can receive information about the client's condition.

3. The nurse should not discuss the situation with the client. This would alert the client to potential breaches in confidentiality.

4. The nurse should remind the volunteer of the HIPAA and confidentiality rules that govern any information concerning clients in a health-care setting.

54. 1. Under shared governance, some nurses become so involved with the management of facilities that they are no longer eligible for representation by a bargaining agent (union), but there are no guarantees.

2. The manager is responsible for disseminating information under a centralized system of organization.

3. Shared governance is an organizational framework in which the nurse has autonomy over the nursing practice. The nurse is given direct input into the working of the unit.

4. Shared governance is a system in which the nurse represents the nursing practice.

55. 1. This might be the second statement for the nurse to make if the client does not calm down and discuss the problems with the nurse. Because it could escalate the anger, it should not be the first statement.

2. The nurse should remain calm and try to allow the client to verbalize his frustrations in a more acceptable manner. The nurse should repeat calmly in a low voice any instructions given to the client.

3. This statement will escalate the situation and could cause the visitor to lash out at the nurse.

4. This statement will escalate the situation and could cause the visitor to lash out at the nurse.

56. 1. The nurse should leave if he determines that the staffing is not now nor ever will be as it was relayed to him in the interview; however, this may be a temporary situation that can be resolved.

2. The nurse should give the manager a chance to discuss the situation before quitting. A temporary problem, such as illness, may be affecting staffing.

3. This action could cause the manager to think of the new nurse as a troublemaker.

4. The nurse should not discuss this with the charge nurse because this may cause a rift between the charge nurse and the new nurse. The nurse should clarify the staffing situation with the unit manager.

57. **Correct order is 1, 5, 2, 3, 4.**
   1. This is the first intervention the nurse should implement. Checking the HCP's order is the priority.
   5. This is the second intervention; the nurse should not administer the antibiotic if it is not compatible with the primary IV.
   2. This is the third intervention the nurse should implement. Determining if the antibiotic is compatible is second, because client allergies won't be assessed if the medication is not compatible.
   3. This is the fourth intervention. The secondary piggyback (antibiotic) must be hung above the primary IV bag so the secondary piggyback will infuse.
   4. This is the fifth intervention. Ensuring the right rate is necessary before starting the infusion.

58. 1. Checking the client's armband is done before actually administering the medications, but it is not the first action for the nurse to take.

2. The nurse should have assessed the client's IV site on first rounds. At this time, all medications to be administered are oral.

3. This is part of the two-identifier system of medication administration implemented to prevent medication errors, but it is not the first action for the nurse to take.

4. The nurse should assess the client's last potassium (K⁺) level because hypokalemia (abnormally low K⁺ level) is the most common cause of dysrhythmias in clients receiving digoxin (Lanoxin) secondary to clients concurrently taking diuretics. Furosemide (Lasix) is a loop diuretic. The nurse should check for digoxin and K⁺ levels and apical pulse (AP) before administering digoxin.

59. 1. This client has been on a medication to control the angina for 2 days and could be discharged.

2. This client is currently completing the amount of care that would be provided in the hospital setting. The client can be taught to continue the warfarin (Coumadin) at home and return to the HCP's office for blood work, or a home health nurse can be assigned to go to the client's home and draw blood for the laboratory work.

3. Because resistant infections are very difficult to treat, this client should remain in the hospital for the required IVPB medication.

4. These blood gases are expected for a client diagnosed with COPD. This client could go home with oxygen and home health follow-up care.

60. 1. The nurse may wish to consult the hospital's attorneys or retain a personal attorney, but this is not the first action for the nurse.
    2. **The nurse should be familiar with the EHR and the situation so that details can be remembered. This should be the nurse's first action.**
    3. It is too late to purchase liability insurance to cover the current situation. The nurse may wish to purchase insurance for any future litigation.
    4. The nurse should refrain from discussing the case with anyone who could be called as a witness or be named in the lawsuit.

61. 1. **One of the many jobs of a manager is to see that performance evaluations are completed on the staff.**
    2. The manager should receive input from many sources to make decisions. Some decisions are made for the manager by administration based on costs or any number of other reasons.
    3. The nurses retain responsibility for their own actions because they practice under the state's nursing practice act. The manager retains responsibility for the functioning of the unit.
    4. The nurse manager attends many meetings pertaining to nursing but attends medical committee meetings only when a nursing issue is being discussed.

62. 1. **Usually, the charge nurse should attempt to settle a conflict at the lowest level possible, in this case, confronting the nurse. However, the charge nurse does not have the authority to require a drug screen, which is the intervention needed in this situation. The charge nurse should notify the unit manager.**
    2. The charge nurse does not have the authority to force the nurse to submit to a drug screening, which is what this behavior will ultimately require. Therefore, the charge nurse should not confront the staff nurse. The charge nurse should notify the supervisor.
    3. Nurses have the right to take breaks with or without their peers. The charge nurse cannot enforce this option.

4. An occurrence report is not used for this type of situation. This is a management or a peer review issue. The nurse can go through the manager or a peer review committee.

63. 1. **Telling jokes with sexual innuendos creates a "hostile work environment" and should be addressed with the HCP. This is a courtesy to allow the HCP to correct the behavior without being embarrassed.**
    2. If the behavior is not corrected, then the nurse should report the HCP to the manager or chief nursing officer (CNO). The manager or CNO may find it necessary to report the behavior to the medical staff committee or president.
    3. The charge nurse should first report the behavior to the manager and then, if the problem is not resolved, to the CNO; in other words, follow the chain of command.
    4. Some facilities have a code for staff to use when an HCP is acting out, but it is rarely, if ever, used.

64. 1. The nurse would not need to notify the surgeon of the client's refusal because this is a situation the nurse should manage.
    2. **Feeling a "pop" after an abdominal hysterectomy may indicate possible wound dehiscence, which is a surgical emergency and requires the nurse to notify the surgeon via telephone.**
    3. This situation indicates that it is time for the nurse to reinfuse the lost blood.
    4. A negative Chvostek sign is normal and indicates the calcium level is within normal limits.

65. 1. The client who had an endotracheal tube would have a sore throat; therefore, the PACU nurse would not assess this client first.
    2. **A pulse oximeter reading of lower than 93% indicates an oxygenation problem; therefore, this client should be assessed first.**
    3. Epidural surgery affects the lower extremities, so a palpable pedal pulse indicates a sufficient blood supply; this client should not be assessed first.
    4. Drainage of green bile from the nasogastric (N/G) tube is normal; therefore, this client should not be seen first.

66. 1. After assessing the client's vital signs, the nurse may need to increase the client's intravenous rate, but it is not the first intervention.

2. The nurse should assess the client's vital signs but not before stopping the bleeding.

3. The nurse should keep a large tourniquet at the client's bedside and should apply it when suspecting arterial bleeding; this is the nurse's first intervention.

4. The nurse will need to notify the client's HCP, but the nurse must first address the immediate concern, hemorrhaging.

67. 1. The nurse should always document the findings in the EHR, but the first intervention is to get help because the client has neurovascular compromise.

2. Elevating the client's right hand will not help neurovascular compromise.

3. The Doppler can be used to assess the radial pulse, but this client is experiencing neurovascular compromise, which requires immediate medical intervention.

4. The client is exhibiting severe neurovascular compromise, which indicates a surgical complication and requires notifying the surgeon immediately.

68. 1. The first time a client ambulates after hip surgery should be with a physical therapist or an RN qualified to evaluate the client's ability to ambulate safely with a walker. The UAP does not have these qualifications.

2. According to the National Council of State Boards of Nursing (NCSBN), collaboration with interdisciplinary team members is part of the Management of Care. Physical therapy is responsible for management of the client's ability to move and transfer.

3. The physical therapist will measure the client and obtain the correct walker for the client.

4. The social worker is not responsible for assisting the client to ambulate, but may assist the client on discharge in obtaining needed medical equipment in the home.

69. 1. The UAP is being paid to assist the RN to care for clients on the surgical unit, not take clients downstairs to smoke.

2. The UAP can take vital signs on a newly admitted client.

3. The client has a tube into the stomach via the abdominal wall that requires assessing the residual to determine whether the stomach is digesting the tube-fed nutrients. This task is not appropriate to delegate to the UAP.

4. If the toes are cold, have a capillary refill time of more than 3 seconds, or are pale, the nurse

must make a judgment as to the circulatory status of the foot; therefore, the RN would not delegate this task.

70. 1. The LPN can bathe a client, but this should be assigned to the UAP, thereby allowing the LPN to perform a higher-level task.

2. The LPN can document the amount of food the client eats, but this should be assigned to the UAP, thereby allowing the LPN to perform a higher-level task.

3. According to the NCLEX-RN® test plan, collaboration with interdisciplinary team members is part of the management of care. The activity director of the long-term care facility would be responsible for this activity.

4. The LPN's scope of practice allows routine sterile procedures on the client who is stable, such as clients in a surgical rehabilitation facility.

71. 1. Any member of the staff can change the sharps container when it is full. There is an OSHA fine if the sharps containers are over the full line.

2. The housekeeping department can change the sharps container as well as any staff member.

3. The nurse should reward appropriate behavior by the other health-care members. Verbal praise is always appreciated by anyone.

4. The RN could let the clinical manager know the UAP was emptying the sharps container, but the best action is to directly praise the UAP.

72. 1. The RN should assess the client's neurovascular status when the UAP reports any abnormality.

2. The client should be repositioned by log rolling, but it is not appropriate when the client has a neurovascular compromise.

3. The nurse should assess the client whenever receiving any information from another member of the health-care team.

4. The nurse should not request another member of the health-care team to assess a client who is exhibiting a possible surgical complication.

73. 1. The client who has just returned from surgery should not be transferred from the ICU because the client may not be stable.

2. A sigmoid colostomy is a surgical procedure that causes major fluid shifts and has the po-

tential for multiple complications; therefore, this client should not be transferred to the surgical unit.

   3. **Although the client is only 1 day postoperative for a total hip replacement, it is an elective procedure, which indicates that the client was stable before the surgery. The incision is also dry and intact. Of the four clients, this client is the most stable and should be transferred to the surgical unit.**
   4. A fat embolism is a potentially life-threatening complication of a fracture; therefore, this client should not be transferred from the ICU.

74. 1. Family members should be asked to stay in the client's room until the lights come back on. This helps ensure safety of the family members.
   2. **During an electrical failure, the red outlets in the hospital run on the backup generator, and all IV pumps and necessary equipment should be plugged into these outlets.**
   3. The hospital may provide tap bells for contacting the hospital staff, but would not provide flashlights to all clients. The hospital staff would need the flashlights.
   4. The charge nurse should not tie up the phone lines during an emergency situation; the phones may not even be working.

75. 1. The charge nurse should contact the laboratory, but the first action should be to address the HCP's behavior in a private area.
   2. **This is the charge nurse's first action because it will diffuse the HCP's anger. Inappropriate behavior at the nurse's station should not occur in an area where visitors, clients, or staff will observe the behavior.**
   3. The HCP can call the laboratory and share concerns, but it is not the first intervention.
   4. The charge nurse has the option to report any HCP's inappropriate behavior, but the immediate situation must be dealt with first.

76. 1. The staff nurse should go through the chain of command pursuant to investigating a problem.
   2. **Increased infection rates among clients with PICCs falls within the infection control nurse's scope of practice, and the infection control nursing staff will have data from all units in the hospital.**

   3. The nurse should follow through with investigating a potential problem, but this problem does not fall within the scope of practice of the employee health nurse.
   4. The staff nurse should be a part of the solution to a problem. Volunteering is a good action to effect change, but it is not the first action. More information—which the infection control nurse can provide—is necessary first.

77. 1. Because there are multiple surgical clients requiring custodial care, the RN charge nurse should not send an experienced UAP to the medical unit.
   2. The charge nurse should not send the experienced RN to the medical unit because this nurse represents the strength of the staff.
   3. **The LPN would be the most appropriate staff to send to the medical unit because the LPN has experience on the unit. Expertise of the LPN is also not required to perform custodial care.**
   4. A new orientee should not be sent to an unfamiliar area.

78. **Correct order is 2, 4, 3, 1, 5.**
   The nurse must remember the acronym RACE(E), which is a recognized national standard for fire safety in health-care facilities.
   2. R is for rescue.
   4. A is for alert.
   3. C is for confine.
   1. E is for extinguish.
   5. E is for evacuate.

79. 1 The nurse should notify the operating room team, but according to The Joint Commission, the first intervention is to call a time-out, which stops the surgery until clarification is obtained.
   2. **According to The Joint Commission, the first intervention is to call a time-out, which stops the surgery until clarification is obtained.**
   3. The nurse should discuss this with the client, but should first initiate the time-out procedure.
   4. Calling the surgeon is a part of the time-out procedure, so the first intervention is to call the time-out.

80. 1. The nurse should initiate a client care conference to discuss the client's feelings, but at this time the most appropriate response is to allow the client to begin the grieving process.

2. The nurse could notify the social worker about the client's situation, but the most appropriate response is to allow the client to begin the grieving process, which the client often goes through when experiencing any type of loss. In this situation, the client is losing her independence and her home.

3. The client does not owe the nurse an explanation for "feelings."

4. **According to the NCLEX-RN® test plan, advocacy is part of Management of Care under Safe and Effective Care Environment client needs. Therapeutic communication involves being an advocate in this situation, because sometimes the nurse cannot prevent a perceived "bad" situation from occurring.**

81. 1. **The client cannot be restrained just as needed. The nurse must have documentation for the need and an HCP's specific order that includes the reason for restraint and the time limited to no more than 24 hours. This HCP order should be clarified.**

2. The client in restraints should be offered fluids at least every 2 hours.

3. Hand mitts are the least restrictive limb restraints and can be used to help prevent the client from pulling out lines.

4. The nurse must check to ensure that restrained limbs have adequate circulation at least every 2 hours.

82. 1. The RN is responsible for assessing clients; therefore, this is an appropriate assignment.

2. **The LPN may be allowed to administer some IVP medications in some facilities, but the word "all" makes this an inappropriate assignment. Many IVP medications are considered high risk, and only RNs should administer such IVP medications.**

3. This option has the word "all," but it is within the scope of the UAP to complete the a.m. care. The RN and LPN can perform a.m. care, but it should be assigned to the UAP.

4. The RN should monitor laboratory values because this requires interpretation, evaluation, and notification of the HCP in some instances.

83. 1. Tardiness information is objective data obtained for all employees in the facility, but it does not specifically provide information about the nurse's performance.

2. The attitude of the nurse is very subjective to evaluate and does not specifically provide information about the nurse's performance.

3. Thank-you notes from the clients are nice for the nurse to receive, but they are not taken into consideration during the evaluation process of the nurse.

4. **The nurse's ability to document client care directly correlates with the nurse's performance; therefore, this data should be included in the yearly evaluation.**

84. 1. The home health-care agency would not be the best referral because comorbid conditions increase the client's recovery time. The client at home does not have access to health care 24 hours a day.

2. A senior citizen center may help the client's psychosocial needs but not the client's rehabilitation needs.

3. **The rehabilitation facility will provide intensive therapy and address the comorbid conditions 24 hours a day. This will assist in the client's recovery.**

4. An outpatient physical therapist does not have the education to address and care for the comorbid issues. The physical therapist is focused on the hip fracture only, and the client may have transportation problems going to an outpatient clinic.

85. 1. The nasogastric tube should be replaced, but this task will require more time and require new equipment; therefore, it should not be done first.

2. **The client scheduled for surgery is the priority and must be ready when the OR calls; therefore, completing the preoperative checklist is the first task the nurse should implement. The preoperative checklist ensures the client's safety.**

3. The client being discharged can wait until the safety needs of the client going to surgery have been addressed.

4. This is a minimal amount of drainage, which can require a dressing change, but not before making sure the client going to surgery is ready.

86. 1. **Antiplatelet medication will increase the client's bleeding time and should be held 5 days before surgery; therefore, clopidogrel (Plavix) should be questioned.**

2. A client with a TKR is at risk for developing deep vein thrombosis (DVT); therefore, enoxaparin (Lovenox), an anticoagulant medication, would not be questioned.

3. The client with a Whipple procedure has had part of the pancreas removed and is placed on insulin; therefore, the nurse would not question administering sliding scale regular insulin.

4. Vancomycin, an aminoglycoside antibiotic, is not in the penicillin family; therefore, the nurse would not question administering this medication.

87. 1. A client who is 4 hours postoperative for abdominal surgery would be expected to have abdominal pain and hypoactive bowel sounds secondary to general anesthesia. This client would not be assessed first.

2. This output indicates the client is voiding at least 30 mL an hour; therefore, the nurse would not assess this client first.

3. The client with an open cholecystectomy frequently has a T-tube that would normally drain green bile. This client would not be assessed first.

4. **The client is exhibiting signs of compromised circulation; therefore, the nurse should assess this client first. The nurse should assess for the 6 Ps: pain, pulse, paresthesia, paralysis, pallor, and polar (cold).**

88. 1. **This situation should be addressed first because the charge nurse is responsible for family and client reports of concerns. If the family contacts the administration, the charge nurse must be aware of the situation.**

2. The evaluation needs to be completed, but it does not take priority over handling an irate family member.

3. The charge nurse could assign this task to another nurse or unit secretary. Dealing appropriately with an irate family member takes priority over calling the laboratory.

4. The charge nurse could assign this task to another nurse or unit secretary. Dealing appropriately with an irate family member takes priority over transferring a client.

89. 1. Notifying the kitchen will only scare the kitchen personnel and will not alert the bomb squad as to the situation.

2. The operator would not be able to trace a phone call that has been disconnected.

3. **The chain of command in a hospital is to notify the security department, and they will implement the hospital procedure for the bomb threat.**

4. The nurse should not directly call the local police department because the hospital security department is responsible for implementing the procedure for a bomb scare.

90. 1. Autocratic managers use an authoritarian approach to direct the activities of others.

2. Laissez-faire managers maintain a permissive climate with little direction or control.

3. **A democratic manager is people oriented and facilitates efficient group functioning. The environment is open and communication flows both ways, and this includes having meetings to discuss concerns.**

4. This statement reflects shirking of responsibility, thus letting someone else address the problem, and is not characteristic of a democratic manager.

91. **Correct order is 2, 4, 1, 3, 5.**

2. **The nurse should always explain the procedure to the client even if the client has had the procedure done before.**

4. **This procedure is very painful and the nurse should premedicate the client 30 minutes before performing wound care.**

1. **Obtaining the needed supplies can be done after premedicating the client because the nurse should wait 30 minutes after medicating the client.**

3. **The nurse should remove the old dressing.**

5. **The nurse should assess the burned area for signs of infection, viable tissue, or any eschar.**

92. 1. This client will require time to adjust to living in an extended care facility. This would be an expected reaction.

2. This client may or may not be allowed a glass of wine at night. Some long-term care facilities do allow the client to have a controlled amount of alcohol with an HCP order and the family supplying the alcohol, but this client is not the priority.

3. **This client may or may not have a valid issue. The nurse should investigate whether or not the report is true. Failure to answer a call light can result in the client's attempting to ambulate without assistance and could be a safety issue. The nurse should speak with this client first.**

4. The nurse is not in control of the client's son and his discharge, but if the son is being

discharged, it can be assumed that the son is in stable condition, and it is not a priority for the charge nurse to see this client.

93. 1. The director of nurses must first understand the extent of the report. Telling staff to ignore preconceived ideas about older adult clients does not work. The director of nurses should have valid information to discuss with the staff.
2. The client has a general concern, and so more than one staff member may have ignored the client's statements. Neglect was not mentioned in the stem of the question. Not treating the client with the dignity that the client deserves is implied.
3. This is a false statement. Some residents in a long-term care facility may not be able to determine their needs, but this is not true of all residents.
4. **The director of nurses should discuss the resident's concerns with the resident and then determine a plan of action to remedy the situation.**

94. 1. This may be a true statement, but this client is exhibiting symptoms of depression. The client may or may not wish to make friends at the facility.
2. This is not acknowledging the client's feelings.
3. **This client is exhibiting symptoms of depression. Therapeutic conversation is implemented to help the client verbalize feelings. This statement acknowledges the client's feeling and offers help.**
4. This action may get the client to interact with other people, but it does not acknowledge the client's feelings.

95. 1. **The RN charge nurse should remind the UAPs not to discuss confidential information in a public place. This is the first action.**
2. The charge nurse may need to inform the manager of the breach of confidentiality, but the first action is to stop the conversation.
3. The RN charge nurse or the manager may need to make sure the UAPs are familiar with confidentiality, but the conversation should be terminated first.
4. This might be a better activity for the UAPs, but the first action is to stop the conversation.

96. 1. **An ombudsman is a representative appointed to receive and investigate**

reports made by individuals of abuses or capricious acts. All Medicare and Medicaid long-term care facilities must have an ombudsman to act as a neutral party in matters of dispute with the facility. This is the best person to investigate a report.
2. The social worker is employed by the facility and is not the best person to investigate the report.
3. The upset family member should attend the conference but should have the ombudsman investigate the report.
4. The director will be biased; the best person to investigate the validity of the issue is the ombudsman.

97. 1. The nurse should not refer the client to a church or volunteer organization to ensure continuity of care. The organization's work may depend on unpaid individuals, and a volunteer may or may not be available to transport the client when needed.
2. **The nurse should refer the client to a home health agency for follow-up care. The nurse will go to the client's home to assess the client and perform dressing changes. The home health agency will also assess the client and the client's home for further needs.**
3. The client is unable to drive and would not be able to get to an outpatient clinic.
4. The client is unable to drive and would not be able to get to the HCP's office.

98. 1. The nurse must assess the cause of the bruises before filing a report of abuse. The nurse would file a report of elder abuse only if it is determined that the client has been abused.
2. **The nurse should ask the client whether there is a reason for the bruises that the nurse should be aware of. This is the first intervention and can be done while the nurse is currently with the client.**
3. The nurse should check the client's MAR to see whether he is currently on a medication, such as warfarin (Coumadin) or a systemic steroid, that would increase the risk for bruising; however, this would be done after talking with the client because the bruising is "new," and bruising from the medications can take several days to weeks to develop.
4. The family may need to be notified but not until the nurse assesses the situation.

99. **1. The client is expressing negative feelings about being placed in the nursing home. Asking about the client's feelings is a therapeutic response that encourages the client to verbalize feelings.**
  2. This is not acknowledging the client's feelings and is nontherapeutic because it is a judgmental statement.
  3. The client does not owe the nurse an explanation. "Why" is never therapeutic.
  4. This is assuming the client is correct in being "trouble at home" and agreeing that the family would punish the client for being a problem.

100. 1. The nurse cannot testify to what preceded the client's fall because the nurse was not on duty at the time.
  2. The nurse was not on duty to assess the client's injuries, so any information about the injuries received from the fall would have to be hearsay or obtained from the EHR.
  3. The nurse cannot testify to the client's mental status before the fall because the nurse was not on duty at the time.
  4. The nurse initiated a policy that is designed to prevent falls from occurring. This is all the nurse can testify to.

101. 1. The registered nurse, experienced or not, can be assigned nursing duties of assessment, planning, teaching, and other duties that cannot be delegated or assigned. The charge nurse has only two RNs for 35 clients. This nurse should not be requested to stay home.
  2. An experienced LPN will be needed by the unit to care for the many IV lines and medications.
  3. The UAP cannot administer medications or care for IVs and has requested to be allowed to stay home. This is the best staff member to request to stay home.
  4. This UAP may be less experienced on the floor but has not worked long enough to receive any paid time off, and this could greatly affect the UAP's pay.

102. **1. The charge nurse does not have a right to interfere with two consenting adults having a relationship. Doing nothing is the correct action for the charge nurse. If one of the residents involved is incapable of giving consent to a relationship, then the charge nurse would need to get involved.**
  2. Two consenting adults have a right to form a bond. The family does not have a right

to interfere with the expression of a basic human need, to form an intimate relationship with another human being.
  3. The residents have the right to companionship. They should be allowed to participate in any activity that they wish, when they wish.
  4. This is a normal situation, and no care plan meeting is needed.

103. 1. The argument should already be in a private area because the argument ensued during report. Report should always be held in a confidential area.
  2. The CNO should evaluate the concerns of each charge nurse and then make a decision as to a plan of care for the resident. The CNO is the next in command over the charge nurses in an extended care facility.
  3. This argument does not involve the family. If, after listening to both sides, the CNO thinks there is a need for a family member's input, then the CNO could contact the family, but a decision should be made until this can occur.
  4. The nurses each have a concern over a resident. This situation should be resolved before continuing report.

104. 1. Calling a time-out when a discrepancy is noted on the surgical permit is an appropriate action to prevent an error during a surgical procedure.
  2. The Joint Commission requires two identifiers be utilized before administering medications. Most hospitals use the client's date of birth for the second identifier. This is an appropriate action to prevent an error during a medication administration.
  3. A quiz during orientation is given to assess whether the new employee understands the information being taught. Giving the answers to the quiz completes the required documentation for the employee's files but does not ensure the new hire understands how to utilize the IV pump. This is a violation of the Patient Safety Goals.
  4. Initiating a fall prevention program for an older adult client to prevent falls is an appropriate action to attempt to ensure client safety.

105. 1. This client should be tagged as black, which means the injury is extensive and chances of survival are unlikely even with definitive care.

Clients should receive comfort measures and be separated from other casualties, but not abandoned.

2. This client should be red tagged (immediate), which means the injury is life threatening but survivable with intervention. These clients can deteriorate rapidly without treatment.

3. This client should be tagged as green, which means the injury is minor and treatment can be delayed hours to days. These clients are considered "walking wounded."

4. The client should be tagged as a yellow, which means the injury is significant and requires medical care, but the client is not in immediate danger of death. Clients in this category receive treatment after red tagged (immediate) casualties are treated.

106. 1. The normal white blood cell count is 4.5 to 11.1 x 10³/microL; therefore, this client does not require immediate intervention.

2. The client's cholesterol level is elevated, but this would not require immediate intervention by the nurse. An elevated cholesterol level is not life threatening and can be discussed at the client's next appointment.

3. The client's calcium level is within the normal range of 8.2 to 10.2 mg/dL; therefore, this client does not require an immediate intervention.

4. The therapeutic range for an INR is 2 to 3. This client is at risk for bleeding and requires immediate intervention by the nurse. The nurse should call the client and instruct the client to stop taking warfarin (Coumadin), an anticoagulant.

107. 1. A spokesperson should address the media away from the victim care area as soon as possible. This could be a nurse in some situations, but it is not the priority intervention when triaging victims.

2. The disaster tag number and the client's name should be recorded in the disaster log book, but it is not the priority intervention. The disaster tag must be attached to the client before logging the client into the disaster log book.

3. Client tracking is a critical component of casualty management. Disaster tags, which include name, address, age, location, description of injuries, and treatments or medications administered, must be securely attached to the client.

4. Family and friends arriving at the disaster must be cared for by the disaster workers, but it is not the first intervention for the nurse who is triaging disaster victims.

108. **1. Parish nursing emphasizes the relationship between spiritual faith and health. A parish nurse (PN) is a registered nurse with a minimum of 2 years' experience who works in a faith community to address health issues of its members as well as those in the broader community or neighborhood.**

2. The parish nurse works in the community, not in an acute care setting.

3. There is no such thing as a parish clinic.

4. The parish nurse can be an RN or an LPN.

109. 1. The client's HCP may need to be notified, but it is not the nurse's first intervention.

2. The nurse must first assess the reddened area to determine the stage of the pressure ulcer and what treatment should be recommended.

3. The reddened area should be documented in the EHR, but this is not the first intervention.

4. The client may or may not need to be referred to a wound care nurse, but it is not the nurse's first intervention. If the reddened area is stage 1 or 2, the wound care nurse probably would not be notified.

110. 1. The occupational therapist assists the client with activities of daily living, not with employment concerns.

2. The NCLEX-RN® test plan lists referrals under Management of Care. After a client has been injured and is unable to return to previous employment because of the injury, the rehabilitation commission of each state will help evaluate the client and determine whether the client is eligible to receive training or education for another occupation.

3. The client is not asking about disability but rather about employment. The nurse needs to refer the client to the appropriate agency.

4. The client should discuss his concerns with his wife, but the nurse should refer the client to an agency that can address his concerns about employment.

111. 1. The mother may want to see her infant before the body is removed from the room.

2. The infant's body will be sent to a funeral home. The parents will not be allowed to take the body home.

3. The body should be treated with the dignity accorded to any human remains.
4. **The nurse can present the parents with a lock of the infant's hair and a set of footprints. Giving the parents something of the infant helps with the grieving process.**

112. 1. **Nasal flaring and grunting indicate the infant is in respiratory distress. The nurse should assess this infant first.**
2. The nurse would not worry about the infant not passing meconium until 20 to 24 hours after birth. The nurse would not assess this infant first.
3. This situation requires teaching the mother and patience, but the infant is not in distress. The nurse would not assess this infant first.
4. This is normal for a newborn. The nurse would not assess this infant first.

113. 1. Because this client is reporting an incident that occurred hours ago and she is not in imminent danger, this client is not the first client the nurse should call.
2. **The nurse should return this call first because the nurse must determine whether the client has a plan for suicide.**
3. Not wanting to eat is part of the anorexia disease process. The nurse does not need to return this call first.
4. Hand trembling is part of the Parkinson's disease process. Control of the symptoms of Parkinson's disease is affected by several factors, including the amount of sleep the client had, fatigue, and the development of tolerance to the medications. Because this client is not at risk for suicide, he is not the first client for the nurse to see.

114. 1. **Pediatric clients in a psychiatric facility must keep up with schoolwork. Clients must be escorted from one building to another. The MHW should be assigned to this task.**
2. The MHW is not qualified for this task to lead a group therapy session.
3. Explaining the purpose of recreation therapy is teaching, and teaching cannot be delegated to an MHW.
4. Clients in a psychiatric facility are expected to meet their own hygiene needs as part of assuming responsibility for themselves. This is not the best task to assign to the MHW.

115. Correct answers are 1, 2, and 5.
1. **Smoking while taking birth control pills increases the risk of adverse reactions such as formation of blood clots.**
2. **The client should take the pill at approximately the same time each day to maintain a blood level of the hormone.**
3. The client should be instructed to take a missed pill as soon as she realizes she missed the dose during the intervening 24 hours. However, if the client doesn't realize she missed the pill until the next day, she should not take two pills at that time.
4. Breakthrough bleeding may indicate a change in dose is needed, but the client should not stop taking the pill.
5. **There may be interactions with other medications. Many antibiotics interfere with the action of the birth control pill, and the client should use other contraceptive methods when on an antibiotic.**

116. 1. Vaginal itching while receiving antibiotics indicates that the good bacterial flora in the vagina is being destroyed. Yogurt contains these bacteria and can help replace the needed bacteria. However, requesting the dietary department to send yogurt each day is not the priority intervention.
2. **The nurse should first explain to the client that this is a side effect of the antibiotic medication ceftriaxone (Rocephin). Then, the nurse should notify the dietitian and HCP. The antibiotic therapy cannot be discontinued because of the need for antibiotic therapy after knee replacement surgery.**
3. The HCP should be notified of the vaginal itching, but it is not an emergency and can wait until the HCP makes rounds.
4. The client's sexual history is not a concern because the vaginal infection is secondary to the antibiotic therapy.

117. 1. The manager should ask for input into the budgetary needs from the staff, but an assessment of the current year's budget is the first step.
2. An assessment of the costs of any new department projects should be done, but the first step is to assess the present budget.
3. **The first step in a budgetary process is to assess the current budget.**
4. Explaining the new budget to the staff is the last step in the process.

118. 1. The nurse should confront the client with the behavior, but this is not the first intervention.
2. The nurse should document the behavior in the client's EHR, but this is not the first intervention.
3. **The nurse should intervene to stop the behavior first before one of the clients is injured. Approaching the client with another staff member shows strength and provides the nurse with the ability to perform a safe "take down."**
4. The client should be told to return to the room, but stopping the behavior is the first intervention.

119. 1. This surgeon should speak with the client, but the first intervention is to stop the procedure.
2. Asking the client to discuss concerns should be done, but the first intervention is to stop the procedure.
3. Continuing to prep the client for the surgery can be done, but is inappropriate when the client no longer is giving consent.
4. **Stopping the surgical procedure is the first intervention for the nurse to implement.**

120. 1. Four episodes of mania in 6 months do not indicate therapy has been effective.
2. **The ability to hold a job for 9 months indicates the client is responding to therapy.**
3. Wearing a nightgown to the day room does not indicate the client is responding to treatment.
4. Three motor vehicle accidents do not indicate the client is responding to treatment.

121. 1. The clients would not understand the importance of the specific tasks. Clients will tell the RN whether the UAP is pleasant when in the room but not whether the delegated tasks have been completed.
2. The nurse retains responsibility for the delegated tasks. The charge nurse may be able to tell the RN that the UAP has been checked off as being competent to perform the care, but would not know whether the care was actually provided.
3. **The nurse retains responsibility for the care. Making rounds to see that the care has been provided is the best method to evaluate the care.**
4. The RN would not have time to complete all the higher-level required nursing functions if the nurse watched the UAP perform all the UAP's work.

122. 1. A client in a crisis should be assigned to a registered nurse (RN).
2. Biliary atresia involves liver failure and multiple body systems. This client should be assigned to an RN.
3. Anaphylaxis is an emergency situation. The client should be assigned to an RN.
4. **The LPN can administer routine medications and care for clients who have no life-threatening conditions.**

123. 1. **Erythropoietin alpha (Epogen), a biological response modifier, stimulates the bone marrow to produce red blood cells. An adverse reaction to Epogen is hypertension, which this client has, with a BP of 200/124. Hypertension can cause the dosage of erythropoietin to be decreased or discontinued.**
2. Erythropoietin alpha (Epogen), a biological response modifier, does not affect the pulse.
3. A hematocrit of 38% would indicate the medication is effective.
4. A side effect of the medication is long bone pain. This can be treated with a non-narcotic analgesic. This is not an adverse reaction.

124. 1. The nurse should assess the client for complications before administering the medication.
2. This should occur, but not before assessing the client for complications.
3. **The first step in administering a PRN pain medication is to assess the client for a complication that may require the nurse to notify the HCP or implement an independent nursing intervention.**
4. This is not the first intervention.

125. 1. The infection can come from kissing someone who has the infection in the mouth as well as from oral sex. This is not the best statement.
2. Smear of oral tissue is not done routinely.
3. Because of frequent partner changes transferring the organism from mucous membranes to mucous membranes via oral sex or kissing, the infection is the fastest rising incidence of causation for head and neck cancers.
4. **Human papillomavirus (HPV) infections are increasing exponentially and many younger persons are developing mouth infections and cancers from HPV.**

126. 1. The AIDS virus can be transmitted during the first exposure to it. The class should be taught that no exposure is safe.
2. The use of condoms is somewhat protective but it does not guarantee protection from transmitting a sexually transmitted disease.
3. **The more exposure there is to blood or body fluids from other individuals (more partners), the greater the chance there is of developing an STI.**
4. Both syphilis and gonorrhea are usually treatable, but long-lasting health problems can result. For example, pelvic inflammatory disease can scar the fallopian tube and cause fertility issues.

127. 1. **The child is stable and the UAP can escort the child to the car. This task can be delegated by the RN.**
2. This is assessment and the RN cannot delegate assessment, teaching, evaluation, medications, or an unstable client to a UAP.
3. This is teaching and the nurse cannot delegate teaching.
4. The UAP may be able to assist the HCP with this task, but of the four options the test taker should select the least invasive, or the task that will require the least amount of nursing knowledge.

Bibliography

American Diabetes Association. (n.d.). Insulin pumps. Retrieved from diabetes.org/living-with
-diabetes/treatment-and-care/medication/insulin/insulin-pumps.html

Bulger-Noto, J. (2018). Leadless pacemakers. *American Nurse Today, 13*(10), 18–21.

Callahan, B. (Ed.). (2015). *Clinical nursing skills: A concept-based approach to learning* (2nd ed.). Boston, MA: Pearson.

Colgrove, K. C. (2017). *Med-surg success* (3rd ed.). Philadelphia, PA: F.A. Davis Company.

Lewis, S. L., Bucher, L., Heitkemper, M. M., & Harding, M. M. (2017). *Medical-surgical nursing: Assessment and management of clinical problems* (10th ed.). St. Louis, MO: Elsevier.

McKinney, E. S., James, S. R., Murray, S. S., Nelson, K. A., & Ashwill, J. W. (2018). *Maternal-child nursing* (5th ed.). St. Louis, MO: Elsevier.

National Council of State Boards of Nursing. (2018). *Strategic practice analysis.* NCSBN Research Brief, 71. Retrieved from https://www.ncsbn.org/NCLEX_Next_Winter18_Eng_05.pdf

National Council of State Boards of Nursing. (2019). 2019 NCLEX-RN test plan. Retrieved from ncsbn.org/2019_RN_TestPlan-English.htm

Story, L. (2018). *Pathophysiology: A practical approach* (3rd ed.). Burlington, MA: Jones & Bartlett Learning.

Treas, L. S., Wilkinson, J. M., Barnett, K. L., & Smith, M. H. (2018). *Basic nursing: Thinking, doing, and caring* (2nd ed.). Philadelphia, PA: F. A. Davis Company.

Vallerand, A. H., & Sanoski, C. A. (2017). *Davis's drug guide for nurses* (16th ed.). Philadelphia, PA: F. A. Davis Company.

Van Leeuwen, A. M., & Bladh, M. L. (2017). *Davis's comprehensive handbook of laboratory & diagnostic tests with nursing implications* (7th ed.). Philadelphia, PA: F. A. Davis Company.

Appendix A: Normal Laboratory Values

These values are obtained from *Davis's Comprehensive Handbook of Laboratory and Diagnostic Tests With Nursing Implications* (7th edition). Laboratory results may differ slightly depending on the resource manual or the laboratory normal values.

Arterial Blood Gas	Adult
pH	7.35 to 7.45
P_{CO_2}	35 to 45 mm Hg
H_{CO_3}	22 to 26 mmol/L
P_{O_2}	80 to 95 mm Hg
O_2 saturation	95% to 99%

Chemistry	Adult
Cholesterol	Less than 200 mg/dL
HDL	40 to 60 mg/dL
LDL	Less than 100 mg/dL
Creatinine	Male: 0.61 to 1.21 mg/dL
	Female: 0.51 to 1.11 mg/dL
Glucose	Fasting: Less than 100 mg/dL
	Random: Less than 200 mg/dL
Potassium	3.5 to 5.3 mEq/L or mmol/L
Sodium	135 to 145 mEq/L or mmol/L
Calcium	8.2 to 10.2 mg/dL
Triglycerides	Less than 150 mg/dL
Blood urea nitrogen	8 to 21 mg/dL
	Adult over 90 years: 10 to 31 mg/dL

Blood Count	Adult
Hematocrit (Hct)	Male: 42% to 52%
	Female: 36% to 48%
Hemoglobin (Hgb)	Male: 14 to 17.3 g/dL
	Female: 11.7 to 15.5 g/dL
Activated partial thromboplastin time (aPTT)	25 to 35 seconds
Prothrombin time (PT)	10 to 13 seconds
Red blood cell count (RBC)	Male: 4.21 to 5.81 × 10^6 cells/microL
	Female: 3.61 to 5.11 (10^6 cells/microL)
White blood cell count (WBC)	4.5 to 11.1 × 10^3/microL
Platelets	140 to 400 × 10^3/microL
Erythrocyte sedimentation rate (ESR)	Adult less than 50 years: 0 to 15 mm/hr
	Adult 50 years and older: 0 to 20 mm/hr

Drug Levels	Adult
Digoxin (Lanoxin)	0.5 to 2.0 ng/mL
International Normalized Ratio (INR)	0.9 to 1.1 without anticoagulation therapy
	2 to 3 with therapy
	2.5 to 3.5 if the client has a mechanical heart valve
Lithium	0.6 to 1.2 mEq/L
Phenytoin (Dilantin)	10 to 20 mcg/mL
Theophylline (Aminophylline)	10 to 20 mcg/mL
Valproic acid (Depakote)	50 to 125 mcg/mL
Vancomycin (trough level)	5 to 15 mcg/mL

Urinalysis	Adult
pH	4.5 to 8
Specific gravity	1.005 to 1.03
Glucose	Negative
Ketones	
Hemoglobin	
Bilirubin	
Nitrite	
Leukocyte esterase	
Urobilinogen	Up to 1 mg/dL
Protein	Less than 20 mg/dL
Microscopic	Adult
RBCs	Less than 5/hpf (high power field)
WBCs	Less than 5/hpf (high power field)
Bacteria	None seen

Appendix B: Common Abbreviations

Abnormal Involuntary Movement Scale (AIMS)

Absolute neutrophil count (ANC)

Acquired immune deficiency syndrome (AIDS)

Activity of daily living (ADL)

Acute respiratory distress syndrome (ARDS)

Advance directive (AD)

Against medical advice (AMA)

Allow natural death (AND)

American Cancer Society (ACS)

American Heart Association (AHA)

Americans with Disabilities Act (ADA)

Aminotransferase (AST)

Amyotrophic lateral sclerosis (ALS)

Angiotensin-converting enzyme (ACE)

Antidiuretic hormone (ADH)

Apical pulse (AP)

Arterial blood gas (ABG)

Attention deficit hyperactivity disorder (ADHD)

Below-the-knee amputation (BKA)

Benign prostatic hypertrophy (BPH)

Blood pressure (BP)

Blood urea nitrogen (BUN)

Cardiopulmonary resuscitation (CPR)

Cerebrospinal fluid (CSF)

Cerebrovascular accident (CVA)

Chief nursing officer (CNO)

Child Protective Services (CPS)

Chronic kidney disease (CKD)

Chronic obstructive pulmonary disease (COPD)

Complementary alternative medicine (CAM)

Complete blood count (CBC)

Computed tomography (CT)

Congestive heart failure (CHF)

Continuous bladder irrigation (CBI)

Continuous glucose monitoring (CGM)

Continuous passive motion (CPM)

Coronary artery bypass graft (CABG)

Coronary artery disease (CAD)

Critical care unit (CCU)

Culture and sensitivity (C&S)

Cystic fibrosis (CF)

Cytomegalovirus (CMV)

Deep vein thrombosis (DVT)

Diabetes insipidus (DI)

Diabetes mellitus (DM)

Diabetic ketoacidosis (DKA)

Disseminated intravascular coagulation (DIC)

Dissociative identity disorder (DID)

Do not resuscitate (DNR)

Durable medical equipment (DME)

Electronic health record (EHR)

Electronic medication administration record (eMAR)

Emergency department (ED)

End-of-life (EOL)

Endotracheal (ET)

End-stage renal disease (ESRD)

Esophagogastroduodenoscopy (EGD)

Evidence-based practice (EBP)

Glomerular filtration rate (GFR)

Graduate nurse (GN)

Health-care provider (HCP)

Health Insurance Portability and Accountability Act (HIPAA)

Hemoglobin and hematocrit (H&H)

Hemolysis elevated liver enzymes and low platelet count (HELLP)

Highly active antiretroviral therapy (HAART)

Home health (HH)

Home health aide (HHA)

Human immunodeficiency virus (HIV)

Human papillomavirus (HPV)

Hyperglycemic hyperosmolar nonketotic coma (HHNC)

Hypertension (HTN)

Ideal body weight (IBW)

Inflammatory bowel disease (IBD)

Intake & output (I&O)

Intensive care unit (ICU)

International Normalized Ratio (INR)

Intimate partner violence (IPV)

Intracranial pressure (ICP)

Intramuscular (IM)

Intravenous (IV)

Intravenous piggyback (IVPB)

Intravenous push (IVP)

Jackson-Pratt (JP)

Kidney ureter bladder (KUB)

Licensed practical nurse (LPN)

Magnetic resonance imaging (MRI)

Medication administration record (MAR)

Mental health worker (MHW)

Methicillin-resistant *Staphylococcus aureus* (MRSA)

Motor vehicle accident (MVA)

Myasthenia gravis (MG)

Myocardial infarction (MI)

Narcissistic personality disorder (NPD)

Nasogastric (NG)

Nasogastric tube (NGT)

National Association for Home Care (NAHC)

National Council Licensure Examination (NCLEX-RN®)

National Council of State Boards of Nursing (NCSBN)

Neonatal intensive care unit (NICU)

Nitroglycerin (NTG)

Nonsteroidal anti-inflammatory drug (NSAID)

Nurse practitioner (NP)

Obstetric (OB)

Occupational Health and Safety Administration (OSHA)

Open reduction and internal fixation (ORIF)

Operating room (OR)

Over the counter (OTC)

Packed red blood cell (PRBC)

Parish nurse (PN)

Parkinson's disease (PD)

Partial thromboplastin time (PTT)

Patient-controlled analgesia (PCA)

Percutaneous endoscopic gastrostomy (PEG)

Peripheral arterial disease (PAD)

Peripherally inserted central catheter (PICC)

Phenylketonuria (PKU)

Physical therapist (PT)

Physician assistant (PA)

Physicians' Desk Reference (PDR)

Post-anesthesia care unit (PACU)

Post-traumatic stress disorder (PTSD)

Premature ventricular contractions (PVC)

Pulmonary embolism (PE)

Purified protein derivative (PPD)

Range of motion (ROM)

Rapid Response Team (RRT)

Red blood cell (RBC)

Registered nurse (RN)

Rheumatoid arthritis (RA)

Rheumatoid factor (RF)

Rule out (R/O)

Sequential compression device (SCD)

Sexual assault nurse examiner (SANE)

Sexually transmitted infection (STI)

Significant other (SO)

Spinal cord injury (SCI)

Sudden infant death syndrome (SIDS)

Syndrome of inappropriate antidiuretic hormone (SIADH)

Systemic lupus erythematosus (SLE)

Telephone order (TO)

Tetralogy of Fallot (TOF)

To keep open (TKO)

Total hip replacement (THR)

Total knee replacement (TKR)

Total parenteral nutrition (TPN)

Transient ischemic attack (TIA)

Transurethral resection of the prostate (TURP)

Traumatic brain injury (TBI)

Unlicensed assistive personnel (UAP)

Urinary tract infection (UTI)

White blood cell (WBC)

Glossary of English Words Commonly Encountered on Nursing Examinations

Abnormality – defect, irregularity, anomaly, oddity

Absence – nonappearance, lack, nonattendance

Abundant – plentiful, rich, profuse

Accelerate – go faster, speed up, increase, hasten

Accumulate – build up, collect, gather

Accurate – precise, correct, exact

Achievement – accomplishment, success, reaching, attainment

Acknowledge – admit, recognize, accept, reply

Activate – start, turn on, stimulate

Adequate – sufficient, ample, plenty, enough

Angle – slant, approach, direction, point of view

Application – use, treatment, request, claim

Approximately – about, around, in the region of, more or less, roughly speaking

Arrange – position, place, organize, display

Associated – linked, related

Attention – notice, concentration, awareness, thought

Authority – power, right, influence, clout, expert

Avoid – keep away from, evade, let alone

Balanced – stable, neutral, steady, fair, impartial

Barrier – barricade, blockage, obstruction, obstacle

Best – most excellent, most important, greatest

Capable – able, competent, accomplished

Capacity – ability, capability, aptitude, role, power, size

Central – middle, mid, innermost, vital

Challenge – confront, dare, dispute, test, defy, face up to

Characteristic – trait, feature, attribute, quality, typical

Circular – round, spherical, globular

Collect – gather, assemble, amass, accumulate, bring together

Commitment – promise, vow, dedication, obligation, pledge, assurance

Commonly – usually, normally, frequently, generally, universally

Compare – contrast, evaluate, match up to, weigh or judge against

Compartment – section, part, cubicle, booth, stall

Complex – difficult, multifaceted, compound, multipart, intricate

Complexity – difficulty, intricacy, complication

Component – part, element, factor, section, constituent

Comprehensive – complete, inclusive, broad, thorough

Conceal – hide, cover up, obscure, mask, suppress, secrete

Conceptualize – to form an idea

Concern – worry, anxiety, fear, alarm, distress, unease, trepidation

Concisely – briefly, in a few words, succinctly

Conclude – make a judgment based on reason, finish

Confidence – self–assurance, certainty, poise, self-reliance

Congruent – matching, fitting, going together well

Consequence – result, effect, outcome, end result

Constituents – elements, components, parts that make up a whole

Contain – hold, enclose, surround, include, control, limit

Continual – repeated, constant, persistent, recurrent, frequent

Continuous – constant, incessant, nonstop, unremitting, permanent

Contribute – be a factor, add, give

Convene – assemble, call together, summon, organize, arrange

Convenience – expediency, handiness, ease

Coordinate – organize, direct, manage, bring together

Create – make, invent, establish, generate, produce, fashion, build, construct

Creative – imaginative, original, inspired, inventive, resourceful, productive, innovative

Critical – serious, grave, significant, dangerous, life threatening

Cue – signal, reminder, prompt, sign, indication

Curiosity – inquisitiveness, interest, nosiness, snooping

Damage – injure, harm, hurt, break, wound

Deduct – subtract, take away, remove, withhold

Deficient – lacking, wanting, underprovided, scarce, faulty

Defining – important, crucial, major, essential, significant, central

Defuse – resolve, calm, soothe, neutralize, rescue, mollify

Delay – hold up, wait, hinder, postpone, slow down, hesitate, linger

Demand – insist, claim, require, command, stipulate, ask

Describe – explain, tell, express, illustrate, depict, portray

Design – plan, invent, intend, aim, propose, devise

Desirable – wanted, pleasing, enviable, popular, sought after, attractive, advantageous

Detail – feature, aspect, element, factor, facet

Deteriorate – worsen, decline, weaken

Determine – decide, conclude, resolve, agree on

Dexterity – skillfulness, handiness, agility, deftness

Dignity – self-respect, self-esteem, decorum, formality, poise

Dimension – aspect, measurement

Diminish – reduce, lessen, weaken, detract, moderate

Discharge – release, dismiss, set free

Discontinue – stop, cease, halt, suspend, terminate, withdraw

Disorder – complaint, problem, confusion, chaos

Display – show, exhibit, demonstrate, present, put on view

Dispose – to get rid of, arrange, order, set out

Dissatisfaction – displeasure, discontent, unhappiness, disappointment

Distinguish – to separate and classify, recognize

Distract – divert, sidetrack, entertain

Distress – suffering, trouble, anguish, misery, agony, concern, sorrow

Distribute – deliver, spread out, hand out, issue, dispense

Disturbed – troubled, unstable, concerned, worried, distressed, anxious, uneasy

Diversional – serving to distract

Don – put on, dress oneself in

Dramatic – spectacular

Drape – cover, wrap, dress, swathe

Dysfunction – abnormal, impaired

Edge – perimeter, boundary, periphery, brink, border, rim

Effective – successful, useful, helpful, valuable

Efficient – not wasteful, effective, competent, resourceful, capable

Elasticity – stretch, spring, suppleness, flexibility

Eliminate – get rid of, eradicate, abolish, remove, purge

Embarrass – make uncomfortable, make self-conscious, humiliate, mortify

Emerge – appear, come, materialize, become known

Emphasize – call attention to, accentuate, stress, highlight

Ensure – make certain, guarantee

Environment – setting, surroundings, location, atmosphere, milieu, situation

Episode – event, incident, occurrence, experience

Essential – necessary, fundamental, vital, important, crucial, critical, indispensable

Etiology – assigned cause, origin

Exaggerate – overstate, inflate

Excel – to stand out, shine, surpass, outclass

Excessive – extreme, too much, unwarranted

Exertion – intense or prolonged physical effort

Exhibit – show signs of, reveal, display

Expand – get bigger, enlarge, spread out, increase, swell, inflate

Expect – wait for, anticipate, imagine

Expectation – hope, anticipation, belief, prospect, probability

Experience – knowledge, skill, occurrence, know–how

Expose – lay open, leave unprotected, allow to be seen, reveal, disclose, exhibit

External – outside, exterior, outer

Facilitate – make easy, make possible, help, assist

Factor – part, feature, reason, cause, think, issue

Focus – center, focal point, hub

Fragment – piece, portion, section, part, splinter, chip

Function – purpose, role, job, task

Furnish – supply, provide, give, deliver, equip

Further – additional, more, extra, added, supplementary

Generalize – to take a broad view, simplify, to make inferences from particulars

Generate – make, produce, create

Gentle – mild, calm, tender

Girth – circumference, bulk, weight

Highest – uppermost, maximum, peak, main

Hinder – hold back, delay, hamper, obstruct, impede

Humane – caring, kind, gentle, compassionate, benevolent, civilized

Ignore – pay no attention to, disregard, overlook, discount

Imbalance – unevenness, inequality, disparity

Immediate – insistent, urgent, direct

Impair – damage, harm, weaken

Implantation – attachment of the early embryo to the maternal uterine wall, to put in

Impotent – powerless, weak, incapable, ineffective, unable

Inadvertent – unintentional, chance, unplanned, accidental

Include – comprise, take in, contain

Indicate – point out, sign of, designate, specify, show

Ineffective – unproductive, unsuccessful, useless, vain, futile

Inevitable – predictable, to be expected, unavoidable, foreseeable

Influence – power, pressure, sway, manipulate, affect, effect

Initiate – start, begin, open, commence, instigate

Insert – put in, add, supplement, introduce

Inspect – look over, check, examine

Inspire – motivate, energize, encourage, enthuse

Institute – implement, initiate, institution

Institutionalize – to place in a facility for treatment

Integrate – put together, mix, add, combine, assimilate

Integrity – honesty

Interfere – get in the way, hinder, obstruct, impede, hamper

Interpret – explain the meaning of, to make understandable

Intervention – action, activity

Intolerance – bigotry, prejudice, narrow-mindedness

Involuntary – instinctive, reflex, unintentional, automatic, uncontrolled

Irreversible – permanent, irrevocable, irreparable, unalterable

Irritability – sensitivity to stimuli, fretful, quick excitability

Justify – explain in accordance with reason

Likely – probably, possible, expected

Liquefy – to change into or make more fluid

Logical – using reason

Longevity – long life

Lowest – inferior in rank

Maintain – continue, uphold, preserve, sustain, retain

Majority – the greater part of

Mention – talk about, refer to, state, cite, declare, point out

Minimal – least, smallest, nominal, negligible, token

Minimize – reduce, diminish, lessen, curtail, decrease to smallest possible

Mobilize – activate, organize, assemble, gather together, rally

Modify – change, adapt, adjust, revise, alter

Moist – slightly wet, damp

Multiple – many, numerous, several, various

Natural – normal, ordinary, unaffected

Negative – no, harmful, downbeat, pessimistic

Negotiate – bargain, talk, discuss, consult, cooperate, settle

Notice – become aware of, see, observe, discern, detect

Notify – inform, tell, alert, advise, warn, report

Nurture – care for, raise, rear, foster

Obsess – preoccupy, consume

Occupy – live in, inhabit, reside in, engage in

Occurrence – event, incident, happening

Odorous – scented, stinking, aromatic

Offensive – unpleasant, distasteful, nasty, disgusting

Opportunity – chance, prospect, break

Organize – put in order, arrange, sort out, categorize, classify

Origin – source, starting point, cause, beginning, derivation

Pace – speed, rhythm, tempo, rate

Parameter – limit, factor, limitation, issue

Participant – member, contributor, partaker, applicant

Perspective – viewpoint, view, perception

Position – place, location, point, spot, situation

Practice – do, carry out, perform, apply, follow

Precipitate – to cause to happen, to bring on, hasten, abrupt, sudden

Predetermine – fix or set beforehand

Predictable – expected, knowable

Preference – favorite, liking, first choice

Prepare – get ready, plan, make, train, arrange, organize

Prescribe – set down, stipulate, order, recommend, impose

Previous – earlier, prior, before, preceding

Primarily – first, above all, mainly, mostly, largely, principally, predominantly

Primary – first, main, basic, chief, most important, key, prime, major, crucial

Priority – main concern, giving first attention to, order of importance

Production – making, creation, construction, assembly

Profuse – a lot of, plentiful, copious, abundant, generous, prolific, bountiful

Prolong – extend, delay, put off, lengthen, draw out

Promote – encourage, support, endorse, sponsor

Proportion – ratio, amount, quantity, part of, percentage, section of

Provide – give, offer, supply, make available

Rationalize – explain, reason

Realistic – practical, sensible, reasonable

Receive – get, accept, take delivery of, obtain

Recognize – acknowledge, appreciate, identify, aware of

Recovery – healing, mending, improvement, recuperation, renewal

Reduce – decrease, lessen, ease, moderate, diminish

Reestablish – reinstate, restore, return, bring back

Regard – consider, look upon, relate to, respect

Regular – usual, normal, ordinary, standard, expected, conventional

Relative – comparative, family member

Relevance – importance of

Reluctant – unwilling, hesitant, disinclined, indisposed, adverse

Reminisce – to recall and review remembered experiences

Remove – take away, get rid of, eliminate, eradicate

Reposition – move, relocate, change position

Require – need, want, necessitate

Resist – oppose, defend against, keep from, refuse to go along with, defy

Resolution – decree, solution, decision, ruling, promise

Resolve – make up your mind, solve, determine, decide

Response – reply, answer, reaction, retort

Restore – reinstate, reestablish, bring back, return to, refurbish

Restrict – limit, confine, curb, control, contain, hold back, hamper

Retract – take back, draw in, withdraw, apologize

Reveal – make known, disclose, divulge, expose, tell, make public

Review – appraisal, reconsider, evaluation, assessment, examination, analysis

Ritual – custom, ceremony, formal procedure

Rotate – turn, go around, spin, swivel

Routine – usual, habit, custom, practice

Satisfaction – approval, fulfillment, pleasure, happiness

Satisfy – please, convince, fulfill, make happy, gratify

Secure – safe, protected, fixed firmly, sheltered, confident, obtain

Sequential – chronological, in order of occurrence

Significant – important, major, considerable, noteworthy, momentous

Slight – small, slim, minor, unimportant, insignificant, insult, snub

Source – basis, foundation, starting place, cause

Specific – exact, particular, detail, explicit, definite

Stable – steady, even, constant

Statistics – figures, data, information

Subtract – take away, deduct

Success – achievement, victory, accomplishment

Surround – enclose, encircle, contain

Suspect – think, believe, suppose, guess, deduce, infer, distrust, doubtful

Sustain – maintain, carry on, prolong, continue, nourish, suffer

Synonymous – same as, identical, equal, tantamount

Systemic – affecting the entire organism

Thorough – careful, detailed, methodical, systematic, meticulous, comprehensive, exhaustive

Tilt – tip, slant, slope, lean, angle, incline

Translucent – see-through, transparent, clear

Unique – one and only, sole, exclusive, distinctive

Universal – general, widespread, common, worldwide

Unoccupied – vacant, not busy, empty

Unrelated – unconnected, unlinked, distinct, dissimilar, irrelevant

Unresolved – unsettled, uncertain, unsolved, unclear, in doubt

Untoward – adverse, unexpected, inappropriate, inconvenient, unforeseen

Utilize – make use of, employ

Various – numerous, variety, range of, mixture of, assortment of

Verbalize – express, voice, speak, articulate

Verify – confirm, make sure, prove, attest to, validate, substantiate, corroborate, authenticate

Vigorous – forceful, strong, brisk, energetic

Volume – quantity, amount, size

Withdraw – remove, pull out, take out, extract

Index

References followed by the letter "f" are for figures and "t" are tables.